American Academy of Orthopaedic Surgeons
American Academy of Pediatrics

ESSENTIALS of
Musculoskeletal Imaging

Edited by
Thomas R. Johnson, MD
Lynne S. Steinbach, MD

Published 2004 by the
American Academy of Orthopaedic Surgeons
6300 North River Road
Rosemont, IL 60018

First Edition

Copyright ©2004 by the
American Academy of Orthopaedic Surgeons

The material presented in *Essentials of Musculoskeletal Imaging* has been made available by the American Academy of Orthopaedic Surgeons for educational purposes only. This material is not intended to present the only, or necessarily best, methods or procedures for the medical situations discussed, but rather is intended to represent an approach, view, statement, or opinion of the author(s) or producer(s), which may be helpful to others who face similar situations.

Some drugs or medical devices demonstrated in Academy courses or described in Academy print or electronic publications have not been cleared by the Food and Drug Administration (FDA) or have been cleared for specific uses only. The FDA has stated that it is the responsibility of the physician to determine the FDA clearance status of each drug or device he or she wishes to use in clinical practice.

The U.S. FDA has expressed concern about potential serious patient care issues involved with the use of polymethylmethacrylate (PMMA) bone cement in the spine. A physician might insert the PMMA bone cement into vertebrae by various procedures, including vertebroplasty and kyphoplasty.

PMMA bone cement is considered a device for FDA purposes. In October 1999, the FDA reclassified PMMA bone cement as a Class II device for its intended use "in arthroplastic procedures of the hip, knee, and other joints for the fixation of polymer or metallic prosthetic implants to living bone." The use of a device for other than its FDA-cleared indication is an off-label use. Physicians may use a device off-label if they believe, in their best medical judgment, that its use is appropriate for a particular patient (eg, tumors).

The use of PMMA bone cement in the spine is described in Academy educational courses, videotapes, and publications for educational purposes only. As is the Academy's policy regarding all of its educational offerings, the fact that the use of PMMA bone cement in the spine is discussed does not constitute an Academy endorsement of this use.

Furthermore, any statements about commercial products are solely the opinion(s) of the author(s) and do not represent an Academy endorsement or evaluation of these products. These statements may not be used in advertising or for any commercial purpose.

ISBN 0-89203-253-7
Printed in the U.S.A.
Second printing, 2007

Library of Congress Cataloging-in-Publication Data

Essentials of musculoskeletal imaging / edited by Thomas R. Johnson, Lynne S. Steinbach.
    p. ; cm.
    Includes index.
    ISBN 0-89203-253-7 (alk. paper)
    1. Musculoskeletal system—Diseases—Diagnosis. 2. Musculoskeletal system—Imaging.
I. Johnson, Thomas R. II. Steinbach, Lynne S. III. American Academy of Orthopaedic Surgeons.
    [DNLM: 1. Musculoskeletal Diseases—radiography. 2. Diagnostic Imaging. WE 141 E781 2003]
RC925.7.E842 2003
616.7'0754—dc22

2003058334

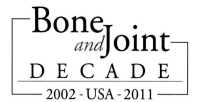

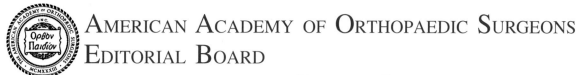

Contributors

Christopher S. Ahmad, MD
Assistant Professor of Orthopaedic Surgery
Department of Orthopaedic Surgery
Center for Shoulder, Elbow and Sports Medicine
Columbia University
New York, New York

Enrico F. Arguelles, MD, FACR, CCD
Clinical Rheumatologist
Arthritis and Osteoporosis Center
Billings, Montana

Aaron A. Bare, MD
Department of Orthopaedic Surgery
Northwestern University
Chicago, Illinois

Gregory C. Berlet, MD
Clinical Assistant Professor
Department of Orthopedics
Ohio State University
Columbus, Ohio

Louis U. Bigliani, MD
Frank E. Stinchfield Professor and Chairman
Director, Orthopaedic Surgery Services
Department of Orthopaedic Surgery
Columbia University
New York, New York

Michael E. Brage, MD
Assistant Professor
Department of Orthopaedics
University of California
San Diego, California

Raymond M. Carroll, MD
Clinical Instructor
Department of Orthopaedic Surgery
Georgetown University Medical Center
Washington, DC

John M. Flynn, MD
Assistant Professor
Division of Orthopaedic Surgery
The Children's Hospital of Philadelphia
University of Pennsylvania
Philadelphia, Pennsylvania

Vincent A. Fowble, MD
Department of Orthopaedic Surgery
Kingsbrook Jewish Medical Center
Brooklyn, New York

Mitch Gallagher, MD
Department of Radiology
St. Vincent Healthcare
Billings, Montana

Jessica Gallina, MD
Chief Resident
Department of Orthopaedics
Mount Sinai Medical Center
New York, New York

Timothy A. Garvey, MD
Associate Professor
Twin Cities Spine Center
Minneapolis, Minnesota

Steven L. Haddad, MD
Assistant Professor of Clinical Orthopaedic Surgery
Illinois Bone and Joint Institute, Ltd.
Northwestern University
Glenview, Illinois

Paul J. Herzwurm, MD
Chief of Orthopaedics
University Hospital
Orthopaedic Associates of Augusta
Augusta, Georgia

Denise T. Ibrahim, DO
Department of Orthopaedic Surgery
Children's Memorial Hospital
Northwestern University
Chicago, Illinois

Thomas H. Lee, MD
Chief, Foot and Ankle Service
Department of Orthopedics
Ohio State University
Columbus, Ohio

Khristinn Kellie Leitch, MD, MBA, FRCS(C)
Pediatric Orthopaedics
Childrens Hospital Los Angeles
Los Angeles, California

Contributors

Gregory N. Lervick, MD
Department of Orthopaedics
The Park Nicollet Clinic
St. Louis Park, Minnesota

William N. Levine, MD
Assistant Professor
Director, Sports Medicine
Orthopaedic Surgery
Columbia-Presbyterian Medical Center
New York, New York

Steven C. Ludwig, MD
Assistant Professor
Orthopedics and Rehabilitation
University of Maryland Medical Systems
Baltimore, Maryland

Richard M. Marks, MD, FACS
Associate Professor
Director, Division of Foot and Ankle Surgery
Department of Orthopaedic Surgery
Medical College of Wisconsin
Milwaukee, Wisconsin

Robert W. Molinari, MD
Chief, Spinal Surgery Service
Assistant Professor of Surgery
Uniformed Services University of the Health Sciences
Madigan Army Medical Center
Tacoma, Washington

Albert D. Olszewski, MD
Flathead Valley Orthopedics
Kalispell, Montana

Raymond A. Pensy, MD
Chief Resident
Orthopaedics Department
University of Maryland Medical Systems
Baltimore, Maryland

Andrew K. Sands, MD
Chief, Foot and Ankle Surgery
Department of Orthopaedics
Saint Vincent's Medical Center, Manhattan
New York, New York

James F. Schwarten, MD
Orthopedic Surgeons, PSC
Billings, Montana

Charles N. Seal, MD
Department of Orthopaedics
University of Maryland Medical System
Baltimore, Maryland

Curtis Settergren, MD, MS
Orthopedic Surgeons, PSC
Billings, Montana

Kern Singh, MD
Chief Resident
Orthopaedic Surgery Department
Rush-Presbyterian-St. Luke's Medical Center
Chicago, Illinois

David L. Skaggs, MD
Associate Professor of Orthopaedic Surgery
University of Southern California
Childrens Orthopaedic Center
Childrens Hospital Los Angeles
Los Angeles, California

Alexander R. Vaccaro
Professor
Co-Chief Spine Surgery
Co-Director Spine Fellowship Program
Co-Director of the Delaware Valley Regional Spinal Cord
  Injury Center
Thomas Jefferson University and the Rothman Institute
Philadelphia, Pennsylvania

Kirkham B. Wood, MD
Associate Professor
Department of Orthopaedic Surgery
University of Minnesota
Minneapolis, Minnesota

Preface

Essentials of Musculoskeletal Imaging is designed as a guide and easy-to-use reference for selecting and interpreting the appropriate imaging modalities to diagnose and evaluate numerous and common musculoskeletal problems. The goal of this text is not to provide in-depth coverage of all imaging modalities for all musculoskeletal conditions but rather to provide the physician with an easy-to-use guide for ordering and interpreting appropriate and cost-effective imaging studies for the most common problems seen in the office. As health care costs escalate, the physician has a responsibility to order only those imaging studies that are cost-effective and have the highest degree of sensitivity and specificity. Our hope is that this book will help accomplish this goal.

This text is the second in the *Essentials* series published by the American Academy of Orthopaedic Surgeons. The structure, organization, and practical approach used in the first book, *Essentials of Musculoskeletal Care*, has proved to be very popular among our readers. This format has been carried forward in this new addition to the series. Most chapters are organized along the following headings: Synonyms, ICD-9 Codes, Definition, History and Physical Findings, Imaging Studies (required for diagnosis, required for comprehensive evaluation, special considerations, and pitfalls), Image Descriptions, and Differential Diagnosis.

The text includes four general sections (Imaging Modalities, General Orthopaedics, Tumors, and Pediatric Orthopaedics) and seven anatomic sections. Each anatomic section begins with an overview, followed by chapters that describe specific musculoskeletal problems. A CD-ROM with more than 700 images from all sections accompanies this book.

The concept for this book was supported by the Publications Committee of the American Academy of Orthopaedic Surgeons (Marilyn Fox, PhD, staff liaison, and Alan Levine, MD, chairman) and approved by the Board of Directors. The American Academy of Pediatrics has reviewed and endorsed this book as they have done for *Essentials of Musculoskeletal Care*. We are grateful for their involvement in the development of the content and for their support in promoting its use to their members.

Several contributors from orthopaedics and radiology made this book possible. Our sincere thanks go to section editors and their authors for unselfishly giving of their time and expertise in the writing of this book. Without the contributions of the following editors, this book would not have been possible: JH Edmund Lee, MD (Imaging Modalities), James Johnston, MD (Tumors), Theodore Blaine, MD (Shoulder and Elbow), Joseph Erpelding, MD (Hip and Thigh), Andrew Haims, MD, and Peter Jokl, MD (Knee and Lower Leg), Daniel Gelb, MD, and Louis Jenis, MD (Spine), Carol Frey, MD (Foot and Ankle), John Sarwark, MD, and Richard Shore, MD (Pediatric Orthopaedics). Thanks also to Jay Lieberman, MD, for offering terrific suggestions on the chapters regarding total joint complications.

Essentials of Musculoskeletal Imaging has been our passion for the past 3 years, but we have shared that passion with Lynne Shindoll, Managing Editor, and David Stanley, Assistant Production Manager, in the Academy's Publications Department. Lynne and Robert Snider, MD, were responsible for developing the concept and format for *Essentials of Musculoskeletal Care* and more than anyone else are responsible for any success this book will enjoy.

Thanks also go to Walter Greene, MD, who set a high standard of excellence with his editorship of the second edition of *Essentials*. David Stanley and Mary Steermann, Manager, Production and Archives, and all the staff in the production area have done their usual expert job in the layout, reproduction, and handling of literally 1,000 images. A most pleasant and expert addition to the publication team has been Senior Editor Laurie Braun, who has done the lion's share of the editing of this book. Her persistence, enthusiasm, and gentle prodding helped to keep us on schedule. Also, we would be remiss if we did not thank Senior Editor Joan Abern for helping us out in crunch time with her usual exceptional editing skills. This book would not have happened without the expertise provided by these professionals. It has been an honor and privilege to work with them.

A first edition of any book leaves room for improvement. We welcome your comments and recommendations. Please take time to fill out the comment card enclosed with this book. Your feedback is invaluable to future editors as the Academy plans subsequent editions. You can also write to us at *Essentials of Musculoskeletal Imaging*, AAOS Publications Department, 6300 North River Road, Rosemont, IL 60018. You may send your comments to us by email at the following addresses: shindoll@aaos.org, ThomasJ502@aol.com, or Lynne.Steinbach@radiology.ucsf.edu.

Thomas R. Johnson, MD
Lynne S. Steinbach, MD
Editors

Table of Contents

SECTION THREE
TUMORS

SECTION FOUR
SHOULDER

Section Five
Elbow and Forearm

Section Six
Hand and Wrist

Section Seven
Hip and Thigh

Section Eight
Knee and Lower Leg

Section Eleven
Pediatric Orthopaedics

To my wife, Judy,
and our children, Brett, Burke, and Paula Rae,
who sacrificed precious time to allow me to be a physician.
And to my mentors,
Ron Losee, MD, Wayne Southwick, MD,
H. Kirk Watson, MD, Perry M. Berg, MD,
and Raymond Johnson, MD,
role models all, worthy of emulation.
—Thomas R. Johnson, MD

To my husband, Eric Tepper, MD,
my son, Mark Tepper,
and my parents, Howard and Ilse Steinbach.
—Lynne S. Steinbach, MD

IMAGING MODALITIES

Section Editor
J.H. Edmund Lee, MD

Contributor
Mitch Gallagher, MD

RADIOGRAPHY

Radiography is a process by which images are obtained by projecting x-ray beams through a subject and onto an image detector. The radiographic image produced is a projectional map of the amount of radiation absorbed by the subject along the course of the x-ray beam. Radiographs have typically been obtained using an analog detector system (ie, a film cassette), although digital detector systems are being used increasingly in clinical settings. When a digital detector system is used, the technique is called digital, or computed, radiography.

On a radiograph, the whiteness of the image is a function of the radiodensities and thicknesses of the various objects or tissues between the source of the x-ray beam and the detector. Because the higher mass density of bones and metal hardware results in greater attenuation of the x-rays projected through the body part, they appear whiter on the radiographic image than do soft tissues or plastic hardware.

Advantages

Radiography remains the most commonly used medical imaging modality because it has several key advantages over other modalities. Radiography is a simple, readily available, relatively inexpensive technique that most physicians can interpret without technical training. In addition, the spatial resolution of radiography far exceeds that of cross-sectional imaging modalities such as ultrasound, CT, or MRI. Radiography can theoretically detect objects as small as 0.05 to 0.1 mm (depending on the equipment), compared with 0.4 to 1 mm for a typical high-resolution CT scan.[1] Although imaging artifacts occur, most are not so serious as to completely prohibit interpretation of the image. Real-time radiographic imaging, or fluoroscopy, provides guidance during invasive medical procedures such as angiography and hardware placement. The excellent bone detail provided by radiography is advantageous in the evaluation of arthritis (Figure 1-1).

Limitations

The greatest drawback of radiography is that radiation is transmitted to the patient and medical personnel. This risk can be minimized by taking proper precautions, as described in a separate chapter on Radiation Safety.

Radiographs also provide relatively poor contrast resolution, especially for soft-tissue imaging, compared with that of other imaging methods. The radiodensities of most human tissues fall within a rather narrow range, resulting in limited contrast on radiographs between different tissues such as muscles and fat. Soft tissues are not visualized well on radiographs unless fat or calcification is present. Fortunately, bone has a relatively high mineral content, allowing good contrast between bones and adjacent soft tissues.

Other limitations of radiography are related to the technology, which involves projection of an x-ray beam onto a two-dimensional detector. First, because the x-ray beams diverge as they leave the source, the projected image is always larger than the actual subject. Therefore, any measurements of length on a radiograph must be calibrated to a physical standard that is placed adjacent to the patient at the time that the image is obtained. Failure to do so can result in the overestimation of fracture length or fragment size. This enlargement, however, can sometimes be used to advantage, such as in magnification radiography of arthritic hands. Second, in contrast to cross-sectional images, on radiographs overlapping objects can be obscured. This problem can be compensated for by the use of several different views.

Radiography requires several pieces of equipment, including an x-ray generator, an image detector, and image processing equipment. Because most physicians are unfamiliar with the use of such equipment, a radiology technician is needed to operate the equipment. The physician therefore depends on the skill of the technician to produce good radiographs, but it must be remembered that the physician bears the ultimate responsibility for obtaining complete, adequate-quality radiographic studies.

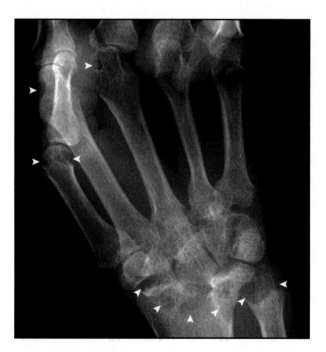

Figure 1-1
PA radiograph of the right hand and wrist of a 50-year-old woman with long-standing rheumatoid arthritis. The arrowheads show articular erosions involving the radiocarpal, ulnar styloid, and metacarpophalangeal joints in a pattern classic for rheumatoid arthritis. The patient's left hand and feet were similarly affected.

Principal Musculoskeletal Indications

Radiography is typically used as the initial diagnostic imaging modality for musculoskeletal conditions. In addition, for fractures, arthritis, bone tumors, and skeletal dysplasia, radiography is frequently sufficient to establish the diagnosis, and other imaging modalities are not needed. Follow-up of musculoskeletal disease also has traditionally been performed with radiographs. A variety of stress maneuvers can be performed while examining joints, providing clues to abnormalities in joint dynamics as well. In summary, radiography forms the basis of primary musculoskeletal imaging and usually should be ordered prior to other imaging modalities.

Contraindications

Unfortunately, radiography frequently cannot evaluate musculoskeletal conditions that primarily involve soft tissues in the earliest stages or conditions that produce minimal or no changes in the bone. An example is chondromalacia, a softening of the articular cartilage of the patella, which cannot be detected on radiographs in the earliest stage because cartilage generally cannot be seen on radiographs but is detectable later, when bone becomes involved. Primarily medullary diseases, especially those involving the mid-diaphyses of long bones, where bone trabeculae are sparse, can be missed altogether because they do not involve bone loss. Abnormalities of unossified growth plates in children cannot be seen except by indirect signs. Joint injuries or soft-tissue spine injuries may be missed if no malalignment is present.

Cautions

Inadequate imaging technique is a common problem. A single view may not provide adequate information. In most situations, at least two views, preferably orthogonal (90° to one another; eg, AP and lateral), should be obtained because structures and abnormalities can be obscured on one view. Improper positioning can result in misinterpretation and omit abnormalities from the field of view. Joint instabilities such as carpal instability or foot deformities may not be seen or adequately characterized without stress maneuvers. Accurate measurements of parameters such as ulnar variance or patellar tilt require views in which the limb is specially positioned. Radiographs taken with portable units, which tend to be of poor quality, should be interpreted with caution, as should radiographs in which the image is obscured by cast material. Finally, as with any medical procedure, the identity of the patient should be carefully verified when ordering, obtaining, and interpreting any radiographic study.

SECTION 1 ■ IMAGING MODALITIES

Principal Views

Routine screening views of various bones and joints are listed in Table 1. Radiographs of long bones such as the humerus should include the adjacent joints so that the entire bone is imaged. Various views for arthritis surveys and other myriad specialized views exist as well but are beyond the scope of this book. A good source for specialized views is *Merrill's Atlas of Radiographic Positions and Radiologic Procedures.*[2]

Table 1
Routine Screening Views

Upper Extremity	
Fingers	PA, lateral, oblique (fingers should be separated)
Hand	PA, oblique, lateral
Wrist	PA, lateral (both with neutral positioning)
Forearm	AP, lateral
Elbow	AP (supinated), lateral (90° flexed). Oblique views may be added for trauma patients
Humerus	AP, lateral
Glenohumeral joint	AP in internal and external rotation, true AP of the scapula, axillary. A 30° caudal tilt view is added for suspected impingement. A transscapular view is helpful in assessing glenohumeral dislocation and acromion morphology.
Acromioclavicular joint	AP, 10° cephalad AP (Zanca view)
Lower Extremity	
Hip	AP internal rotation, frog-lateral (or cross-table lateral)
Femur	AP, lateral
Knee	AP, lateral (30° flexion)
Knee, arthritis	Add AP weight-bearing views or PA flexed weight-bearing views, lateral weight bearing views, and occasionally Merchant axial views
Knee, intercondylar notch	Tunnel view (angulated PA or AP 45° flexed)
Knee, patellofemoral joint	Merchant view
Tibia/fibula	AP, lateral
Ankle	AP, lateral, mortise
Foot	AP, lateral, medial (internal) oblique (weight-bearing AP and lateral for foot alignment abnormality)
Subtalar joint	Lateral view, posterior tangential
Calcaneus	Lateral, AP, axial
Toes	AP, lateral, AP oblique
Axial Skeleton	
Cervical spine	AP and lateral views. A lateral flexion-extension view can be added in patients with rheumatoid arthritis and suspected instability. A trauma spine series should include an open mouth odontoid view and a swimmer's view if C7 is not visualized.
Thoracic spine	AP, lateral
Lumbar spine	AP, lateral
Sacrum	30° cephalad angulated AP, lateral
Coccyx	10° caudal angulated AP, lateral
Sacroiliac joints	30° cephalad angulated AP (Ferguson view)
Pelvis	AP (Judet views and/or inlet/outlet views for pelvic ring fractures)

References

1. Curry TS III, Dowdey JE, Murry RC Jr: *Christensen's Physics of Diagnostic Radiology*, ed 4. Malvern, PA, Lea & Febiger, 1990.

2. Ballinger PW, Frank ED, Merrill V: *Merrill's Atlas of Radiographic Positions and Radiologic Procedures,* ed 9. St Louis, MO, Mosby-Year Book, 1999.

COMPUTED TOMOGRAPHY

CT uses x-rays to produce tomographic images, or images that show slices of the subject. In transmission tomography, a thinly collimated x-ray beam is transmitted through the subject and received by the detector. The amount of x-ray radiation received at the detector is a function of the amount of radiation absorbed or scattered by tissues and objects along the course of the beam. The transmission data are manipulated mathematically and reconstructed by computer to form an image, which is typically then adjusted, using various algorithms depending on the type of tissue being evaluated (eg, bone, soft tissue), to enhance detail or minimize image noise. Typically, multiple contiguous slices of data are obtained. The resulting images form a computed map of the x-ray densities of the various tissues and objects that were scanned.

In CT, x-ray densities are measured in Hounsfield units (HUs) or CT numbers, where water is assigned a value of 0 HU and air a value of –1,000 HU, fixing the scale for other densities. These values are a function of the technique used to obtain the CT scan and can vary. Images are typically displayed in grayscale, with denser objects appearing lighter. The grayscale can be modified, or "windowed," to show only those data that fall within a fixed range of densities, such as bone or lung windows. Because CT uses x-ray beams to obtain images, iodinated material, barium suspension, or air can be used as a contrast medium, producing modified images that show vascular flow, extracellular diffusion (through the use of delayed enhancement), or joint anatomy.

Advantages

The greatest advantages of CT over plain radiography are the tomographic nature of the imaging and the higher contrast resolution of the images (Figures 1-2 and 1-3). Tomographic images allow the anatomy to be seen in slices without intervening tissues that can obscure the area of interest. Contrast resolution refers to the ability of an imaging modality to distinguish between two objects based on a physical parameter such as radiographic density. Both CT and plain radiography produce good images of bones and lungs, which contain tissues with large differences in x-ray densities. These imaging methods are relatively less effective, however, at differentiating among soft tissues, which is why contrast media are frequently used to enhance the radiographic distinctions between soft tissues. An additional advantage of CT is that its digital nature allows data from multiple images to be reconstructed to produce images in planes other than the one in which the original images were obtained.

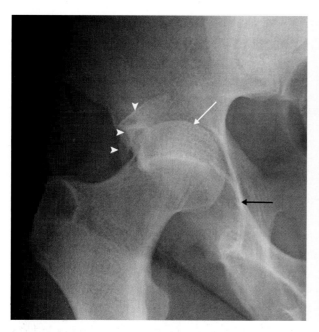

Figure 1-2

Posterior hip dislocation in a 30-year-old man who sustained multiple trauma. AP radiograph shows the femoral head (white arrow) dislocated posteriorly from the acetabulum (black arrow). Several fracture fragments (arrowheads) lie adjacent to the joint, but none is clearly intra-articular.

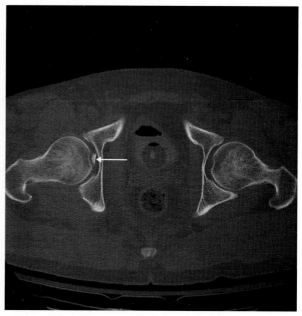

Figure 1-3

An axial CT scan through the middle of the hips of the same patient shown in Figure 1-2 was taken after joint reduction, and the resulting data were "windowed" to enhance bone detail, producing this bone window representation. It shows a large, comminuted intra-articular fragment (arrow) that was not visible on postreduction plain radiographs. The fragment was subsequently removed to prevent accelerated joint degeneration. Note that excellent bone detail is demonstrated. Similarly, soft-tissue windows can be used to evaluate muscle and fat.

CT scanners are widely available in the United States, and many physicians have experience in interpreting the images. The cost of CT is higher than that of plain radiography, but it is certainly lower than MRI. Imaging times range from 5 to 10 minutes, and the procedure is generally tolerated well by cooperative patients.

Indications

Combined with injection of contrast medium into anatomic spaces, CT can be used for imaging joints (CT arthrography) and the dural sac (CT myelography), although MRI has replaced CT in many of these instances. With the help of a stereotactic frame, CT can produce precisely mapped images that can be used to guide surgery or radiation therapy. Modern, fast CT scanners combined with timed intravenous contrast medium injection can produce angiographic images, such as for arteriography, and perfusion images, such as for assessment of tissue viability. Fast CT scanners also can image the motion of joints (kinematic CT) such as the patellofemoral joint. Biopsies can be performed using CT guidance; this can be especially useful in the biopsy of small lesions. Using specialized tools, three-dimensional models can be created to facilitate prosthesis fitting. Angles can be measured, as in the evaluation of lower limb torsion. Finally, CT can be used to measure dimensions accurately, as in pelvimetry, without the magnification artifacts that occur in plain radiography.

Limitations

CT can produce a variety of artifacts. The most common is blurring caused by patient movement. Whereas plain radiographic images are typically obtained in substantially less than 1 second, most CT slices are obtained in about 1 second, which is long enough for motion to disrupt the acquisition of data. A second type of motion artifact occurs when the patient moves between the imaging of different slices, resulting in potential misregistration of slices, which in turn can lead to misinterpretation and inaccurate images.

Much orthopaedic hardware contains metal, which is of sufficiently high x-ray density to prevent sufficient x-rays from being transmitted through the body part. This results in an artifact called "beam hardening." Beam hardening appears as streaks of white or black that obscure anatomy adjacent to the hardware. This artifact is much more severe than the artifact produced by metal in plain film tomography, to the extent that the images can be worthless for diagnosis. Therefore, the amount of metal hardware near the area of interest should be considered prior to ordering CT.

CT provides more limited soft-tissue contrast resolution than do MRI and ultrasonography, so CT scans may reveal few identifying characteristics, especially in tissues where fat is not present to provide a natural contrast to soft tissues. CT does not usually provide a direct scan in several different planes, though such images can be reconstructed digitally, whereas both MRI and ultrasonography can do this readily. Also, CT relies on a single physical parameter (x-ray density) to produce images, whereas MRI can examine many different parameters. In addition, the osmolality of the contrast medium used with CT makes it inappropriate for use with patients with renal insufficiency.

CT scanners require a large physical site. Most scanners cannot accommodate patients larger than approximately 300 to 400 lb. Although the cost of a CT examination is not as high as MRI, initial costs to purchase and install the equipment are relatively high. Finally, as with radiography, CT exposes the patient to potentially harmful ionizing radiation. In fact, the evolution and proliferation of fast CT scanners has led to greater use, increasing radiation doses to patients and the population in general.

Principal Musculoskeletal Indications

Common musculoskeletal uses for CT include the staging of complex or comminuted fractures, the detection of small intra-articular fragments, the evaluation of fracture healing in suspected nonunion, the confirmation of fractures suspected on plain radiography (eg, spine injuries), and the evaluation of bone tumors. Although CT can detect and stage soft-tissue tumors, MRI is generally superior for this purpose. The best modality for the evaluation of loose bodies in the joint is a CT arthrogram, which requires intra-articular injection of contrast medium and/or air. Intravenous contrast medium is useful for the evaluation of soft-tissue disease or destructive bone tumors, but it is unnecessary for the evaluation of fractures or skeletal deformities. MRI and scintigraphy (bone scan) detect nondisplaced or incomplete fractures with higher sensitivity than does CT.

Cautions

The principal misuses of CT typically fall into one of two categories. The first misuse is ordering CT for a condition that is well evaluated by plain radiography or in situations where CT does not provide additional useful information. This results in unnecessary expense and radiation exposure to the patient. As with all diagnostic tests, before ordering secondary diagnostic tests such as CT or MRI, the physician should have in mind a well-formed question that can be answered by the particular imaging modality.

The second category of misuse is ordering CT when it is very unlikely to produce diagnostic-quality images. Examples include ordering CT for patients who cannot tolerate temporary immobilization, patients with significant amounts of metal hardware near the site to be scanned, and conditions that cannot be differentiated on the basis of CT examination, such as cystic versus solid lesions.

CT may be impractical for obese patients. Each scanner is rated to handle patients up to a certain weight. Above this weight, the table that carries the patient through the scanner ring may not move, and it may actually break. Specialized CT scanners that can handle very large patients may be available by special arrangement.

Pregnant women should generally not undergo CT, except in life-threatening circumstances, because of the potential for damage to the fetus from radiation. For more information, see the chapter on Radiation Safety.

MAGNETIC RESONANCE IMAGING

MRI is similar in concept to CT in that images are produced by reconstruction of a data set. Unlike CT, which uses an x-ray beam with multiple detectors to record differences in tissue attenuation, MRI applies a strong magnetic field with radiofrequency (RF) pulses to record differences in tissue signal intensity. Because MRI does not employ radiation, it does not have the tissue-damaging properties of radiation-based imaging modalities. The MRI scanner consists of a very large, powerful magnet that generates a static magnetic field and multiple coils that send and receive RF signals. These tiny RF signals are obtained from the area of the body being imaged and are then processed and reconstructed by computer.

MRI fundamentally images the protons in hydrogen atoms, which are present in all human tissues. The protons in hydrogen exist in many different atomic microenvironments (bone, fluid, muscle, fat, etc) and concentrations in the body, and the MRI technique images these differences.

When protons are subjected to a strong magnetic field, they line up like countless compasses. A brief (milliseconds) RF pulse is applied to the tissue, essentially deflecting the protons. When this pulse is terminated, the protons realign, or "relax," along the dominant strong magnetic field. The protons relax at different rates that depend on the atomic microenvironment. The basic principle of MRI is that, during relaxation, protons emit a weak signal with

Table 1			
Relative Signal Intensities of Selected Structures on Spin Echo Sequences in Musculoskeletal MRI			
Structure	Sequence		
	T1-weighted; short TR/short TE	**Proton-density; long TR/short TE**	**T2-weighted; long TR/long TE**
Fat[*]	bright	bright	intermediate
Fluid[†]	dark	intermediate	bright
Fibrocartilage[‡]	dark	dark	dark
Ligament, tendon§	dark	dark	dark
Muscle	intermediate	intermediate	dark
Bone marrow	bright	intermediate	dark
Nerve	intermediate	intermediate	intermediate

TR = repetition time. Short = < 600 to 700 ms; long = > 2,000 ms

TE = echo time. Short = < 20 to 30 ms; long = >90 ms

*Includes yellow marrow. Signal will be dark if fat-suppression techniques (eg, fat-saturation, STIR) are used

†Includes edema, most tears, and most cysts

‡Includes labrum, menisci, triangular fibrocartilage

§Signal may be increased because of artifacts (eg, magic angle artifact seen in the rotator cuff or the ankle tendons)

properties distinct to each type of tissue: a magnetic resonance "signature" (Table 1). The MRI scanner receives and records these signals and ultimately reconstructs them into a highly accurate anatomic image. Many disease processes alter the proton relaxation characteristics within normal tissues; these changes become visible as areas of abnormal signal intensity. The strength of the magnet is often expressed in tesla (T) units. MRI equipment is currently clinically available with magnet strengths from 0.2 to 3.0 T.

Advantages

The greatest advantage of MRI is its superior contrast resolution, particularly with regard to distinguishing differences among soft tissues such as fat and muscle. CT and radiography provide better spatial resolution than does MRI, but in many circumstances, the superior contrast resolution of MRI yields more valuable clinical information (Figures 1-4 and 1-5). Although CT remains the technique of choice in detailed cortical bone imaging, MRI is superior to CT in the diagnosis of early pathologic processes within bone marrow. Stress fractures, osteomyelitis, malignancy, and marrow-infiltrating diseases are clearly seen on MRI scans as areas of high signal intensity within bone marrow. Although somewhat limited with regard to specificity, MRI offers a very high degree of sensitivity in the evaluation of diseases that affect bone marrow.

Contrast materials, primarily gadolinium-based compounds, can be used with MRI to enhance the imaging of disease processes in a variety of tissues. Gadolinium behaves much like iodinated contrast mediums, accumulating in highly vascular and metabolically active tissues. Gadolinium compounds are also safer than iodine-based contrast mediums and can be safely administered to patients with renal insufficiency.

Limitations

Compared with CT, MRI is prone to a larger number of and more severe types of artifacts. Motion blurring and metal artifacts can occur with both MRI and CT, but others are unique to MRI and are frequently difficult to understand and eliminate. For example, the size of a metal artifact in MRI is a function of the type as well as the quantity of metal; therefore, a tiny shotgun pellet can produce a huge artifact, obscuring anatomic information. However, MRI-compatible surgical implants are safe and produce insignificant artifacts.

The strong magnetic field created inside and in the vicinity of an MRI scanner must be carefully considered. Electrical appliances such as pacemakers and mechanical pumps can malfunction, with potentially disastrous consequences. In a small subset of patients, metal cardiac valves can be held open or

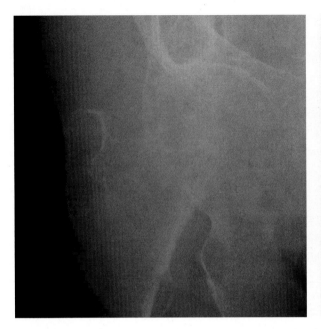

Figure 1-4
AP radiograph of the right hip of a 76-year-old woman who reported sudden pain after a fall shows poor bone detail because of extreme osteopenia. No fracture is apparent.

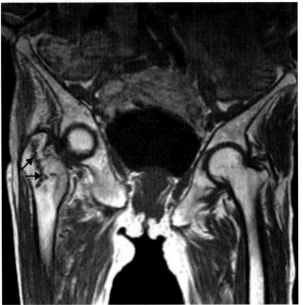

Figure 1-5
Coronal T1-weighted MRI of the right hip of the same patient in Figure 1-4 was ordered subsequently because the patient was unable to bear weight, raising a high clinical suspicion for a radiographically occult fracture. The dark line through part of the intertrochanteric right femur (arrows) indicates an area of low signal intensity, characteristic of an incomplete fracture. MRI is exquisitely sensitive to conditions such as this that affect bone marrow.

closed. Other metal objects can be turned into dangerous projectiles. For example, non–MRI-compatible oxygen containers can fly through the magnet bore, seriously injuring the patient or nearby staff members. Metal foreign bodies within the eye can migrate and cause ocular injury and blindness. Tattoos and cosmetics containing metal can absorb energy and burn the skin seriously. Therefore, careful screening of each patient's medical, surgical, and social history is necessary for the safety of the staff and the patients.

Other complications can arise as well. Some patients who are claustrophobic cannot tolerate the procedure, which typically involves being confined in a small space for 20 to 60 minutes. These patients can be pretreated with anti-anxiety medication or scanned in open MRI units. Early open MRI units produced images that were inferior to those from closed scanners, but newer models with improved image quality are now available. Some patients cannot tolerate prolonged immobilization if they are experiencing pain. In some patients, undergoing MRI induces muscle twitching, visual scotomata, or elevated body temperature due to energy absorption. These effects are far more common with systems with high magnetic field strength (1.5 to 3.0 T).

An additional disadvantage of MRI is cost. MRI is perhaps the most expensive imaging modality in routine use. Contributing factors include the cost of the large, shielded imaging suite necessary to accommodate the unit and the fact that fewer MRI studies can be performed in a given day compared with CT studies. These cost factors have limited the availability of MRI, especially outside the United States.

Finally, although MRI has generally high sensitivity and high negative predictive value, its specificity varies, depending on the condition. For example, a normal MRI scan can effectively exclude an incomplete bone fracture, but an abnormal bone marrow signal may be caused by a variety of conditions including fracture, stress reaction, infection, or marrow infiltration from tumor. Interpretation of an MRI scan is generally more difficult than with other imaging modalities.

Principal Musculoskeletal Indications

MRI typically should not be used as an initial screening study but as a problem-solving tool, so careful clinical evaluation and radiography should be ordered prior to MRI. Common musculoskeletal indications for MRI include the evaluation of intra-articular structures (eg, meniscus, cartilage, loose bodies), musculotendinous injury, joint instability, osteomyelitis, suspected fracture, stress injury, vertebral disk disease, soft-tissue tumors, and skeletal malformations. MR arthrography (see also the chapter on Arthrography) can increase accuracy in the evaluation of joint instability, suspected loose bodies, and the postoperative status of joints. MR angiography can be useful for patients who are unable to undergo conventional catheter angiography because of renal insufficiency or a history of idiosyncratic reactions to iodinated contrast media.

Whole-body screening, such as for metastatic cancer, should be performed by bone scan and/or CT; MRI is not of proven value in such situations, and it is more expensive. MRI does, however, play an important role in screening the brain and spine in patients with acute neurologic symptoms and known or suspected malignancy. Although MRI can detect foreign bodies in soft tissues, a combination of radiography and ultrasound can accomplish the same result more expeditiously and with less expense.

SCINTIGRAPHY

Scintigraphy is a form of nuclear medicine imaging. Radioisotope-labeled, biologically active drugs administered to the patient serve as tracers of biologic activity. The drug then distributes itself according to the targeted metabolic mechanism. Technetium Tc 99m, for example, is incorporated into metabolically active bone. The images produced by scintigraphy are a collection of the radiation emissions from the radioisotopes and are obtained with a special camera.

With scintigraphy, both single-projection images (planar images) and cross-sectional images (single-photon emission computed tomography, or SPECT) can be obtained. A variety of radioisotopes of various energies and a wide assortment of drugs with different biodistributions are used. Some isotopes, such as iodine-131, are given as therapy but also produce x-ray emissions that can be captured to produce images. Nuclear medicine tracers usually are eliminated from the body metabolically, as well as by spontaneous decay.

Positron-emission tomography (PET) is performed similarly to SPECT, but PET uses positron-emitting radioisotopes that produce high-energy photons that can be easily localized within the patient. The images on PET scans are generally of higher spatial resolution than those produced with SPECT; unfortunately, most PET agents have very short half-lives and are thus difficult to administer and image. PET agents are costly to manufacture as well.

Bone scintigraphy, commonly referred to as bone scanning, is generally performed using diphosphonates labeled with radioactive technetium. These compounds distribute in the body in three phases. In the initial, or transient, phase, the tracer is delivered to perfused tissues; images obtained during this phase are referred to as perfusion images. The second, or blood-pool, phase follows shortly after the initial phase. Finally, in the delayed phase, the tracer accumulates in tissues with active turnover of phosphates, mostly in bone undergoing turnover or growth. Images obtained in single-phase examinations come from this final phase. Images from all three phases are acquired in three-phase bone scintigraphy (Figure 1-6).

Other radiopharmaceutical agents also distribute in bone. Labeled sulfur colloid distributes within organs with reticuloendothelial tissue such as red bone marrow, the liver, and the spleen: these scans are referred to as liver-spleen scans or bone marrow scans, depending on the clinical indication. In white cell scintigraphy, labeled white cells are injected; they eventually distribute normally to the spleen, liver, and bone marrow, but abnormal accumulation is seen in areas of acute inflammation. In

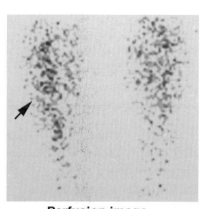
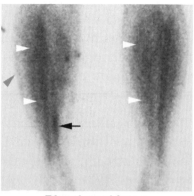
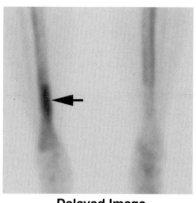

Perfusion image **Blood-pool image** **Delayed Image**

Figure 1-6

Anterior views from a technetium Tc 99m monodiphosphate three-phase bone scan in a 35-year-old woman with pain in the distal right tibia clinically suspected to be a stress fracture. Perfusion image shows relatively increased radiotracer flow (arrow) to the symptomatic right leg. Blood-pool image shows relatively increased tracer delivery (gray arrowhead) to the right leg. Note extensive soft-tissue activity (white arrowheads) during this phase and early accumulation of radiotracer in the right tibial stress fracture (black arrow). Delayed image shows clearance of the soft-tissue uptake compared to the blood-pool image. The stress fracture is clearly visible as a linear band of increased uptake in the tibia (arrow). (Figures courtesy of Bijan Bijan, MD)

gallium scintigraphy, radioactive gallium citrate is used to show regions of both acute and chronic inflammation. In addition, new agents such as labeled monoclonal antibodies show promise in imaging very specific tissues or disease processes.

Advantages

The principal strength of scintigraphy lies in its ability to image metabolic activity. Unfortunately, most normal metabolic processes involving bone have relatively slow metabolic activity compared with organs such as the liver or kidneys. Fortunately, most radioisotopes, with the exception of PET agents, are relatively long-lived (ie, they emit detectable radiation for several hours) and provide ample time for imaging various organs, making delayed whole-body bone scintigraphy possible. Bone scintigraphy is also exquisitely sensitive to many bone conditions such as fractures and tumors. In fact, a negative bone scan is frequently assumed to exclude fractures, osteomyelitis, and metastases. Although the specificity is not as high as the sensitivity, bone scan coupled with radiography frequently results in an accurate diagnosis.

In the past, bone marrow scintigraphy was used for imaging bone infarcts, but MRI is currently used for this reason. Bone marrow scans are sometimes used for comparison with white cell scans in the evaluation of osteomyelitis.

White cell scintigraphy and gallium scintigraphy are frequently used for the evaluation of osteomyelitis, especially in areas in which previous surgery or hardware placement renders the bone scan nonspecific and therefore less useful. White cell scintigraphy is more specific but less sensitive than gallium scintigraphy in the detection of osteomyelitis.

Last, radioactive isotopes can be used to localize lesions with a Geiger counter or other appropriate detector during surgery. This can be helpful in guiding resection of small bone tumors.

Limitations

The most significant limitation of scintigraphy is the lack of detail in the image. This arises from a relative paucity of signal compared to radiography, CT, and MRI. Thus, images obtained by scintigraphy have relatively poor spatial resolution, making small lesions (1 to 2 cm) difficult to detect. White cell and gallium scans have even poorer detail compared to bone scans.

As described above, low specificity can be a problem in situations where incidental disease such as osteoarthritis or disk degeneration overlaps a region of suspected disease. Sites of hardware placement can remain abnormal for several years, making exclusion of infection at the site impossible or difficult without the use of white cell or gallium scans.

Another potential problem is caused by the limited early sensitivity of scintigraphy to fractures in patients with very slow bone metabolism/turnover, such as elderly patients. In these patients, fractures may require several days to show up as abnormal uptake on a bone scan. Low sensitivity can also occur with lytic diseases such as multiple myeloma. Finally, bone scans are less sensitive than MRI in detecting medullary lesions because of the relative paucity of bone trabeculae in this area of the bone.

Principal Musculoskeletal Indications

Scintigraphy is used for screening of skeletal metastases, in the evaluation of focal bone tumors, for screening of stress and insufficiency fractures, and for screening of osteomyelitis. Radiography should be used for skeletal survey for multiple myeloma and dysplasia. Because early insufficiency fractures may not be seen on bone scans, MRI may be needed to rule out these fractures.

Contraindications/Cautions

Scintigraphy exposes patients to ionizing radiation. Although the radiation dose is relatively low with bone scintigraphy, other studies such as gallium scintigraphy can deliver relatively high doses to various organs. Therefore, children and pregnant women should be very carefully screened to ensure that scintigraphy is indicated.

ARTHROGRAPHY

Arthrography is the imaging of joints or any other synovial-lined space, including tendon sheaths (tenography) and bursae (bursography), following injection of a contrast medium into the area under study. Tears and defects of ligaments and tendons can be diagnosed by noting abnormal extension of the contrast medium into spaces. For example, extension of the contrast medium from the glenohumeral joint into the subdeltoid bursa indicates a rotator cuff tear. The use of conventional arthrography has become less common since the advent of cross-sectional imaging (CT and MRI).

The injection is typically performed percutaneously, referred to as direct arthrography. Frequently the injection is done in conjunction with some type of imaging guidance such as fluoroscopy, CT, or ultrasonography, but it also can be done by palpation. The type of contrast medium varies, depending on the type of study: it can be an iodinated medium and/or air with fluoroscopy and CT arthrography; saline or dilute gadolinium chelate with MR arthrography; or any type of fluid with ultrasonography. Local anesthetic and/or corticosteroids can be injected at the same time for diagnosis and/or therapy as well.

In indirect arthrography, gadolinium chelate is injected intravenously in conjunction with MRI. Discussion of this technique, however, is beyond the scope of this text.

Advantages

Direct arthrography produces two advantages when accompanied by cross-sectional imaging. First, the addition of contrast medium into the joint can highlight intra-articular soft-tissue structures such as ligaments, tendons, and fibrocartilaginous structures (Figures 1-7 and 1-8). Cartilaginous joint structures can be seen better as well. Second, the joint distention that occurs on injection stretches the joint capsule, forcing fluid into defects such as ligament, labrum, and meniscus tears. These combined effects allow CT to evaluate intra-articular disease[1] and improve the accuracy of MRI for diagnosing several musculoskeletal conditions, such as shoulder instability.[2]

Arthrography performed in conjunction with fluoroscopy still has many advantages over cross-sectional imaging. Arthrography can be very accurate, matching or exceeding the accuracy of MRI alone in some circumstances, such as the diagnosis of intrinsic wrist ligament tears. The high spatial resolution of fluoroscopy allows for highly accurate analysis of fine anatomic detail. This is particularly advantageous in small joints such as the wrist, where arthrography allows overlapping structures to be clearly distinguished. High temporal resolution allows for tracking the flow of the contrast medium and can help localize the site of a tear. Kinematic

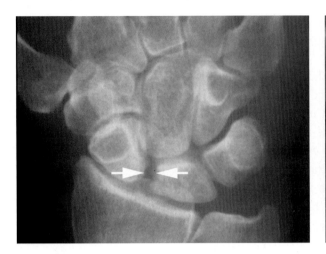

Figure 1-7

A 57-year-old man presented with radial-sided wrist pain. Preinjection PA view shows a wide scapholunate interval (arrows), suspicious for scapholunate dissociation and tear.

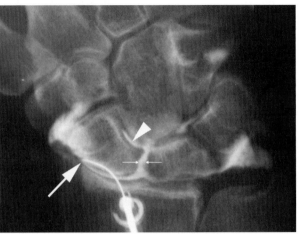

Figure 1-8

PA view taken after injection of iodinated contrast medium into the radiocarpal joint (long arrow) of the same wrist shown in Figure 1-7 shows flow of the contrast medium through the defect in the scapholunate ligament (short arrows) into the midcarpal joint (arrowhead), diagnostic of scapholunate ligament disruption.

evaluation can be performed simultaneously in patients with joint instability or other motion abnormalities.

Other advantages include lower cost and greater availability than either CT or MR arthrography. Diagnostic injection of anesthetics can help localize pain, and corticosteroid injection can provide pain relief (eg, spinal nerve root injection, facet block, epidural injection). Aspiration of joint fluid can be performed to evaluate for septic arthritis or crystalline arthropathy. Finally, arthrography is free of many of the artifacts that plague CT and MRI.

Limitations

The most obvious limitation of arthrography is that it is an invasive procedure. Percutaneous injection carries the risks of introducing infection and causing bleeding. The procedure also can be painful despite the use of local anesthetics. If fluoroscopy or CT is used, the patient receives radiation. Allergic reactions to the sterilizing preparation, contrast medium, and local anesthetic can occur. The needle can damage nerves, blood vessels, and other soft tissues. Needles can inadvertently pass through viscera as well, such as perforation of the bowel in an inguinal hernia. In fact, the drawbacks associated with the invasive nature of procedures such as arthrography led to the growth of noninvasive cross-sectional imaging.

The lack of cross-sectional images is a major limitation of arthrography with fluoroscopy. Certain structures such as the labrum in the shoulder are difficult, if not impossible, to evaluate with fluoroscopy. Structures that are not outlined by contrast are not seen at all, and those that overlap bones or other contrast-filled spaces can be obscured. In these circumstances, CT or MR arthrography can be used; these modalities offer the advantages of both arthrography and cross-sectional imaging.

A radiologist who lacks knowledge and experience can make the procedure especially painful and prolonged. Also, lack of experience in interpreting arthrograms can result in inadequate evaluation or misinterpretation.

Principal Musculoskeletal Indications

As mentioned before, arthrography has been replaced in large part by cross-sectional imaging for routine joint screening. Arthrography can be used in conjunction with both CT and MRI. It is also frequently used for patients who are unable to undergo MRI. Diagnostic anesthetic and/or steroid injections and aspirations for evaluation of infection or crystal analysis are also indications for arthrography. Dynamic evaluation of joint kinematics, such as evaluation of carpal instability and dynamic stress imaging of joints, can be performed as well. Bursography and tenography are indicated for patients with pain that is localized to the appropriate space, frequently as a follow-up to an abnormal noninvasive imaging study that showed characteristic abnormalities.

Common indications for MR arthrography include postoperative assessment of joints, suspected recurrent knee meniscus tear, shoulder instability, ankle impingement, suspected hip or shoulder labrum tear, wrist ligament and triangular fibrocartilage complex tear, and suspected joint body. Some orthopaedic surgeons prefer MR arthrography to routine MRI for rotator cuff tear assessment.

Contraindications

Because of the risk of septic arthritis, arthrography should not be performed if the needle entry site is infected. Bleeding diathesis is also a contraindication, especially in situations where even a small volume of hemorrhage can result in nerve compression, such as epidural injections. Patients with allergies to iodinated or gadolinium chelate contrast medium should not undergo arthrography if MRI or ultrasonography can answer the clinical question. In these cases, saline or air can sometimes serve as an adequate contrast agent, especially if arthrography is performed only to verify needle positioning during anesthetic or steroid injections.

Precautions

Although arthrography is a relatively "old" imaging study, it requires technical skill and knowledge of joint anatomy to perform and interpret correctly. In fact, the recent increase in cross-sectional imaging of joints has led to an overall decline in the number of radiologists with experience in arthrography. Inadequate needle positioning can lead to incorrect diagnoses and incorrect placement of injected contrast agents. Inadvertent injection into two separate compartments can make it appear that a communicating defect exists between the compartments, leading to an incorrect diagnosis of a tear. The radiologist should be aware that some defects, as in the wrist, will not leak contrast unless the appropriate provocative maneuvers are performed.

References

1. Hunter JC, Blatz DJ, Escobedo EM: SLAP lesions of the glenoid labrum: CT arthrographic and arthroscopic correlation. *Radiology* 1992;184:513-518.
2. Lill H, Lange K, Reinbold WD, Echtermeyer V: [MRI arthrography—improved diagnosis of shoulder joint instability]. *Unfallchirurg* 1997;100:186-192.

ULTRASONOGRAPHY

Ultrasonography, or ultrasound, uses high-frequency sound waves to produce images, analogous to sonar images of the ocean floor. A transducer produces the sound waves, which are transmitted into the patient and reflected back by different tissues. The same transducer detects the reflected sound waves, and then a computer synthesizes the time that the sound waves traveled and the amplitude of the reflected sound waves into a tomographic, or body slice, image. Recent developments make three-dimensional imaging of objects possible as well. Ultrasonography, in a broad sense, also includes modalities in which sound waves are measured using other methods, but these methods are not commonly used for anatomic imaging.

The echogenicity of a structure, or the degree to which the structure reflects sound waves, determines the brightness of objects on ultrasound, resulting in measurement of entirely different physical parameters of objects than those measured by plain radiography, CT, or MRI. Echogenicity is a function of the frequency of the sound waves and the homogeneity of the object. In general, objects with low echogenicity, such as cysts, are more homogeneous: they possess few sharp interfaces of acoustic impedance that reflect sound waves. Highly echogenic structures, such as solid masses, generally appear white on ultrasound. The frequency of the sound waves is fixed by the transducer that is used and generally ranges from 2.5 to 20 mHz. High-frequency transducers provide better detail, whereas low-frequency transducers can image deeper tissues. Sound frequencies higher than those used for imaging are used therapeutically to heat tissues.

Doppler ultrasonography can be used to image motion. When objects move, their sound frequency shifts (Doppler effect); the direction and magnitude of these shifts can be correlated with flow. These measurements are used routinely for imaging blood vessels and can be presented graphically as plots of flow velocity against time (pulse-wave) or as color maps (color Doppler).

Advantages

Ultrasound is noninvasive at the frequencies used for diagnostic imaging and has no known harmful effects, other than the theoretically harmful effects in fetuses caused by heating of sensitive tissues. Because it is noninvasive and does not emit ionizing radiation, ultrasound is commonly used in the imaging of children and pregnant women. In addition, ultrasound can show nonossified structures in children, such as the femoral head, that are not directly seen with radiography. It is also relatively inexpensive compared to other tomographic imaging modalities such as CT and MRI. The equipment is highly portable, with recently introduced book-sized devices making imaging possible even in very remote locations. This attribute also allows for real-time surgical guidance. Most transducers are hand-held devices that can be positioned in any plane and allow visualization of objects in multiple views.

The spatial resolution of ultrasound is very high compared to that of CT and MRI and allows imaging of small structures such as ligaments and tendons. Doppler techniques can provide information about the speed, direction, and amount of blood flow. Manipulative techniques can be performed during imaging, such as compression in deep venous thrombosis evaluation, providing additional diagnostic information. Images of motion can be readily obtained to evaluate conditions such as snapping tendons. Highly echogenic structures such as foreign bodies in soft tissues are easily detected with ultrasonography, which can image foreign bodies that are not visible on radiography.

Limitations

The use of ultrasound in musculoskeletal imaging is relatively uncommon, despite its advantages, principally because it cannot image inside bone. Bone cortex reflects almost all of the sound, making imaging of deeper structures impossible. A fracture can be seen as a disruption in the echogenic cortex, but fracture identification is much more accurate with radiography. Similarly, ossified epiphyses prevent evaluation of most joints, although unossified epiphyses in children allow evaluation of joints such as the hip. Air obscures deeper tissues as well.

Another limitation of ultrasound is the relatively small field of view that is available compared to all other imaging methods; this makes global survey of an extremity time-consuming. Deep objects are poorly imaged in large patients, and this can result in poor or incorrect diagnoses.

The accuracy of ultrasound depends greatly on the skill of the technician, both in image acquisition ("scanning") and image interpretation. Most physicians who are not radiologists find ultrasound images to be confusing, perhaps even more so than MRI scans. This limits their use in preoperative planning. Ultrasound

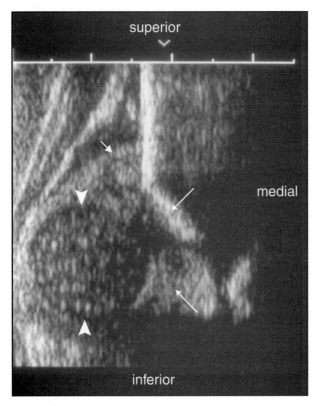

Figure 1-9
Coronal ultrasound image of the right hip of a 1-month-old infant with a history of breech delivery. The image shows lateral displacement of the femoral head (arrowheads) out of the acetabulum (long arrows), which is diagnostic of developmental dysplasia of the hip. The bone cortex is highly echogenic and appears as a bright line (upper long arrow). The labrum (short arrow) is thickened and dysplastic. (Figure courtesy of Sandra Gorges, MD)

also produces many artifacts, which can reduce sensitivity and specificity.

Principal Musculoskeletal Indications

Whenever possible, ultrasonography is routinely the study of choice in children (younger than 1 year) for the evaluation of developmental dysplasia of the hip, joint effusion, and spinal dysraphism (Figure 1-9). In adults, its use is generally limited to soft tissues, such as evaluation of tendon pathology (eg, rotator cuff tears, Achilles tendon rupture, patellar tendon tears, snapping hip, tenosynovitis), ligament tears (eg, ankle and hand), soft-tissue tumors, and vascular disease (arterial and venous). Although fractures can be seen on ultrasound, plain radiography is the imaging modality of choice. The same is true of any condition that primarily involves bone, such as bone tumors and osteomyelitis. Some intra-articular pathology such as meniscal tears and shoulder labral tears can be seen, but MRI is preferred for global screening of intra-articular pathology.

Ultrasound is also used widely for guiding procedures such as biopsy and soft-tissue drainage. Novel uses include ultrasound-guided compression and ablation of femoral arteriovenous fistula.

Contraindications

Only a theoretical contraindication for ultrasound exists: heating of sensitive developmental tissues in fetuses with techniques that deposit large amounts of energy (such as power Doppler imaging). This is not of practical concern in orthopaedic imaging.

RADIATION SAFETY

Medical imaging contributes greatly to musculoskeletal and other types of medical care, but it should be performed with care to minimize the potentially harmful effects of ionizing radiation used in some imaging modalities. Children and pregnant women are especially susceptible to the deleterious effects of ionizing radiation. In addition, medical personnel should follow safety guidelines rigorously to minimize their own radiation exposure. Following good principles can reduce, though not completely eliminate, the risks posed by the use of ionizing radiation.

Imaging methods that use ionizing radiation, such as plain radiography, CT, and bone scintigraphy, produce ions and free radicals that can deposit energy in organs and tissues. The deposited energy can damage molecules such as DNA, with potentially detrimental effects. The total deposited energy (dose) and the radiation type determine the extent and type of damage. Large particles, such as alpha particles, produce more biologic damage than do smaller particles, such as x-ray beams, for the same dose deposited in the patient. Diagnostic imaging is generally performed using the latter (ie, x-ray beams or x-ray–producing radionuclides). Data on the effects of ionizing radiation in humans are extrapolated from studies of atomic bomb survivors, radiation workers, and radiation therapy patients.

Radiation exposure from scintigraphy primarily affects the patient. Typically, the target organ of the pharmaceutical agent and the organs that excrete the agent receive the highest doses. Scintigraphy doses are carefully designed, however, to balance image quality with the lowest possible radiation dose to the patient. Some scintigraphy agents (eg, iodine-131) have half-lives of several days and can concentrate in excreted body fluids and breast milk; patients who receive these agents may require partial or full isolation from others for a short period of time.

Table 1
Threshold Acute Exposure Doses for Effects in Humans

Organ Exposed	Dose* (in Gy)†	Effect
Ocular lens	2	Cataracts
Bone marrow	2 to 7	Marrow failure with infection, death
Skin	3	Temporary hair loss
Skin	5	Erythema
Testes	5 to 6	Permanent decrease in sperm count
Skin	7	Permanent hair loss
Intestines	7 to 50	Gastrointestinal failure, death
Brain	50 to 100	Cerebral edema, death

*Doses are approximate. Some effects such as neoplasm induction, congenital defects, and genetic mutations are thought to have no thresholds; ie, there is no exposure level that is determined to be harmless.
†1 Gy = 100 rad

Table 2
Typical Doses in Musculoskeletal Imaging

Type	Dose (in mSv)*
Plain radiography	0.1 to 2.0
Bone scintigraphy	5
CT	5 to 15

*1 milliSievert (mSv) = 1 millirem (mrem); dose is effective dose equivalent.

Types of Damage

Some types of damage to humans are deterministic or nonstochastic, meaning they occur only above a certain dose, whereas others (stochastic effects) are thought to occur at any dose, although they are more likely at higher doses. Deterministic effects include skin erythema, development of cataracts, hair loss, sterility, acute radiation sickness, and decreased sperm and lymphocyte counts. These effects can be prevented if the total radiation dose is kept below a specific threshold. The doses at which these problems develop are measured in terms of the target organ involved (Table 1). Stochastic effects include carcinogenesis and genetic damage, and minimizing the radiation dose can reduce but not eliminate the risk of their occurrence. Rapidly dividing tissues are the most susceptible to radiation-induced neoplasia; these include bone marrow, breast tissue, gastrointestinal mucosa, gonads, and lymphatic tissue. The risk of cancer is estimated to be approximately 4% per Sievert (100 rems) by the US National Academy of Sciences Committee on the Biological Effects of Ionizing Radiation.[1] The risk of fetal malformation is greatest in the first trimester and with doses greater than 0.1 Gy (10 rad). Later in pregnancy (150 days or more after conception), the greatest risk is an increase in childhood malignancies such as leukemia, with 10 mGy (1 rad) of administered dose increasing childhood leukemia risk as much as 40% (from 3.6 in 10,000 to 5 in 10,000).[2] Typical doses administered during musculoskeletal imaging are listed in Table 2.

Protection

Protection against radiation-induced effects should be applied to both patients and medical personnel. Patients can be shielded to protect sensitive organs such as the gonads, but the best protection is to follow the principle of ALARA (as low as reasonably achievable) dosing, especially in the case of children and pregnant women. When radiography is indicated, such reduction of exposure can be effected by limiting the number of radiographic studies performed, by reducing the total times for fluoroscopy, and by the effective use of collimators. In some circumstances, a different imaging modality such as ultrasound may be substituted to eliminate the radiation exposure altogether.

Medical personnel can reduce the dose they receive during radiologic procedures in several ways. First, exposure time can be minimized, such as by reducing fluoroscopy time. Second, because exposure to radiation decreases as an inverse square of the distance from the source, maintaining as great a distance as possible from the radiation source is quite effective in reducing dose. Third, use of shielding material such as lead aprons, thyroid shields, leaded glasses, and lead gloves can reduce the dose, but it should be remembered that these do not provide complete protection. Rooms used for radiologic procedures must be designed to minimize radiation exposure and require shielded walls. Finally, radiation dose to medical personnel should be monitored using devices such as film badges.

Another consideration in ordering imaging studies is the effect of medical radiation use on the population in general. Any consideration of population screening for disease should take into account the potentially deleterious effects of radiation dosing on a population. This issue has piqued interest recently with the increased use of high-speed CT scanners, since CT delivers the highest contribution of radiation dose to the US population among all medical imaging procedures (Table 2).

References

1. Committee on Biological Effects of Ionizing Radiation: Board on Radiation Effects Research, Commission on Life Sciences, National Research Council. Health effects of exposure to low levels of ionizing radiation: BEIR V. Washington, DC, National Academy Press, 1990.

2. Brent RL, Gorson RO: Radiation exposure in pregnancy, in *Current Problems in Radiology: Technic of Pneumoencephalography.* Chicago, IL, Year Book Medical, 1972, pp 1-47.

GENERAL ORTHOPAEDICS

Section Editor
Thomas R. Johnson, MD

Contributors
Enrico F. Arguelles, MD, FACR, CCD
James F. Schwarten, MD

FRACTURE HEALING

DEFINITION

To better interpret fracture healing on radiographs, understanding how fractures heal is of key importance. Following a fracture, a complex series of events is initiated. These events are typically described as three somewhat overlapping phases: inflammation, repair, and remodeling. The phases of fracture healing are shown in the figure below.

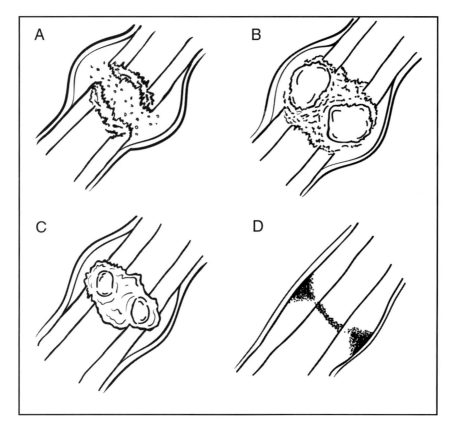

Phases of fracture healing. **A,** Inflammatory phase. **B,** Reparative phase (early). **C,** Reparative phase (late). **D,** Remodeling phase. (Adapted with permission from the Mayo Foundation, Rochester, MN.)

The inflammatory response begins immediately after injury and lasts for 1 to 3 days. A hematoma forms between the fracture ends and under the torn periosteum. Injured tissues and platelets release vasoactive mediators, growth factors, and substances called cytokines. These substances direct new vessel formation and cellular differentiation at the fracture site. Macrophage and polymorphonuclear cells begin the process of cleaning up the necrotic debris. The inflammatory phase occupies about 10% of the healing cycle.

The reparative phase begins 2 to 3 days after injury. As the dead tissue is resorbed, fibroblasts and chondrocytes appear between the bone ends in the fracture hematoma and produce a matrix called callus. This callus is transformed into cartilage and woven bone. The amount of callus that is formed is related to the degree of stability at the fracture site. The more rigidly a fracture is stabilized, the smaller the amount of callus that is formed. The reparative phase occupies about 40% of the healing cycle.

The remodeling phase actually begins during the reparative phase and is the longest phase, occupying 70% of the healing cycle. During this phase, the fracture callus becomes mineralized and woven bone forms between the fracture ends. As healing progresses, the woven bone is replaced by lamellar bone and the medullary canal is reconstituted. This type of healing is called secondary healing because intermediate callus is formed in the fracture gap and secondarily replaced by bone.

How a fracture heals depends on how it is stabilized. Fractures that are not rigidly stabilized heal by secondary healing, as described above. Fractures that are rigidly fixed heal by primary or gap healing. With primary healing, the fracture line disappears by endosteal (or internal) callus formation. This direct type of bone healing occurs without external callus formation. When the cortical bone ends are in direct contact with one another, contact healing can occur in which lamellar bone forms across the fracture site. Special cells called osteoclasts cut across the fracture site, followed by an invasion of blood vessels and osteoblasts, which lay down new bone. These are often referred to as cutting cones. As these cutting cones cross the fracture site, they establish new haversian systems that allow for the passage of new blood vessels with their specialized osteoprogenitor and mesenchymal cells, which lead to new bone formation. For primary healing to occur, anatomic reduction of the fracture is necessary, the fixation rigid, and an adequate blood supply ensured.

Several factors influence bone healing. Systemic factors that delay fracture healing include malnutrition, diabetes mellitus, cigarette smoking, anemia, and use of certain medications including oral steroids and nonsteroidal anti-inflammatory drugs such as ibuprofen. Local factors that delay fracture healing include an open fracture with significant soft-tissue injury, bone loss, radiation, presence of infection, pathologic lesion, the specific bone fractured, and the presence of a vascular injury.

On radiographs, fractures fixed anatomically with a compression plate will not show callus as the fracture heals. Fractures fixed with intramedullary devices that allow for some motion or fractures fixed with external fixators that are not rigid will show some callus formation during the healing process. Fractures treated with casting only may show the greatest amount of callus.

IMAGE DESCRIPTIONS

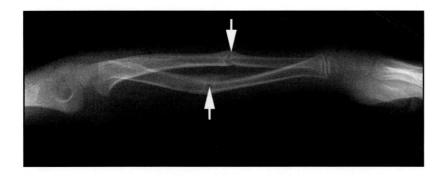

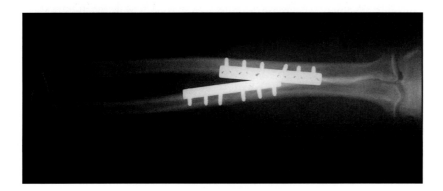

Figure 2-1

Both-bone fracture (forearm)—Lateral view

Both-bone fracture of the forearm in a child treated with cast immobilization demonstrates exuberant callus formation (arrows).

Figure 2-2

Both-bone fracture (forearm)—AP view

AP view shows a both-bone fracture of a forearm treated with rigid anatomic fixation. Note the absence of callus formation.

SECTION 2 ■ GENERAL ORTHOPAEDICS

FRACTURE NONUNION

ICD-9 Code

733.82
Nonunion of fracture;
pseudoarthrosis (bone)

SYNONYM
Pseudarthrosis

DEFINITION
A fracture nonunion is said to occur when solid union is not present after an arbitrary time period, frequently, 6 to 9 months. From a functional standpoint, fracture nonunion may be said to exist when there is no sign of healing and the treating physician does not anticipate healing without additional treatment, typically surgery. Within 6 weeks after the injury, many fractures show resorption at the fracture site, signaling the likelihood of a nonunion. For a fracture to heal satisfactorily, there must be good bone apposition, the blood supply to the fractured bone must be adequate, and there must be a certain degree of mechanical stability.

Several anatomic factors contribute to fracture nonunion. Poor bone contact may result from an inadequate closed reduction with soft-tissue interposition. Loss of bone that sometimes occurs with an open fracture can create a wide gap across which the healing process must occur. Open fractures also lead to periosteal stripping and interruption of blood supply at the fracture site. Poor blood supply to the fracture site also may exist normally, such as in fractures of the scaphoid in which the proximal fracture fragment is devoid of blood supply or in fractures of the femoral neck. Tibial shaft fractures are also at increased risk for nonunions because of a lack of muscle coverage over the anteromedial portion of the tibia. Excessive motion at the fracture site can result from inadequate external or internal fixation or fixation failure.

Age is also a factor; nonunions are uncommon in children. Poor nutrition is a contributing factor, as is a history of cigarette smoking, use of oral steroids, and a history of metabolic bone disease. Whether nonsteroidal anti-inflammatory drug (NSAID) use delays fracture healing remains controversial, although some NSAIDs such as ibuprofen do appear to cause some delay. Infection always has been considered a potential cause of nonunion.

HISTORY AND PHYSICAL FINDINGS
Persistent pain at the fracture site after a period of time in which a fracture is normally expected to heal should raise the suspicion of a nonunion. Deformity at the fracture site also suggests a nonunion. Documenting a history of any medication use, particularly NSAIDs and corticosteroids, and tobacco use is critical in any suspected nonunion. Any history of fever, swelling, redness, or drainage from

the fracture site needs to be noted as well. The way in which the fracture was originally treated (ie, open or closed) has an impact on further treatment decisions.

Physical examination will reveal tenderness on palpation at the fracture site. Any motion at the fracture site should be assessed because the adjacent joints may become stiff. The fracture site also must be carefully inspected for any signs of infection such as erythema or drainage.

IMAGING STUDIES

Required for diagnosis

AP and lateral radiographs of the fracture site, including the joints above and below the fracture, will reveal a nonunion in most cases. If the degree of healing is in question, an oblique view should be added. These three views should be compared with previous radiographs, if available, to evaluate healing activity at the fracture site.

The key to radiographic evaluation of a fracture nonunion is to assess the viability of the nonunion to heal. In one classification system, nonunions are considered either viable (capable of some healing activity) or nonviable (incapable of biologic activity). A viable nonunion will show callus formation, indicating adequate blood supply. If a large amount of callus formation is present, the term "elephant-foot type" is often used, as this describes the radiographic appearance. When a lesser amount of callus is present, the term "horse-hoof type" is used. Viable nonunions are also divided into two additional categories: hypertrophic and oligotrophic. Oligotrophic nonunions have little callus formation but still have adequate blood supply to achieve bone healing.

Radiographs of nonviable nonunions fail to reveal any callus formation, and a gap is clearly visible between the fracture ends. The term atrophic nonunion is often used to describe this type of nonunion. Resorption of the bone ends at the fracture site is observed, and the bones appear osteopenic.

A broken component usually is a sign of a nonunion. Most components are designed to provide stability at the fracture site until bony union has occurred. These components are not designed to hold up indefinitely, however, and are subject to fatigue and failure over time if the fracture does not heal. Loose screws suggest that motion has occurred at the fracture site and that union has not occurred.

Required for comprehensive evaluation

Radiographs may not always identify a fracture nonunion. In this situation, CT is useful to visualize a cross-sectional area to determine if bone is bridging across the fracture site. A nonunion typically will have less than 10% of the fracture site bridged by bone.

Bone scans are useful in studying the vascularity of nonunions, particularly technetium Tc 99m scans because they show increased uptake in viable nonunions. This type of bone scan will also differentiate a synovial pseudarthrosis from a nonunion. In a synovial pseudarthrosis, fluid is found between the two medullary bone ends, which are sealed. A pseudocapsule holds the fluid in place. The bone scan will show a cold cleft (ie, no uptake) at the nonunion site, whereas the bone ends will show increased uptake. Gallium scans can be useful in the diagnosis of chronic infections at nonunion sites.

Special considerations
None

Pitfalls
None

IMAGE DESCRIPTION

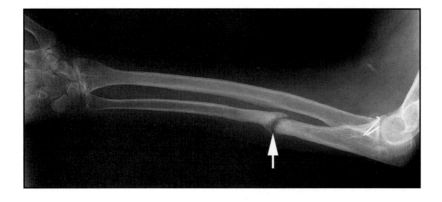

Figure 2-3

Fracture nonunion— AP view

AP view of the left forearm shows a viable nonunion of a fracture of the ulna. Note the widened area of the distal fracture end (arrow), indicating an attempt at callus formation and fracture healing.

DIFFERENTIAL DIAGNOSIS

Congenital pseudarthrosis (present in young children)

Infected nonunion (positive gallium scan, increased erythrocyte sedimentation rate)

Synovial pseudarthrosis (no uptake on bone scan)

FRACTURE PATTERNS

DEFINITION

A fracture is a complete or incomplete disruption in the continuity of bone or cartilage that occurs as a result of a direct blow to the bone or an indirect force applied to the limb. Most fractures result in gross interruption of the bone matrix. Fractures, however, may occur at a microscopic level, as seen in stress fractures. A dislocation is the complete separation of the cartilage surfaces of a joint so that they are no longer in contact. A subluxation is the partial separation of the joint surfaces. A fracture involving cartilage is called a chondral fracture, whereas a fracture involving bone and cartilage is called an osteochondral fracture. A fracture-dislocation is a combination of a fracture near a joint with a dislocation of the adjacent joint. Diastasis refers to the separation of a joint that ordinarily has only minimal movement. Examples of such joints are the distal tibiofibular syndesmosis, the symphysis pubis, and the sacroiliac joint.

HISTORY AND PHYSICAL FINDINGS

The classic symptoms of acute fractures are swelling, deformity, decreased function, and pain that is aggravated by movement. Nondisplaced fractures may not exhibit any obvious deformity. Stress fractures often present with the indolent onset of mild swelling and tenderness and pain with weight bearing. Table 1 lists the defining characteristics of specific types of fractures.

Examination reveals localized tenderness, swelling, and often deformity. A complete examination should include an evaluation of the surrounding skin integrity, stability of the adjacent joints, and function of the nerves and vessels distal to the site of injury. Any laceration or abrasion of the skin should be considered an open fracture. All suspected open fractures require further evaluation for exploration and débridement.

IMAGING STUDIES

Required for diagnosis

Radiographs usually identify an acute fracture. With stress fractures and some nondisplaced fractures, the injury may not be visible on radiographs until bone resorbs from the fracture ends (1 to 4 weeks). Carpal navicular fractures often are missed for this reason. Tomography, CT, and MRI usually are not indicated in the initial assessment of fractures unless the diagnosis cannot be confirmed with radiographs.

Table 1
Fracture Classification

Location of bone

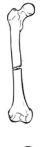

Epiphyseal
The end of the bone, forming part of the adjacent shaft

Metaphyseal
The flared portion of the bone at the ends of the shaft

Diaphyseal
The shaft of a long bone

Integrity of skin and soft-tissue envelope around fracture

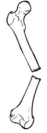

Closed
The skin over and near the fracture is intact

Open
The skin over and near the fracture is lacerated or abraded by the injury

Amount of Displacement

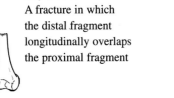

Nondisplaced
A fracture in which the fragments are in anatomic alignment

Displaced
A fracture in which the fragments are no longer in their usual alignment

Angulated
A fracture in which the fragments are malaligned

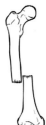

Bayonetted
A fracture in which the distal fragment longitudinally overlaps the proximal fragment

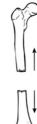

Distracted
A fracture in which the distal fragment is separated from the proximal fragment by a gap

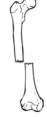

Orientation/Extension of fracture line

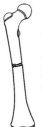

Transverse
A fracture that is perpendicular to the shaft of the bone

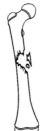

Comminuted
A fracture in which there is more than two fracture fragments

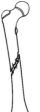

Oblique
An angulated fracture line

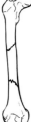

Segmental
A type of comminuted fracture in which a completely separate segment of bone is bordered by fracture lines

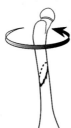

Spiral
A multiplanar and complex fracture line

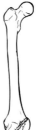

Intra-articular
The fracture line crosses the articular cartilage and enters the joint

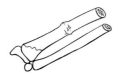

Torus
An incomplete buckle fracture of one cortex, often seen in children

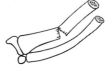

Greenstick
An incomplete fracture with angular deformity, seen in children

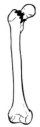

Impaction
A fracture that occurs when one bone hits or "impacts" an adjacent bone

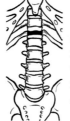

Compression
A type of impaction fracture that occurs in the vertebrae, resulting in depression of the end plates

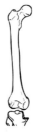

Depression
A type of impaction fracture that occurs in the knee when the femoral condyle strikes the softer tibial plateau

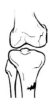

Stress (Fatigue)
A fracture in normal bone that has been subjected to repeated or cyclical loads that in and of themselves are not sufficient to cause a fracture

Stress (Insufficiency)
A fracture in weakened bone that has been subjected to a load insufficient to fracture normal bone

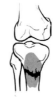

Pathologic
A fracture through bone weakened by tumor, metabolic bone disease, or osteoporosis

Required for comprehensive evaluation
MRI is helpful in diagnosing stress fractures not visualized on radiographs. CT is useful in defining the characteristics of intra-articular and comminuted fractures.

Special considerations
None

Pitfalls
None

DIFFERENTIAL DIAGNOSIS

Dislocation (marked deformity, disruption of normal joint alignment on radiographs)

Infection (fever, elevated erythrocyte sedimentation rate, no history of trauma)

Sprain (normal radiographs)

Tumor (gradual onset, bone destruction evident on radiographs)

Hematoma

Synonym
Blood clot

ICD-9 Codes

923
Contusion of upper limb

924
Contusion of lower limb and of other and unspecified sites

Definition

The accumulation of blood, usually clotted, into the soft tissues, an organ, or space within the extremities or trunk as a result of a broken vessel wall is called a hematoma. A history of trauma to an extremity is common. The trauma may be minimal in patients who take anticoagulants or have a history of a bleeding disorder. Occasionally, spontaneous bleeding into a muscle may occur without any known traumatic episode.

Hematomas may simulate soft-tissue masses and must be differentiated on imaging studies from benign or malignant tumors. The red blood cells (erythrocytes) contain hemoglobin, which in the presence of a hematoma breaks down into methemoglobin and hemosiderin. Because of this changing state of hemoglobin and its iron-containing degradation products, findings on MRI will vary over time as the hematoma progresses from acute to the chronic stage.

History and Physical Findings

Swelling and a palpable soft-tissue mass are common on physical examination. These areas may or may not be tender. If the hematoma is superficial, red-blue skin discoloration may be seen as well as an abrasion of the skin. With a deep hematoma, a discrete mass may not be palpable, but the circumference of the extremity will be increased. Active motion of the affected extremity also may be painful.

Imaging Studies

Required for diagnosis
Frontal and lateral radiographs should be ordered first to identify any soft-tissue swelling or calcification.

Required for comprehensive evaluation

MRI should be ordered to evaluate the extent of the soft-tissue mass and to rule out a tumor. The presence of iron affects the images, particularly the T1 relaxation times. Therefore, the age of the hematoma, because its degradation products contain iron, will affect the image. The subacute hematoma is characterized by increased signal intensity on all imaging sequences caused by the accumulation of methemoglobin. In chronic hematoma, hemosiderin presents with characteristic low signal intensity on all imaging sequences. Hematomas can contain many different stages of blood within the same mass and are often heterogeneous in signal intensity.

Special considerations

None

Pitfalls

Hematomas may be difficult to differentiate from hemorrhage into a tumor because both may show hemorrhagic characteristics. Tumors tend to have a more solid mass associated with the hemorrhagic component.

IMAGE DESCRIPTIONS

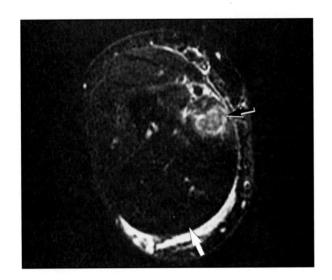

Figure 2-4

Hematoma—Axial MRI

Axial fast inversion recovery MRI image of a proximal forearm shows a mass of high signal intensity (black arrow) surrounded by high signal intensity within the extensor muscle, consistent with a chronic hematoma containing hemosiderin. Note also the increased signal intensity between the fascia and the subcutaneous tissue (white arrow), indicating the presence of fluid.

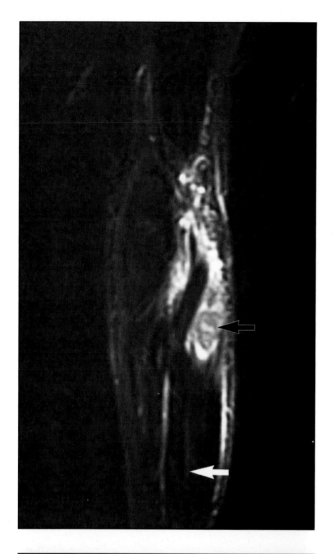

Figure 2-5

Hematoma—Coronal MRI

Coronal fast inversion recovery MRI image of a proximal forearm shows a mass of low signal intensity surrounded by high signal intensity within the extensor muscle (black arrow), which clearly delineates the longitudinal dimension of the hematoma. Note also the fluid between the fascia and the subcutaneous tissue (white arrow).

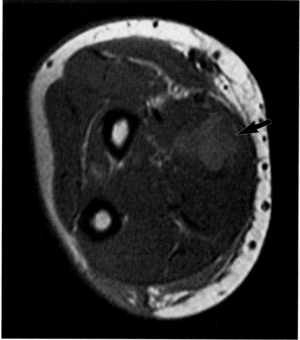

Figure 2-6

Hematoma—Axial MRI

Axial T1-weighted MRI scan shows characteristic increased signal intensity related to methemoglobin within the muscle mass (arrow), suggesting a hematoma.

DIFFERENTIAL DIAGNOSIS

Hemorrhage into tumor (angiography may differentiate)

Tumor (no history of trauma, bleeding disorder, anticoagulants, or surgery)

Myositis Ossificans Traumatica

Synonyms

Heterotopic ossification
Myositis ossificans circumscripta
Myositis ossificans progressiva
Posttraumatic myositis ossificans
Sterner's tumor

ICD-9 Code
728.12
Traumatic myositis ossificans

Definition

Myositis ossificans, the most common type of heterotopic ossification, occurs in muscle, with 80% of cases occurring in the large muscles of the extremities. The term myositis ossificans is a misnomer in that the condition does not involve a primary inflammatory process. Adults are most commonly affected, and incidence is not related to race or sex. The localized form of myositis, often referred to as myositis ossficans circumscripta, sometimes develops after trauma but also is seen in patients with no history of injury. Predisposing factors include tissue injury such as blunt trauma, fractures, burns, surgery, and stab wounds. Neurologic conditions, such as stroke, traumatic brain injury, and paraplegia, and bleeding disorders, such as hemophilia, also predispose to the development of myositis ossificans. Other predisposing conditions include ankylosing spondylitis and diffuse idiopathic skeletal hyperostosis (DISH).

The mechanism is understood to be as follows: Following trauma with hemorrhage into the muscle, fibroblasts and osteoblasts appear, and the osteoblasts deposit osteoid in a centripetal manner. Ultimately, a shell of lamellar bone forms around a core of cancellous bone. The characteristic appearance of this formation on imaging studies helps to differentiate this condition from neoplastic or inflammatory processes with which it may be confused. Myositis ossificans progressiva is a genetic disorder seen in children older than age 5 years. With this condition, ossific masses tend to form in the sternocleidomastoid, paraspinal, shoulder, and pelvic girdle muscles.

History and Physical Findings

Approximately 75% of patients will report a history of trauma, usually to the large muscles of the extremities and especially the proximal extremity. Typically, the patient will report pain and swelling along with loss of motion of the adjacent joints. Rarely, fever is present. On physical examination, a firm, tender mass in the affected extremity may be noted. Active and passive range of motion of the adjacent joints also may be noted.

IMAGING STUDIES

Required for diagnosis

AP and lateral views are typically sufficient to establish the diagnosis. A flocculent calcific mass may appear from 11 days to 6 weeks following the injury and may be confused with a soft-tissue sarcoma. Therefore, radiographs should be repeated 4 weeks after the initial series. The characteristic progression of myositis ossificans will make the diagnosis apparent; its benign nature is suggested by its lack of continuity with adjacent bone. By 6 to 8 weeks after the injury, a layer of new bone is sharply defined at the periphery. Progression to maturity occurs in a centripetal pattern, with the center ossifying last. This pattern of ossification, with a central radiolucent marrow-filled area surrounded by a dense layer of lamellar bone, is characteristic of myositis ossificans and allows for diagnosis based on imaging studies. Maturity of the mass occurs within 6 to 12 months. In younger patients, the mass may shrink over time.

Required for comprehensive evaluation

CT will show the characteristic features of myositis ossificans and, more importantly, will show the peripheral rim of mineralization and a radiolucent band or zone between the lesion and underlying bone that distinguishes it from a parosteal osteosarcoma. Serial bone scans have been used to help in timing surgical planning. Decreased isotope uptake is felt to be an indicator of decreased bone formation activity, making it safer to intervene surgically; however, this remains controversial.

Special considerations

None

Pitfalls

Early in the course of the disease, myositis ossificans may be confused with an osteosarcoma. MRI is nonspecific for myositis ossificans.

Image Description

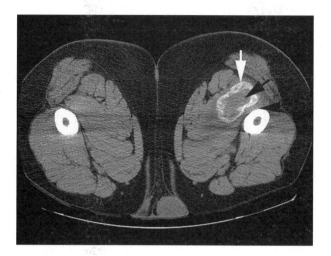

Figure 2-7

Myositis ossificans—CT

CT scan of the thigh in a collegiate football player shows a well-circumscribed mass with a sharply marginated ossified rim (white arrow) and a central lucent area (black arrow). Note that there is no contact with the femur (arrowhead).

Differential Diagnosis

Juxtacortical chondroma (soft-tissue calcification and excavation of bone)

Osteochondroma (arises from and connects to underlying bone)

Osteoma (arises from outer surface of the cortex)

Parosteal osteosarcoma (incomplete or absence of lucency between the mass and underlying metaphyseal bone; centripetal ossification)

Periosteal osteosarcoma (arises in the cortex of diaphyseal bone)

STRESS FRACTURES

SECTION 2 ■ GENERAL ORTHOPAEDICS

ICD-9 Codes

733.93
Stress fracture of tibia or fibula

733.94
Stress fracture of the metatarsals

733.95
Stress fracture of other bone

SYNONYMS

Fatigue fracture
Insufficiency fracture

DEFINITION

Two types of stress fractures occur: fatigue fractures and insufficiency fractures. Fatigue stress fractures occur in response to repeated low-level forces or stress on normal bone. This single load or stress may be insufficient to cause a fracture of normal bone, but after repeated cyclic loading, this stress ultimately leads to fracture. The term insufficiency stress fracture refers to a fracture that occurs through weakened bone caused by a load insufficient to fracture a normal bone. A pathologic fracture is one that occurs through a bone usually weakened by tumor.

Stress fractures tend to occur in specific locations: (1) the proximal medial tibial shaft, (2) the proximal or middle femoral shaft along the medial cortex, (3) the medial femoral neck, (4) the metatarsal bones (march fractures), and (5) the pars interarticularis portion of a lumbar vertebra (which can lead to spondylolisthesis). Long-distance runners such as those training for marathons are prone to stress fractures in the lower extremities. Basketball and soccer players are also at risk during preseason workouts. Military personnel are at risk for march fractures, as are professional dancers.

HISTORY AND PHYSICAL FINDINGS

Stress fractures occur most commonly as a result of a new athletic or recreational activity, such as training for a marathon, or beginning practice for a seasonal sport. Physical examination will reveal localized tenderness at the site of the fracture. Occasionally, swelling and warmth may be present. Radiographs are often normal when symptoms first appear. Only 10% to 15% of radiographs will show the stress fracture during the first week of symptoms. Even several weeks after the onset of symptoms, fewer than 60% of radiographs will show a stress fracture; therefore, a high index of suspicion is necessary to make this diagnosis, and further imaging studies are indicated.

IMAGING STUDIES

Required for diagnosis

Even though the yield is low in diagnosing a stress fracture, AP and lateral radiographs should be ordered first because a fracture or a bone lesion may be visualized. Early radiographic changes in stress fractures include a subtle irregularity in the cortex (cortical lucency). Stress fractures in cancellous bone are even more difficult to detectand present with linear sclerosis. If there is no urgency, a second radiograph should be obtained in 14 days.

Required for comprehensive evaluation

If radiographs are normal and the index of suspicion for a stress fracture remains high given the patient's history and the location of the pain, a bone scan or MRI can be ordered. Although the bone scan has been the gold standard for diagnosing stress fractures for many years, MRI has slowly replaced it as the study of choice if radiographs are normal and a stress fracture is suspected. A limited series of sequences in the appropriate plane will show the stress fracture and reduce the overall cost of the MRI. Although bone scans show increased activity early after symptoms develop, they lack specificity. Synovitis, arthritis, tumor, infection, and stress reaction may all look similar to stress fractures on a bone scan.

Special considerations

None

Pitfalls

Radiographs that appear normal, especially for the first few weeks after onset of symptoms, should not be assumed to rule out a stress fracture. MRI should be ordered.

IMAGE DESCRIPTIONS

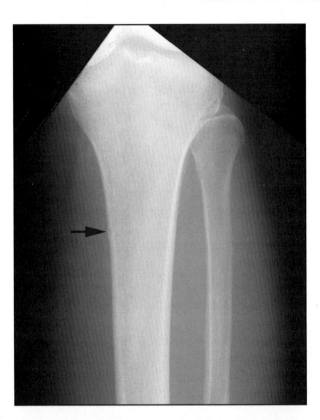

Figure 2-8

Stress fracture—AP view

AP view of the left tibia in a 56-year-old man who was training for a marathon shows subtle cortical irregularity in the proximal medial tibial diaphysis (arrow). This finding corresponded to the area of maximal tenderness.

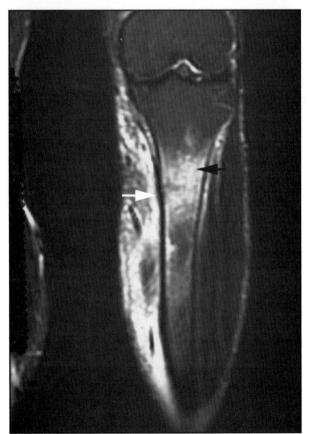

Figure 2-9

Stress fracture—MRI

Coronal fat-suppressed T2-weighted MRI scan shows marrow edema (black arrow) and a transverse stress fracture in the proximal medial tibial diaphysis (white arrow).

Differential Diagnosis

Metastatic carcinoma (history of a primary malignancy; usually more geographic without a fracture line)

Osteoid osteoma (no history of excessive exercise; pain at night relieved by aspirin)

Osteomyelitis (increased erythrocyte sedimentation rate and white blood cell count)

GAS GANGRENE

ICD-9 Code

040.0
Gas gangrene

SECTION 2 ■ GENERAL ORTHOPAEDICS

SYNONYM
Clostridial myonecrosis

DEFINITION
Gas gangrene is a severe, life-threatening infection involving muscle necrosis caused by toxins produced by *Clostridia*, usually *Clostridium perfringens*, but other *Clostridia* species (*C tetani*, *C septicum*, *C novyi*) may be involved as well. *Streptococcus*, coliform, *Staphylococcus*, and *Bacteroides* organisms may also produce gas-forming infections.

Gas gangrene infections occur following trauma, penetrating wounds, surgery, septic abortions, burns, and in association with cancer, especially cancers of the gastrointestinal tract. Hypoxia and vascular insufficiency contribute to the development of these infections. Thus, gas gangrene infections commonly occur as a result of untreated diabetic foot infections. The incubation period for a gas gangrene infection is less than 3 days; often, it occurs within 6 to 8 hours after inoculation. The mortality rate, estimated at 25%, increases to more than 50% within a day and a half after the onset of the infection. Therefore, this represents a medical emergency and must be treated aggressively.

HISTORY AND PHYSICAL FINDINGS
Symptoms of toxic shock syndrome, particularly tachycardia and hypotension, are not uncommon, as is pain that is out of proportion to the appearance of the wound. Palpation of the limb may reveal crepitation from the gas in the soft tissues. The patient's temperature may be slightly elevated. The odor of a clostridial infection is distinctive, often described as the somewhat sweet odor of rotting fruit. A Gram stain will show dumbbell-shaped, gram-positive rods.

IMAGING STUDIES

Required for diagnosis
PA and lateral radiographs are adequate to reveal gas in the subcutaneous, intramuscular, and intermuscular planes. The gas has a linear or netlike radiolucent appearance. Cortical destruction and osteopenia may be present in the diabetic foot. Loss of cartilage may also be present.

Required for comprehensive evaluation
None

Special considerations
None

Pitfalls
Gas in the soft tissues can have many causes. It is not specific for clostridial infections.

IMAGE DESCRIPTIONS

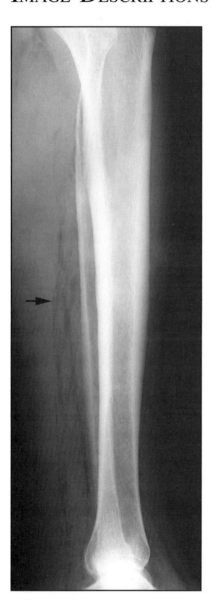

Figure 2-10

Gas gangrene—Lateral view

Lateral view of a left leg shows linear, radiolucent streaking in the calf muscles (arrow) in a patient with diabetes, consistent with a gas gangrene infection.

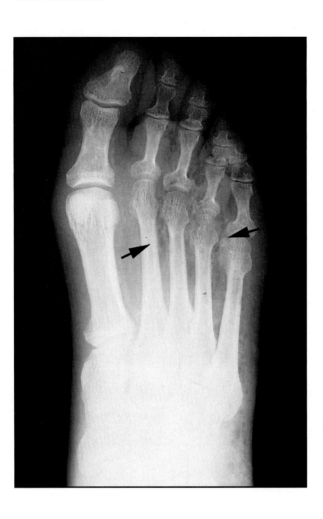

Figure 2-11

Gas in the soft tissues—AP view

AP view of the foot in a patient with diabetes mellitus shows gas in the soft tissues (arrows). In this case, the causative organism was *Escherichia coli*.

Differential Diagnosis

Open fracture (fracture seen on radiograph)

Skin laceration (negative Gram stain)

Visceral rupture (Gram stain and cultures negative for clostridial organisms)

NECROTIZING FASCIITIS

SYNONYMS

Flesh-eating disease
Hemolytic streptococcal gangrene

ICD-9 Code

728.86
Necrotizing fasciitis

DEFINITION

Necrotizing fasciitis is a rare but life-threatening and rapidly spreading soft-tissue infection characterized by necrosis that predominantly affects the superficial fascia and subcutaneous fat with local coagulopathy and vessel thrombosis in the extremities. Secondary involvement of muscle is not uncommon. It is more commonly found in association with drug addiction, alcoholism, HIV infection, and other conditions that compromise the immune system.

Type I necrotizing fasciitis involves at least one anaerobic species, most commonly *Bacteroides* and *Peptostreptococcus,* in combination with one or more facultative anaerobic species such as *Streptococcus* other than group A. Type II is hemolytic streptococcal gangrene caused by group A *Streptococcus.*

HISTORY AND PHYSICAL FINDINGS

Necrotizing fasciitis occurs after penetrating wounds, especially in individuals with diabetes mellitus or peripheral vascular disease or those who are immunocompromised. Common signs and symptoms include a syndrome similar to toxic shock with chills, fever, or profound hypothermia and shock, confusion, nausea, vomiting, tachycardia, hypotension, and multiple-organ failure.

Physical examination reveals that the affected limb is swollen, erythematous without sharp margins, exquisitely tender, and painful. Progression typically is rapid, occurring over several days and characterized by sequential color changes from red-purple to patches of blistering. Within 3 to 5 days of onset, skin breakdown and bullae formation progress to frank gangrene. By this time, destruction of superficial sensory nerves occurs and anesthesia may be present, antedating the appearance of frank gangrene. Blood cultures are positive.

Imaging Studies

Required for diagnosis

PA and lateral radiographs should be ordered initially and will show soft-tissue swelling and gas, if present. However, gas in the soft tissues may not be present initially; therefore, additional imaging studies such as CT are needed. CT, especially with injection of a contrast medium, will show fascial thickening, edema in the muscle and soft tissue, and gas along fascial planes.

Required for comprehensive evaluation

MRI can be used to evaluate the extent of the infection in both the superficial and deep tissues but will not be specific for gas. If MRI does not show deep fascial involvement, then the diagnosis of necrotizing fasciitis is in doubt.

Special considerations

If the diagnosis is in doubt, needle aspiration of the affected site should be obtained.

Pitfalls

Gas may not be present, especially early in the course of the disease. Therefore, radiographs alone are not a dependable means of confirming the diagnosis. Advanced imaging studies are needed but should not delay aggressive surgical treatment for more than 1 or 2 hours.

IMAGE DESCRIPTIONS

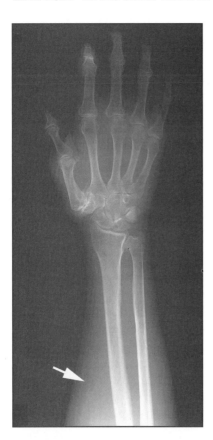

Figure 2-12

Necrotizing fasciitis—AP view

AP view of the forearm of a 50-year-old man with diabetes mellitus and a history of a puncture wound shows soft-tissue swelling (arrow), consistent with necrotizing fasciitis.

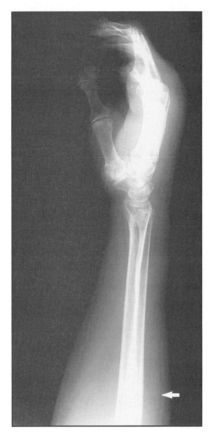

Figure 2-13

Necrotizing fasciitis—Lateral view

Lateral view of the same patient shown in Figure 2-12 shows gas in the soft tissues (arrow), consistent with necrotizing fasciitis.

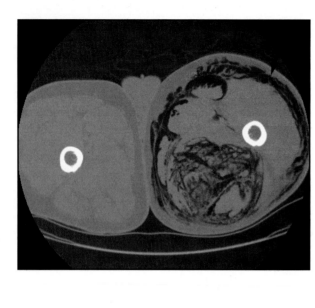

Figure 2-14

Necrotizing fasciitis—Axial CT

Axial CT scan of the thighs in a 70-year-old man on chemotherapy with a draining knee wound shows soft-tissue swelling and gas in the soft tissues (arrow).

DIFFERENTIAL DIAGNOSIS

Cellulitis (lack of toxic shock symptoms)

Clostridial cellulitis (odor)

Clostridial myonecrosis (lack of characteristic odor, involvement of deep and superficial soft tissues)

Septic Arthritis

Synonyms
Infectious arthritis
Pyemic arthritis
Pyogenic arthritis

ICD-9 Code
711.0
Pyogenic arthritis

Definition
Septic arthritis is an infection in a synovial joint; it is considered to be the most destructive and dangerous form of arthritis. Usually, only a single joint is involved. The hip and knee are most commonly affected, followed by the ankle, wrist, and shoulder. Septic arthritis is considered an emergency, with immediate treatment required to prevent destruction of the articular cartilage both by the bacteria and by the host immune response to the bacteria. In addition to possible destruction of the articular cartilage, increased pressure within the hip joint can lead to osteonecrosis, femoral head destruction, and physeal arrest.

Organisms can enter the joints by hematogenous spread, by spread from a contiguous site such as epiphyseal osteomyelitis, by direct inoculation from an object penetrating a joint, or by contamination at the time of surgery. *Staphylococcus aureus* is the most common inciting organism. A wide variety of organisms, including *Pseudomonas aeruginosa* and *Serratia marcescens*, are isolated in IV drug users. In young children, *Haemophilus influenzae* is commonly found in septic hips. Known HIV infection raises the possibility of fungi or mycobacteria. Tuberculous arthritis can affect the hip and knee (most commonly) in children and young adults.

An existing underlying inflammatory arthritis such as rheumatoid arthritis can predispose to bacteremia localizing in an affected joint. In this situation, an acute inflammatory response is created, depositing bacteria in the synovial membrane, followed by the release of cytokines and proteases that cause cartilage degradation and inhibit cartilage synthesis. The large synovial effusion that results from uncontrolled infection and inflammation can lead to pressure necrosis that further destroys cartilage and bone.

History and Physical Findings
A single acute, painful, and swollen joint is the most typical presentation, involving the knee in more than half of patients. Patients with systemic inflammatory or connective tissue disease are more likely to have multiple joint involvement. Typical

presentations include fevers and chills, though elderly and immunocompromised patients may be afebrile. Children with septic arthritis generally appear gravely ill. Pain with weight bearing is common.

Clues to the infecting organism can include associated skin, respiratory, or urinary tract infection. The use of certain drugs including immunosuppressive medications such as steroids can increase predisposition to septic arthritis as well as minimize inflammatory response to infection.

On physical examination, swelling, tenderness, redness, and warmth of the affected joint are common findings. Regional lymph nodes may be enlarged. Motion of the affected joint is limited and painful. Children typically refuse to move the involved joint or walk on an affected lower limb. Even short-arc range of motion is resisted. Laboratory studies including erythrocyte sedimentation rate, white blood count, and C-reactive protein level are abnormal. Synovial fluid aspirate is positive in most patients with infection. Negative cultures are seen in those previously exposed to antimicrobials, as well as with some fastidious streptococci or *Mycoplasma*. Joint aspiration with Gram stain and culture of the joint fluid is needed for a definitive diagnosis.

IMAGING STUDIES

Required for diagnosis
AP and lateral views of the affected joint are the first studies to order. However, radiographic changes other than a joint effusion may not be seen for 2 to 3 weeks. Late changes (after 3 weeks) seen on radiographs include periarticular osteopenia and cartilage destruction leading to joint space narrowing. Marginal and central osseous erosions can be seen late as well. Marginal erosions with preservation of joint space are typical of tuberculous infections.

Required for comprehensive evaluation
MRI is useful to demonstrate an effusion, localized abscesses, osteomyelitis adjacent to the joint, extent of involvement, and any internal derangement of the joint.

Special considerations
Aspiration of the affected joint with Gram stain and joint fluid culture is needed for a definitive diagnosis. Gonadal shielding is recommended for children on follow-up images.

Pitfalls

Bone scans or MRI can show changes of osteomyelitis before they are evident on radiographs. The availability of MRI and ultrasound, however, should not delay the urgent aspiration and analysis of synovial fluid. In most cases, findings on radiographs and joint aspiration will direct treatment.

IMAGE DESCRIPTIONS

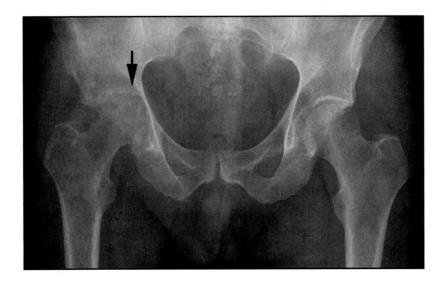

Figure 2-15

Septic arthritis (adult)—AP view

AP view of a pelvis with an infected right hip shows osteopenia and diffuse joint space narrowing of the right hip joint (arrow), consistent with septic arthritis.

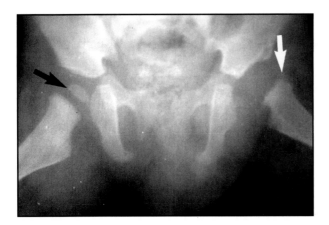

Figure 2-16

Septic arthritis (pediatric)— AP view

AP view of the hips and pelvis in an infant shows a femoral ossific nucleus on the unaffected side (black arrow) but none on the affected side. The femoral metaphysis also appears slightly more laterally displaced (white arrow) compared to the unaffected side, suggestive of an intra-articular collection of fluid or other material.

SECTION 2 ■ GENERAL ORTHOPAEDICS

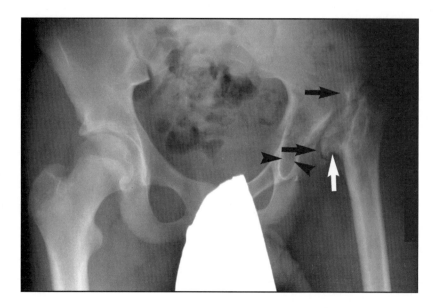

Figure 2-17

Septic arthritis (pediatric)— AP view

AP view shows severe late sequelae of septic arthritis. The left proximal femur is subluxated superiorly (black arrows). There is loss of joint space, coxa breva, and deformation of the femoral head (white arrow). The acetabular teardrop is widened (arrowheads), suggesting that the relationship between the femur and acetabulum has been abnormal for some time.

DIFFERENTIAL DIAGNOSIS

Calcium pyrophosphate dihydrate (CPPD) crystal deposition disease (urate or calcium pyrophosphate crystals seen on aspiration)

Gonococcal arthritis (migratory polyarthritis and tenosynovitis in a young, sexually active adult)

Gout (elevated serum uric acid level, urate crystals found on joint aspiration)

Lyme disease (acute monoarthritis, characteristic rash, a history of a visit to an endemic area)

Mycobacterial and fungal arthritis (significantly immunocompromised patient, such as HIV infection)

Reiter's syndrome (reactive arthritis, single or multiple joint involvement in the setting of uveitis and urethritis)

Rheumatoid arthritis (negative joint aspirate, multiple joint involvement, positive rheumatoid factor)

Transient synovitis of the hip (children aged 4 to 8 years; the child appears less ill; joint aspirate will show no bacteria and few white cells; radiographs will be normal)

CALCIFICATION OF THE SOFT TISSUES

SYNONYMS

Calcinosis
Calcinosis circumscripta
Calcinosis universalis
Chondrocalcinosis
Heterotopic ossifications
Tumoral calcinosis

ICD-9 Codes

275.9
Unspecified disorder of mineral metabolism

709.3
Degenerative skin disorders: Calcinosis circumscripta

710.3
Dermatomyositis

DEFINITION

Calcific deposits in the soft tissues are an abnormal finding, but their presence on radiographs is not definitive for any one diagnosis. The location and characteristics of calcifications, however, help narrow the differential diagnosis. For example, it is helpful to differentiate calcific deposits from ossific deposits. In large deposits, trabecular patterns may be seen, whereas in smaller lesions the differentiation may be more difficult to see. Calcification within joint capsules, menisci, or bursae suggests calcium pyrophosphate dihydrate (CPPD) crystal deposition disease as a possibility. Hemangiomas will often have phleboliths (circular areas of calcification with a radiolucent center). Periarticular calcifications can be seen in hyperparathyroidism, collagen vascular diseases, and renal osteodystrophy.

Three main types of calcific deposits have been described in the soft tissues: (1) metastatic calcification, (2) calcinosis, and (3) dystrophic calcification.

Metastatic calcification is caused by an abnormality in calcium and/or phosphorus metabolism and is seen in milk-alkali syndrome, hyperparathyroidism or hypoparathyroidism, renal osteodystrophy, hypervitaminosis D, sarcoidosis, leukemia, plasma cell myeloma, and skeletal metastases. Metastatic calcification shows a predilection for periarticular tissues.

Calcinosis describes calcium deposits in the skin and subcutaneous tissues in the presence of normal calcium metabolism. This type of deposition occurs in scleroderma, dermatomyositis, idiopathic tumoral calcinosis, and idiopathic tumoral calcinosis universalis. Tumoral calcinosis occurs primarily in young and adolescent blacks and is characterized by the development of large calcific masses about the shoulders, hips, and elbows. This diagnosis is made by ruling out other diseases such as chronic renal disease, hyperparathyroidism, and collagen vascular disease.

Dystrophic calcification refers to calcium deposited in damaged tissue (such as burns and muscle injury) with normal calcium metabolism. Damaged tissues produce an environment of decreased carbon dioxide concentration and higher pH, which is conducive to calcium deposition. Many traumatic, inflammatory, and neoplastic conditions result in calcium deposition because of the relative alkalinity of the local tissues. Dystrophic calcification makes up 95% to 98% of soft-tissue calcification. Richardson developed the mnemonic VINDICATE (vascular, infection, neoplasm, drugs, inflammatory, congenital, autoimmune, trauma, endocrine/metabolic) to help remember the many causes of dystrophic calcification.

HISTORY AND PHYSICAL FINDINGS

The medical history may include one of the many conditions described above. In rare cases, the cause of the calcification is not known. Soft-tissue calcification usually is not of functional significance but rather is a reflection of a potentially more serious underlying medical condition. Calcific deposits are sometimes palpable and may be tender to palpation. Joint motion can be restricted if the deposits occur in sufficient volume around a joint.

IMAGING STUDIES

Required for diagnosis

PA and lateral radiographs of the affected structure will show the calcifications. However, laboratory studies and a clinical history are needed to make a definitive diagnosis.

Required for comprehensive evaluation

When evaluating tumors, CT is better at imaging calcifications than MRI.

Special considerations

None

Pitfalls

None

IMAGE DESCRIPTIONS

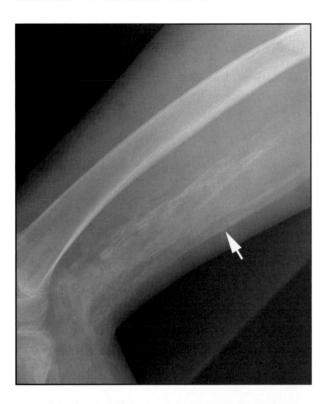

Figure 2-18

Dermatomyositis (thigh)— Lateral view

Lateral view of a thigh shows sheetlike calcification in the soft tissues posterior to the femur and knee (arrow).

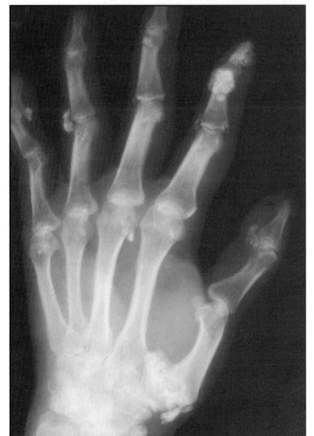

Figure 2-19

Scleroderma (hand)—PA view

PA view of a hand shows scattered soft-tissue calcification throughout the hand. Note also diffuse subluxation and narrowing in the metacarpophalangeal, proximal interphalangeal, and distal interphalangeal joints.

SECTION 2 ■ GENERAL ORTHOPAEDICS

SECTION 2 ■ GENERAL ORTHOPAEDICS

DIFFERENTIAL DIAGNOSIS

Collagen vascular disease (subcutaneous calcifications in scleroderma, CREST [calcinosis cutis, Raynaud's phenomenon, scleroderma, and telangiectasis])

Dietary causes (excessive vitamin D intake) (amorphous masses of calcium in periarticular region, excessive intake of milk or alkali)

Metaboliccauses (periarticular calcifications; abnormal serum calcium, phosphate, and uric acid levels; abnormal renal function)

Trauma (calcification about joints; history of injury, head injury, or burn)

Tumor (dystrophic calcification seen on CT of malignant tumor masses such as malignant fibrous histiocytoma [MFH])

CPPD CRYSTAL DEPOSITION DISEASE

SYNONYMS

Calcium pyrophosphate arthropathy
Chondrocalcinosis
CPPD
Crystal deposition disease
Pseudogout syndrome

ICD-9 Codes

275.49
Other disorders of calcium metabolism

712.2
Chondrocalcinosis due to pyrophosphate crystals

DEFINITION

The term calcium pyrophosphate dihydrate (CPPD) crystal deposition disease encompasses several clinical syndromes that have in common the precipitation of CPPD crystals, usually intra-articularly and less commonly in periarticular tissue. Certain joints are at risk, most commonly the knee, wrist (radiocarpal joint), index and middle metacarpophalangeal (MCP) joints, symphysis pubis, shoulder, elbow, and hip. The presence of calcium pyrophosphate crystals in the joint causes pain and ultimately joint destruction.

Patients with CPPD crystal deposition disease may have one or some combination of any of the following three conditions: chondrocalcinosis, pseudogout, or pyrophosphate arthropathy. Thus, the clinical spectrum of CPPD crystal deposition disease varies and can mimic virtually any type of arthritis, including osteoarthritis, gout, rheumatoid arthritis, inflammatory osteoarthritis, and neuropathic joint disease. Chondrocalcinosis (cartilage calcification) may be symptomatic or asymptomatic. When symptomatic, the term pseudogout is often used. Pseudogout refers to acute crystalline-induced painful synovitis secondary to CPPD crystals that are positively birefringent. Patients with pseudogout do not respond to colchicine, which usually is helpful in treating gout. When structural damage to the joint is apparent, the condition is referred to as calcium pyrophosphate arthropathy.

The knee joint is most commonly affected, accounting for more than 80% of all acute cases. Chondrocalcinosis tends to occur in the triangular fibrocartilage complex (TFCC) of the wrist and the MCP joints of the index and middle fingers; the reason for the latter is unclear. Chondrocalcinosis within the scapholunate ligament may result in a scapholunate advanced collapse (SLAC) wrist, characterized by narrowing of the radioscaphoid joint and damage to the scapholunate ligament.

Masses of CPPD crystals resembling tophi, referred to as tumoral calcium pyrophosphate deposition disease, are rare. Occasionally urate crystals and CPPD crystals coexist in a single inflammatory effusion. In CPPD crystal deposition disease, bone density usually is normal, and large subchondral cysts are common.

History and Physical Findings

Joint pain and swelling in characteristic locations in a middle-aged or elderly patient suggest the possibility of CPPD crystal deposition disease. Episodes of pain may be acute and self-limited or chronic and progressive. The joint pain may be similar to that of gout; in fact, as previously stated, gout may occur simultaneously with CPPD crystal deposition disease. Patients with a history of gout, hyperparathyroidism, or hemochromatosis are at greater risk for CPPD.

Patterns of CPPD crystal deposition disease that are similar to rheumatoid arthritis or osteoarthritis may also be present. A pattern similar to rheumatoid arthritis (5% of patients) occurs in the elderly. The clinical picture in these patients includes leukocytosis, fever, and inflammatory symmetric polyarthritis along with mental confusion. This condition is reversible with anti-inflammatory treatment. A pattern similar to osteoarthritis (30% to 60% of patients) is a possibility when the joints typically affected in osteoarthritis are seen together with calcification on radiographs. With this pattern of CPPD crystal deposition disease, the joints most commonly affected are the knees, the wrists, the MCP joints, the shoulders, and the hips. Less commonly, the elbows and spine are affected.

Subtle clues on physical examination include joint contractures and valgus deformities of the knees. Examination of the joints in advanced disease will show decreased range of motion and tenderness to palpation. CPPD crystal deposition disease is confirmed by the presence of CPPD crystals in joint aspirate seen with a polarizing microscope, particularly with intracellular crystals seen in acute pseudogout. The crystals show weak or no positive birefringence, unlike gout, which demonstrates positive birefringence.

Imaging Studies

Required for diagnosis
AP and lateral radiographs of the knee and PA and lateral radiographs of the wrists and hands are the imaging studies of choice. Chondrocalcinosis is commonly seen in the TFCC of the wrist and in the ligaments and hyaline cartilage of the proximal carpal row. A SLAC wrist deformity may be present, as may erosion of the scaphoid into the radius.

Required for comprehensive evaluation
MRI is useful to evaluate the degree of cartilage and bone destruction, as well the amount of synovial involvement.

Special considerations
None

Pitfalls

Chondrocalcinosis has many causes that may not be identified on radiographs. Diagnosis is based on identification of positively birefringent crystals on a polarizing microscope. CPPD crystal deposition disease is easily confused with gout, rheumatoid arthritis, and osteoarthritis.

IMAGE DESCRIPTIONS

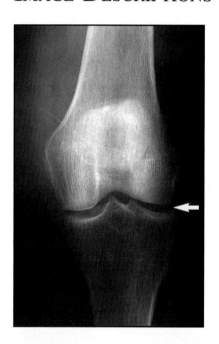

Figure 2-20

Chondrocalcinosis (knee)—AP view

AP view of a knee shows calcification of the meniscus. Note there is little destruction of the joint space (arrow). Clinically, the patient did not experience the severe pain typical of pseudogout.

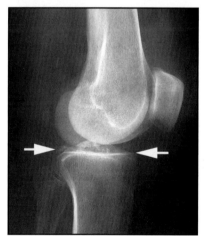

Figure 2-21

Chondrocalcinosis (knee)—Lateral view

Lateral view of the same patient shown in Figure 2-20 shows the calcification even more clearly (arrow).

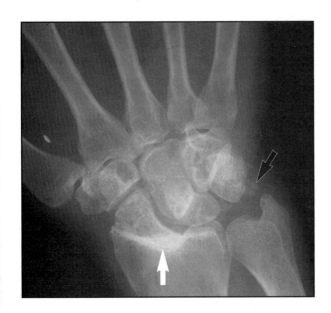

Figure 2-22

SLAC wrist deformity—PA view

PA view of the right hand of a 50-year-old woman shows a SLAC wrist deformity. Note the cartilage calcification within the TFCC (black arrow) and erosion of the scaphoid into the radius (white arrow); the latter is common with CPPD crystal deposition disease.

DIFFERENTIAL DIAGNOSIS

Collagen vascular disease (no chondrocalcinosis)

Degenerative joint disease (no crystals on joint aspiration, no calcification, involvement of the carpometacarpal joint of the thumb rather than the radiocarpal joint and MCP joints)

Gout (presence of urate crystals, great toe involvement, elevated serum uric acid)

Hyperparathyroidism (subchondral, subperiosteal bone resorption, serum calcium abnormalities)

Osteochondritis dissecans (apparent underlying cartilage defect, no calcification)

Renal osteodystrophy (no chondrocalcinosis, history of renal failure)

Rheumatoid arthritis (erosive changes seen on radiographs, no calcification)

Scleroderma (subcutaneous rather than intra-articular calcifications)

HYPERPARATHYROIDISM

SYNONYM

Generalized osteitis fibrosis cystica

ICD-9 Code

252.0
Hyperparathyroidism

DEFINITION

Hyperparathyroidism is a condition characterized by elevated levels of serum parathyroid hormone (PTH). There are three types of hyperparathyroidism: primary, secondary, and tertiary.

In primary hyperparathyroidism, increased secretion of PTH results from a parathyroid adenoma (80%), diffuse hyperplasia (10% to 20%), or carcinoma (< 1%). Hypercalcemia is common. Women in their 30s and 40s are three times more likely to be affected than men. Secondary hyperparathyroidism results from increased PTH in response to hypocalcemia. The hypocalcemia may be caused by chronic renal failure or malabsorption. Bony changes of osteomalacia can also occur, in which case the condition is called renal osteodystrophy. In tertiary hyperparathyroidism, serum calcium levels become elevated, and the parathyroid glands appear to act autonomously. This condition is seen in patients with chronic renal failure.

PTH and vitamin D are the major regulators of calcium and phosphate metabolism. Parathyroid dysfunction can present as asymptomatic hypercalcemia, symptomatic hypercalcemia, symptomatic renal calculi (nephrolithiasis), bone disease, or rarely as parathyroid crisis. Nephrolithiasis secondary to hyperparathyroidism occurs in 15% to 20% of patients, with chronic hyperparathyroidism leading to significant bone disease. Bone disease can include, though now rare, findings of osteitis fibrosa cystica and brown tumor. These findings are generally associated with prolonged and severe hyperparathyroidism. Cortical bone loss occurs more rapidly than trabecular bone loss, affecting the forearm, hip, and spine. Women with hyperparathyroidism are at increased risk for fractures of the ribs, vertebrae, pelvis, and distal radius.

HISTORY AND PHYSICAL FINDINGS

Most patients are asymptomatic, with up to 80% of cases found on regular biochemical screening. Nonspecific symptoms include fatigue, weakness, anorexia, depression, and cognitive or neuromuscular dysfunction that is associated with hypercalcemia. Up to 25% of patients may have bone pain and tenderness. A history of gastric or duodenal ulcers may be present.

Imaging Studies

Required for diagnosis

PA views of the hand should be obtained to screen for hyperparathyroidism. Typical radiographic findings include subperiosteal (lace-like) bone resorption on the radial aspect of middle phalanges, tuft resorption, and soft-tissue calcification.

PA and lateral views of the shoulder, skull, and lumbar spine should be obtained if these areas are symptomatic. Generalized osteopenia is more usual in primary hyperparathyroidism, whereas increased bone density is seen in secondary hyperparathyroidism. Soft-tissue calcification is also more common in secondary hyperparathyroidism. Patients with chronic renal failure with secondary hyperparathyroidism may have osteitis fibrosa cystica, characterized by focal aggregates of osteoclasts resorbing bone, osteoblasts forming bone, and peritrabecular fibrosis deposition in the marrow. The spine adjacent to the end plates may appear to have increased bone density. This appearance is referred to as a "rugger jersey" spine because of the horizontally striped appearance, like a rugby shirt. Skull findings include trabecular resorption, commonly seen as a "salt-and-pepper" skull. Erosion of the lateral end (acromial end) of the clavicle can be seen in the shoulder.

Required for comprehensive evaluation

MRI is seldom indicated but can be useful in the evaluation of brown tumors.

Special considerations

None

Pitfalls

The cause of the osteopenia may not be evident from radiographs. In these patients, the history and laboratory findings are essential.

IMAGE DESCRIPTION

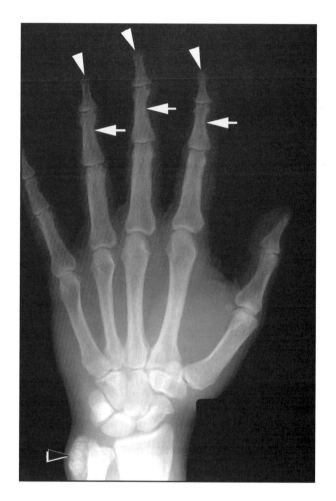

Figure 2-23

Hyperparathyroidism—PA view

PA view of a left hand demonstrates several findings typical of hyperparathyroidism. Acroosteolysis can be seen in the tufts of the index, middle, and ring fingers (white arrowheads); subperiosteal reabsorption is apparent along the radial side of the middle phalanges of the index, middle and ring fingers (white arrows); and a calcified soft-tissue mass is seen about the distal ulna (black arrowhead).

SECTION 2 ■ GENERAL ORTHOPAEDICS

DIFFERENTIAL DIAGNOSIS

Hypercalcemia of malignancy (usually evident clinically at the time of diagnosis, most often caused by PTH-related protein hypersecretion)

Milk-alkali syndrome (calcium carbonate supplementation)

Overuse of thiazide diuretics (history of thiazide diuretic use)

OSTEOMALACIA/RICKETS

SECTION 2 ■ GENERAL ORTHOPAEDICS

ICD-9 Codes

268.0
Rickets, active

268.2
Osteomalacia, unspecified

SYNONYMS

Infantile rickets
Vitamin D–resistant rickets

DEFINITION

Inadequate mineralization of osteoid leads to rickets in children and osteomalacia in adults. Vitamin D is a prohormone that functions to maintain normal serum calcium and phosphate levels and normal bone mineralization. Any abnormality in the vitamin D metabolism chain can result in rickets or osteomalacia. Other etiologies include gastrointestinal malabsorption, liver disease, renal disease, medication use (some anticonvulsants), some types of tumor, and parathyroid disorders. Laboratory studies typically reveal decreased serum and urine calcium and phosphate levels plus an elevated alkaline phosphatase level.

HISTORY AND PHYSICAL FINDINGS

Osteomalacia may be asymptomatic, or it may be characterized by diffuse bone pain and tenderness. The patient may have a history of liver or kidney disease. Premature infants who require prolonged periods of parenteral feeding are at risk for rickets. Infants with rickets tend to be restless with poor sleep patterns. The costochondral junctions may become enlarged, creating a deformity called a "rachitic rosary." The skull is affected as well, with softening of the cranium. In older children, a waddling gait occasionally may be seen, as can muscle wasting and muscle weakness that is present more proximally than distally. Insufficiency fractures occur frequently in both osteomalacia and rickets, most commonly involving the ribs, vertebrae, and long bones.

IMAGING STUDIES

Required for diagnosis

AP and lateral radiographs of symptomatic areas are needed to establish the diagnosis. Characteristic radiologic findings in osteomalacia include Looser transformation zones, described as pseudofractures, or narrow radiolucent lines up to 5 mm in width with sclerotic borders. Typical sites include the axillary margin of the scapula, the femoral neck, the medial aspect of the femoral shaft, the lesser trochanter, and the pubic and ischial rami. Nonspecific findings include osteopenia with cortical thinning, loss of radiologic sharpness of the vertebral body caused by defective mineralization of osteoid, and loss of secondary trabeculae. Bone softening that occurs with more advanced disease can lead to a biconcave shape of the vertebral bodies, termed "codfish vertebrae." Shortening and bowing of the tibia and insufficiency fractures may occur with more severe disease. Rickets is characterized by widening of growth plates with metaphyseal fraying and cupping. Bones may be bowed.

Required for comprehensive evaluation

If the initial radiographs are normal and the patient has bone pain, MRI should be ordered to identify insufficiency fractures.

Special considerations

None

Pitfalls

The etiology of osteomalacia often cannot be determined by radiographs alone; therefore, the medical history and results of laboratory studies are necessary.

IMAGE DESCRIPTIONS

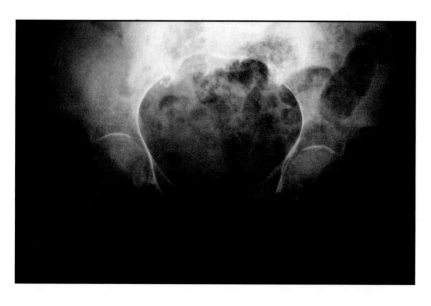

Figure 2-24

Osteomalacia— AP view

AP view of the pelvis in a patient with osteomalacia reveals mild varus of the hips (arrows) and coarsening of the trabeculae.

SECTION 2 ■ GENERAL ORTHOPAEDICS

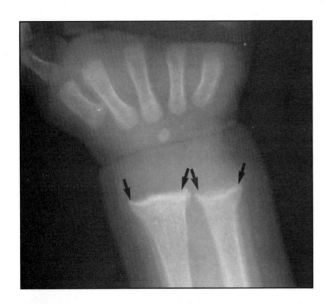

Figure 2-25

Rickets—PA view

PA view of the wrist in a child with rickets shows radial and ulnar metaphyseal fraying and cupping (arrows).

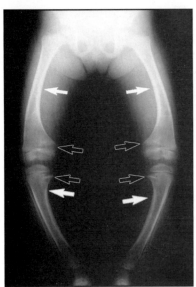

Figure 2-26

Rickets—AP view

AP view of the lower extremities in a child with rickets demonstrates bowing of the femurs and tibias (white arrows) as well as metaphyseal widening and irregularity (black arrows).

DIFFERENTIAL DIAGNOSIS
Osteoporosis (normal laboratory studies)

OSTEOPOROSIS

SYNONYMS

Generalized osteoporosis
Regional osteoporosis

DEFINITION

Osteoporosis is a metabolic bone disease characterized by decreased bone mass leading to microarchitectural deterioration. The bone that is present, however, is fully mineralized and appears normal histologically. Trabecular bone is resorbed more rapidly than cortical bone, which causes the bone to become more fragile and susceptible to fracture.

Osteoporosis may be generalized, regional, or local in distribution. The most common types of the generalized form are postmenopausal (type I) and senile (type II). Type I osteoporosis is six times more common in women than in men. Vertebral fractures and distal radius fractures are common with this type. In type II osteoporosis, hip and pelvic fractures are common. Women older than age 70 years are twice as likely as men to have type II osteoporosis. Common causes of generalized osteoporosis include medication use (steroids and heparin); alcohol abuse and chronic liver disease; history of smoking; malnutrition, anemia, and calcium deficiency; and endocrine diseases such as diabetes mellitus, hyperparathyroidism, hyperthyroidism, testosterone deficiency, and Cushing's syndrome (hyperadrenocorticism). An idiopathic juvenile form is seen occasionally in prepubescent children. Causes of regional or localized osteoporosis include disuse of an extremity such as occurs following cast immobilization, reflex sympathetic dystrophy, and a transient form that occurs around joints in the lower extremity. Transient osteoporosis of the hip can occur in women during the last trimester of pregnancy and in young to middle-aged men.

Osteoporosis occurs in one of two women and in one of eight men. Race is also a factor. Both whites and Asians are more commonly affected. Of the 1.3 million osteoporotic fractures that occur each year, 50% are vertebral fractures, 25% are hip fractures, and the remainder are fractures of the distal radius and proximal humerus. Pelvic and hip fractures lead to higher risk for mortality—up to 25% of women and 40% of men die within the first year after hip fractures.

ICD-9 Codes

731.0
Osteitis deformans without mention of bone tumor

733.00
Osteoporosis, unspecified

733.01
Senile osteoporosis

733.02
Idiopathic osteoporosis

733.03
Disuse osteoporosis

733.09
Drug-induced osteoporosis

SECTION 2 ■ GENERAL ORTHOPAEDICS

HISTORY AND PHYSICAL FINDINGS

Osteoporosis may not be symptomatic until a fracture occurs. Compression fractures of the spine may occur in a context of little or no obvious trauma. A patient may notice the sudden onset of back pain when getting up from a chair. Similarly, a hip fracture may occur first, causing the patient to fall, rather than a fall causing the hip fracture. Usually a fall on an outstretched hand is the cause of distal radius fractures. Physical examination will reveal obvious deformity of the wrist in the case of wrist fractures and external rotation of the hip in the case of femoral neck or intertrochanteric fractures. Localized tenderness over the involved vertebrae is found with compression fractures of the spine. Laboratory studies usually are normal.

IMAGING STUDIES

Required for diagnosis

For patients with suspected compression fractures, PA and lateral radiographs of the spine are sufficient to establish the diagnosis. The lateral views will identify the fracture and any loss of vertebral height. Increased radiolucency in the spine and long bones will be seen in advanced osteoporosis. Mild to moderate osteoporosis, however, is difficult to diagnose with radiographs.

Required for comprehensive evaluation

MRI is useful in differentiating compression fractures secondary to vertebral body metastases in patients with a history of malignancy from fractures related to osteoporosis. Quantitative analysis of bone density or bone density testing is required to make a definitive diagnosis. A dual-energy x-ray absorptiometry (DEXA) scan is useful in documenting osteoporosis in the axial skeleton. DEXA scans are indicated in women older than age 65 years and are also recommended for postmenopausal women with one additional risk factor such as a fracture, steroid use, alcohol abuse, history of smoking, or family history of osteoporosis insufficiency fracture. Testing bone density in the forearm is useful in the context of nephrolithiasis and hyperparathyroidism to differentiate cortical from trabecular bone loss.

Special considerations

None

Pitfalls

Failure to recognize a pathologic (metastatic) compression fracture as opposed to a benign osteoporotic fracture is possible.

IMAGE DESCRIPTION

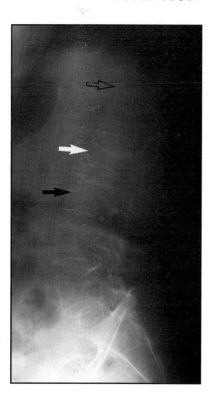

Figure 2-27

Osteoporosis (spine)—Lateral view

Lateral view of an 83-year-old woman shows three characteristic findings of osteoporosis in the spine: (1) the "empty box" appearance of a vertebra (black arrow); (2) a "codfish" (biconcave) vertebra (white arrow); and (3) a wedge-shaped fracture (open arrow). The empty box appearance is caused by a relative increase in the density of the vertebral end plates as a result of resorption of the bony trabeculae. The codfish appearance is caused by expansion of the nucleus pulposus into the weakened vertebral end plates, causing collapse of the central position of the end plate.

DIFFERENTIAL DIAGNOSIS

Metastatic disease (positive MRI)

Osteomalacia (difficult to differentiate on radiographs; tissue biopsy may be needed; metaphyseal changes in children with rickets)

PAGET'S DISEASE

ICD-9 Code

731.0
Osteitis deformans without
mention of bone tumor

SYNONYM
Osteitis deformans

DEFINITION

Paget's disease of bone is a focal skeletal disorder characterized by an increased rate of bone turnover. The accelerated formation and resorption of bone results in a "mistake" pattern of lamellar bone with an associated increase in blood flow to the bone, fibrous tissue, and adjacent bone marrow. The incidence of Paget's disease, based on autopsy studies and radiographs, varies from 3% to 4% in persons older than age 40 years. It affects men and women equally, increasing in frequency with age.

The exact etiology is unknown, but genetic factors appear to play a significant role. The risk of disease is increased sevenfold in first-degree relatives of patients with Paget's disease. It is more common in Caucasians and is rare in Asian populations. Viral infection may also play a role in its development, as osteoclasts contain viral particles. Current literature suggests that Paget's disease may result from latent viral infection of osteoclasts in a genetically susceptible individual.

Pathologic and stress fractures are common complications of Paget's disease. The subtrochanteric region is the most common femoral site for pathologic fractures, whereas stress fractures commonly occur in the femoral neck and upper anterior one third of the tibial shaft. These fractures generally heal, but the healing may be slow.

Osteogenic sarcomas rarely occur but are the most common tumors of bone that arise in association with Paget's disease. These tumors are manifested by increased local pain at affected sites, typically the pelvis, femur, humerus, skull, and facial bones. Giant cell tumors, lymphomas, and plasma cell myeloma also have been reported in association with Paget's disease.

Most cases of vertebral Paget's disease are asymptomatic, but with advanced stages of Paget's disease, neurologic complications may develop because of bony changes in the spine and at the base of the skull. Neurologic dysfunction may be caused either by pathologic fracture of the vertebra or by enlargement of the vertebra that causes encroachment on the spinal canal or nerve roots. Ischemia of the neural elements may be caused by direct compression or by a vascular steal phenomenon secondary to shunting of blood into the hypermetabolic bone.

HISTORY AND PHYSICAL FINDINGS

Paget's disease of bone is generally asymptomatic. In patients who report symptoms, pain and deformity are common. Paget's disease is sometimes diagnosed with the accidental finding of elevated serum alkaline phosphatase levels on routine laboratory studies.

The pain associated with Paget's disease generally occurs at the most common sites of skeletal involvement—the pelvis, spine, skull, and proximal and distal areas of the femur, tibia, and humerus. Pain resulting from complications is caused by abnormal bone that leads to symptoms of degenerative arthritis involving the hip and knee, entrapment neuropathy, fracture, and sometimes (but rarely) osteosarcoma. Medical management can relieve mechanical bone pain, as well as bone pain that is worse at night. Long bone deformity results from the enlargement and abnormal contour of affected bones, which leads to lateral bowing of the femur and anterior bowing of the tibia.

IMAGING STUDIES

Required for diagnosis

PA and lateral views of the affected part(s) of the skeleton are sufficient to make the diagnosis. Typically, radiographs will show lytic changes, sclerotic changes, and a mixture of both with coarsened trabeculae, cortical thickening, enlarging bones, and bowing of long bones. The radiographic hallmark of vertebral Paget's disease is enlargement of the diameter of the vertebral body both anteroposteriorly and transversely with no increase in the vertical height. Changes in bone density lead to a characteristic "picture frame" appearance on radiographs.

Required for comprehensive evaluation

Bone scans can be useful in the evaluation of Paget's disease because abnormalities may be seen on bone scans before radiographic changes are evident. In the presence of an elevated serum alkaline phosphatase level and normal radiographs, a bone scan is helpful in diagnosing early Paget's disease. CT and MRI are not needed to diagnose the disease, but MRI can be helpful in evaluating any sarcomatous changes in affected bone and for evaluating spinal stenosis related to Paget's disease.

Special considerations

In rare instances of new nonspecific radiographic findings, occurring years after onset of Paget's disease, bone biopsy may be necessary to exclude malignant degeneration, metastatic bone disease, or myeloma.

Pitfalls

Transformation to a sarcoma may easily be missed.

IMAGE DESCRIPTIONS

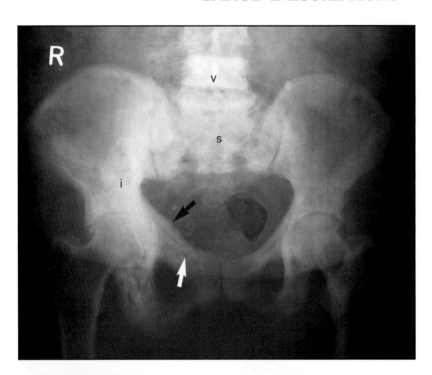

Figure 2-28

Paget's disease (hip)—AP view

AP view of a pelvis demonstrates cortical thickening. Note the thickened iliopectineal line (black arrow); sclerosis of the right ilium (i), sacrum (s), and L5 vertebral bodies (v); and trabecular coarsening (white arrow). Note also the narrowing and osteophytosis of both hip joints consistent with osteoarthritis.

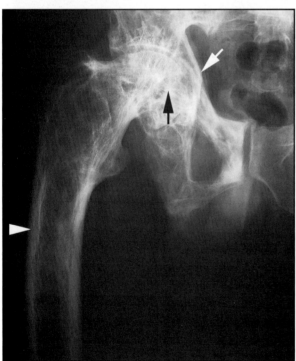

Figure 2-29

Paget's disease—AP view

AP view of a right hip shows trabecular coarsening (black arrow), deformities of bone softening including abnormal bowing of the femur (arrowhead), and protrusion of the acetabulum (white arrow).

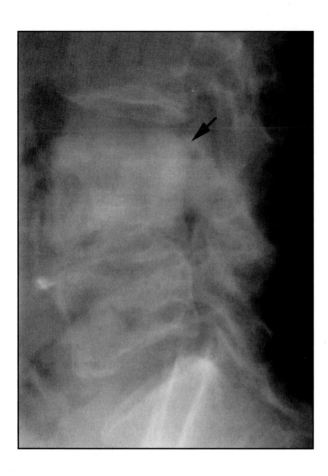

Figure 2-30

*Paget's disease (spine)—
Lateral view*

Lateral view of a lumbar spine shows sclerosis
and expansion of the L4 vertebra (arrow)
consistent with Paget's disease.

DIFFERENTIAL DIAGNOSIS

Fibrous dysplasia ("ground glass" appearance of bone lesion)

Metastatic prostate cancer (elevated prostate-specific antigen
level, prostate mass)

Renal osteodystrophy (subchondral bone resorption)

TOTAL JOINT REPLACEMENT— DISLOCATION/SUBLUXATION

ICD-9 Code

996.4
Mechanical complication of internal orthopedic device, implant, and graft

SYNONYMS
None

DEFINITION
Dislocation of a total joint prosthesis almost always involves the components of a total hip arthroplasty. Subluxation occurs following total knee arthroplasty and total shoulder arthroplasty as well as total hip arthroplasty. Hip components are especially susceptible to dislocation, principally posterior dislocation, during the first 6 to 8 weeks following surgery, before the body has formed a tight soft-tissue capsule around the prosthesis. Additional risk factors for dislocation after a revision total hip arthroplasty are lax tissues and improperly placed components, such as an acetabular cup that is too anteverted or retroverted or a femoral component that is too anteverted.

HISTORY AND PHYSICAL FINDINGS
Patients may report pain and a sensation of the hip partially slipping out of joint (subluxating) or dislocating following activities such as crossing the legs, getting up from a toilet seat or a low chair, or rolling over in bed. If the hip has dislocated posteriorly, the leg assumes a characteristic position in which the hip is flexed and internally rotated. With an anterior dislocation, the leg is extended and externally rotated. Frequently, the hip can be reduced in the emergency department with mild sedation, especially if the hip has dislocated several times. Multiple dislocations indicate the need for surgical revision of the components.

IMAGING STUDIES

Required for diagnosis
An AP view of the hip will readily show the dislocation but not necessarily the direction of displacement, which is more reliably determined by clinical observation of the position of the leg. A cross-table lateral view of the hip is helpful for assessing dislocation.

Required for comprehensive evaluation
CT may be indicated if the hip cannot be reduced, suggesting that either soft tissue or bone cement may be preventing the reduction. However, all dislocations should be referred to a specialist for treatment planning.

Special considerations

If a hip cannot be reduced, most often the surgeon will do an open reduction rather than resort to additional imaging studies.

Pitfalls

A frog-lateral view may not be possible because positioning the leg for this view will cause pain.

IMAGE DESCRIPTION

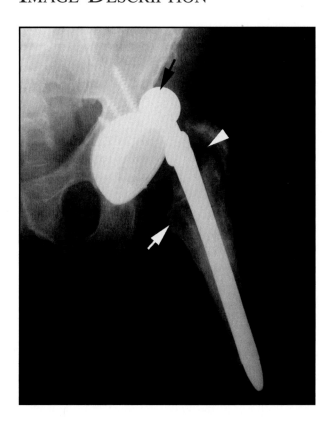

Figure 2-31

Dislocation after total joint replacement (hip)—AP view

AP view of the left hip in a 74-year-old woman shows a dislocation of a total hip prosthesis (black arrow). This is probably an anterior dislocation because the lesser trochanter is in full view (white arrow), suggesting the leg is externally rotated. Note also the nonunion of the greater trochanteric osteotomy (arrowhead). Note that neither the acetabular nor the femoral component shows signs of loosening (no lucent zone around the components).

DIFFERENTIAL DIAGNOSIS

Periprosthetic fracture (fracture seen on radiographs)

TOTAL JOINT REPLACEMENT— HETEROTOPIC OSSIFICATION

ICD-9 Code

755.8
Other specified anomalies of
unspecified limb

SYNONYMS

Ectopic bone formation
Heterotopic bone formation
Myositis ossificans circumscripta
Myositis ossificans traumatica

DEFINITION

Heterotopic ossification (HO) is the development of mature lamellar bone in soft tissues. Myositis ossificans is the formation of mature bone in muscle. HO differs from ectopic calcification, which is the mineralization of soft tissues without bone formation. The specific cause of HO is unknown, but the basic defect involves the transformation of certain cells of unknown origin into osteoblasts (bone-forming cells). HO is a fairly common complication following total joint arthroplasty, especially after a total hip replacement, having been reported in as many as one half of patients who undergo this procedure. HO is less common after total knee or total shoulder arthroplasties. This is in contrast to HO that is secondary to brain and spinal cord injury or burns, which occurs around the elbow, knee, and shoulder, as well as the hip. With HO following total joint arthroplasty, ectopic bone formation can be seen as early as 5 weeks after surgery and matures over an 8- to 12-month period.

Risk factors for developing HO after total hip arthroplasty include male sex, age older than 65 years, history of previous hip surgery, and lack of preoperative prophylaxis with nonsteroidal anti-inflammatory drugs (NSAIDs). In the knee, the most important risk factor appears to be infection. Fully mature heterotopic bone may cause a complete bony ankylosis about the hip. HO does not seem to significantly affect the outcome of total knee and total shoulder surgery. NSAIDs and low-dose radiation (700 rad) given during the first 3 days postoperatively or preoperatively have been successful in preventing HO.

HISTORY AND PHYSICAL FINDINGS

Patients typically are asymptomatic during the first few weeks following surgery. Hip pain and stiffness develop as the ectopic bone matures. Radiographs taken 4 weeks postoperatively may show faint, ill-defined opaque areas about the hip. Physical examination will reveal decreased range of hip motion late in the course of the disease but little physical restriction in the early phases.

IMAGING STUDIES

Required for diagnosis

AP and lateral views of the hip are adequate to establish the diagnosis, but until 4 or 5 weeks postoperatively, no radiographic changes may be evident. Only after that time may faint areas of opacification be seen about the hip. Serial AP views are useful to follow the progression of the disease. After a few months, fully mature bone with trabeculae may be seen adjacent to the joint.

Required for comprehensive evaluation

If the patient experiences decreased range of motion and pain in the hip, the patient should be referred to a specialist for further imaging studies. Bone scans have been used to follow the progress of maturation as an aid to timing surgical intervention to remove the mature heterotopic bone. Once the bone scan shows decreased uptake (usually 8 months to 1 year after surgery), suggesting that the ossification process has slowed or stopped, the ectopic bone can be more safely removed.

Special considerations

None

Pitfalls

None

IMAGE DESCRIPTIONS

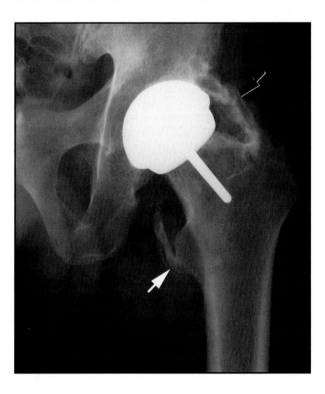

Figure 2-32

Total joint complications (heterotopic ossification)—AP view

AP view of the left hip of a 72-year-old man who underwent a surface replacement hip arthroplasty 14 months earlier shows mature bone bridging the hip joint from the greater trochanter to the acetabulum (black arrow). HO can also be seen arising from the lesser trochanter in the iliopsoas tendon (white arrow). This bone is sufficiently mature that surgical excision can be carried out safely.

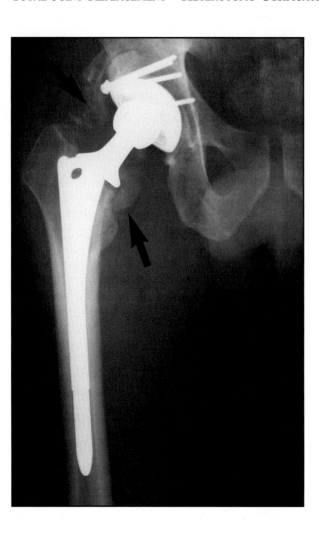

Figure 2-33

Total joint complications (heterotopic ossification)— AP view

AP view of a right total hip arthroplasty shows HO about the lesser trochanter and lateral to the acetabulum (arrows). In this patient, joint motion was not restricted.

DIFFERENTIAL DIAGNOSIS

None

TOTAL JOINT REPLACEMENT—INFECTION

SYNONYMS

Septic total joint
Total joint sepsis

DEFINITION

Infection following total joint arthroplasty is devastating for the patient and clinician alike. Although the rate of infection has been reduced from 10% in the 1960s to 2% or less, because of the consequences for the patient and the large number of procedures performed, infection remains a serious medical and economic problem. In the United States alone, more than 4,000 infections occur yearly following total hip arthroplasty, and the annual cost of treating these infections exceeds $200 million.

The incidence of infection after primary total joint (hip and knee) arthroplasty is in the range of 1% to 2%, and the incidence after revision hip or knee arthroplasty is three to four times as high. The most commonly used classification of infection after total hip arthroplasty is that of Coventry and Fitzgerald, who recognize three types of infections. Type I infections occur during the immediate postoperative period. These infections are caused by infected hematomas or superficial wound infections that ultimately spread to the joint space. Type II infections are believed to start at the time of surgery but do not become manifest until 6 to 24 months after the initial operation. Symptoms suggesting infection at the time are an increase in pain accompanied by a decrease in function. Type III infections, which are not common, are caused by hematogenous spread from a distant source to a previously asymptomatic hip or knee, often 2 years or more after the initial surgery. Patients who are immunocompromised are most at risk for a type III infection.

Sources of total joint infection include contamination at the time of surgery, seeding from drains or catheters, and hematogenous spread from dental procedures or distant sites of infection. Patients at risk of hematogenous spread include immunocompromised patients; patients with type I diabetes, rheumatoid arthritis, or skin lesions; patients who have undergone total joint arthroplasty within the past 2 years; and patients with poor nutrition. *Staphylococcus epidermidis* and *Staphylococcus aureus* are the organisms that account for most infections, with *S epidermidis* being the most frequently isolated organism. Several preventive measures are usually taken to prevent infection after hip arthroplasty, including administration of antibiotics preoperatively, elimination of any urinary obstructions, the use of hoods and specially ventilated operating rooms, and limited use of drains.

ICD-9 Code

996.67
Infection and inflammatory reaction due to other internal orthopedic device, implant, and graft

SECTION 2 ■ GENERAL ORTHOPAEDICS

HISTORY AND PHYSICAL FINDINGS

Symptoms of infection should prompt referral to a specialist. Joint pain is the primary presenting symptom in patients with infection related to total joint arthroplasty. The typical symptoms of infection, such as fever and chills, may be absent in these patients. Pain at rest or at night suggests an underlying infection. Infection should also be suspected if the patient has a history of wound problems postoperatively; a history of a recent infection in another part of the body; a loose implant within 2 years of surgery, suggested by pain with weight bearing; or intermittent or persistent pain following the initial surgery. Antibiotics should be withheld until appropriate cultures have been obtained. An elevated erythrocyte sedimentation rate (ESR) and C-reactive protein (CRP) level are suggestive of an underlying infection. These are the most useful laboratory screening procedures that the primary clinician should order. The white blood cell count rarely is abnormal and is not helpful in ruling out infection as a cause of joint pain. The onset of pain may precede radiographic changes by at least 6 months. Hip or knee aspiration with culture of the joint fluid is the most definitive study to diagnose an infected total joint arthroplasty. This is done by the radiologist or orthopaedic specialist.

IMAGING STUDIES

Required for diagnosis

Serial PA and lateral radiographs are required for diagnosis. Radiographs should be obtained initially but are of limited value in the diagnosis of infection. Early on in the course of an infection, the plain radiographs frequently are normal. Later, classic findings of loosening secondary to infection include resorption around the stem of the components with a wide cement-bone lucent zone seen within the first 2 years after surgery, a scalloped border on the inner surface of the cortex, and marked periosteal reaction. Periosteal new bone formation is an indication of infection. This may be present with or without signs of loosening. Resorption about the lateral third of the acetabular component suggests an infection. Early loosening and progression of radiolucent lines are also suggestive of infection. Any of the above signs should prompt an immediate referral to a specialist.

Required for comprehensive evaluation

Differentiation between aseptic and septic loosening can be difficult to differentiate on radiographs. Joint arthrography with aspiration and culture will help to differentiate infection from loosening. Joint aspiration and culture remains the gold standard for diagnosing an infection after total joint arthroplasty. This can also be useful in determining loosening if the contrast medium can be seen to penetrate between the bone and methylmethacrylate. Other features on arthrography that suggest infection include an irregular contour of the joint capsule, sinus tracts, and filling of nonbursal cavities.

Special considerations

Arthroscintigraphy can be helpful to determine if any loosening of the femoral stem is present. Injection of an isotope (technetium Tc 99m sulfur colloid) into the joint at the time of arthrography can detect femoral component loosening. Extension of the isotope beyond the joint capsule along the stem of the femoral component indicates loosening. These studies would typically be ordered by the radiologist or orthopaedic specialist. Occasionally, none of the preoperative studies yield a definitive diagnosis, in which case a final diagnosis can be made only on histologic examination of frozen sections of deep tissue specimens taken at the time of surgery.

Pitfalls

Bone scans have a limited role in the diagnosis of septic total joints. A negative scan does not absolutely exclude loosening or infection. Likewise, a positive scan does not necessarily indicate loosening or infection. Also, the pattern of uptake is not specific for loosening or infection. On arthrography, a lack of penetration of contrast medium between the bone and cement does not rule out a loose prosthesis because a soft-tissue membrane between the cement and the bone may block the passage of the contrast medium.

IMAGE DESCRIPTION

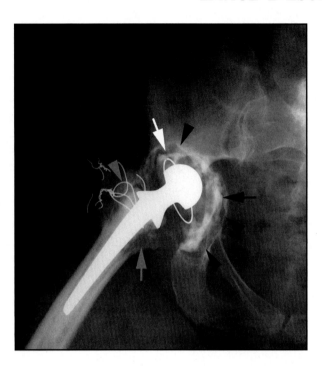

Figure 2-34

Infection after total joint replacement—Frog-lateral view

Frog-lateral view of a right total hip arthroplasty shows medial migration of the acetabulum (black arrow) with a wide cement-bone lucent zone seen about the lateral aspect of the acetabulum (white arrow), which is highly suggestive of infection. Note the scalloped appearance of the cortex about the acetabular component (black arrowheads). Resorption can also be seen about the lesser trochanter of the femur (gray arrow). Broken wires can be seen about the greater trochanter (gray arrowhead).

DIFFERENTIAL DIAGNOSIS

Aseptic loosening (normal erythrocyte sedimentation rate and C-reactive protein level, negative joint aspirate)

Cement disease (granulomatous disease) (extensive resorption around the proximal femoral stem)

TOTAL JOINT REPLACEMENT— OSTEOLYSIS, WEAR, AND LOOSENING

SYNONYMS

Aseptic loosening
Cement disease
Particle disease
Polyethylene wear

ICD-9 Code

996.4
Mechanical complication of internal orthopedic device, implant, and graft

DEFINITION

Osteolysis is the most common complication in total joint arthroplasty and the most common cause of prosthetic loosening and failure. Other causes are infection and inadequate fixation. Osteolysis occurs over time as a result of an inflammatory reaction to particle debris—most commonly polyethylene particulate debris—at the cement-bone or metal-bone interface. The result is bone loss about the prosthesis. Osteolysis may or may not result in loosening. Loosening that results from osteolysis is sometimes called "aseptic loosening."

Osteolysis has been reported to occur in up to 30% of total hip arthroplasties where femoral stems were inserted without cement. Current cementing techniques, however, have reduced the incidence to less than 4%. In total knee arthroplasties, osteolysis is more likely to occur around the tibial component and is seen in up to 15% of knees. In total shoulder arthroplasties, osteolysis about the glenoid component has been reported in more than 10% of patients.

Osteolysis results from and is mediated by macrophage response to wear debris. The debris usually is polyethylene, but it may also be polymethylmethacrylate (bone cement) or metal, including titanium and ceramic materials. The wear particles initially are captured within cells in the joint capsule. However, over time the amount of wear debris exceeds the capacity of the joint capsule to contain these particles. The excess debris infiltrates the interfaces about the prosthesis (bone-cement, prothesis-bone, or prosthesis-cement). The result is bone resorption and, ultimately, loosening of the prosthesis.

Polyethylene wear of tibial and acetabular components remains among the most serious challenges to long-term survival of total hip and total knee arthroplasties. In total hip arthroplasties, polyethylene wear has many causes, including the size of the femoral head, the implant design, and the presence of surface abrasions. The acetabular cup has been shown to wear at an average rate of 1 mm/year. Different approaches to decrease this wear have been tried, such as using a smaller femoral head, using metal-on-metal components or ceramic materials, and varying the polyethylene thickness. Nonsteroidal anti-inflammatory drugs may also slow the process of osteolysis.

Initially, radiolucency about a total joint prosthesis may be asymptomatic. However, when the zone of radiolucency exceeds 2 mm and extends circumferentially around the prosthesis, the prosthesis probably is loose. Any migration greater than 4 mm is a sign of loosening, as is a fracture of the component. Likewise, a fracture of the bone cement is an indication of loosening. Osteolysis can be seen as early as 1 year after total joint arthroplasty. Osteolysis tends to be progressive, and if the prosthesis becomes loose, the rate of osteolysis increases.

History and Physical Findings

Significant osteolysis can occur following total joint arthroplasty without the development of symptoms, so the physical examination may be normal in the presence of osteolysis. For this reason, periodic radiographs, at least every 2 years, should be considered. With loosening of the prosthesis, the patient may report feeling something "slip" or move in the hip or knee. Pain with ambulation is a common symptom with a loose prosthesis, and should prompt referral to a specialist. A history of a change in limb length or the development of varus or valgus angulation at the knee also suggests a loose prosthesis. Pain that persists longer than 2 weeks after surgery may be a sign of loosening or infection. The patient should be questioned about any recent infections or flulike symptoms, which might indicate periprosthetic infection.

On physical examination, antalgic gait or limb length differences may be noted, and pain with passive and active range of motion of the joint may be present; these are signs of loosening. With the patient standing, any varus or valgus angulation of the knee may be seen.

IMAGING STUDIES

Required for diagnosis

AP and lateral views are sufficient to identify osteolysis and polyethylene wear in the hip and knee. Oblique views of the acetabulum are helpful in identifying osteolysis about an acetabular component. In the knee, the tibial component is most often involved with loosening, which occurs at the cement-bone interface. Signs of loosening in total knee arthroplasties include an enlarging lucent zone wider than 2 mm, fracture of the cement or fracture of the prosthesis, changes in the component position into valgus or varus, and changes in alignment of the knee seen on weight-bearing AP and lateral views.

Required for comprehensive evaluation

A bone scan can be helpful in differentiating a loose prosthesis secondary to infection from one secondary to mechanical factors. A normal scan suggests that the prosthesis is not loose.

Special considerations

The specialist may try an anesthetic injection into the joint to help differentiate pain arising from within the joint from pain arising from an extra-articular source such as the back. Although less commonly used now, arthrography of the affected joint has been used to evaluate loosening when radiographs are inconclusive. Aspiration and culture of joint fluid at the hip is also indicated to rule out an infection.

Pitfalls

A negative bone scan does not always rule out loosening or infection; false-negative results occasionally occur. Osteolysis may be present without loosening, and loosening may be present without osteolysis.

IMAGE DESCRIPTIONS

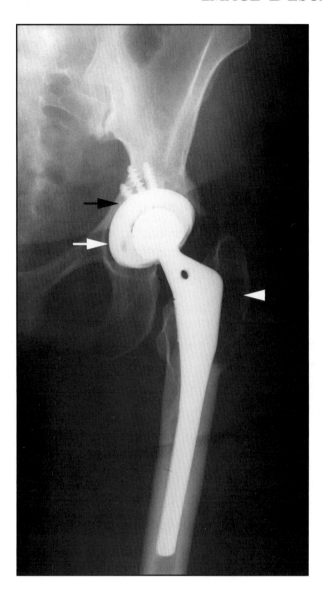

Figure 2-35

Loosening and osteolysis of total hip arthroplasty components— AP view

AP view of the left hip in a 68-year-old woman shows a wide area of radiolucency about the acetabular component (black arrow) with subsidence of the cup (white arrow). Note also the large cyst in the greater trochanter (arrowhead) related to osteolysis.

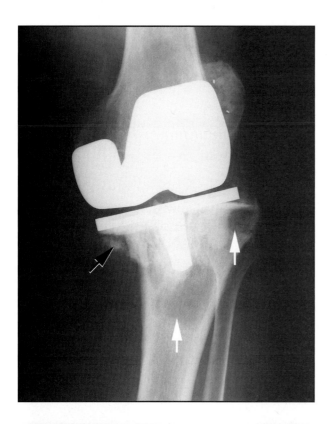

Figure 2-36

Loosening and osteolysis of total knee arthroplasty components— AP view

AP view of the left knee in a 74-year-old man shows settling of the prosthesis on the medial side with varus angulation (black arrow), suggesting loosening of the tibial component. Note the presence of lytic lesions below the central tibial peg and the lateral subchondral region of the tibia (white arrows).

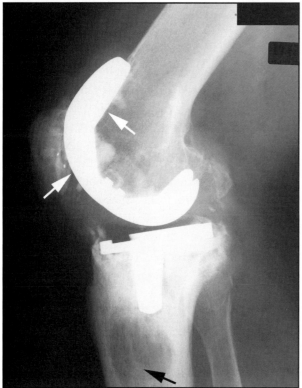

Figure 2-37

Loosening and osteolysis of total knee arthroplasty components—Lateral view

Lateral view of the same patient in Figure 2-36 shows a lytic lesion below the peg of the tibial component (black arrow). Note the absence of lucent zones about the femoral or patellar components (white arrows) suggesting that these components are not loose.

SECTION 2 ■ GENERAL ORTHOPAEDICS

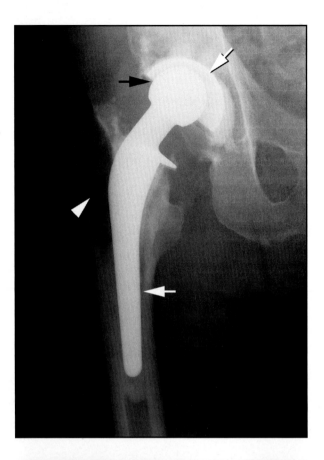

Figure 2-38

Wear of total hip arthroplasty components—AP view

AP view of the right hip in a 92-year-old man who had had a hip prosthesis for the past 20 years shows that the femoral component is riding high and laterally (black arrow) consistent with wear of the polyethylene liner. Note that there is no radiolucent line along the shaft of the femoral component or about the acetabular cup (white arrows), but there is an area of bone resorption about the area of the greater trochanter (arrowhead).

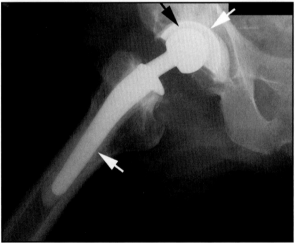

Figure 2-39

Wear of total hip arthroplasty components—Lateral view

Lateral view of the same patient shown in Figure 2-38 shows thinning of the superior and lateral portion of the acetabular cup (black arrow). No radiolucent zones can be seen around either the femoral or acetabular components (white arrows) despite the long time since surgery (20 years).

DIFFERENTIAL DIAGNOSIS

Infection (positive joint aspirate, elevated white blood cell count and erythrocyte sedimentation rate, fever)

Low back pain (pain not relieved by intra-articular injection of an anesthetic agent; MRI shows nerve root impingement)

Trochanteric bursitis (pain relieved by a lateral hip injection of an anesthetic agent into the trochanteric bursae)

TOTAL JOINT COMPLICATIONS— PERIPROSTHETIC FRACTURES

SYNONYMS
None

DEFINITION

Fractures about total joint prostheses occur in three patterns: just proximal to the tip of the prosthesis, distal to the tip of the prosthesis, and extending along the shaft of the prosthesis. Periprosthetic fractures are uncommon but have increased with the advent of press-fit femoral components. Risk factors for periprosthetic fractures include osteoporosis, infection, rheumatoid arthritis, notching or perforation of the femur at the time of surgery, varus position of the stem of the femoral hip component, osteolysis about the components, and drill holes in the femur.

In the hip, more periprosthetic fractures occur about the femoral component than about the acetabular component. Fractures that occur in the middle region of the shaft are associated with prosthetic loosening, whereas those that occur distal to the tip are associated with a high incidence of nonunion.

With total knee arthroplasties, periprosthetic fractures occur in only a small percentage of patients. Most of these fractures occur about the femoral component; fractures about the tibial component and patellar component are much less common. Women older than age 70 years are at particular risk for fractures about a total knee prosthesis.

Fractures associated with total shoulder arthroplasty are even less common than those about the hip and knee. These fractures occur below the tip of the humeral prosthetic stem.

Stress fractures can occur about total joint prostheses and may be difficult to diagnose. Treatment of periprosthetic fractures usually involves a surgical procedure in which a plate and screws with allograft struts or a longer stemmed prosthesis is inserted, often with allograft struts, or a plate with screws and cerclage wires is applied.

HISTORY AND PHYSICAL FINDINGS

Patients with osteoporosis and rheumatoid arthritis, especially those on steroid medication, are at increased risk for fractures about total joint prostheses. A clear history of trauma usually is present, with a fall being the usual mechanism of injury. On physical examination, pain and tenderness at the fracture site are noted. The extremity may appear deformed, and any movement of the extremity is painful. Weight bearing is impossible without crutches or a walker.

ICD-9 Codes
812.21 Fracture of shaft of humerus, closed
820.22 Fracture of neck of femur, subtrochanteric section, closed
821.01 Fracture of shaft of femur, closed
821.23 Supracondylar fracture of femur, closed
822.0 Fracture of patella, closed
823.20 Fracture of tibia and fibula, shaft, closed, tibia alone

SECTION 2 ■ GENERAL ORTHOPAEDICS

However, on occasion the patient may just have a stress fracture around the femoral prosthesis. These patients will report thigh pain with ambulation.

IMAGING STUDIES

Required for diagnosis
AP and lateral views usually are adequate to diagnose a periprosthetic fracture. Long-leg views of the involved limb are useful in evaluating fractures about a total knee arthroplasty. Oblique images can be added if a fracture is suspected but is not visible on AP and lateral views.

Required for comprehensive evaluation
If radiographs are negative and a stress fracture is suspected, a bone scan may show localized uptake at the site of the fracture.

Special considerations
None

Pitfalls
Stress fractures may easily be missed.

IMAGE DESCRIPTIONS

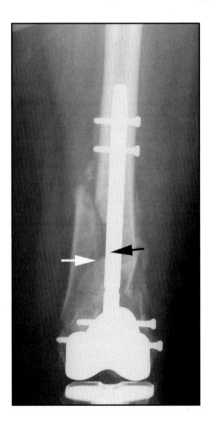

Figure 2-40

Periprosthetic fracture (femur)—AP view

AP view of the left femur in a 70-year-old woman who fell 3 months after a left total knee arthroplasty shows a comminuted supracondylar fracture of the femur (white arrow). The fracture has been fixed with a locked intramedullary rod (black arrow).

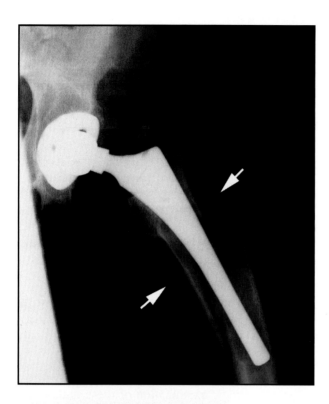

Figure 2-41

Periprosthetic fracture (femur)—AP view

AP view of a left hip demonstrates a comminuted fracture surrounding the femoral component of a press-fit total hip replacement (arrows).

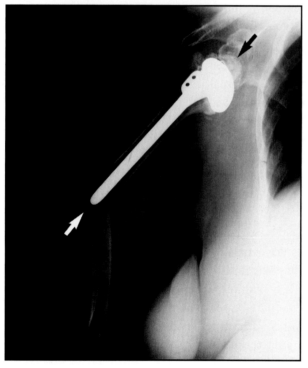

Figure 2-42

Periprosthetic fracture (humerus)—AP view

AP view of a right humerus demonstrates a comminuted fracture located at the tip of the humeral component of the total shoulder replacement (white arrow). Note the loosening of the cemented glenoid component (black arrow).

DIFFERENTIAL DIAGNOSIS

Infected prosthesis (lucent zone, positive joint aspirate, no fracture seen on radiographs)

Loose prosthesis (lucent zone, no fracture line)

TOTAL JOINT REPLACEMENT— SILICONE SYNOVITIS

ICD-9 Code

996.67
Infection and inflammatory reaction due to other internal orthopedic device, implant, and graft

SYNONYMS

Implant synovitis
Inflammatory synovitis
Particle synovitis

DEFINITION

Silicone synovitis is a chronic, progressively destructive process that results from the shedding of silicone particles caused by shear and compression forces on a silicone implant. When abraded, silicone polymers break up. These shed particles incite an inflammatory response in the synovium, with invasion of the subchondral bone and cyst formation in the adjacent carpal bones. Microscopic examination will reveal intracellular silicone particles within macrophages at the implant site. In addition, silicone particles can be transported to regional lymph nodes by the lymphoreticular system. Histologic examination of these nodes has shown giant cell foreign body reaction, with silicone particles seen within the cells. Silicone particulate debris has also been reported in bone marrow distant from the implant site.

Silicone prostheses have been used primarily in the hand and upper extremity to replace carpal bones (scaphoid, trapezium, and lunate), metacarpophalangeal and interphalangeal joints, the radiocarpal joint, and the radial head. The metatarsophalangeal joint of the great toe has also been replaced with silicone rubber prostheses. Silicone synovitis is more common after lunate and scapholunate silastic replacements (occurring in 75% of patients) and scaphoid replacements (occurring in 50% of patients) and less common after metacarpophalangeal, proximal interphalangeal, and trapezium replacements. With carpal implants, the greatest compressive forces are across the lunate, causing deformity and fibrillation of the implant. Less deformity is found with scaphoid implants, and still less with trapezium implants.

Silicone synovitis may be seen months to years after surgery. The condition requires surgical removal of the implant, synovectomy, and joint reconstruction. Once the diagnosis is made, referral to a specialist is appropriate.

HISTORY AND PHYSICAL FINDINGS

Typically, a patient with a history of a silicone joint implant will report pain and swelling at that joint. Limitation of joint motion is common. Synovitis from silicone debris may act like active rheumatoid arthritis. Therefore, the condition may be missed initially when implants have been inserted in patients with rheumatoid arthritis. Onset of symptoms usually does not occur until at least 3 years after surgery. A few patients will remain asymptomatic despite the presence of extensive synovitis and radiographic changes. On physical examination, the affected joint is usually swollen, warm, and tender to palpation, and range of motion is decreased. Lymphadenopathy caused by silicone particle debris is typically painless and is characterized by enlarged nodes that occur at least 3 years after implant surgery. These enlarged nodes have been seen in the upper and lower extremities and must be distinguished from tumor and adenopathy secondary to infection. The primary care physician should always ask about surgery in which silicone prostheses have been implanted when a patient presents with enlarged lymph nodes.

IMAGING STUDIES

Required for diagnosis

AP and lateral views of the affected joints are adequate to make the diagnosis. Typical radiographic findings include subchondral lucent defects with thin sclerotic margins, soft-tissue swelling, and fracture of the prosthesis. The silicone prosthesis may be difficult to see, however, as its radiographic density is close to that of the soft tissues. Unlike with an infection, with silicone synovitis, the cartilage spaces are usually preserved, and osteopenia is not seen about the cysts.

Required for comprehensive evaluation

MRI has been used to make this diagnosis but is necessary only very rarely.

Special considerations

None

Pitfalls

Enlarged regional lymph nodes secondary to silicone debris may be mistaken for a malignancy.

IMAGE DESCRIPTIONS

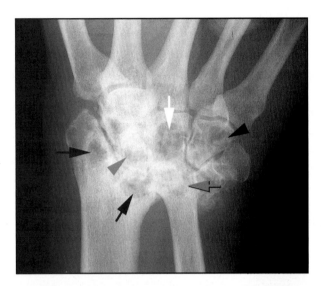

Figure 2-43

Silicone synovitis (wrist)—AP view

AP view of a right wrist shows large cysts in the radius (black arrows), capitate (white arrow), and hamate (black arrowhead) and erosive changes in the distal ulna (gray arrow) following a lunate silicone replacement 7 years earlier. The prosthesis is not well visualized on this view. Also, the radioscaphoid joint space is markedly narrowed (gray arrowhead).

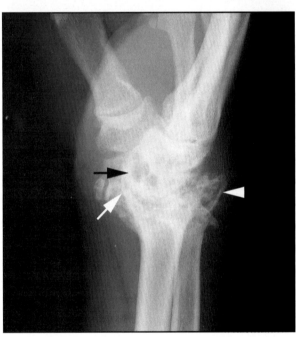

Figure 2-44

*Silicone synovitis (wrist)—
Lateral view*

Lateral view of the same wrist shown in Figure 2-43 demonstrates large cysts in the scaphoid (black arrow) and radius (white arrow). Erosive changes are also seen in the ulna (arrowhead).

DIFFERENTIAL DIAGNOSIS

Amyloidosis (history of renal dialysis, no implant seen)

Infection (usually more osteopenia)

Pigmented villonodular synovitis (no silicone prosthesis seen)

Rheumatoid arthritis (presence of an implant plus extensive cystic changes around the prosthesis)

TUMORS

Section Editor
James O. Johnston, MD

IMAGING TUMORS—AN OVERVIEW

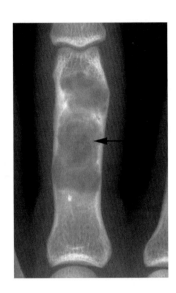

Figure 1

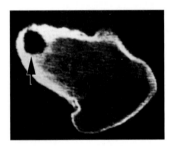

Figure 2

IMAGING MODALITIES

Radiographs

Until the 1980s, AP and lateral radiographs constituted the principal modality for imaging of musculoskeletal tumors. Even today, this simple and inexpensive study should always be the starting point in the total staging process for all bone and soft-tissue neoplasms. Only after this initial radiographic study has been evaluated and correlated with the significant clinical data should the physician determine what further studies, if any, might effectively produce a working differential diagnosis. Based on this differential diagnosis, the need for a diagnostic tissue biopsy can be determined. For example, an asymptomatic enchondroma (Figure 1) identified as an incidental finding would not require further imaging studies or a biopsy to make a diagnosis.

Today the physician has the luxury of a multitude of diagnostic imaging tools readily available for the evaluation of bone and soft-tissue lesions. These studies include CT, MRI, bone scintigraphy (bone scanning), ultrasound, and positron emission tomography (PET).

Computed tomography

CT is most valuable for obtaining a detailed cross-sectional image of a lesion located in dense cortical bone, such as the nidus of an osteoid osteoma (Figure 2). Even with heavily mineralized soft-tissue lesions, CT may prove superior to MRI, such as in the differential diagnosis of myositis ossificans versus soft-tissue osteosarcoma versus tumoral calcinosis. However, CT is not helpful for diagnosing poorly mineralized lesions in fatty bone marrow, such as metastatic carcinoma. Likewise, for nonmineralized soft-tissue tumors, CT is inferior to a good MRI study. In staging for metastatic disease to the lung, CT is superior.

Magnetic resonance imaging

Since the 1990s, MRI has proved to be the gold standard for identifying soft-tissue lesions with minimal calcification and has nearly eliminated the need for angiography, which was used previously to study the relationship between soft-tissue tumors and adjacent large blood vessels. MRI is also needed to evaluate intraosseous and extracortical portions of primary bone tumors, especially when considering limb salvage versus amputation. Gadolinium contrast is not indicated in all MRI studies but can be beneficial when evaluating the degree of vascular perfusion of a lesion, especially as it relates to the effect of chemotherapy on a malignant tumor. Gadolinium contrast can discriminate between solid and viable lesions versus cystic lesions such as a solitary bone cyst, tumor necrosis, or a gelatinous Baker's cyst.

Bone scan

Bone scans utilizing the radioactive isotope technetium Tc 99m to detect areas of rapid bone turnover have been used since the 1980s to stage bone tumors and metastases to bone. The problem with isotope bone scans is that they are very sensitive for any reactive process involving new bone formation, including trauma, infection, metabolic disorders, and tumors, both benign and malignant. However, a negative bone scan for a lesion visible on plain radiographs can be assumed to indicate an asymptomatic, benign process. The only exception to this is multiple myeloma and other purely lytic lesions, which can cause extensive destruction without a reactive reparative bone response.

Positron emission tomography

PET scanning has evolved into an effective tool for grading soft-tissue tumors, analyzing tumor response to chemotherapy, and evaluating possible tumor recurrence. However, the PET scan is inferior to the chest CT in detecting lung metastases. In addition, a PET scan is a very expensive procedure, and medical insurers may refuse to cover it. Ultrasound, being rapid and inexpensive, is a better choice than a PET scan to assess the size and the cystic or solid nature of a soft-tissue mass.

STAGING OF TUMORS

Blastic versus lytic

When staging a bone tumor using plain radiographs, a radiologist will refer to lesions as either blastic or lytic to help arrive at a logical differential diagnosis (Table 1). The word blastic, or sclerotic, suggests a dense, heavily mineralized bony lesion that appears white on the radiograph and that in most cases will turn out to be a benign condition such as a bone island, an osteoid osteoma, or monostotic fibrous dysplasia. However, Figure 3 shows a blastic lesion in the proximal tibial metaphysis of a teenaged boy that on biopsy was found to be a blastic form of malignant osteogenic sarcoma. In this situation,

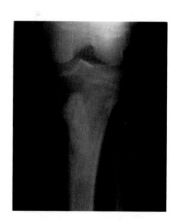

Figure 3

Table 1 Blastic Versus Lytic Lesions	
Blastic	Also called "sclerotic"; indicates a dense, heavily mineralized bony lesion that appears white on radiographs. Blastic lesions are more often benign than malignant.
Lytic	Indicates a region of loss of mineralized bony structure that appears black on radiographs. Lytic lesions can be either benign or malignant.

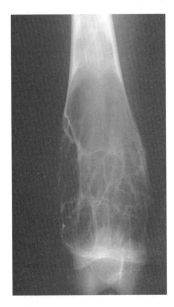

Figure 4

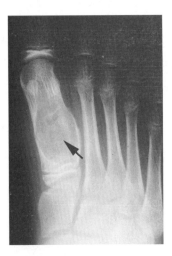

Figure 5

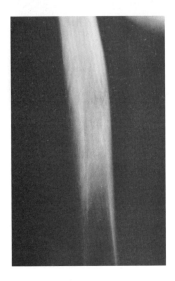

Figure 6

an MRI study would be indicated to evaluate the extension of tumor into the surrounding soft tissue and the edematous response in adjacent bone marrow, which cannot be appreciated on a plain radiograph.

In contrast to blastic lesions, lytic lesions appear black on radiographs because of a loss of mineralized bony structure. Lytic lesions can be either benign or malignant. One example of a benign lytic process is a unicameral bone cyst. Figure 4 shows a unicameral bone cyst in the distal femoral metaphysis of a teenaged boy. The chronically thinned and slightly dilated cortex with a "soap-bubble" pattern suggests a benign diagnosis such as solitary bone cyst, fibrous dysplasia, or Gaucher's disease. However, a lytic lesion where the lysis is more acute, with a poorly defined zone of transition between the tumor and the surrounding cortical structure, can be indicative of malignant disease such as lymphoma or Ewing's sarcoma.

In the case of metastatic carcinoma to bone, blastic lesions are more frequently associated with a diagnosis of prostate carcinoma, whereas lung, renal, and thyroid carcinoma demonstrate a more lytic destructive pattern. With breast cancer, the most common metastatic carcinoma, a mixture of lytic and blastic changes is common.

STAGING TERMS

Geographic, permeative, moth-eaten, and periosteal response are staging terms commonly used by radiologists when describing radiographs of bone tumors (Table 2). The word geographic is used to describe a sharply defined lytic lesion in bone such as a bone cyst, fibrous dysplasia, or enchondroma, all of which have a well-defined narrow and sclerotic zone of transition between the lytic tumor and the surrounding bone. Figure 5 shows a geographic lesion in the first metatarsal of a teenaged girl. The cortex is thinned and chronically dilated, and there is a well-defined sclerotic margin at the periphery of the lesion. The smoky appearance of the

Table 2 Staging Terms	
Geographic	Describes a sharply defined lytic lesion in bone with a well-defined narrow and sclerotic zone of transition between the lytic tumor and the surrounding bone.
Permeative	Opposite of geographic. Describes a more diffuse lytic process in bone.
Moth-eaten	Used to describe lesions with a lytic appearance halfway between sharply margined geographic lesions and diffuse permeative lesions. Can indicate either benign or malignant conditions.
Reactive periosteal response	Reaction of periosteal bone to a pathologic condition, either benign or malignant. Descriptions of various types of reaction include "hair-on-end" and "onion-skin."

matrix of the lesion suggests a diagnosis of fibrous dysplasia, which was borne out by biopsy. A "popcorn" or "arcs and rings" calcification of the matrix would have suggested enchondroma. No matrix calcification at all would suggest a unicameral bone cyst.

Permeative is the opposite of *geographic*. The radiologist uses the term permeative to describe a more diffuse lytic process in bone suggestive of a high-grade round cell sarcoma such as a lymphoma, Ewing's sarcoma, or leukemia. Figure 6 shows permeative lysis of the midshaft of the femur in a middle-aged man with chronic lymphocytic leukemia. There is a very fine granular cortical lysis with a diffuse sclerotic reparative response and slight cortical thickening. Note the fuzzy and poorly defined zone of transition at both the upper and lower medullary margins. However, permeative lysis is also associated with a multitude of benign pathologic bone conditions, such as acute osteomyelitis, hyperparathyroidism, radiation osteitis, the early lytic phase of Paget's disease, and early Langerhans' cell histiocytosis.

The term moth-eaten describes lesions that on radiographs have a lytic appearance halfway between the sharply marginated geographic lesions and the diffuse permeative conditions. This includes a wide spectrum of disease processes, including malignant diseases such as breast carcinoma and multiple myeloma. In Figure 7, the arrow indicates a typical "punched-out" lesion very suggestive of multiple myeloma. However, moth-eaten lysis can also be found in benign bone diseases such as hemangioma and giant cell tumor. In addition, nonneoplastic diseases (eg, chronic osteomalacia) and chronic low-grade infectious diseases (eg, tuberculous osteomyelitis) can produce a moth-eaten lysis.

A reactive periosteal response to pathologic conditions of bone is also seen in a wide spectrum of disease processes, both malignant and benign. One example is the typical "hair-on-end" reactive bone seen bridging the gap between the elevated periosteum and subadjacent bone in Ewing's sarcoma (Figure 8). A similar periosteal response seen frequently in Ewing's sarcoma is the laminated "onion-skin" periosteal reaction (Figure 9, arrow). However, this pattern can also be seen in nonneoplastic, inflammatory conditions of bone such as infectious osteomyelitis and eosinophilic granuloma. In addition, reactive periosteal new bone is seen in young patients with stress fractures or traction periosteal reaction, which is caused by excessive repetitive muscle pull on bone.

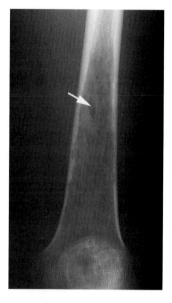

Figure 7

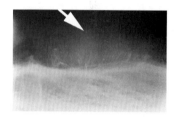

Figure 8

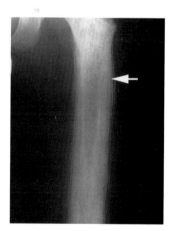

Figure 9

SECTION 3 ■ TUMORS

REFERRAL

As soon as a physician becomes concerned about the diagnosis of a malignant tumor based on the initial imaging studies, an appropriate referral to a local oncologist should be considered. The oncologist will then order the necessary cost-effective staging studies for the given clinical problem.

ENCHONDROMA

SYNONYMS
None

DEFINITION
Enchondromas are solitary or multiple benign bone tumors
originating from cartilage. Solitary enchondromas commonly
present as hamartomatous, or developmental, geographic lesions in
the small tubular bones of the hands and feet. They commonly
develop in children between the ages of 5 and 15 years but,
because they are asymptomatic, may not be discovered until years
later, as an incidental finding on radiographs obtained following
trauma. Multiple enchondromatosis can be unilateral, in which case
the condition is referred to as Ollier's disease. When multiple
enchondromatosis is associated with soft-tissue hemangiomas, the
condition is referred to as Maffucci's syndrome.

HISTORY AND PHYSICAL FINDINGS
Most cases of solitary enchondroma of the hands or long bones are
not discovered until the patient sustains a pathologic fracture
through one of the lesions or until an asymptomatic lesion is seen
as an incidental finding. Enchondromas in the hand are sometimes
aneurysmal, creating a firm, nontender lump that can be felt
through the skin. Multiple enchondromatosis can cause gross limb
deformity, with shortening more pronounced on one side of the
body than the other. In Maffucci's syndrome, soft-tissue
hemangiomas overlie the bones involved with the enchondromas.

IMAGING STUDIES

Required for diagnosis
With enchondromas in the hands or feet, AP and oblique lateral
radiographs are frequently sufficient to establish a diagnosis.
However, with larger lesions in the ends of long bones such as the
femur or humerus, MRI is helpful in considering the differential
diagnosis of central chondrosarcoma and metaphyseal bone infarcts,
which can have a similar appearance on radiographs.

Required for comprehensive evaluation
MRI is helpful in visualizing any hemangiomas associated with
enchondromatosis.

ICD-9 Codes

213
Benign neoplasm of bone
and articular cartilage

213.5
Benign neoplasm of short
bones of upper limb

SECTION 3 ■ TUMORS

SECTION 3 ■ TUMORS

Special considerations
None

Pitfalls
None

IMAGE DESCRIPTIONS

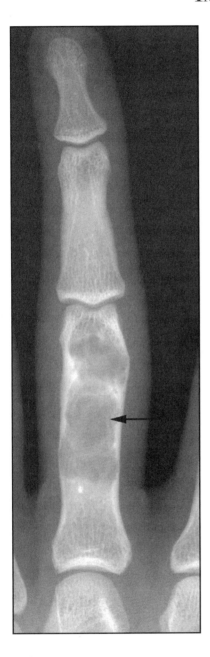

Figure 3-1

Solitary enchondroma—AP view of middle finger

AP view of a geographic multilobulated lytic lesion centrally located in the distal two thirds of the proximal phalanx of the middle finger of a young man. There is marked cortical thinning with a sharp, well-defined zone of transition between the lesion and the surrounding cortex. Note the matrix of the lesion (arrow), which is smoky in appearance and has calcified arcs and rings distally, features that strongly suggest an enchondroma.

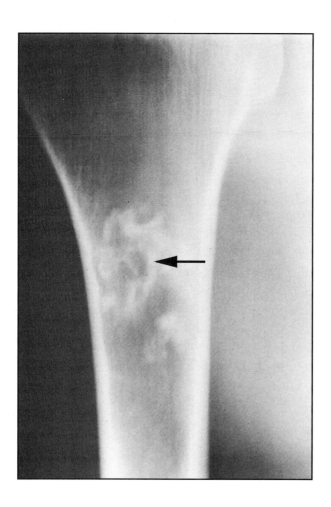

Figure 3-2

Enchondroma—
AP view of proximal humerus

AP view of the proximal humerus of a
middle-aged man with shoulder pain
secondary to rotator cuff tendinitis. Note the
heavily calcified, lobulated centrally located
metadiaphyseal lesion but no evidence of
endosteal cortical scalloping or permeation
that would suggest a chondrosarcoma. Note
the arcs-and-rings calcific matrix pattern
(arrow) characteristic of a low-grade
chondroid neoplasm.

DIFFERENTIAL DIAGNOSIS

Bone cyst of the hand (no matrix calcification)

Giant cell reparative granuloma of the hand (no matrix
calcification)

Giant cell tumor of the hand (no matrix calcification)

Low-grade central chondrosarcoma (malignant; rare in the
hand but not unusual in larger bones)

Malignant chondrosarcoma of larger bones (cortical thinning
and scalloping)

Metaphyseal infarct (MRI will differentiate)

FIBROUS DYSPLASIA

ICD-9 Code

733.29
Fibrous dysplasia

SYNONYMS
None

DEFINITION
Fibrous dysplasia is a fairly common developmental disorder of bone seen most often in the first three decades of life, with females affected more often than males. The most common form is monostotic (affecting a single bone), occurring centrally in metadiaphyseal bone. The polyostotic (affecting multiple bones) form tends to be unilateral, with the greatest involvement in the pelvis and lower extremity. Limb-length discrepancy can result from a varus "shepherd's crook" deformity of the proximal femur. Five percent of patients with polyostotic fibrous dysplasia have Albright's syndrome, which is characterized by café au lait spots and precocious puberty.

HISTORY AND PHYSICAL FINDINGS
Most patients with the common monostotic form of fibrous dysplasia are asymptomatic unless stress pain or a pathologic fracture in the weakened bone develops. In the less common polyostotic forms, including Albright's syndrome, clinical findings include rough, serrated-edge café au lait spots in the overlying skin and shortening deformity of the leg. In more severe cases, unilateral hyperostotic deformation of the craniofacial bones associated with orbital exophthalmos may be present.

IMAGING STUDIES

Required for diagnosis
AP and lateral radiographs are the gold standard for localizing and diagnosing the monostotic forms of fibrous dysplasia.

Required for comprehensive evaluation
In the case of polyostotic fibrous dysplasia, a bone scan will help identify other asymptomatic lesions. In rare cases where aneurysmal bone cysts or even associated myxomas in surrounding muscle can be seen, MRI might be beneficial because the myxomas are not apparent on radiographs.

Special considerations
None

Pitfalls

A solitary bone cyst will sometimes look like a fibrous dysplastic lesion on radiographs, in which case a bone scan is indicated: the bone scan will show high uptake in fibrous dysplasia but none in a bone cyst.

IMAGE DESCRIPTIONS

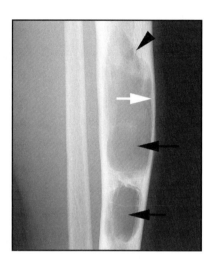

Figure 3-3

Fibrous dysplasia—Lateral view of lower leg

Lateral view of the lower leg of a young woman, taken after an injury. The patient reported no preinjury pain. Note the large, multiloculated geographic lytic lesion located centrally in the middiaphysis of the tibia (black arrows). The surrounding cortex is chronically thinned and slightly dilated, with a sharply defined sclerotic narrow zone of transition (white arrow) typical of a benign tumor. The "smoky" appearance of the upper portion of the lesion (arrowhead) is caused by fibro-osseous tissue typically found in the lytic core of fibrous dysplastic lesions. This feature is not seen in solitary bone cysts, which appear darker because of the lack of such tissue.

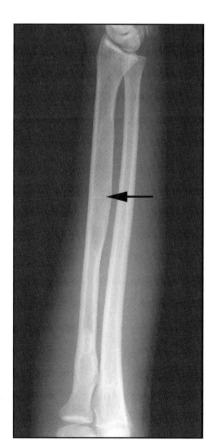

Figure 3-4

Fibrous dysplasia—AP view of forearm

AP view showing fibrous dysplasia involving the entire radius of a young woman who reported no pain. Note the "smoky" area of fibro-osseous matrix calcification surrounded by a thinly dilated cortex (arrow).

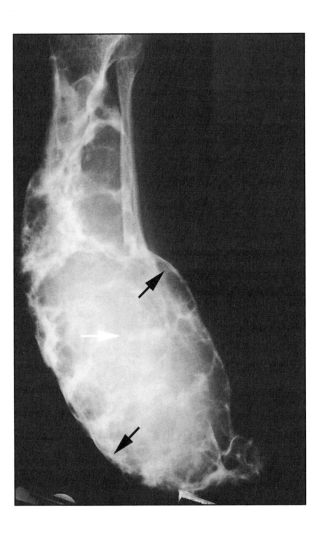

Figure 3-5

*Severe fibrous dysplasia—
AP view of lower leg*

AP view showing evidence of severe deformation of the entire tibia in a young man with extensive polyostotic fibrous dysplasia. Note the extensive cortical dilatation, a "soap-bubble" appearance (black arrows), and the classic "smoky" matrix calcification (white arrow). Because of severe bone stock deficiency associated with bowing and shortening, this patient elected to have his leg amputated at the knee.

DIFFERENTIAL DIAGNOSIS

Nonossifying fibroma (dark central core on radiograph; wider zone of sclerotic transition; no cortical thinning)

Solitary bone cyst (no uptake on bone scan)

GIANT CELL TUMOR

SYNONYM
Osteoclastoma

DEFINITION
The giant cell tumor of bone is a common benign lytic tumor that occurs in young adults, more often in women than in men, and accounts for 20% of all benign bone tumors. Giant cell tumors and chondroblastomas are the only tumors found in the epiphyseal-metaphyseal area. Fifty percent of these tumors occur about the knee joint; the sacrum and distal radius represent other common locations. A number of so-called variants are seen typically in children that, with the exception of hemorrhagic osteosarcoma, are benign. These variants include the chondroblastoma, osteoblastoma, aneurysmal bone cyst, and giant cell reparative granuloma. In an unusual process of benign metastasis, 2% of primary giant cell tumors metastasize to the lung, as do 6% of recurrent lesions. The prognosis for patients with these metastases is good, with an 85% survival rate.

HISTORY AND PHYSICAL FINDINGS
Patients will report a history of spontaneous onset of dull, aching pain in the joint adjacent to the tumor, which may be partially relieved by nonsteroidal anti-inflammatory drugs. Because of the early cortical breakthrough typical of these tumors, deep palpation over the lytic process will elicit local tenderness. Severe destruction of articular bone sometimes leads to early pathologic fracture, resulting in severe pain and acute hemarthrosis of the adjacent joint.

IMAGING STUDIES

Required for diagnosis
AP and lateral radiographs are usually sufficient to make the diagnosis because they have two distinct characteristics that are apparent on radiographs: the unique epiphyseal location, and the absence of matrix calcification.

Required for comprehensive evaluation
The more aggressive stage 3 lesions may have a large aneurysmal destructive appearance, in which case MRI is indicated to differentiate them from large aneurysmal bone cysts or malignant hemorrhagic osteosarcomas.

ICD-9 Codes

213.4
Benign neoplasm of scapula and long bones of upper limb

213.6
Benign neoplasm of pelvic bones, sacrum, and coccyx

213.7
Benign neoplasm of long bones of lower limb

SECTION 3 ■ TUMORS

Special considerations
None

Pitfalls
None

IMAGE DESCRIPTION

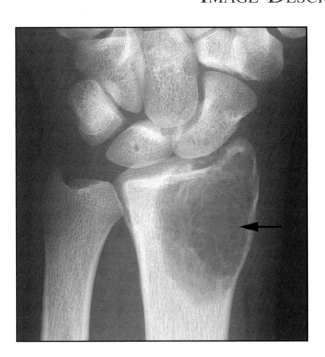

Figure 3-6

Giant cell tumor—AP view of wrist

AP view of the wrist of a young woman with a fairly well marginated lytic lesion (arrow) in the distal epiphyseal-metaphyseal area of the radius, lying directly on the distal articular surface of the radius. Extensive cortical erosion (arrow) suggests an aggressive lytic process but no evidence of matrix calcification.

DIFFERENTIAL DIAGNOSIS

The classic location of the giant cell tumor in the epiphyseal area of the distal radius rules out an otherwise extensive list of similar-appearing lesions:

Aneurysmal bone cyst (metaphyseal location)

Brown tumor of hyperparathyroidism (usually polyostotic)

Giant cell rich osteogenic sarcoma (aggressive appearance)

Infection (rare in epiphyseal bone)

Lymphoma (rare epiphyseal location)

Metastatic carcinoma (usually polyostotic)

Nonossifying Fibroma

Synonyms

Fibroma
Fibrous cortical defect
Fibrous cortical desmoid
Metaphyseal fibrous defect
Xanthofibroma

ICD-9 Codes

213.7
Benign neoplasm of long
bones of lower limb

213.8
Benign neoplasm of short
bones of lower limb

Definition

Nonossifying fibromas (NOFs) and the morphologic variants listed
as synonyms above are considered benign fibrotic hamartomatous
(developmental) lesions. They occur commonly in growing children
as peripheral metaphyseal lesions, usually about the knee and ankle.
These asymptomatic lesions are found in one third of normal
children at age 4 years. As the child matures, the lesions tend to
remodel out of existence or can enlarge and become more central in
location, resulting in a high incidence of pathologic fracture. In
some cases, the lesions are multiple and are associated with café au
lait spots on the skin, suggesting a relationship to fibrous dysplasia.

History and Physical Findings

NOFs tend to be asymptomatic, but because the NOF acts as a
stress riser, it increases the risk of fracture through the lesion.
Typically, a patient who has become active in sports will present
with an acute fracture from a single injury or, less frequently, a
stress fracture, and the NOF will be an incidental finding on
radiographs. If the patient had no pain prior to the fracture the
lesion should be considered benign.

Imaging Studies

Required for diagnosis
AP and lateral radiographs are usually sufficient to establish the
diagnosis. Diagnostic biopsy is not necessary.

Required for comprehensive evaluation
None

Pitfalls
None

Section 3 ■ Tumors

IMAGE DESCRIPTION

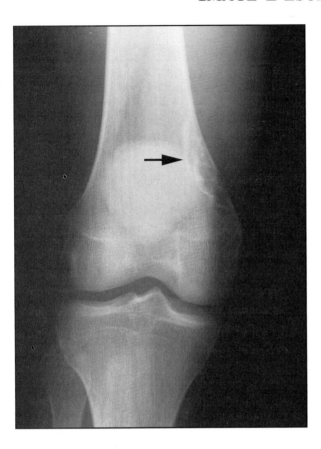

Figure 3-7

*Nonossifying fibroma—
AP view of knee*

AP view of the knee of a young woman with a well-defined peripheral lytic lesion in the distal femoral metaphysis. Note the sharply defined narrow sclerotic zone of transition (arrow) with no evidence of surrounding permeation or periosteal reaction. This is a common location for a fibrous cortical defect that is most likely one of the variants of the NOF.

DIFFERENTIAL DIAGNOSIS

Chondromyxoid fibroma (usually seen in proximal tibia)

Hand-Schuller-Christian disease (multiple osseous disease involving the skull)

Hyperparathyroidism (multiple lytic lesions of bone)

Monostotic fibrous dysplasia ("smoky" matrix calcification)

OSTEOBLASTOMA

SYNONYM
Giant osteoid osteoma

ICD-9 Code

213.2
Benign neoplasm of vertebral
column, excluding sacrum
and coccyx

DEFINITION
Osteoblastomas are generally considered the same benign osteoid-producing tumors as osteoid osteomas but with a more aggressive lytic nidus measuring larger than 1.5 cm in diameter. Osteoblastoma occurs in the same population (age 10 to 25 years, males more frequently affected than females) as osteoid osteoma, but it is less common, accounting for only 1% of all bone tumors. Unlike osteoid osteomas, osteoblastoma lesions are found most often in the posterolateral aspects of the thoracolumbar spine and occasionally about the wrist and ankle, but they rarely occur in the cortical structure of long bones.

HISTORY AND PHYSICAL FINDINGS
Typical symptoms include dull, aching pain that is worse at night. Because it is typically located in the posterolateral aspects of the thoracolumbar spine, osteoblastoma is associated with symptoms of radiculopathy secondary to irritation of adjacent nerve roots, and occasionally cord compression causes paraparesis. Pain is relieved somewhat by aspirin and nonsteroidal anti-inflammatory drugs, but relief is typically not as dramatic as with osteoid osteomas.

IMAGING STUDIES

Required for diagnosis
AP and lateral radiographs can usually identify an osteoblastoma because of the dense blastic peripheral reaction in bone. For a spinal lesion, MRI might be useful because osteoblastoma has a larger nidus than does osteoid osteoma.

Required for comprehensive evaluation
CT can help to define the exact anatomic location to facilitate surgery. MRI is especially useful when an aneurysmal cyst is associated with the osteoblastoma or in cases where the spinal cord is compromised.

Special considerations
None

Pitfalls
None

IMAGE DESCRIPTION

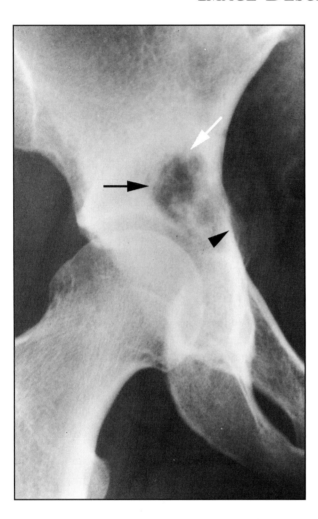

Figure 3-8

Osteoblastoma—AP view of hip

AP view of the hip of a young woman that shows a 2-cm moth-eaten nidus (black arrow) in the supra-acetabular area of the hip. Note also a 1-cm halo of surrounding inflammatory sclerotic osteitis (white arrow) and a slight periosteal reactive change (arrowhead) on the medial cortex of the ilium.

DIFFERENTIAL DIAGNOSIS

Eosinophilic granuloma (presence of eosinophils and specific Langerhans-type histiocytes in biopsy specimen)

Infectious inflammatory granuloma (inflammatory cells might have positive culture for bacteria)

Osteosarcoma (numerous atypical mitotic figures seen in malignant osteoblasts found in biopsy material)

OSTEOCHONDROMA

SYNONYMS

Bone spur
Osteocartilaginous exostosis

DEFINITION

Osteochondroma is one of the most common types of
hamartomatous (developmental) bone tumors. It arises as an ectopic
separation from the outer edge of the enchondral growth plate,
resulting in lateral (rather than longitudinal) growth from the
metaphyseal bone. The lesion can be pedunculated, as seen
typically about the knee joint, or sessile, seen commonly in the
proximal humerus. The pedunculated exophytic mass points away
from the adjacent joint, medullary fat extends into the bony base,
and there is a cauliflower-like cartilaginous cap at the peak of the
exostosis.

Multiple osteochondromas are called hereditary multiple
exostoses, an autosomal dominant inherited condition that is only
one tenth as common as the solitary disorder, which is not
inherited. The chance that hereditary multiple exostoses will convert
to secondary peripheral chondrosarcoma in an adult is about 1%,
compared with a very slight conversion rate for the solitary lesion.

HISTORY AND PHYSICAL FINDINGS

Osteochondromas usually present in childhood as painless,
nontender bony spurs felt beneath the skin of the knee. In runners,
their presence can create mechanical problems, resulting in painful
bursae over the cartilaginous cap that sometimes require surgical
removal. With multiple exostoses, shortening and deformity of the
extremities might necessitate surgical osteotomy. A lesion that starts
to grow after skeletal maturity is cause for concern because it might
develop into a secondary chondrosarcoma.

IMAGING STUDIES

Required for diagnosis
AP and lateral radiographs are usually adequate to establish the
diagnosis and location of osteochondromas.

Required for comprehensive evaluation
If the presence of a bursa adjacent to the osteochondroma or the
possible conversion to secondary chondrosarcoma is a concern,

ICD-9 Codes
213.4
Benign neoplasm of scapula and long bones of upper limb
213.7
Benign neoplasm of long bones of lower limb

SECTION 3 ■ TUMORS

MRI is helpful. If the cartilaginous cap grows larger than 2 cm in thickness or demonstrates multiple satellite lesions, chondrosarcoma must be considered a possibility.

Special considerations
None

Pitfalls
None

IMAGE DESCRIPTIONS

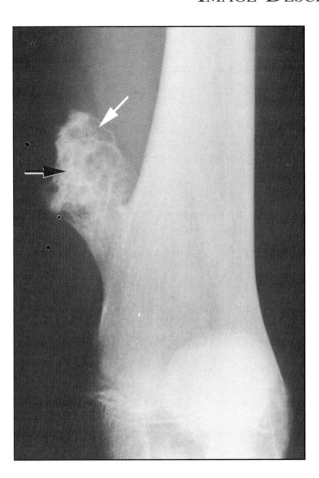

Figure 3-9

Osteochondroma—AP view of distal femur

AP view of the distal femur of a teenaged boy showing an osteochondroma. Note the bony exophytic mass (black arrow) arising from the medial cortex of the distal femoral metaphysis with a benign-appearing cartilaginous cap (white arrow) that points away from the knee joint. Medullary fat extends into the bony base.

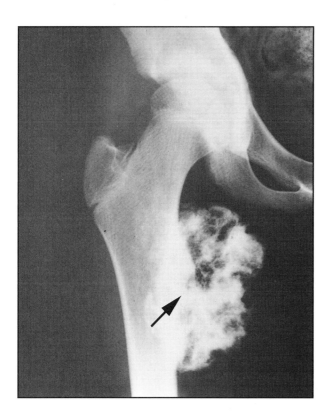

Figure 3-10

Osteochondroma—AP view of proximal femur and hip

AP view of the proximal femur and hip of a young man showing a large, pedunculated, cauliflower-shaped solitary osteochondroma (arrow) arising from the lesser trochanter. A lesion of this type must be periodically evaluated, with the assistance of MRI, for possible conversion to a secondary chondrosarcoma.

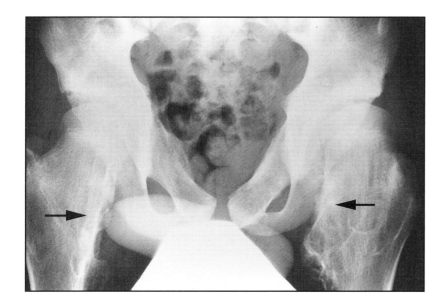

Figure 3-11

Multiple exostoses— AP view of pelvis

AP view of the pelvis of a young man with hereditary multiple exostoses. Note the diffuse circumferential and symmetric involvement of the proximal inter-trochanteric portions of both femurs (arrows), resulting in a widening and thinning of the cortical structures not seen in the solitary form of the same disease.

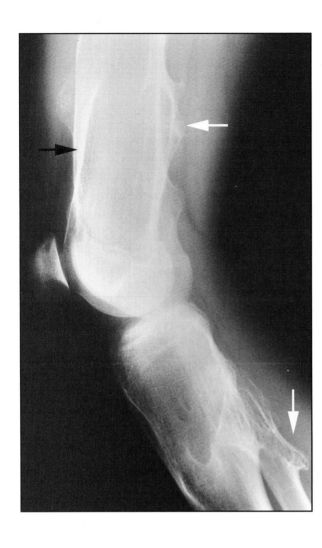

Figure 3-12

Multiple exostoses—Lateral view of knee

Lateral view of the knee of a young man with hereditary multiple exostoses. Note that the metaphyseal cortices are widely distended (black arrow), with several small exostoses arising from the surface of the bone (white arrows).

DIFFERENTIAL DIAGNOSIS

Periosteal chondroma

Periosteal chondrosarcoma

Surface osteosarcoma

Traumatic reaction bone spurs

(None of the above will have a benign cartilaginous cap on a bony exostosis.)

OSTEOID OSTEOMA

SYNONYMS

None

DEFINITION

Osteoid osteomas are the most common types of osteoid-forming neoplasms, accounting for 10% of all benign bone tumors. They are more common in males than in females and occur most often in patients between the ages of 10 and 25 years. These lesions typically develop in the bone cortex in the ends of long bones, most often in the femur and tibia. When osteoid osteomas occur in the spine, the most common location is the pedicle area of the thoracolumbar vertebrae. The least common location is an intra-articular area such as the hip, where the lesion causes a painful synovitis that could be mistaken for pyarthrosis.

HISTORY AND PHYSICAL FINDINGS

Patients typically present with a history of dull, aching pain in the back or lower extremity that is worse at night. Aspirin or nonsteroidal anti-inflammatory drugs reduce the pain, which is caused by inflammation resulting from the high concentrations of prostaglandins found in the center, or nidus, of an osteoid osteoma. The prostaglandins are a product of the large population of macrophages found in the nidus tissue. In the spinal area, the inflammatory pain can cause asymmetric muscle spasms, which can result in scoliosis. With intra-articular lesions, the clinical picture will be that of monoarticular arthritis. Because of the long history of pain and corresponding decreased activity, muscle atrophy will be present in the area of the tumor.

IMAGING STUDIES

Required for diagnosis

Because of the dense sclerotic reaction in the cortical bone around the nidus of the lesion, AP and lateral radiographs can usually make the diagnosis. However, in cases where the nidus is very small and surgical removal is being considered, CT will help identify the exact location of the nidus. MRI is not a good choice for locating a small nidus.

ICD-9 Codes

213.2
Benign neoplasm of vertebral column, excluding sacrum and coccyx

213.7
Benign neoplasm of long bones of lower limb

SECTION 3 ■ TUMORS

Required for comprehensive evaluation
A bone scan is helpful in the differential diagnosis of an osteoid osteoma because the scan is always positive with an active painful lesion. A negative scan most likely indicates an asymptomatic, burned-out lesion or an asymptomatic incidental finding such as a large bone island or osteoma.

Special considerations
None

Pitfalls
None

IMAGE DESCRIPTION

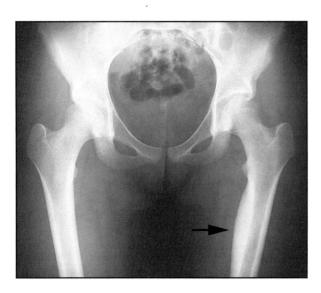

Figure 3-13

Osteoid osteoma—AP view of pelvis

AP view of the pelvis and proximal femurs of an adolescent girl. Note the typical fusiform sclerotic thickening of the medial femoral cortex just below the lesser trochanter (arrow), the most common location for an osteoid osteoma.

DIFFERENTIAL DIAGNOSIS

Intracortical Brodie's abscess (the nidus tissue will demonstrate inflammatory cells and may culture positive for bacteria)

Stress-reactive lesions (no nidus on CT)

Unicameral Bone Cyst

ICD-9 Code

733.21
Solitary bone cyst

Synonyms

Simple bone cyst
Solitary bone cyst

Definition

The unicameral bone cyst is considered to be a developmental anomaly of growing enchondral bone. It occurs centrally in the metaphysis of skeletally immature children and is filled with serous fluid produced by a thin fibrous membrane located beneath a thinned-out and slightly dilated metaphyseal cortex. Fifty percent of unicameral bone cysts occur in the proximal humerus, and 25% occur in the upper femur. In younger children, ages 5 to 13 years, the cyst is in direct contact with the growth plate and is more active, which leads to a high failure rate when bone grafts are attempted. In children age 14 years and older, the lesions become inactive, grow away from the growth plate, and respond better to bone grafting. Steroid injections are considered standard treatment for active lesions in the younger age group.

History and Physical Findings

The unicameral bone cyst is the most common cause of pathologic fracture in children. In most cases, the patient will report no pain prior to the fracture. Fractures in the proximal femur caused by these cysts can result in varus deformity if not treated properly.

Imaging Studies

Required for diagnosis

In most cases, AP and lateral radiographs are sufficient to make the diagnosis, even if a fracture has occurred through the cyst.

Required for comprehensive evaluation

If clear serous fluid cannot be obtained at the time of steroid injection, MRI might be indicated to rule out other conditions such as fibrous dysplasia or even more aggressive conditions such as desmoplastic fibroma or osteosarcoma.

Special considerations

None

Pitfalls

None

IMAGE DESCRIPTION

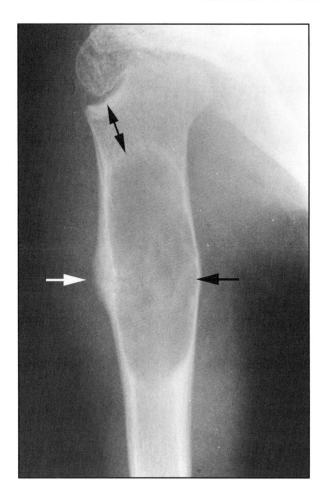

Figure 3-14

Unicameral bone cyst—AP view of proximal humerus

AP view of the proximal humerus of a 12-year-old girl showing a large, centrally located lytic lesion in the metadiaphyseal area. The lesion is surrounded by a thinned-out and slightly dilated cortex (black arrow) without matrix calcification. Note the callus formation from a prior fracture through the cyst wall (white arrow). This lesion is starting to migrate away from the growth plate (double-headed arrow), suggesting that the cyst is in an early latent stage or that the cystic process has arrested.

DIFFERENTIAL DIAGNOSIS

Aneurysmal bone cyst (peripheral location in metadiaphyseal bone, large dilated aneurysmal component with florid periosteal reactive bone formation)

Early osteosarcoma (further imaging, including MRI, indicated)

Fibrous dysplasia, monostotic form (absence of "smoky" matrix calcification)

Low-grade malignant fibrous histiocytoma (further imaging, including MRI, indicated)

CHONDROSARCOMA

SYNONYMS
None

DEFINITION
Chondrosarcoma has many variants but most commonly is a low-grade primary sarcoma of bone that is rare in children and more common in middle-aged or older adults. It represents about 10% of all bone sarcomas. Typical locations are the pelvis, femur, and proximal humerus, where the tumor is most likely to occur in the metaphysis. Because chondrosarcoma is generally not responsive to chemotherapy and has a low metastatic potential, it is rarely treated with chemotherapy, but it requires aggressive surgical treatment to prevent local recurrence.

HISTORY AND PHYSICAL FINDINGS
Because chondrosarcomas are slow growing and there is little inflammatory response to the tumor, patients experience minimal pain, which can delay their seeking treatment. Often a large tumor mass has developed by the time a diagnostic imaging study is ordered.

IMAGING STUDIES

Required for diagnosis
AP and lateral radiographs can usually identify a low-grade chondroid tumor.

Required for comprehensive evaluation
With a central primary lesion, MRI should also be ordered to evaluate medullary extension and cortical permeation. For peripheral secondary lesions arising from osteochondromas with heavy calcification, CT may be adequate, though if there is minimal calcification, MRI may be more beneficial. Because chondrosarcomas can metastasize to the lung, CT of the chest is indicated.

Special considerations
None

Pitfalls
None

ICD-9 Codes
170.4 Malignant neoplasm of scapula and long bones of upper limb
170.6 Malignant neoplasm of pelvic bones, sacrum, and coccyx
170.7 Malignant neoplasm of long bones of lower limb

SECTION 3 ■ TUMORS

IMAGE DESCRIPTIONS

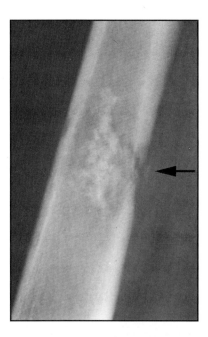

Figure 3-15

Chondrosarcoma—AP view of femoral diaphysis

AP view of the femoral diaphysis of an elderly man. The centrally located, moth-eaten, heavily calcified lesion with lytic permeation into the adjacent cortex (arrow) strongly suggests a low-grade central primary chondrosarcoma of the femur.

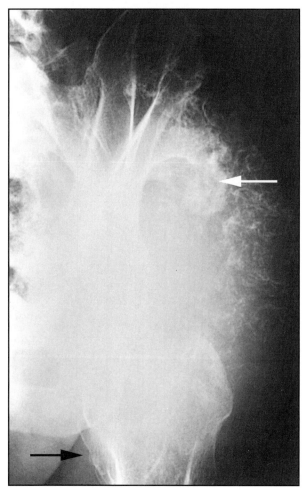

Figure 3-16

Secondary chondrosarcoma— Oblique view of pelvis

AP oblique view of the pelvis of a middle-aged man with known hereditary multiple exostoses, as can be seen by the dilated irregular pattern of the proximal femur (black arrow). A large, extracortical, calcifying, low-grade chondroid mass appears to be arising from a bony exophytic (growing outward from the surface of the ilium) mass (white arrow). This represents a pre-existing osteochondroma. The histologic diagnosis was a grade I secondary chondrosarcoma, which carries an excellent prognosis for survival.

DIFFERENTIAL DIAGNOSIS

Benign osteochondroma (thin cartilaginous cap)

Bone infarct (outer edge of reactive sclerosis)

Enchondroma (minimal cortical erosion in large bones)

EWING'S SARCOMA

SYNONYMS
None

DEFINITION
Ewing's sarcoma is the most malignant primary sarcoma of bone. It occurs in children and young adults, with males affected more often than females, and accounts for 10% of all primary bone sarcomas. A marrow sarcoma, Ewing's can be found in nearly every bone in the skeleton. The pelvis is a common site. In the long bones such as the femur, tibia, and proximal humerus, the tumor arises from the medullary portion of the metaphysis-diaphysis. Ewing's sarcoma is part of a larger family of neuroectodermal tumors, including neuroblastoma and primitive neuroectodermal tumor, all of which carry a poor prognosis and require chemotherapy.

HISTORY AND PHYSICAL FINDINGS
Patients with Ewing's sarcoma frequently have localized pain, a low-grade fever, weight loss, and an elevated erythrocyte sedimentation rate that might suggest infectious disease. A tumor mass, tender to palpation, may not appear until the late stages of the disease.

IMAGING STUDIES

Required for diagnosis
As with osteosarcoma, Ewing's sarcoma usually can be seen on AP and lateral radiographs as a permeative lytic lesion in bone. However, because the differential diagnosis is considerable, additional imaging studies are necessary.

Required for comprehensive evaluation
Local MRI with contrast medium, a whole-body bone scan to assess for multifocal disease, and CT of the chest and abdomen to look for metastatic disease are advisable. Oncology consultation is suggested when the primary lesion suggests malignant disease.

Special considerations
None

Pitfalls
Both the radiographic and clinical findings in Ewing's sarcoma are similar to those found in patients with osteomyelitis.

IMAGE DESCRIPTION

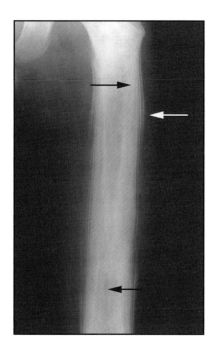

Figure 3-17

Ewing's sarcoma—AP view of femur

AP view of the femur in a teenaged girl that shows a diffuse, permeative lysis of the entire femoral diaphysis (black arrows) and extensive circumferential onion-skin reaction (white arrow). The onion-skin reaction is a multilaminated periosteal reactive bone formation that is evident on radiographs and is very characteristic of Ewing's sarcoma. Note the laminated periosteal response on the lateral cortex (white arrow).

DIFFERENTIAL DIAGNOSIS

Langerhans histiocytosis (or eosinophilic granuloma) (less destructive)

Leukemia (minimal bone destruction; negative bone scan)

Lymphoma (older age group)

Metastatic neuroblastoma (patient younger than age 5 years)

Osteomyelitis (metaphyseal location)

LEUKEMIA

SECTION 3 ■ TUMORS

ICD-9 Code

205.9
Unspecified myeloid leukemia

SYNONYMS
None

DEFINITION
Leukemia is a diffuse myelogenous (produced in bone marrow) sarcoma that spills into the peripheral blood; as a result, it can be detected on a peripheral blood smear. The most common type is acute lymphoblastic leukemia, which affects children. This form can produce abnormalities that can be seen on skeletal radiographs such as generalized osteopenia, radiolucent metaphyseal bands, diffuse periostitis, and localized permeative lytic changes in cortical structures. In the chronic forms of myelogenous leukemia found in adults, radiologic abnormalities are less common and, when present, are less severe than in the acute lymphogenous type seen in children.

HISTORY AND PHYSICAL FINDINGS
Patients with leukemia present with nonspecific symptoms of low-grade fever, generalized aches and pain, and weight loss. Presenting symptoms sometimes include painful joint swelling that might suggest a rheumatoid synovitis associated with anemia.

IMAGING STUDIES

Required for diagnosis
AP radiographs that show radiolucent metaphyseal bands and generalized osteopenia of all skeletal structures are characteristic. In these cases, a complete blood count should be ordered; if findings are suspicious, the patient should be referred to a hematologist.

Required for comprehensive evaluation
None

Special considerations
None

Pitfalls
None

IMAGE DESCRIPTION

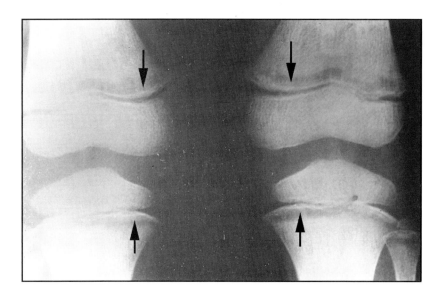

Figure 3-18

Acute lymphoblastic leukemia—AP view of knees

AP view of both knees of a child with acute lymphoblastic leukemia. Note the radiolucent metaphyseal bands in the femurs and tibias (arrows) and generalized osteopenia of all skeletal structures. These are, however, nonspecific findings in many diseases, including scurvy, that affect the general nutrition of a growing child. Biopsy material from such lytic metaphyseal bands may not demonstrate leukemic infiltrates.

DIFFERENTIAL DIAGNOSIS

Diffuse histiocytosis X (geographic lesions with sharp edges)

Osteomyelitis (usually localized to one site)

Renal failure (elevated serum P2 phosphates and creatinine)

Scurvy (history of nutritional deficiency)

Sickle cell disease (family background)

Lymphoma of Bone

Synonym
Reticulum cell sarcoma

Definition
Lymphomas of bone occur in several forms, but the most common is a systemic sarcoma that originates in the bone marrow. This form can present as a solitary lytic process in a single bone without involving other lymphatic organs such as the lymph nodes, liver, and spleen, but later it may become more generalized. Lymphomas of bone account for 7% of all bone sarcomas. Most lymphomas are of the non-Hodgkins type. They can affect all age groups, but the highest incidence is in men older than age 25 years. The lytic process produces a permeative cortical destruction that is associated with a high incidence of pathologic fracture. The spine, pelvis, femur, humerus, and proximal tibia are the usual sites of occurrence. In cases of primary involvement of a single bone, chemotherapy results in an excellent 5-year survival rate of nearly 70%.

History and Physical Findings
In primary bone lymphoma, the most common presenting symptom is localized bone pain in the proximal skeleton that is worse at night; frequently, pathologic fracture is an associated finding. In some patients, a tender, localized tumor mass is the presenting symptom. With more generalized involvement, the lymph nodes, liver, and spleen may be enlarged.

Imaging Studies

Required for diagnosis
AP and lateral radiographs of the painful area should always be ordered first, but because of the likelihood of extensive marrow involvement and extracortical tumor masses, MRI is strongly indicated as well. Because of the potential for multiple bone involvement, a total-body bone scan is also important. Referral to an oncologist is advisable when the initial radiographs suggest malignant disease. Routine staging for lymphoma should include CT of the chest and abdomen to rule out involvement of other organs.

Required for comprehensive evaluation
None

Special considerations
None

Pitfalls
None

IMAGE DESCRIPTION

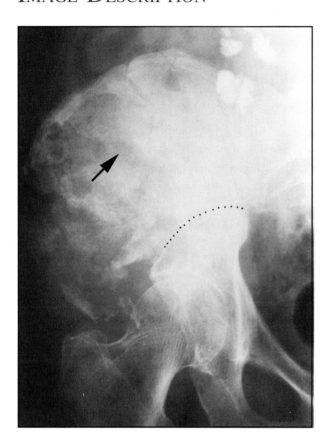

Figure 3-19

Lymphoma—AP view of right hip

AP view of the right hip of a middle-aged woman with a large, destructive, permeative lytic lesion of the body of the ilium (black arrow) and an associated pathologic fracture (dotted line). The large soft-tissue mass that overlies the fracture could be better visualized on an MRI scan.

DIFFERENTIAL DIAGNOSIS

Metastatic carcinoma from renal cell, lung, or breast (no extracortical mass)

Multiple myeloma (punched-out lytic lesions)

Plasmacytoma (geographic lysis)

METASTATIC CARCINOMA

Section 3 ■ TUMORS

ICD-9 Code

198.5
Secondary malignant neoplasm of bone and bone marrow

SYNONYMS
None

DEFINITION
Advanced terminal cancer metastasizes to bone in approximately 70% of patients. The overall incidence of metastatic carcinoma of bone is 15 times the total of all other bone tumors. The primary tumors most likely to metastasize to bone are those of the prostate, breast, kidney, thyroid, and lung. The spine is the most common site of metastasis. The next most common sites of metastasis, in descending order of frequency, are the pelvis, femur, rib, proximal humerus, and skull. Metastases distal to the elbow or knee are rare; when present, they are most likely to have originated in the lung. Metastases from the prostate are usually blastic in nature and carry a better prognosis and a low incidence of fracture. The more lytic metastases, including those from the kidney, thyroid, and lung, have a worse prognosis and are associated with a high incidence of pathologic fracture.

HISTORY AND PHYSICAL FINDINGS
Most patients with metastatic carcinoma have a history of carcinoma of a primary organ within the last 5 years. They present with skeletal pain with or without a pathologic fracture in the spine, pelvis, or long bones. Physical examination is unlikely to reveal a tumor mass.

IMAGING STUDIES

Required for diagnosis
AP and lateral radiographs of the painful area are advised initially. If there is a pathologic fracture in a long bone such as the femur, the entire bone should be imaged to identify possible multiple lesions. In the spinal area, sagittal MRI is indicated to identify multiple lesions with multiple sites of spinal cord compromise. A total-body bone scan is essential for identifying early asymptomatic lesions. However, in 9% of patients, metastatic carcinoma will be solitary. CT of the chest and abdomen is required to rule out metastatic disease to the lung as well as to locate the primary tumor, for example, in the lung or kidney. Mammograms are routine when looking for breast carcinoma. Referral to an oncologist is advised if the initial radiograph suggests malignant disease.

Required for comprehensive evaluation
None

Special considerations
None

Pitfalls
None

IMAGE DESCRIPTION

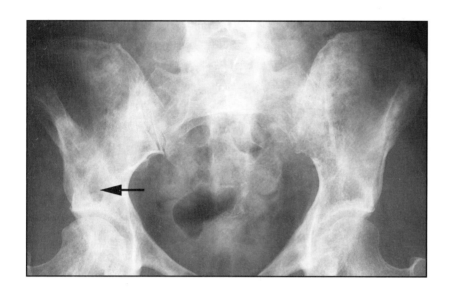

Figure 3-20

Metastatic carcinoma— AP view of pelvis

AP view of the pelvis of a middle-aged woman with extensive metastatic breast carcinoma. Extensive moth-eaten lytic lesions of the entire pelvis are apparent. Note the supra-acetabular lytic lesion (arrow) with a fair amount of blastic response at the periphery; such lesions are typical of metastatic breast carcinoma.

DIFFERENTIAL DIAGNOSIS

Ewing's sarcoma (metadiaphyseal lesions in children)

Hyperparathyroidism (elevated serum calcium and parathyroid hormone levels)

Lymphoma (extracortical mass)

Malignant fibrous histiocytoma (solitary lesion)

Multiple myeloma (punched-out lesions)

MULTIPLE MYELOMA

ICD-9 Code

238.6
Neoplasm of uncertain
behavior of plasma cells

SYNONYMS
None

DEFINITION
Multiple myeloma is a sarcoma that originates in the bone marrow, arising from malignant monoclonal plasma cells. It occurs in patients older than age 40 years and accounts for 45% of all primary bone sarcomas. Multiple myeloma presents most commonly in the axial skeleton, the pelvis, and the proximal ends of the femur and humerus; involvement distal to the knee or elbow is rare. Elevated monoclonal immunoglobulin levels in the blood or urine are usually diagnostic. However, the solitary form of plasmacytoma is found in a younger age group and usually evolves into multiple myeloma within 3 years. In less than 2% of patients with multiple myeloma, the bone changes are sclerotic instead of lytic and can be associated with polyneuropathy. This latter syndrome is referred to as POEMS to designate the most important characteristics—polyneuropathy, organomegaly, endocrinopathy, M protein, and skin changes—found in this myeloma variant.

HISTORY AND PHYSICAL FINDINGS
Patients with multiple myeloma of the spine have a history of back pain associated with anemia, an elevated erythrocyte sedimentation rate, and protein in the urine. Pathologic fractures in long bones are common, and excessive bleeding is observed at the fracture site at the time of surgery. Because of excessive osteolysis in bone, the serum calcium level may be elevated, resulting in lethargy or coma.

IMAGING STUDIES

Required for diagnosis
AP and lateral radiographs frequently will reveal punched-out lytic lesions in the cortical bone of the proximal skeleton, which are typical of multiple myeloma.

Required for comprehensive evaluation
MRI is helpful in evaluating the extent of marrow involvement; in addition, a sagittal MRI scan can help the neurosurgeon locate a focus of spinal cord compression.

Special considerations
None

Pitfalls
Bone scans are often nonreactive early in the course of the disease, when the bone disease is purely lytic in nature.

IMAGE DESCRIPTIONS

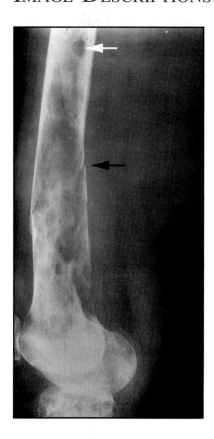

Figure 3-21

Multiple myeloma—Lateral view of distal femur

Lateral view of the distal femur of a middle-aged man showing a pathologic fracture in the distal diaphysis (black arrow) secondary to extensive moth-eaten and punched-out lytic lesions in the cortices (white arrow). Periosteal response and soft-tissue cortical mass are absent, further evidence of multiple myeloma.

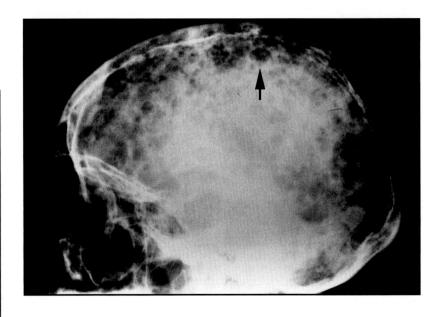

Figure 3-22

Multiple myeloma—
Lateral view of skull

Lateral view of the skull of a middle-aged woman showing multiple punched-out lytic lesions (arrow), diagnostic of multiple myeloma. Note again the absence of periosteal reaction or extra-cortical soft-tissue mass.

DIFFERENTIAL DIAGNOSIS

Hyperparathyroidism (decreased serum phosphate levels and elevated parathyroid hormone)

Lymphoma (usually demonstrates extra-cortical mass)

Metastatic carcinoma from breast, kidney, or lung (absence of punched-out lesions)

Paget's disease, early lytic phase (usually solitary)

OSTEOSARCOMA

SYNONYM
Osteogenic sarcoma (OGS)

DEFINITION
Osteosarcoma is a malignant osteoid-producing tumor of children and young adults, more commonly seen in males. Excluding multiple myeloma, osteosarcoma is the most common primary tumor of bone, accounting for 20% of all primary bone sarcomas. It is typically found in the metaphyses of long bones, with about 50% of cases occurring about the knee. Other locations include the hip, pelvis, and proximal humerus. The so-called classic form of osteosarcoma is a high-grade tumor located in the metaphyses of long bones, most often in teenagers. However, there are numerous variants of osteosarcoma, including the low-grade parosteal, periosteal, and intramedullary forms and the higher grade pagetic and radiation-induced forms. The higher grade variants carry a strong potential for pulmonary metastasis and are likely to be treated with chemotherapy.

HISTORY AND PHYSICAL FINDINGS
Osteosarcoma is a fast-growing tumor characterized by pain that begins 1 to 3 months before the onset of a firm and tender mass associated with a major joint such as the knee. Dilated veins in the skin overlying the mass are common.

IMAGING STUDIES

Required for diagnosis
AP and lateral radiographs usually can localize the tumor and make the diagnosis.

Required for comprehensive evaluation
Unlike benign bone tumors, osteosarcoma requires additional imaging studies to stage the disease. Note that a patient should be referred to an oncologist when the initial primary lesion is suspected to be malignant. The oncologist will order the appropriate staging studies, which include local MRI with gadolinium contrast to evaluate the medullary and soft-tissue involvement, a total-body bone scan to look for multifocal disease, and a chest CT to look for metastatic disease to the lung. MRI with contrast medium should be repeated after two or three cycles of chemotherapy to evaluate the effectiveness of the chemotherapy protocol and help determine the

ICD-9 Codes
170.4 Malignant neoplasm of scapula and long bones of upper limb
170.6 Malignant neoplasm of pelvic bones, sacrum, and coccyx
170.7 Malignant neoplasm of long bones of lower limb

SECTION 3 ■ TUMORS

feasibility of limb salvage surgery. Lung imaging should be continued every 3 months up to 5 years after diagnosis to rule outmetastases.

Special considerations
None

Pitfalls
None

IMAGE DESCRIPTION

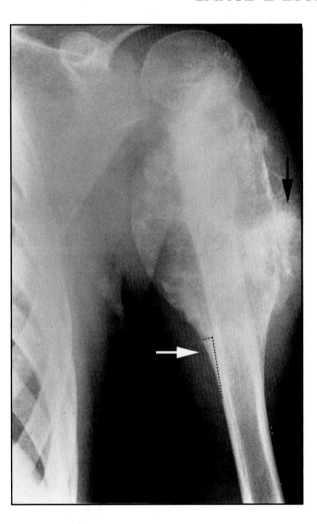

Figure 3-23

Osteosarcoma—AP view of proximal humerus

AP view of the proximal humerus of a teenaged boy showing a large, aggressive-appearing, osteoblastic, centrally located metaphyseal lesion that has broken out circumferentially for a great distance under the periosteum. There is evidence of chaotic neoplastic osteoid formation outside the cortex (black arrow). Codman's reactive triangle (white arrow), nonneoplastic reparative bone formed at the diaphyseal pole of the tumor as a response to periosteal lifting by the tumor and the hallmark of classic osteosarcoma, is outlined by a dotted line.

DIFFERENTIAL DIAGNOSIS

Aneurysmal bone cyst (minimal bone formation in early stages)

Eosinophilic granuloma (diaphyseal location)

Ewing's sarcoma (minimal blastic activity)

Lymphoma (older age groups and minimal blastic response)

Osteomyelitis (minimal osteoblastic activity)

BENIGN NERVE SHEATH TUMOR

SECTION 3 ■ TUMORS

SYNONYMS

None

DEFINITION

Peripheral nerve sheath tumors are common, particularly in young adults. The most common type is the fusiform solitary neurofibroma, a benign lesion found in the center of the smaller peripheral nerves. The combination of multiple neurofibromas, smooth-edged café au lait spots, and soft pedunculated cutaneous fibroma molluscum lesions with large surface plexiform neurofibromas is known as neurofibromatosis, an autosomal dominant disorder that carries a 10% chance of conversion to a malignant schwannoma. The less common form of nerve sheath tumor is the benign neurilemmoma, or neurilemoma, a round tumor found eccentrically located on nerve roots of the spine or in superficial nerves on the flexor surfaces of the upper and lower extremities. The neurilemmoma is located on the surface of the nerve, can be easily removed surgically, and rarely causes neurologic deficiency.

HISTORY AND PHYSICAL FINDINGS

A peripheral nerve sheath tumor usually presents in a young adult as a painless, soft mass in an extremity. Neurologic findings are minimal. Deep palpation or tapping on the mass may elicit a positive Tinel's sign with tingling down the limb along the sensory distribution of the nerve. Multiple neurofibromatosis will be accompanied by café au lait spots or superficial cutaneous fibroma molluscum lesions.

IMAGING STUDIES

Required for diagnosis

Most nerve sheath tumors cannot be seen on radiographs. However, a neurilemmoma in a spinal nerve root can cause dilatation of the bony neural foramen, and neurofibromatosis may be associated with bony deformity, changes that can be seen on radiographs. Nevertheless, MRI is the best way to image most nerve sheath tumors. A T2-weighted image will reveal an area of very high signal intensity on a peripheral nerve. This is best visualized on a sagittal or coronal view.

Special considerations
None

Pitfalls
Because the nerve sheath tumor is rarely calcified and has the
same radiodensity as the surrounding muscle, it cannot be
visualized on radiographs.

IMAGE DESCRIPTION

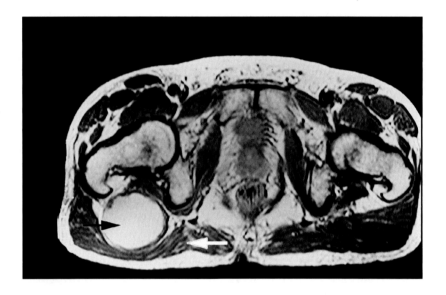

Figure 3-24

*Benign nerve sheath
tumor—MRI of pelvis*

T2-weighted MRI scan
through the pelvis of a
young man. Note the 5-cm
area of increased signal
intensity (black arrow) that
indicates a neurilemmoma
just beneath the gluteus
maximus muscle (white
arrow) on the surface of the
sciatic nerve.

DIFFERENTIAL DIAGNOSIS

Intramuscular myxoma (benign; frequently asymptomatic)

SECTION 3 ■ TUMORS

DESMOID TUMOR

SYNONYM

Aggressive fibromatosis

DEFINITION

The desmoid tumor is a very aggressive fibroblastic tumor seen in older children or young adults. It acts like a low-grade fibrosarcoma but does not metastasize. Abdominal wall desmoids occur in postpartum women, whereas extra-abdominal desmoids are more common in men and are found in fascial planes about the large muscles of the shoulder, hip, and knee. Desmoids are very infiltrative tumors that can engulf neurovascular structures, making the tumor difficult to remove. They can be multifocal, and when they are associated with polyposis (multiple polyps) of the large intestine and craniofacial osteomas, the condition is referred to as Gardner's syndrome.

HISTORY AND PHYSICAL FINDINGS

In women, the desmoid frequently presents after pregnancy as a firm, painless mass in the rectus abdominus muscle fascia. In men, a desmoid usually occurs after a muscle injury, growing very rapidly into a very firm, painless mass suggestive of a soft-tissue sarcoma.

IMAGING STUDIES

Required for diagnosis

The desmoid tumor is composed of very dense collagen tissue. Although it has no calcification, it will frequently appear on radiographs because it is denser than normal muscle. CT will also clearly delineate the lesion from the surrounding muscle and vascular structures. MRI is the best choice for imaging a desmoid tumor because it can differentiate it from soft-tissue sarcomas; the desmoid is characterized by a lower signal intensity on T2-weighted images because of its low water content.

Required for comprehensive evaluation

None

Special considerations

None

Pitfalls

More aggressive desmoids can produce a high signal intensity on T2-weighted images, similar to high-grade sarcomas.

IMAGE DESCRIPTION

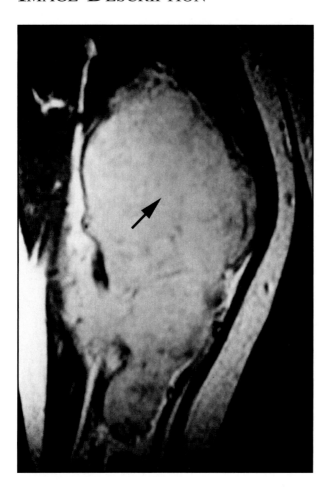

Figure 3-25

Desmoid tumor—Coronal MRI of posterior thigh

Coronal T2-weighted MRI scan of the posterior thigh of a teenaged boy. A large desmoid (arrow) in the posterior compartment engulfs the sciatic nerve. This lesion demonstrates a high T2 signal intensity, similar to that produced by a sarcoma, indicating that the tumor is very aggressive. In fact, the tumor did recur after removal and postoperative radiation therapy.

SECTION 3 ■ TUMORS

DIFFERENTIAL DIAGNOSIS

Low-grade sarcoma such as a fibrosarcoma (higher signal intensity on T2-weighted MRI)

Muscle tear that progresses to myositis ossificans (calcification seen in lesion)

HEMANGIOMA

ICD-9 Code

228.00
Hemangioma of unspecified
site

SYNONYMS
None

DEFINITION
Hemangiomas are the most common soft-tissue neoplasm in
children, accounting for 7% of all benign tumors in all age groups.
Hemangiomas are hamartomatous (developmental) lesions that
appear in a variety of clinical forms. The solitary capillary
cutaneous hemangioma is the most common and occurs more often
in females. This type of hemangioma presents in early infancy as
an elevated, red-to-purple cutaneous lesion about the head or neck.
A less common form that also occurs more often in females is the
cavernous hemangioma, which develops either subcutaneously or in
deep muscle bellies and has the appearance of a large cluster of
purple grapes. In the arteriovenous hemangioma, arteriovenous
shunting associated with increased pulse pressure can occur, causing
heart failure in some cases.

HISTORY AND PHYSICAL FINDINGS
Most patients will report that the hemangioma has been present
since childhood. The capillary cutaneous form is noticed several
weeks after birth and may disappear spontaneously by the time the
patient is 8 years old. However, with the larger and deeper
cavernous hemangioma, there may be no discoloration of the
overlying skin; presenting symptoms may be a vague fullness in the
area that occurs intermittently as the hemangioma enlarges with
dependency of the limb. Pain may accompany spontaneous
hemorrhage into the fragile tumor, which typically occurs once or
twice a year.

IMAGING STUDIES

Required for diagnosis
With a deep, cavernous hemangioma in muscle, AP and lateral
radiographs will show characteristic small punctate calcifications
known as phleboliths that are considered diagnostic for the
condition.

Required for comprehensive evaluation
In cases where no skin discoloration or phleboliths are present,
MRI with contrast medium is necessary to make the diagnosis. MRI

reveals a characteristic mixed-signal serpiginous pattern seen best on T1-weighted images.

Special considerations

With an arteriovenous malformation, angiography may be necessary if embolization treatment is being considered.

Pitfalls

None

IMAGE DESCRIPTIONS

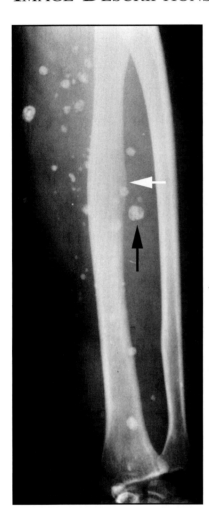

Figure 3-26

Cavernous hemangioma—AP view of forearm

AP view of the forearm of a young woman with a large intramuscular cavernous hemangioma of the entire volar compartment. Note the characteristic phlebolith (black arrow) and the slight thickening of the subadjacent radius (white arrow); the latter is caused by increased warmth and increased blood flow to the surrounding tissue.

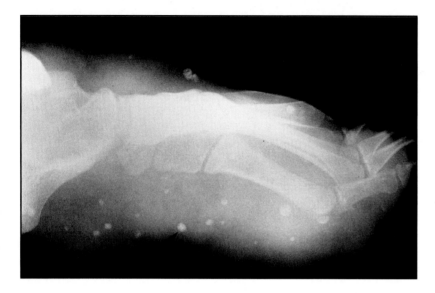

Figure 3-27

Cavernous hemangioma— Lateral view of foot

Lateral view of the foot of a teenaged girl showing a large subcutaneous cavernous hemangioma and extensive soft-tissue swelling about the midtarsal and forefoot area. Note the diagnostic phlebolith (arrow). In such cases, MRI is not necessary for diagnosis.

DIFFERENTIAL DIAGNOSIS

Hygroma (endothelial cell tumor; contains lymphatic fluid instead of blood)

Lymphangioma (no phleboliths; no blood in tumor)

Plexiform neurofibroma (similar to vascular neoplasm but with tan-like discoloration of the skin)

LIPOMA

SYNONYMS
None

DEFINITION
The benign lipoma is by far the most common of the soft-tissue tumors. Most frequently seen as a subcutaneous lesion in older patients, it affects both sexes equally and presents spontaneously without pain. Benign lipomas may appear in multiple locations. They may grow fast at first but then stop growing and never turn malignant. The second most common form is the intramuscular lipoma, which is seen more often in men and occurs in the large muscles of the limbs. Other variants include the spindle cell lipoma, angiolipoma, diffuse lipomatosis, and lumbosacral lipoma; the latter is usually seen in children.

HISTORY AND PHYSICAL FINDINGS
Patients typically present with a fairly large but asymptomatic soft-tissue mass that develops spontaneously, grows rapidly, and then stops with no further changes for many years. On physical examination, the lipoma is soft and nontender and has no adverse effects on adjacent neurovascular structures.

IMAGING STUDIES

Required for diagnosis
Although intramuscular lipomas of the limbs can be seen on AP and lateral radiographs because the lipoma is the only soft-tissue tumor that is less radiodense than the surrounding muscle, CT and MRI scans provide better soft-tissue detail. Either MRI or CT can confirm the diagnosis of lipoma without the need for a biopsy.

Required for comprehensive evaluation
None

Special considerations
None

Pitfalls
None

ICD-9 Codes

215.2
Other benign neoplasm of connective and other soft tissue of upper limb, including shoulder

215.3
Other benign neoplasm of connective and other soft tissue of lower limb, including hip

SECTION 3 ■ TUMORS

IMAGE DESCRIPTIONS

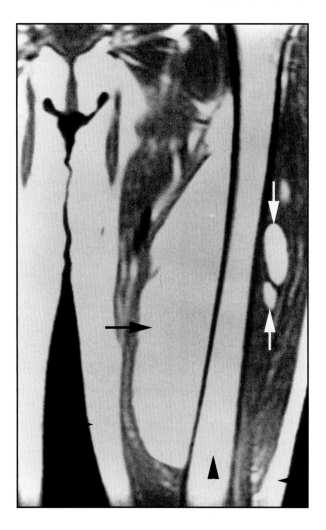

Figure 3-28

Lipoma—Coronal MRI of thigh

Coronal T1-weighted MRI scan of the thigh of an elderly woman showing the increased signal of a large intramuscular abnormality (black arrow) arising from the vastus medialis muscle. Smaller satellite lesions are seen lateral to the femur as well (white arrows). The abnormal area of increased signal intensity is the same as that of the subcutaneous fat and the fatty marrow of the femur (arrowheads), confirming the diagnosis of intramuscular lipoma.

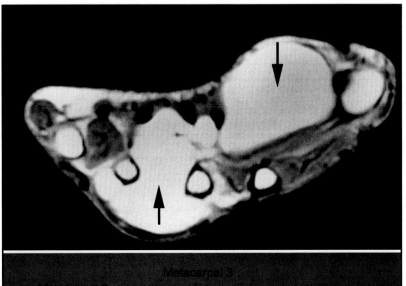

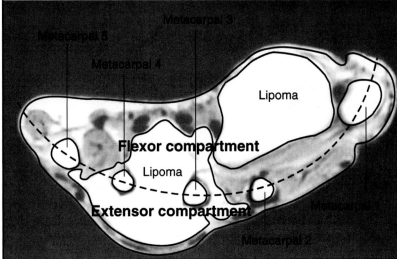

Figure 3-29

Lipoma—Axial MRI of hand

Axial T1-weighted MRI scan of the hand of an elderly man showing a large, multilobulated, soft-tissue mass involving the thenar space, as well as both the flexor and extensor compartments with communication through the interosseous ligaments between the third and fourth metacarpals. Note the areas of high signal intensity (arrows), diagnostic for lipoma.

DIFFERENTIAL DIAGNOSIS

Atypical lipoma (minor histologic variation; MRI images the same)

Intramuscular myxoma (decreased signal intensity on T1-weighted MRI)

Myxoid liposarcoma (decreased signal intensity on T1-weighted MRI)

Plexiform neurofibroma (decreased signal intensity on T1-weighted MRI)

Well-differentiated liposarcoma (appears as lipoma but has a much higher local recurrence rate)

LIPOSARCOMA

SECTION 3 ■ TUMORS

ICD-9 Codes

171.2
Malignant neoplasm of connective and other soft tissue of upper limb, including shoulder

171.3
Malignant neoplasm of connective and other soft tissue of lower limb, including hip

SYNONYMS
None

DEFINITION
Liposarcoma is the second most common type of soft-tissue sarcoma, after malignant fibrous histiocytoma. Liposarcomas are frequently seen in men age 40 to 70 years. These sarcomas may be slow growing and cause minimal pain; they are found in the large muscles about the hip, thigh, knee, shoulder, and retroperitoneal area. The most common type of liposarcoma is the low-grade myxoid type, followed by the well-differentiated form. The latter takes on the clinical appearance of a slow-growing, painless lipoma and carries a similarly excellent prognosis. Both the round cell and pleomorphic variants, however, are high-grade liposarcomas that have a poor prognosis.

HISTORY AND PHYSICAL FINDINGS
The common low-grade liposarcoma usually presents in older patients as a painless, slow-growing mass that is soft and nontender on palpation. The high-grade round cell and pleomorphic types grow faster, are painful, and exhibit a firm, tender mass on deep palpation.

IMAGING STUDIES

Required for diagnosis
MRI with gadolinium contrast is the study of choice to help distinguish the tumor from surrounding muscle tissue. The gadolinium contrast helps to differentiate liposarcomas from cystic lesions, like the larger popliteal Baker's cyst, which demonstrate decreased signal intensity in the gelatinous center. Because of the potential for pulmonary metastasis, CT of the chest is indicated. The patient should be referred to an oncologist if local MRI suggests a malignant tumor.

Required for comprehensive evaluation
None

Special considerations
None

Pitfalls
None

IMAGE DESCRIPTION

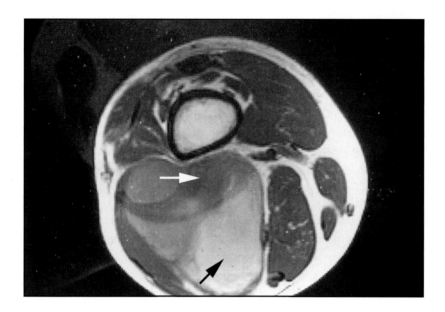

Figure 3-30

Myxoid liposarcoma—Axial MRI of thigh

Axial T1-weighted MRI scan of a 40-year-old man with a myxoid liposarcoma in the lateral hamstring muscles in the posterior compartment of the thigh. Note the area of increased signal intensity, where the tumor looks like a benign lipoma (black arrow); however, the remaining portion shows intermediate signal intensity (white arrow), which indicates a myxoid portion, diagnostic of a low-grade sarcoma.

SECTION 3 ■ TUMORS

DIFFERENTIAL DIAGNOSIS

Lipoma (entire tumor shows increased signal intensity on T1-weighted MRI)

Myxoma (decreased signal intensity on T1-weighted MRI; increased signal intensity on T2-weighted MRI)

Well-differentiated liposarcoma (entire tumor shows increased signal intensity on T1-weighted MRI)

Malignant fibrous histiocytoma (most of tumor will show high signal intensity on T2-weighted MRI)

MALIGNANT FIBROUS HISTIOCYTOMA

ICD-9 Codes

158.0
Malignant neoplasm of retroperitoneum

171.2
Malignant neoplasm of connective and other soft tissue of upper limb, including shoulder

171.3
Malignant neoplasm of connective and other soft tissue of lower limb, including hip

SYNONYM
Malignant fibrous xanthoma

DEFINITION
The most common soft-tissue sarcoma in adults is malignant fibrous histiocytoma (MFH), seen most often in men between the ages of 50 and 70 years. The tumor mass usually occurs deep within the larger muscles about the hip, shoulder, thigh, and retroperitoneum. The most common type is the storiform pleomorphic MFH, which consists of anaplastic fibroblasts and histiocytes and which carries a 45% chance of pulmonary metastasis. Less malignant variants include the myxoid, giant cell, and inflammatory MFH.

HISTORY AND PHYSICAL FINDINGS
MFH usually presents as a fast-growing, painful mass in an extremity, either subcutaneously or in a deep intramuscular position. The mass is firm and tender to palpation.

IMAGING STUDIES

Required for diagnosis
Radiographs are of little help in the staging workup of a soft-tissue MFH because these tumors rarely demonstrate calcification densities and have little effect on adjacent bony structures. For this reason, T2-weighted MRI with gadolinium contrast is the best choice. The mass appears as an area of increased signal intensity, and the gadolinium contrast helps to identify the amount of central necrosis, which is seen in most high-grade MFHs. If local MRI suggests a malignant tumor, the patient should be referred to an oncologist. Because of the high potential for pulmonary metastasis, CT of the chest is an essential part of the initial staging process.

Required for comprehensive evaluation
None

Special considerations
None

Pitfalls
None

IMAGE DESCRIPTION

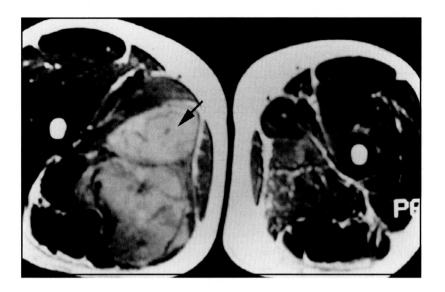

Figure 3-31

Malignant fibrous histiocytoma—Axial MRI of thighs

Axial T2-weighted MRI scan of a 60-year-old man with a high-grade MFH that fills almost the entire adductor compartment of the left thigh (arrow). Note the appearance of the normal right thigh in comparison.

DIFFERENTIAL DIAGNOSIS

Liposarcoma (increased signal intensity on T1-weighted MRI)

Pseudotumors resulting from muscle injury with associated hematoma (site of muscle tear; younger age group)

Rhabdomyosarcoma (younger age group)

Synovial sarcoma (younger age group)

NERVE SHEATH SARCOMA

ICD-9 Codes

171.2
Malignant neoplasm of connective and other soft tissue of upper limb, including shoulder

171.3
Malignant neoplasm of connective and other soft tissue of lower limb, including hip

SYNONYMS

Malignant schwannoma
Malignant neurofibrosarcoma

DEFINITION

A nerve sheath sarcoma can arise from a solitary neurofibroma in adults over age 40 years, in which case it carries a good prognosis with a 5-year survival rate of 75%. In the 10% of patients with neurofibromatosis who develop malignant nerve sheath tumors, however, the prognosis is much worse, with a 5-year survival rate of only 25%. The latter condition usually affects patients around age 30 years. Malignant nerve sheath tumors are usually larger than 5 cm in diameter and tend to arise from large nerve structures such as the sciatic nerve or spinal nerve roots.

HISTORY AND PHYSICAL FINDINGS

Patients may have a known history of a solitary neurofibroma or have neurofibromatosis, in which case symptoms may include café au lait spots over the site of the tumor mass and a tumor that has recently increased in size and become painful. There may be minimal loss of nerve function.

IMAGING STUDIES

Required for diagnosis

A sagittal T2-weighted MRI is the study of choice because the increased signal intensity of the malignant tumor will contrast with the low signal intensity produced by the surrounding muscles. The sagittal view best demonstrates the position of the tumor in a major nerve structure. Because of the high potential for metastatic lung disease, chest CT is indicated as well. The patient should be referred to an oncologist if MRI suggests a malignant tumor.

Required for comprehensive evaluation
None

Special considerations
None

Pitfalls
None

IMAGE DESCRIPTION

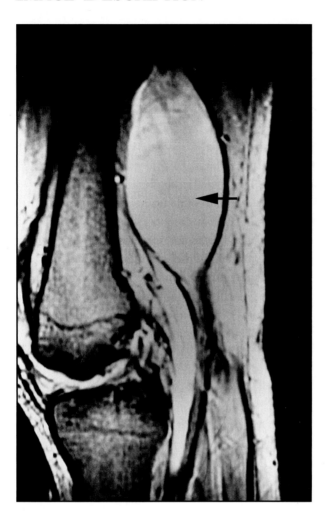

Figure 3-32

Nerve sheath sarcoma—Sagittal MRI of knee

Sagittal gradient echo MRI scan of a 35-year-old woman with a fusiform nerve sheath sarcoma (arrow) centrally located in the sciatic nerve just proximal to its bifurcation above the knee joint.

DIFFERENTIAL DIAGNOSIS

Neurofibroma (usually smaller than 5 cm)

Neurilemmoma (spherical and smaller than 5 cm)

SECTION 3 ■ TUMORS

SYNOVIAL SARCOMA

SECTION 3 ■ TUMORS

SYNONYM
Synovioma

DEFINITION
Synovial sarcoma is the fourth most common soft-tissue sarcoma in young adults between the ages of 15 and 35 years. It occurs slightly more often in males than in females. Despite its name, the tumor is rarely found in joints; it usually arises from juxta-articular structures, fascial planes, and deep muscle about the knee, shoulder, thigh, wrist, and ankle. It is the most common sarcoma of the foot except for melanoma.

HISTORY AND PHYSICAL FINDINGS
Synovial sarcoma differs from other high-grade sarcomas in that it presents slowly in young patients, often after an injury, and causes minimal pain. Approximately 40% of these tumors demonstrate calcification, which can suggest a benign diagnosis and thus sometimes delay tissue biopsy by 2 to 4 years. Despite the slow-growing nature of the synovial sarcoma, the 5-year survival rate is only 50%.

IMAGING STUDIES

Required for diagnosis
Because of the high likelihood of degenerative calcification or even bone formation, AP and lateral radiographs of the area should be ordered initially.

Required for comprehensive evaluation
MRI with gadolinium contrast will show better detail of the soft-tissue extension of the tumor and will help differentiate among cystic, necrotic, and hemorrhagic conditions. Because of the 50% chance of pulmonary metastasis, a chest CT is indicated.

Special considerations
None

Pitfalls
None

IMAGE DESCRIPTION

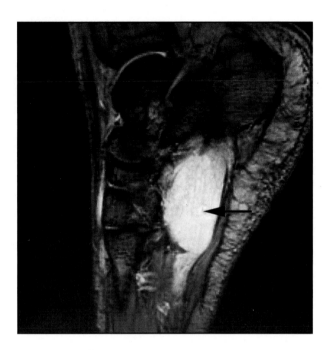

Figure 3-33

*Synovial sarcoma—
Sagittal MRI of foot and ankle*

Sagittal T2-weighted MRI scan of the foot and ankle of a young man. Note the area of increased signal intensity (arrow) in the soft tissue beneath the midtarsal area of the foot.

DIFFERENTIAL DIAGNOSIS

Baker's cyst (low signal intensity in lesion on MRI with gadolinium contrast)

Calcific tendinitis (located directly inside tendon anatomy)

Ganglion cyst (low signal intensity in lesion on MRI with gadolinium contrast)

Heterotopic ossification (usually in the muscle belly soon after significant injury)

Ischemic calcification (seen in the muscle belly in the area of an old hematoma)

SHOULDER

Section Editor
Theodore Blaine, MD

Contributors
Christopher S. Ahmad, MD
Louis U. Bigliani, MD
Raymond M. Carroll, MD
Gregory N. Lervick, MD
William N. Levine, MD

IMAGING THE SHOULDER— AN OVERVIEW

ANATOMY

The shoulder girdle suspends the arm from the thorax and consists of the humerus, scapula, clavicle, and thorax. These bones form four articulations: the glenohumeral, scapulothoracic, acromioclavicular (AC), and sternoclavicular (SC) joints. Of these, the glenohumeral joint is the principal articulation in the shoulder. The proximal humerus consists of a ball-shaped head that articulates with the glenoid portion of the scapula. The glenoid is a shallow, disk-shaped structure that covers only 20% of the humeral head. The glenoid labrum is a fibrous structure attached to the peripheral rim of the glenoid that serves to minimally deepen the socket. Tears of the anterior labrum result from anterior dislocations of the shoulder.

Glenohumeral stability depends on strong capsular ligaments that are attached to the glenoid rim and the proximal humerus. There are three glenohumeral ligaments: superior, middle, and inferior. The rotator cuff muscles (supraspinatus, infraspinatus, subscapularis, and teres minor) provide further dynamic stability, maintain the humeral head centered in the glenoid fossa, and provide rotational movement to the joint. Rotator cuff tears can involve any of these muscles or combinations thereof; however, the supraspinatus is the one most commonly torn. The rotator cuff muscles are covered by the deltoid muscle, which contributes to extension, flexion, and abduction.

Several bursae are found about the shoulder, but the subacromial bursa is important clinically because thickening and inflammation of this bursa contribute to impingement syndrome. The AC joint is formed by the acromion and the lateral end of the clavicle separated by a fibrocartilaginous disk. A series of strong ligaments runs between the clavicle and acromion to stabilize the joint. These ligaments are disrupted with a complete AC separation. The SC joint is composed of the medial end of the clavicle and the sternum, held together by a strong capsule and ligaments. Both of these joints stabilize the scapula to the chest wall. The scapulothoracic articulation consists of the thin body of the scapula and the chest wall. This joint is stabilized by a strong group of muscles that helps to position the scapula so that the glenoid is properly oriented for optimum glenohumeral function.

OSSIFICATION CENTERS

The ossification centers in the shoulder develop as follows. In the clavicle, there are two centers, the medial and lateral; both form during the 5th week of gestation. In the scapula, the coracoid

SECTION 4 ■ SHOULDER

ESSENTIALS OF MUSCULOSKELETAL IMAGING ■ AMERICAN ACADEMY OF ORTHOPAEDIC SURGEONS 171 process has two or three centers; the first center, in the center of the coracoid, forms at 1 year, the second, at the base of the coracoid, forms at 10 years, and the third, at the tip of the coracoid, forms during puberty. The ossification centers in the acromion form during puberty. In the glenoid fossa, the ossification center at the inferior aspect forms at 10 years, while at the superior aspect, it forms during puberty. The proximal humerus has three ossification centers: at the humeral head, which forms during year 1; at the greater tuberosity, which forms during year 3; and at the lesser tuberosity, which forms at year 5.

STANDARD IMAGING VIEWS

Radiographs

Shoulder complaints are common reasons to seek medical attention. Despite the many technological advances in diagnostic aids such as MRI and arthroscopy, most shoulder problems can be diagnosed with a careful history, physical examination, and plain radiographs. To arrive at an accurate diagnosis, however, the correct radiographs must be ordered. It is also important to know when to order additional imaging studies such as MRI.

The standard radiographic series for the shoulder includes five views: three AP views taken in the plane of the scapula with the proximal humerus in (1) neutral (true AP), (2) external rotation, and (3) internal rotation; (4) the scapular lateral view (Y or transscapular view), which is orthogonal to the AP view; and (5) the axillary view.

The AP series reveals the glenohumeral joint, the AC joint, the proximal humeral shaft, and the greater and lesser tuberosities of the proximal humerus. In external rotation, the greater tuberosity is seen on profile. In the internal rotation view, the shape of the proximal humerus is similar to a light bulb. An impaction fracture (Hill-Sachs lesion), often associated with anterior shoulder dislocation, may be visualized with the internal rotation view.

The transscapular view shows the profiles of the body of the acromion, the scapular spine, the scapular body, and the coracoid process. The proximal humeral shaft and the lesser tuberosity are also well visualized. The greater tuberosity is seen en face. The humeral head should be centered over the glenoid in this view. A displaced distal clavicle can also be seen.

The axillary view is taken with the x-ray beam perpendicular to the horizontal axis of the glenohumeral joint. This view is excellent for demonstrating the relationship of the humeral head to the glenoid (eg, particularly helpful in identifying subluxations and dislocations) and for assessing glenoid pathology. The anterior-to-posterior relationship of the distal clavicle at the AC joint is also

seen on this view. An os acromiale, when present, is also
evident on this view.

Computed tomography

CT is helpful in evaluating complex intra-articular fractures of
the proximal humerus and fractures of the scapula.
Sternoclavicular dislocations are also nicely visualized with CT.
Thin-cut CT scans with air contrast also can be used to diagnose
labral tears.

Magnetic resonance imaging

MRI has replaced arthrography as the imaging modality of
choice to diagnose rotator cuff tears. The advantage of MRI is
that it is noninvasive and allows visualization of the soft tissues
in all planes. In addition, the humeral head, glenoid, and lateral
end of the clavicle can be visualized. MRI is also helpful in the
diagnosis of impingement syndrome, especially in the early
phases when a subacromial effusion (defined as inflammatory
changes in the supraspinatus tendon and bursal thickening) can
be visualized. MRI and MR arthrography are used to image
lesions of the glenoid labrum such as a superior labrum anterior
to posterior (SLAP) tear. For patients who cannot undergo MRI
(eg, patients with pacemakers), shoulder CT arthrography can be
substituted to diagnose rotator cuff tears and labral lesions.

Ultrasound

Ultrasound is gaining increasing acceptance in imaging of the
shoulder. The potential advantages are decreased cost, less
discomfort, and real-time imaging. The disadvantage is that only
a few medical centers have mastered this technique with
acceptable accuracy. The primary application has been in
diagnosing rotator cuff tears.

SPECIAL RADIOGRAPHIC VIEWS

Scapular outlet view

This view is taken in the same manner as the transscapular view,
with the exception of a 10° caudal tilt of the x-ray tube. This
specialized view reveals the outlet of the supraspinatus tendon
as it exits inferior to the coracoacromial arch and will show
acromial morphology.

Zanca view

In this view, the x-ray beam is aimed at the AC joint with a 10°
to 15° cephalic tilt. With this view, an unobstructed view of the
AC joint and distal clavicle is provided.

SECTION 4 ■ SHOULDER

30° caudal tilt view

With the patient standing, the x-ray beam is directed at the shoulder with a 30° caudal tilt. This view shows anterior-inferior subacromial spurs in patients with impingement syndrome or rotator cuff tears.

West Point axillary view

To obtain this view, the patient is prone, with the affected shoulder resting on a pad that elevates it 8 cm from the top of the table. The x-ray beam is directed 25° down from the horizontal and 25° medially (from the midline). This view is useful for evaluating the anteroinferior rim of the glenoid. Following anterior dislocations of the shoulder, fractures of this rim or calcifications about the rim may be seen.

EMERGENCIES

Four conditions about the shoulder are considered emergencies and demand urgent attention. (1) Scapulothoracic dissociation is seen after high-energy trauma and requires referral to a trauma specialist. (2) "Floating shoulder" is characterized by a scapular fracture in combination with either a proximal humerus fracture or a clavicle fracture or dislocation; this condition also requires specialty referral. (3) Glenohumeral dislocations are considered relative emergencies. Injury to neurovascular structures may be exacerbated by prolonged dislocation of the glenohumeral joint. (4) A special type of dislocation, luxatio erecta, is a traumatic dislocation of the humeral head inferior to the glenoid. In this condition, the arm is locked in an abducted position. The neurovascular structures are at increased risk with this dislocation; therefore, surgical treatment is required.

NORMAL VARIANTS

A number of findings on imaging studies can appear to be a result of trauma or another type of problem when, in fact, they are simply normal variants of anatomy. In the shoulder there are a number of normal variants worth mention. On the internal rotation AP view, the bicipital groove can be mistaken for an impaction fracture and what appears to be a large cyst is, in fact, a normal finding. In children ages 10 to 16 years, notches may be seen about the upper inner aspect of the humerus and are sometimes mistaken for a malignancy. These are a normal variant and most disappear with skeletal maturity. Deltoid muscle insertions onto the humerus may simulate periostitis. In the proximal humerus, severe osteoporosis may present with multiple lytic lesions that are easily confused with a malignancy. Multiple benign cortical defects also can be seen in the proximal humerus, simulating a malignant process. An os acromiale is a secondary ossification center in the acromion that persists into adulthood and can be mistaken for a fracture. If the ring apophysis of the glenoid fails to close, it may simulate a fracture or a Bankart-type lesion. An end-on projection of the coracoid will look like a lucent lesion in the neck of the scapula. The canal in the clavicle for the supraclavicular nerve may look like a fracture, and the distal end of the clavicle may be quite large and appear cystlike.

Imaging Tips

1. Transscapular lateral views of the shoulder always should be obtained in any patient with a suspected glenohumeral dislocation. Posterior dislocations are easily missed on an AP view.

2. True AP and axillary views will show joint space narrowing of the glenohumeral joint.

3. An os acromiale, which is a normal variant, may be mistaken for a fracture. These are seen on an axillary view.

4. If the distance between the undersurface of the acromion and the top of the humeral head is less than 7 mm, a rotator cuff tear is likely present.

5. An AP view may not show a subacromial spur; if this problem is suspected, the 30° caudal tilt view is helpful.

6. SC dislocations are difficult to visualize on radiographs; if this problem is suspected, CT should be obtained.

7. Rotator cuff tears can be diagnosed by MRI or shoulder arthrography. MRI has become the procedure of choice, if tolerated by the patient.

8. Labral tears can be imaged by MR arthrography or thin-cut CT with air contrast.

9. Radiographs of patients with adhesive capsulitis usually are normal. However, an arthrogram will show decreased capacity of the joint capsule.

10. A Hill-Sachs impaction fracture of the humeral head can be seen on an internal rotation AP view, and a Bankart fracture is seen on an axillary view. Both are pathognomonic of a previous anterior shoulder dislocation.

Section 4 ■ Shoulder

Acromioclavicular Instability

ICD-9 Code

831.04
Dislocation of shoulder, closed, acromioclavicular (joint)

Synonyms

Acromioclavicular joint separation/dislocation
Separated shoulder

Definition

The acromioclavicular (AC) joint is one of the most common sites of shoulder dislocation, second only to the glenohumeral joint. The AC and coracoclavicular (CC) ligaments support the AC joint; disruption of either may lead to displacement of the clavicle where it joins the acromion. This injury most commonly occurs in men and in athletes who participate in contact sports.

History and Physical Findings

Most injuries to the AC joint occur as a result of a fall onto an adducted arm, when the lateral aspect of the shoulder strikes the ground. They can also occur as a result of a fall onto an outstretched hand, but this mechanism of injury is much less common. Patients will report pain over the AC joint, and examination will reveal a characteristic abrasion over the posterolateral corner of the acromion.

AC joint injuries are classified according to the degree of ligamentous disruption and the direction of displacement of the clavicle.

In type I injuries (no ligamentous disruption), the AC joint will be tender on palpation, but radiographs are normal.

With type II injuries, the clavicle will be somewhat elevated relative to the acromion (AC joint disruption, CC ligaments intact).

Type III injuries are characterized by elevation of the clavicle above the acromion, which represents disruption of the CC ligaments.

Type IV injuries are usually diagnosed by the posterior displacement seen on an axillary view.

Type V injuries are characterized by disruption of not only the AC and CC ligaments but also the deltotrapezial fascia.

A type VI injury is characterized by dislocation below the coracoid process.

Typically, types IV, V, and VI injuries are irreducible and require surgical reconstruction.

IMAGING STUDIES

Required for diagnosis

A trauma series, consisting of a true AP view (in the scapular plane), a transscapular view, and an axillary view, should be obtained for all AC joint injuries. On the true AP view, AC joint instability, any fractures of the base or the tip of the coracoid, and the status of the glenohumeral joint can be seen. The degree of displacement of the clavicle from the acromion may be mild. An axillary radiograph will show the acromion and clavicle in the axial plane and demonstrate the relationship of the clavicle to the acromion in the AP plane.

Required for comprehensive evaluation

True AP and axillary radiographs of the opposite, uninjured shoulder should be obtained for comparison. This comparison can be quite helpful in making the diagnosis, especially in type IV dislocations (posterior). It is also helpful to measure the normal coracoclavicular distance for comparison with the injured side in type III and V dislocations. An AP view with both shoulders on the film is the most accurate means of comparing this distance.

Special considerations

CT and MRI are not necessary as they are typically used only to assess physeal injuries in children. Occasionally, these studies may be useful late in the treatment of AC joint injuries if pain persists and arthrosis or soft-tissue injury is suspected.

Pitfalls

Weighted radiographs, which are often painful, may not be necessary and should not be ordered without consultation with a radiologist.

IMAGE DESCRIPTIONS

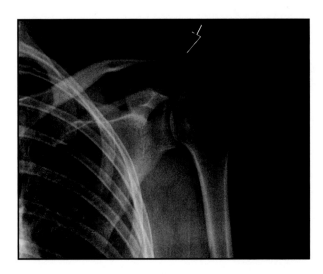

Figure 4-1

Acromioclavicular separation (type II)—AP view

AP view of the left shoulder shows minimal displacement (type II) of the AC joint (black arrow).

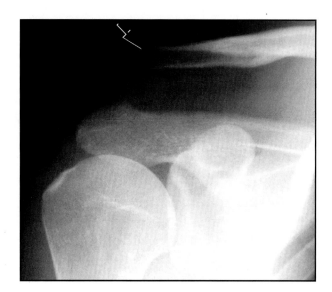

Figure 4-2

Acromioclavicular separation (type III)—AP view

AP view shows a type III AC separation of the right shoulder. Note the location of the clavicle far superior to the acromion (black arrow).

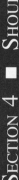

DIFFERENTIAL DIAGNOSIS

AC joint arthritis (osteophytes and AC joint narrowing; bone edema and synovitis)

AC joint osteolysis (focal lytic erosions; AC joint widening)

Fracture of the base of the coracoid (fracture of the coracoid process of the scapula)

Lateral clavicle fracture (fracture distal to the CC ligament insertion)

Rotator cuff tear (tendon injury; no radiographic abnormality except for occasional high-riding shoulder)

SECTION 4 ■ SHOULDER

FRACTURE OF THE CLAVICLE

SECTION 4 ■ SHOULDER

ICD-9 Code

810.00
Fracture of clavicle, closed,
unspecified part

SYNONYM
Broken collarbone

DEFINITION
Fractures of the clavicle are very common, accounting for
approximately 5% of all fractures, and can occur from a fall onto
an outstretched hand or onto the tip of the shoulder. More
commonly, however, these fractures occur in contact sports.
Fractures of the clavicle are classified anatomically as distal,
middle, and medial third. Most fractures are the latter type and
often can be treated nonsurgically.

HISTORY AND PHYSICAL FINDINGS
Crepitus and motion at the fracture site, along with pain, are the
hallmark findings on physical examination. The patient typically has
an obvious deformity and reports pain over the fracture site, along
with the inability to use the arm because of pain. Inspection of the
skin is important during examination because tenting (blanching of
the skin) may compromise the skin's integrity, which can be an
indication for surgical treatment. Vascular examination is especially
critical in widely displaced medial third clavicle fractures because
axillary artery or vein injuries can occur. Auscultation of the chest
is necessary to rule out an associated pneumothorax.

IMAGING STUDIES

Required for diagnosis
AP and 45° cephalic tilt views are needed to make the diagnosis.
The AP view often shows superior displacement of the proximal
fragment and inferior displacement of the distal fragment. The 45°
cephalic tilt view more accurately demonstrates the anteroposterior
relationship of the proximal and distal fragments. For distal third
fractures, anterior and posterior 45° oblique views should be
obtained in addition to the AP view.

Required for comprehensive evaluation
If an intra-articular extension is suspected in a distal third fracture,
CT may be helpful. MRI is rarely indicated for clavicle fracture,
although it may be indicated if associated soft-tissue injuries such
as a rotator cuff tear are suspected. Angiography may be necessary
for medial third clavicle fracture to assess the integrity of the
axillary artery.

Special considerations
None

Pitfalls
In grossly displaced clavicle fractures, it is important to rule out more severe injuries (see Scapulothoracic Dissociation).

IMAGE DESCRIPTIONS

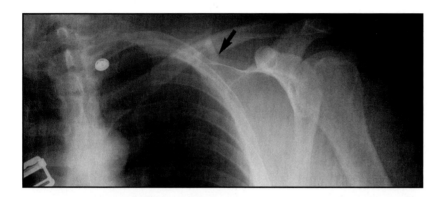

Figure 4-3

Clavicle fracture— AP view

AP view of the left shoulder shows a displaced middle third fracture of the clavicle with comminution (arrow).

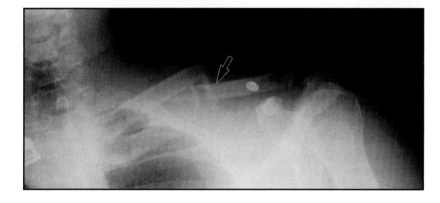

Figure 4-4

Clavicle fracture— 45° cephalic tilt view

This 45° cephalic tilt view of the left shoulder shows a displaced midshaft fracture of the clavicle with comminution (arrow). This view clearly demonstrates the inferior displacement of the distal fragment, which was not seen on the initial AP view.

DIFFERENTIAL DIAGNOSIS

Acromioclavicular instability (displacement of acromion on clavicle at acromioclavicular joint)

Proximal humeral fracture (clavicle in continuity; humeral fracture occurs more distally)

Sternoclavicular instability (displacement of clavicle at sternoclavicular joint)

SECTION 4 ■ SHOULDER

Fracture of the Glenoid

Synonyms

Bony Bankart lesion
Glenoid articular fracture
Shoulder fracture

Definition

Glenoid articular fractures occur as a result of trauma. Fractures of the anterior glenoid rim occur by the same mechanism that causes shoulder instability, with the upper extremity forced into abduction, extension, and external rotation. These are intra-articular fractures and can be displaced, with or without an associated humeral head dislocation. Glenoid fractures may also occur from an axial load to the arm or with high-energy trauma, similar to isolated nonarticular scapular body fractures.

History and Physical Findings

Patients with a glenoid rim fracture will present with the shoulder in slight abduction and external rotation. If the humeral head is dislocated, physical examination will reveal squaring of the shoulder with relative prominence of the acromion. With these fractures, a neurovascular examination is required, with particular attention to the status of the axillary nerve.

Glenoid intra-articular fractures that occur in combination with scapular body fractures are typically associated with other injuries given the high energy and violent nature of the mechanism of injury.

Evaluation of the trauma ABCs (airway, breathing, and circulation) is required, as is neurologic examination of the brachial plexus. Priority in management goes to the potential life-threatening injuries, including pneumothorax, pulmonary contusion, brachial plexus injuries, spinal column injuries, vascular injuries, and other shoulder girdle injuries.

Imaging Studies

Required for diagnosis

A trauma series consisting of AP, transscapular, and axillary views is needed to make the diagnosis. A Velpeau axillary view should be obtained if a standard axillary view cannot be obtained because of pain. To obtain this view, the patient's arm is placed in a sling and then the patient is leaned obliquely backward 45° over the cassette to avoid shoulder manipulation.

Required for comprehensive evaluation

CT with two- or three-dimensional reconstructions may help assess fracture size and identify any displacement, both of which are critical in the evaluation of the intra-articular component of the fracture.

Special considerations

None

Pitfalls

Glenoid articular fractures are commonly seen with glenohumeral dislocations, and the joint congruity should always be evaluated.

IMAGE DESCRIPTIONS

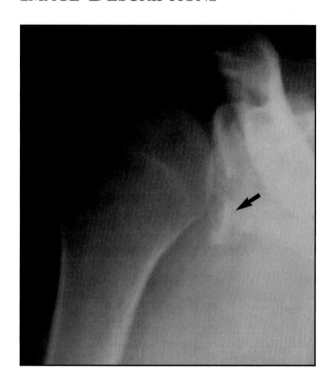

Figure 4-5

Bankart fracture—AP view

AP view of the right shoulder demonstrates an anteroinferior glenoid articular fracture, or bony Bankart fracture (arrow).

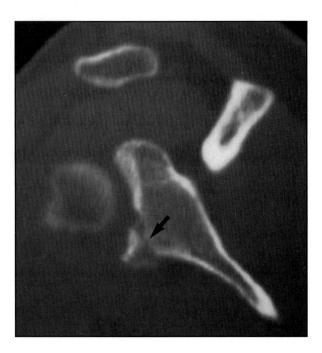

Figure 4-6

Bankart fracture—Axial CT

Axial CT scan of the right shoulder demonstrates a posterior glenoid articular fracture (arrow). These fractures are typically seen in association with posterior glenohumeral dislocation.

DIFFERENTIAL DIAGNOSIS

Acromioclavicular instability (displacement of clavicle at acromioclavicular joint)

Coracoid fracture (cortical disruption of the coracoid bone, best seen on the axillary view)

Glenohumeral instability (labral tear on MRI)

Proximal humeral fracture (disruption of cortex of proximal humerus)

Scapular body fracture (disruption of cortex of scapula)

Sternoclavicular instability (displacement of clavicle at sternoclavicular joint)

FRACTURE OF THE HUMERAL SHAFT

SYNONYM
Fracture of the arm

ICD-9 Code

812.21
Fracture of shaft of humerus, closed

DEFINITION
Fractures of the humeral shaft are classified by their location in the proximal, middle, or distal third of the shaft. The mechanism of injury is either direct or indirect. Trauma from a direct blow is more common and results in transverse or comminuted fracture patterns. Indirect trauma typically results from a fall onto the outstretched hand, resulting in spiral or oblique fracture patterns.

HISTORY AND PHYSICAL FINDINGS
Patients present with pain, swelling, and deformity of the affected arm. A careful neurovascular evaluation is essential with special attention to radial nerve function. Physical examination reveals gross instability and crepitus with gentle manipulation.

IMAGING STUDIES

Required for diagnosis
AP and lateral views of the humerus are needed to make the diagnosis. The joints above and below the fracture site should be included in each view to assess whether the fracture extends beyond the humeral shaft.

Required for comprehensive evaluation
CT and MRI are rarely indicated except for suspected pathologic fracture or established fracture nonunion.

Special considerations
None

Pitfalls
Fractures of both the humeral shaft and the shoulder or elbow result in a floating elbow or shoulder. These are more serious injuries that require immediate attention.

SECTION 4 ■ SHOULDER

IMAGE DESCRIPTION

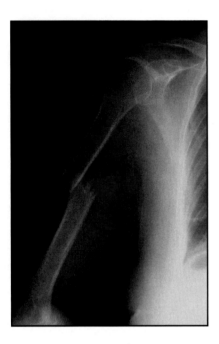

Figure 4-7

Fracture of the humeral shaft—AP view

AP view of the right shoulder shows a midshaft fracture of the humerus. Note the medial displacement of the distal fragment (black arrow).

DIFFERENTIAL DIAGNOSIS

Pathologic fracture (bone neoplasm) (bone resorption seen adjacent to or at the fracture site)

Proximal humeral fracture (disruption of cortex of proximal humerus)

Supracondylar humeral fracture (location of fracture, in the distal third of the humerus)

FRACTURE OF THE PROXIMAL HUMERUS

SYNONYM
Shoulder fracture

ICD-9 Code

812.00
Fracture of humerus, upper end, unspecified part, closed

DEFINITION
Proximal humeral fractures are relatively common shoulder fractures. In older patients with osteoporosis, the mechanism of injury tends to be a low-velocity injury; in younger patients, a high-velocity injury is more common. One common mechanism of injury is a fall onto an outstretched hand.

The bony anatomy of the proximal humerus consists of four major components: the humeral head, the greater tuberosity, the lesser tuberosity, and the humeral shaft. Fractures are classified according to which parts are fractured and the amount of displacement (Fig. 4-8). The humeral head is normally retroverted approximately 30° to 35° and tilted upward 45° in relation to the humeral shaft. The anatomic neck is the junction between the head and the tuberosities, while the surgical neck is just below the tuberosities and the shaft. Proximal humeral fractures are those that occur at or above the surgical neck, which lies just inferior to the tuberosities. All fractures distal to this level down to the elbow are considered humeral shaft fractures.

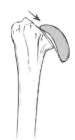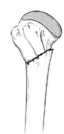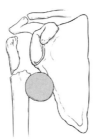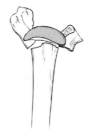

2 Part Fracture
Anatomic neck

2 Part Fracture
Surgical neck

3 Part Fracture
Surgical neck
Greater tuberosity
Shaft

4 Part Fracture
Humeral head
Greater tuberosity
Lesser tuberosity
Shaft

Figure 4-8
Fracture patterns for displaced fractures of the proximal humerus (Neer classification).

(Adapted with permission from Neer CS II: Displaced proximal humeral fractures: I. Classification and evaluation. J Bone Joint Surg Am 1970;52:1077-1089.)

HISTORY AND PHYSICAL FINDINGS
Patients typically report severe pain and may have swelling and bruising around the affected area. They may also report neurologic symptoms depending on the fracture type. Care should be taken to avoid manipulating the affected arm to prevent potential

displacement of a nondisplaced or minimally displaced fracture. The neurovascular examination is also critical, especially in elderly patients, as injuries to the axillary artery, vein, or brachial plexus can occur.

IMAGING STUDIES

Required for diagnosis

Proximal humeral fractures require a trauma series, consisting of a true AP view, a transscapular view, and an axillary view, to make the diagnosis. If the axillary view cannot be obtained because of pain or because movement of the extremity may displace the fracture, a Velpeau axillary view (which is obtained without moving the arm by leaning the patient back over the cassette) should be obtained. This view is important in identifying displacement of the fracture fragments and for excluding concomitant dislocation of the humeral head.

When evaluating radiographs, care should be taken to identify each of the four parts of the proximal humerus, the presence or absence of fracture, and the positions of the fragments. Surgical and anatomic neck fractures are easily identified on AP views. However, these fractures often appear on radiographs similar to an inferior glenohumeral dislocation because of deltoid atony and/or a large intra-articular effusion, which causes pseudosubluxation. Therefore, transscapular and axillary views must be obtained to avoid confusion with a glenohumeral fracture-dislocation. Fractures of the greater tuberosity are best seen on the external rotation AP, transscapular, or axillary views. Isolated greater tuberosity fractures are often seen in association with anterior glenohumeral dislocations, whereas isolated lesser tuberosity fractures are often associated with posterior dislocations.

Required for comprehensive evaluation

If the initial trauma series does not adequately visualize the fracture fragments and pattern, CT or MRI may provide additional information. CT may be helpful in further delineating fracture patterns in more complex, comminuted fractures of the proximal humerus. MRI is best for evaluating occult fractures.

Special considerations

The opposite, uninjured shoulder should be imaged whenever questions arise about subtle abnormalities or when surgical treatment is planned. A true AP view is usually all that is required for preoperative planning purposes. Special tests such as ultrasound are not necessary. Three-dimensional CT reconstructions are rarely required.

Pitfalls

Pseudosubluxation may be mistaken for a true dislocation.

IMAGE DESCRIPTIONS

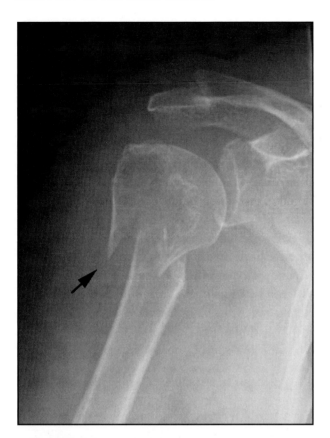

Figure 4-9

Proximal humeral fracture (surgical neck)—AP view

AP view of the right shoulder shows a comminuted fracture of the surgical neck of the proximal humerus (arrow). Note that the fracture extends into the humeral head.

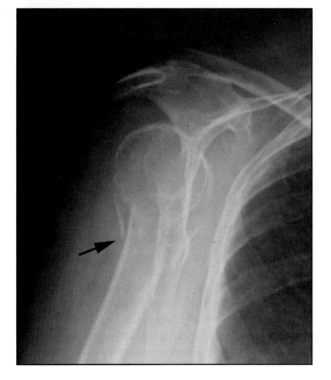

Figure 4-10

Proximal humeral fracture (surgical neck)—Transscapular view

Transscapular view of the right shoulder shows a comminuted fracture of the surgical neck of the proximal humerus (arrow).

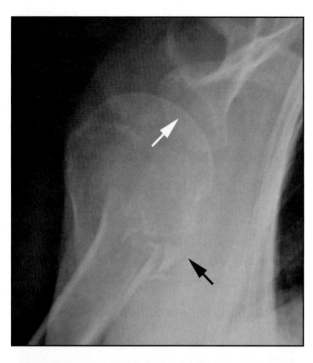

Figure 4-11

Proximal humeral fracture (surgical neck)—Velpeau axillary view

Velpeau axillary view of the right shoulder shows a fracture of the surgical neck of the proximal humerus (black arrow). Note that the humeral head is reduced in the glenoid (white arrow) and no glenohumeral dislocation has occurred.

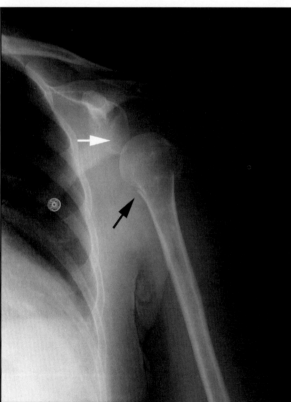

Figure 4-12

Proximal humeral fracture (surgical neck)—AP view

AP view of the left shoulder shows a fracture of the surgical neck of the proximal humerus (black arrow). Note that the humeral head is slightly inferior to the glenoid fossa (white arrow), indicating pseudosubluxation of the humeral head commonly seen as a result of deltoid atony and/or a large intra-articular effusion.

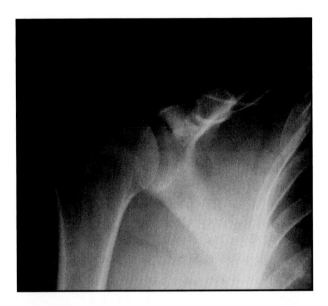

Figure 4-13

*Proximal humeral fracture
(greater tuberosity)—AP view*

AP view of the right shoulder shows a fracture
of the greater tuberosity of the proximal
humerus (arrow).

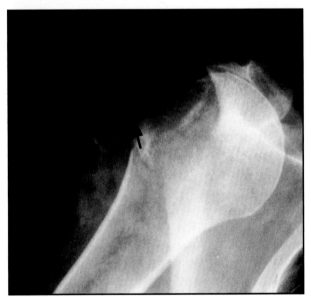

Figure 4-14

*Proximal humeral fracture
(greater tuberosity)—AP view*

AP view of the right shoulder shows an
obviously displaced fracture of the greater
tuberosity of the proximal humerus (arrow).

SECTION 4 ■ SHOULDER

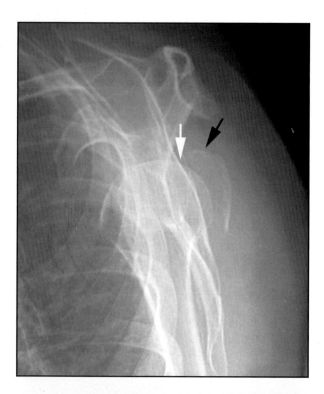

Figure 4-15

Proximal humeral fracture (greater tuberosity)—Transscapular view

Transscapular view of the left shoulder shows a displaced fracture of the greater tuberosity of the proximal humerus (black arrow). Note the fracture fragment is posterior to the humeral head (white arrow).

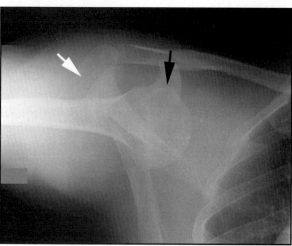

Figure 4-16

Fracture-dislocation of the proximal humerus—AP view

AP view of the right shoulder shows a fracture-dislocation of the proximal humerus. Note that the humeral head is displaced under the coracoid (black arrow) and there is a displaced fracture of the greater tuberosity lateral to the humeral head (white arrow).

DIFFERENTIAL DIAGNOSIS

Glenohumeral instability (bony defect on the anterior glenoid on axillary view)

Humeral shaft fracture (fracture that occurs distal to the proximal third of the humerus)

Pathologic fracture (bone neoplasm) (bone resorption seen adjacent to or at the fracture site)

Rotator cuff tear (no bony injury present)

Scapular fracture (intra- or extra-articular) (disruption of the normal scapular cortex)

FRACTURE OF THE SCAPULA (NONARTICULAR)

SYNONYMS

Acromion fracture
Coracoid fracture
Glenoid neck fracture
Scapular body fracture

ICD-9 Codes

811.00
Fracture of scapula, upper end, unspecified part, closed

811.09
Fracture of other parts of scapula, closed

DEFINITION

Scapular body fractures are not common injuries, but when they occur, they usually result from a high-energy direct blow to the posterior shoulder girdle. Less often, contraction of divergent muscles from electrocution or seizure may fracture the scapular body. Nonarticular fractures occur through the thin, flat triangular portion of the bone that serves as the attachment for the scapular muscles. Fractures may also occur through the scapular spine, coracoid process, or acromion; however, acromial fractures are rare.

HISTORY AND PHYSICAL FINDINGS

Patients with scapular fractures have a high incidence (up to 80% in some studies) of associated injuries because of the high energy and violent nature of these injuries. Therefore, management priorities begin with attention to the trauma ABCs (airway, breathing, and circulation). Neurologic examination of all components of the brachial plexus is required, and a careful vascular assessment is needed because the periscapular collateral circulation may hide a vascular injury. Management focuses on caring for potential life-threatening injuries first, including pneumothorax, pulmonary contusion, spinal column injuries, vascular injuries, and brachial plexus injuries, followed by other shoulder girdle injuries.

IMAGING STUDIES

Required for diagnosis

A trauma series, consisting of a true AP view, a transscapular view, and an axillary view, are needed to make the diagnosis. A chest radiograph is essential to identify associated chest wall injuries, including pneumothorax. The os acromiale is best seen on the axillary view or occasionally on the transscapular view.

Required for comprehensive evaluation

CT with two- or three-dimensional reconstructions improves the assessment of the fracture pattern, displacement, and angulation. MRI can assist in the assessment of soft-tissue injuries, including rotator cuff tears and brachial plexus injuries. Angiography is indicated when vascular injury is suspected.

Special considerations

None

Pitfalls

Scapular fractures are high-energy injuries often seen in association with other life-threatening injuries such as pneumothorax and pericardial effusion. These injuries should always be considered and ruled out.

On radiographs, an os acromiale (unfused acromial apophysis, a normal anatomic variant) appears similar to and is often confused with an acromial fracture. An os acromiale will have a sclerotic margin at the synchondrosis with the rest of the acromion, unlike an acute fracture.

IMAGE DESCRIPTIONS

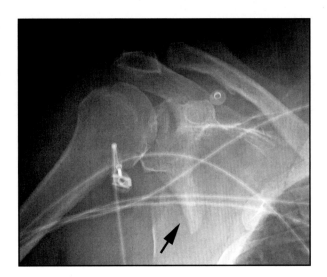

Figure 4-17

Fracture of the scapular body— AP view

AP view of the shoulder of a patient with a fracture of the scapular body shows lack of continuity (arrow) between the proximal and distal portions of the scapular body.

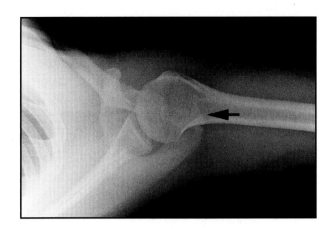

Figure 4-18

Os acromiale—Axillary view

Axillary view of a right shoulder shows an os acromiale at the anterior portion of the acromion (arrow). The os acromiale has a more chronic appearance, with sclerotic margins unlike an acute fracture.

DIFFERENTIAL DIAGNOSIS

Acromioclavicular instability (lateral end of the clavicle higher than the acromion)

Glenohumeral dislocation (humeral head not reduced in the glenoid)

Glenoid articular fracture (disruption in the cortex of the glenoid articular margin)

Proximal humeral fracture (disruption of the cortex of the proximal humerus)

Scapulothoracic dissociation (increased distance from the spinous process to the medial scapular border on the affected side seen on a nonrotated AP view of chest)

Sternoclavicular instability (disruption of the sternoclavicular joint apparent on CT scan)

Glenohumeral Instability

SECTION 4 ■ SHOULDER

Synonyms

Shoulder dislocation
Shoulder subluxation

Definition

The glenohumeral joint is a shallow ball-and-socket joint wherein stability is maintained by the glenohumeral ligaments. Glenohumeral instability occurs when these structures or their bony attachments are torn, resulting in subluxation or dislocation of the humeral head from the glenoid. Radiographs are valuable for diagnosing glenohumeral instability because they can visualize the fractures that are commonly associated with glenohumeral disruption. Examples are Bankart fractures, which result from a disruption of the anteroinferior glenohumeral ligament at its labral attachment to the glenoid rim, and Hill-Sachs lesions, which are posterosuperior fractures of the humeral head that occur in association with anterior dislocations as the humeral head impacts the glenoid rim. Anterior dislocations are far more common than posterior dislocations. Glenohumeral dislocations can occur in patients of all ages. In young athletes, the mechanism of injury typically involves a violent, forceful injury to the arm, while dislocations in the elderly may result from a low-impact fall.

History and Physical Findings

Findings on physical examination will suggest both the mechanism of injury and the direction of the dislocation. Anterior dislocations typically occur with an abduction external rotation force, while posterior dislocations result from violent internal rotation and adduction, as may occur in football blocking or from seizures. The appearance and contour of the injured shoulder will be abnormal compared with the uninjured, opposite shoulder. The hallmark finding of shoulder dislocation is the inability of the examiner to move the arm passively through a full range of motion. Typically, flexion is limited in anterior dislocations, while external rotation is limited in posterior dislocations. Immediate reduction of an acute dislocation is indicated to prevent irreversible damage to the nerves or articular cartilage. Examination of neurologic status may reveal an injury to the axillary nerve.

IMAGING STUDIES

Required for diagnosis

The trauma series, consisting of a true AP, a transscapular view, and an axillary view, is required to confirm the diagnosis and to assess the direction of dislocation as well as the presence of associated fractures. The Hill-Sachs lesion is best seen on the internal rotation AP view, although the West Point or Stryker notch axillary view may also reveal the fracture. Fractures of the anterior or posterior glenoid rim also can be seen best on the axillary view.

Required for comprehensive evaluation

If fractures of the anterior glenoid rim (Bankart fracture) or posterior glenoid rim (posterior Bankart fracture) are suspected in association with an anterior dislocation, CT or MRI may aid in diagnosis. The size of the Bankart fragment (glenoid) and associated Hill-Sachs lesion (humeral head) are important factors in planning treatment. In patients with chronic glenohumeral instability or in acute situations where surgery is contemplated, MRI will reveal the capsuloligamentous integrity and the presence of labral tears (Bankart lesion). MRI is also indicated in patients older than 40 years of age with glenohumeral dislocations because there is a high incidence of rotator cuff tears in this age group.

Special considerations

None

Pitfalls

Missed glenohumeral dislocations can have disastrous consequences, including pain, instability, loss of motion, osteonecrosis, nerve damage, and early degenerative arthritis. Posterior dislocations are the most commonly missed. Glenohumeral dislocations should not be missed if the three views of the trauma series are obtained.

IMAGE DESCRIPTIONS

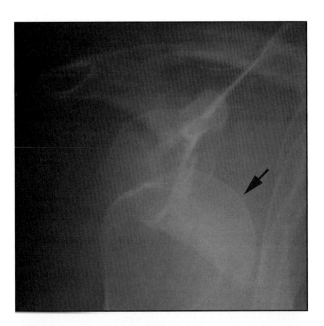

Figure 4-19

*Glenohumeral dislocation
(anterior)—AP view*

AP view of the right shoulder shows an
anterior dislocation of the humeral head
(arrow). Note that the humeral head is inferior
and medial to the glenoid fossa.

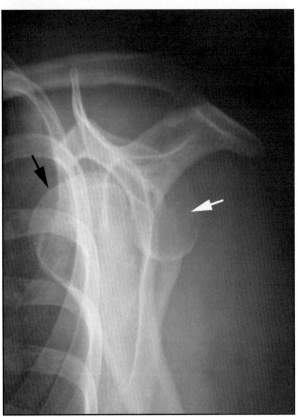

Figure 4-20

*Glenohumeral dislocation
(anterior)—Transscapular view*

Transscapular view shows anterior dislocation
of the humeral head (black arrow). Note that
the entire glenoid is "empty" and is seen in
profile (white arrow).

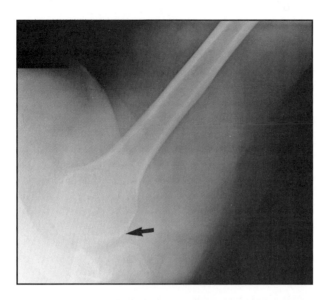

Figure 4-21

Glenohumeral dislocation (anterior)—West Point axillary view

West Point axillary view shows anterior dislocation of the humeral head (arrow). This is the most reliable view for diagnosing anterior glenohumeral dislocations.

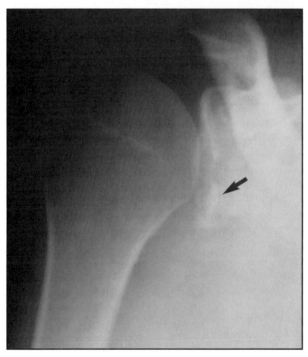

Figure 4-22

Bankart fracture—AP view

AP view of the right shoulder shows an anteroinferior glenoid fracture (bony Bankart lesion). Note that while the humeral head is reduced in the glenoid fossa (arrow) in this image, these fractures are commonly seen in association with anterior dislocations.

SECTION 4 ■ SHOULDER

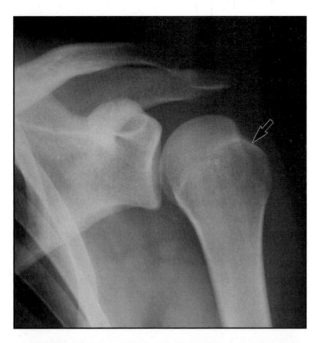

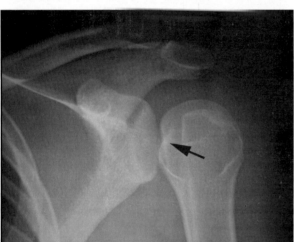

Figure 4-23

Hill-Sachs lesion—AP internal rotation view

AP internal rotation view of the left shoulder shows a superolateral compression fracture, or Hill-Sachs lesion (arrow), which is characteristic of an anterior dislocation of the humeral head.

Figure 4-24

Hill-Sachs lesion (reverse)—AP view

AP view of the left shoulder shows a posterior dislocation of the humeral head. Note that the indentation in the anterior humeral head corresponds to a compression fracture (reverse Hill-Sachs lesion) (arrow). The head may become locked on the rim, rendering the shoulder irreducible. Note the slight overlap of the humeral head on the glenoid. This view is often misread as normal; therefore, with this finding, an axillary view is mandatory.

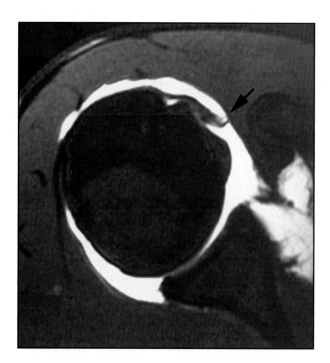

Figure 4-25

Labral Bankart tear—Axial MRI

Axial MRI scan of the right shoulder shows an avulsion of the anteroinferior glenoid labrum. This lesion is typically seen in association with anterior glenohumeral dislocations.

DIFFERENTIAL DIAGNOSIS

Neurologic injury (anteroinferior dislocation on AP view; axillary nerve injury)

Proximal humeral fracture (disruption of cortex of proximal humerus)

Rotator cuff tear (acromial spur; proximal migration of humeral head on radiographs; full-thickness tearing with or without tendon retraction and muscle atrophy on MRI)

Scapular fracture (articular and nonarticular) (disruption of the cortex of the scapula)

OSTEOLYSIS OF THE DISTAL CLAVICLE

ICD-9 Code

715.11
Osteoarthrosis, localized,
primary, shoulder region

SYNONYM

Weight lifter's shoulder

DEFINITION

Osteolysis of the distal clavicle is characterized by resorption of the lateral end of the clavicle. Onset is often insidious and may take many months to complete its course. The etiology is unknown, but some have proposed that it is caused by stress or osteonecrosis. It is much more common in men, especially those who have a history of repetitive microtrauma (eg, wrestlers, weight lifters).

HISTORY AND PHYSICAL FINDINGS

Patients often have a vague recollection of repetitive microtrauma. Physical examination often reveals pain to palpation over the acromioclavicular (AC) joint that increases with a cross-body adduction maneuver. Palpation of the AC joint during the maneuver is necessary to confirm that it is the source of pain. Extension and internal rotation also typically exacerbate the symptoms.

IMAGING STUDIES

Required for diagnosis

AP, transscapular, and axillary views of the shoulder are needed to thoroughly visualize the AC joint. Focal cystic erosions, soft-tissue calcification, and apparent widening of the AC joint space are typical findings.

Required for comprehensive evaluation

Bone scans have been used in the past but are rarely, if ever, necessary. Likewise, MRI is rarely indicated for this diagnosis but may be useful if other diagnoses are suspected.

Special considerations

None

Pitfalls

Osteolysis of the distal clavicle is seldom considered and commonly missed. The AC joint should be carefully assessed in patients with this clinical history.

IMAGE DESCRIPTION

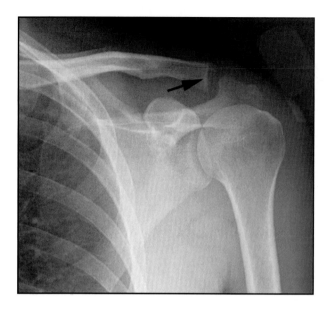

Figure 4-26

Osteolysis of the distal clavicle—AP view

AP view of the left shoulder shows resorption and fragmentation at the lateral end of the clavicle (arrow).

DIFFERENTIAL DIAGNOSIS

AC joint arthritis (osteophytes and narrowing of the AC joint on radiographs; bone edema and synovitis on MRI)

Bone neoplasm (bone resorption involving more than the first few millimeters adjacent to the AC joint)

Impingement syndrome (acromial spur on radiographs; tendinosis or subacromial/subdeltoid edema on MRI)

Rotator cuff tear (acromial spur, proximal migration of humeral head on radiographs; full-thickness tearing with or without tendon retraction and muscle atrophy on MRI)

Septic conditions (AC sepsis) (presence of intra-articular effusion and/or marrow and soft-tissue abnormality in the affected regions on MRI)

SCAPULOTHORACIC DISSOCIATION

ICD-9 Code

726.2
Other affections of shoulder
region, not elsewhere
classified

SYNONYMS
Closed forequarter amputation
Shoulder girdle injury

DEFINITION
Scapulothoracic dissociation is a closed lateral displacement of the
scapula that results from high-energy trauma and is associated with
clavicle fracture and severe soft-tissue injuries. Many patients do
not survive the associated injuries, so the condition is rarely seen
for treatment. Vascular and brachial plexus injuries are very
commonly associated as well, with vascular disruption occurring
most frequently at the level of the subclavian artery and complete
avulsion of the brachial plexus being common. Bony injuries may
include acromioclavicular or sternoclavicular separation or clavicle
fracture. Ipsilateral upper extremity fractures may also be present.

HISTORY AND PHYSICAL FINDINGS
The mechanism of injury is high-energy direct trauma such as
occurs during motorcycle or motor vehicle accidents. Extremities
may be deformed, flail, or pulseless depending on the extent of
brachial plexus and vascular injury.

IMAGING STUDIES

Required for diagnosis
A nonrotated chest radiograph will demonstrate lateral displacement
of the affected scapula compared with the contralateral side.
Displacement can be measured in terms of the distance from the
sternal notch or spinous process of the vertebrae to the coracoid,
glenoid margin, or medial scapular border.

Required for comprehensive evaluation
Neurovascular injury is an unfortunate complication in this severe
injury, which may be described as a closed forequarter amputation.
This is a serious injury that requires immediate consult with an
orthopaedic surgeon. Angiogram may be required in these cases, but
the decision to order this study is left to the surgeon. CT of the
chest may provide additional information in cases where associated
shoulder girdle fractures are suspected. MRI may also reveal severe
soft-tissue injuries at the scapulothoracic articulation.

Special considerations
None

Pitfalls

A rotated radiograph of the chest may incorrectly appear to demonstrate scapulothoracic dissociation. It is imperative to obtain a nonrotated radiograph or a CT scan if necessary.

IMAGE DESCRIPTION

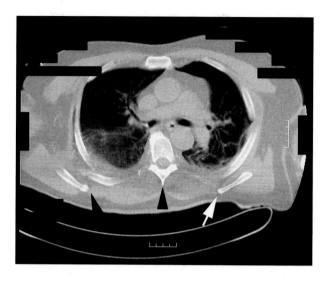

Figure 4-27

Scapulothoracic dissociation— CT scan

CT scan of the chest at the level of the scapulae shows a greater distance from the spinous process (arrowhead) to the medial border of the right scapula (black arrow) than to the left scapula (white arrow), indicating scapulothoracic dissociation on the right side.

DIFFERENTIAL DIAGNOSIS

AC joint instability (displacement of the acromion on the clavicle at the acromioclavicular joint)

Clavicle fracture (disruption of the cortex of the clavicle)

Scapular fracture (disruption of the cortex of the scapula)

Sternoclavicular instability (displacement of the clavicle at the sternoclavicular joint)

SECTION 4 ■ SHOULDER

STERNOCLAVICULAR INSTABILITY

ICD-9 Code

839.61
Dislocation of the sternum,
closed

SYNONYMS

Physeal fracture of the medial clavicle
Sternoclavicular joint separation/dislocation

DEFINITION

The sternoclavicular (SC) joint is the least commonly injured joint
of the shoulder girdle, but when injuries to it do occur, they are
potentially the most severe. Posterior SC dislocations may represent
true musculoskeletal emergencies because compression of the great
vessels, trachea, or esophagus can occur. The mechanism of injury
usually is either a direct blow or an indirect force such as a violent
compression of the shoulder toward the midline. Fortunately, most
SC dislocations occur anteriorly and can be treated with benign
neglect. Misdiagnosis can occur in patients younger than age 25
years because SC dislocations can have the same appearance as
medial clavicular physeal fractures. This physis is the last to fuse,
so these injuries will remodel and rarely require surgical
intervention.

HISTORY AND PHYSICAL FINDINGS

Findings on physical examination are obvious in anterior SC
dislocations given the visible, palpable displacement of the medial
clavicle. However, posterior SC dislocations are not so obvious;
therefore, a careful history, including questions about difficulties
with breathing or swallowing, is imperative to make the diagnosis.
Tenderness to palpation over the SC joint is universally found in
patients with these injuries. Neurovascular examination is usually
normal.

IMAGING STUDIES

Required for diagnosis

An AP view of the chest can sometimes demonstrate the injury
because the relative position of the medial clavicles can be
compared. A 40° cephalic tilt view of both SC joints is needed as
well. With this view, the clavicle will appear larger when dislocated
anteriorly and smaller when dislocated posteriorly. The congruence
of the SC joint should also be assessed, as the superior or inferior
position of the medial clavicle relative to the opposite, uninjured
side may indicate dislocation.

Required for comprehensive evaluation

CT is the imaging modality of choice when SC dislocations are suspected because it allows for thorough evaluation of both joints. Axial CT views are most useful and will define the presence of anterior or posterior dislocation. CT is also helpful in identifying physeal injuries in patients age 25 years and younger.

Special considerations

None

Pitfalls

Posterior SC dislocations can easily be missed. AP, transscapular, and axillary views alone are inadequate for evaluating SC dislocations. MRI is not necessary in these patients.

IMAGE DESCRIPTION

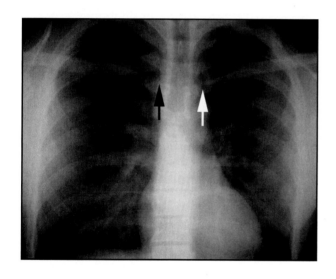

Figure 4-28

Sternoclavicular dislocation— AP view

AP view of the chest shows the superior location of the right medial clavicle (black arrow) compared with that of the left clavicle (white arrow), characteristic of an SC dislocation.

DIFFERENTIAL DIAGNOSIS

Bone neoplasm (bone resorption [lytic lesions] or new bone formation [blastic lesions])

Osteitis of the clavicle (sclerosis of the medial clavicle)

Rheumatoid arthritis (marginal bony erosion, symmetric joint space narrowing, periarticular osteopenia)

Sternoclavicular joint sepsis (history of immunocompromise; bone resorption)

Sternoclavicular osteoarthritis (osteophytes, cysts, loss of joint space)

Neuropathic Shoulder

ICD-9 Codes

336.0
Other diseases of spinal cord, syringomyelia and syringobulbia

713.5
Arthropathy associated with neurologic disorders

716.81
Unspecified arthropathy, shoulder region

Synonym
Charcot arthropathy

Definition
Neuropathic arthropathy is a rare disease of the shoulder that produces extensive and rapid destruction of the proximal humerus and glenoid. Neuropathic arthropathy of the shoulder is often associated with syringomyelia. However, other etiologies have been identified, such as neuropathy related to alcoholism and postoperative neuropathy.

History and Physical Findings
The most frequent presenting symptom is swelling; pain and stiffness are also common. Obvious swelling of the shoulder is sometimes present, and not infrequently, the patient will present with a dislocation of the shoulder. Most patients have neurologic symptoms. On physical examination, decreased range of motion is the most common finding, especially loss of active forward elevation, and decreased passive range of motion is also noted. Deltoid muscle weakness is also a common finding. The neurologic examination often reveals sensory changes in addition to motor weakness. Upper extremity reflexes are often asymmetric. Occasionally, weakness and abnormal neurologic reflexes are evident in the lower extremities.

Imaging Studies

Required for diagnosis
The standard shoulder series, including AP (in the scapular plane) views in neutral, internal, and external rotation and transscapular and axillary views, should be obtained. The most common finding is resorption of the humeral head. Resorption of the glenoid and osseous debris in the soft tissues are additional findings. Dislocations are apparent on the axillary view. Pathologic fractures of the humeral shaft have been described.

Required for comprehensive evaluation
When neuropathic shoulder is suspected and neurologic findings are present, MRI of the cervical spine is appropriate to identify the presence of a cystic lesion, or syrinx, within the spinal cord, characteristic of syringomyelia.

Special considerations

None

Pitfalls

None

IMAGE DESCRIPTION

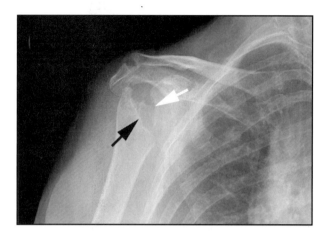

Figure 4-29

Neuropathic shoulder—AP view

AP view demonstrates a pseudosurgical appearance to the humerus with absence of the humeral head (black arrow) and a hypoplastic glenoid (white arrow), consistent with a neuropathic shoulder.

DIFFERENTIAL DIAGNOSIS

Adhesive capsulitis (frozen shoulder) (no radiographic abnormalities)

Bone neoplasm (benign, malignant, or metastatic) (severe cystic erosion with associated soft-tissue mass)

Cervical spondylosis and/or radiculopathy (narrowing of disk spaces and foramen seen on cervical radiographs)

Glenohumeral osteoarthritis (primary or secondary) (osteophyte formation, asymmetric narrowing of glenohumeral joint space, subchondral sclerosis, subchondral cysts)

Gorham disease (vanishing bone disease) (complete absence of bone without associated soft-tissue mass)

Osteonecrosis (subchondral lucency of the humeral head)

Proximal humeral fracture (disruption of the cortex of the proximal humerus)

Rheumatoid arthritis (marginal bony erosion, symmetric joint space narrowing, periarticular osteopenia)

Septic conditions (glenohumeral sepsis, subacromial septic bursitis, AC sepsis) (evidence of intra-articular effusion, joint space narrowing, fluid, or edema on MRI)

Osteoarthritis of the AC and SC Joints

ICD-9 Code

715.11
Osteoarthrosis, localized,
primary, shoulder region

Section 4 ■ Shoulder

Synonyms

Degenerative joint disease
OA

Definition

Osteoarthritis (OA) of the acromioclavicular (AC) and sternoclavicular (SC) joints is a degenerative disease of the articular cartilage. These joints are characterized by the presence of a fibrocartilaginous disk between the articular cartilage surfaces. The AC joint is the articulation of the lateral clavicle with the acromion of the scapula and allows approximately 40° to 50° of rotation through synchronous scapuloclavicular motion. The AC joint itself is relatively incongruous, and degenerative changes have been noted as early as the second decade. The SC joint is the articulation of the medial clavicle with the sternum. Only 50% of the bulbous medial portion of the clavicle articulates with the sternum, giving it the least bony stability of any joint in the body. The SC joint allows 35° of upward motion; a 35° arc of anteroposterior motion; and 50° of rotation around the long axis of the clavicle. OA of the SC joint is typically a result of trauma to the joint and is relatively uncommon.

History and Physical Findings

Pain is the presenting symptom in both types of OA. In patients with OA of the AC joint, the pain is typically reported in the anterior and superior aspects of the shoulder. Often, patients will recall some traumatic event, but it may not have a causal relationship. They often also report pain with activity, specifically when moving the arm across the front of the body (adduction and elevation). A thorough history and physical examination are key in making the diagnosis, because many asymptomatic individuals will have imaging studies that reveal AC joint degeneration.

In patients with OA of the SC joint, pain can be precipitated by any motion of the upper extremity, given the obligate motion at the SC joint. The pain is generally located medially in the region of the joint. Most patients with this type of OA will report a history of a traumatic injury to the joint.

Physical examination should include a thorough evaluation of the shoulder girdle. Direct palpation of the joint (AC or SC) will elicit pain. For the AC joint, cross-body adduction (moving the arm across the front of the body in 90° of elevation) causes discomfort and may reproduce symptoms. Unfortunately, there is no good provocative test for reproducing SC joint symptoms, although the joint may be relatively prominent compared to the unaffected side.

IMAGING STUDIES

Required for diagnosis

A standard five-view series, including AP (in the plane of the scapula) in neutral, external rotation, and internal rotation; transscapular; and axillary views, should be obtained to make the diagnosis. While this joint is best seen on the AP views, its obliquity varies among patients. A criticism of the AP view is that the scapular spine obstructs the view of the inferior aspect of the AC joint. A Zanca view, an AP view taken with a 10° to 15° cephalic tilt, gives an unobstructed view of the AC joint. Joint space narrowing and irregularity, subchondral sclerosis, and the formation of osteophytes and subchondral cysts are findings characteristic of OA.

Routine views of the shoulder are not helpful in diagnosing OA of the SC joint. Special views include the serendipity view, which is taken with the patient supine and the x-ray beam 40° off the vertical, caudad, centered over the sternum. Radiographs will show joint space narrowing, osteophytes, subchondral sclerosis, and cysts. Most of the wear occurs at the inferior aspect of the medial clavicle, and, thus, most degenerative changes are identified in this region.

Required for comprehensive evaluation

MRI can be helpful in the evaluation of a patient with OA of the AC joint. Findings consistent with OA are capsular distention, joint space narrowing and irregularity, subacromial fat effacement, marginal osteophyte formation, and edema of the adjacent subchondral bone. MRI is very sensitive, and many asymptomatic patients will show AC joint changes with this modality. The presence of edema in the adjacent subchondral bone has been correlated with symptomatic OA of the AC joint.

Degenerative changes of the SC joint are best seen on CT or tomography. While tomography is not commonly used, having been largely replaced by CT, it is superior to radiographs in evaluating traumatic and degenerative changes to the SC joint. Findings characteristic of OA in these studies include joint space narrowing, subchondral sclerosis or cyst formation, and osteophyte formation.

Special considerations
None

Pitfalls
Infections are seen more commonly in the SC and AC joints than in the glenohumeral joint, and this diagnosis should always be considered.

IMAGE DESCRIPTIONS

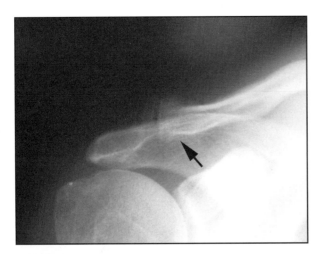

Figure 4-30

Osteoarthritis of the AC joint— AP view

AP view of the right shoulder shows osteophyte formation (black arrow) consistent with a diagnosis of OA. Note that these findings are also common in the general population of asymptomatic individuals; therefore, these findings should be interpreted within a clinical context.

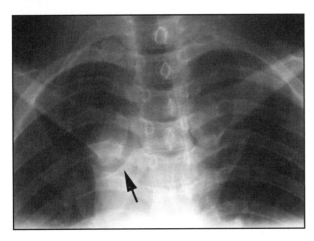

Figure 4-31

Osteoarthritis of the SC joint— AP view

AP view of the SC joints in a patient with OA shows the increased size of the right medial clavicle (black arrow) compared with the left, a characteristic finding of the productive changes and osteophyte formation common in OA.

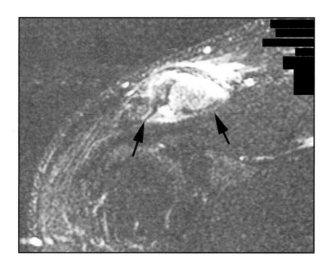

Figure 4-32

Osteoarthritis of the AC joint— Coronal oblique MRI

Coronal oblique T2-weighted MRI scan of the right shoulder in a patient with OA of the AC joint shows increased signal intensity, which indicates edema, in the distal clavicle and medial acromion (black arrows), consistent with a diagnosis of OA.

SECTION 4 ■ SHOULDER

DIFFERENTIAL DIAGNOSIS

Bone neoplasm (benign, malignant, or metastatic) (lytic lesion on plain radiographs)

Calcific tendinitis (calcium in tendons of rotator cuff on plain radiographs; homogeneous abnormally low signal intensity within the tendons on MRI)

Cervical spondylosis and/or radiculopathy (narrowing of disk spaces and foramen on cervical radiographs)

Condensing osteitis of the medial clavicle (occurs in women; productive changes on the medial clavicle)

Impingement syndrome (subacromial spur on plain radiographs; tendinosis or subacromial/subdeltoid edema on MRI)

Rheumatoid arthritis (marginal bony erosion, symmetric joint space narrowing, periarticular osteopenia on radiographs)

Rotator cuff tear (acromial spur, proximal migration of humeral head on radiographs; full-thickness tearing with or without tendon retraction and muscle atrophy on MRI)

Septic conditions (glenohumeral sepsis, subacromial septic bursitis, AC or SC sepsis) (presence of intra-articular effusion, evidence of fluid or edema on MRI)

Seronegative arthropathies (Reiter's syndrome) (conjunctivitis, urethritis)

SLAP (superior labrum anterior and posterior) lesion (tear in superior labrum; best seen on MR arthrogram)

Sternoclavicular hyperostosis (occurs in women; productive changes on the medial clavicle)

OSTEOARTHRITIS OF THE SHOULDER

ICD-9 Code

715.11
Primary osteoarthritis,
shoulder

SYNONYMS

Degenerative arthritis
Degenerative joint disease
Osteoarthrosis

DEFINITION

Degenerative joint disease of the shoulder may result from abnormal forces on a normal shoulder or normal forces on an abnormal shoulder. The overall incidence of osteoarthritis (OA) in an older population ranges from 15% to 20%. Primary OA of the shoulder does occur but less commonly than in the hip or knee, both of which are weight-bearing joints. More typically, OA of the shoulder occurs as a result of an injury such as recurrent dislocations or an intra-articular fracture. Surgical repair for recurrent dislocations in which the anterior capsule is made too tight can result in OA (capsulorrhaphy arthropathy). The typical wear pattern of the glenoid cartilage and bone is posterior.

HISTORY AND PHYSICAL FINDINGS

Patients typically report pain and loss of glenohumeral motion. They also often report a "catching" in their shoulder with certain movements and a history of recurrent dislocation or of a fracture. Any history of steroid use should be noted. Less commonly the history is of insidious onset of pain and loss of motion with no history of injury. In these instances, patients often report difficulty reaching into the back pocket of their pants.

Palpation of the shoulder may reveal anterior or posterior joint line tenderness. Range of motion on the affected side is typically decreased compared with the unaffected side. Crepitation may be present with active and passive motion.

IMAGING STUDIES

Required for diagnosis

A standard five-view series is needed to make the diagnosis, including AP views of the glenohumeral joint in the plane of the scapula in neutral, internal rotation, and external rotation; a transscapular view; and an axillary view. The four primary findings of OA are loss of joint space, subchondral sclerosis, formation of osteophytes, and formation of subchondral cysts. Osteophytes typically form on the inferior surface of the glenoid and proximal humerus. Loose bodies may also be seen. In later stages, posterior wear of the glenoid and posterior subluxation of the humeral head are seen on the axillary view.

Required for comprehensive evaluation

CT may be helpful to assess bony changes such as posterior erosion of the glenoid or to identify loose bodies within the joint. MRI is useful for evaluation of concomitant rotator cuff and labral injury, and to assess potential cartilage damage, if treatment is being considered.

Special considerations

None

Pitfalls

None

IMAGE DESCRIPTIONS

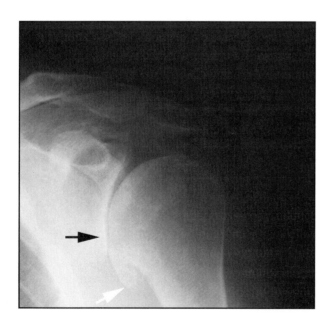

Figure 4-33

Osteoarthritis of the glenohumeral joint—AP view

AP view of the left shoulder shows OA of the glenohumeral joint. Note the characteristic signs of OA, including joint space narrowing, osteophyte formation (white arrow), and subchondral sclerosis (black arrow).

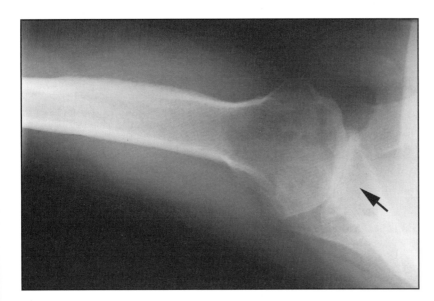

Figure 4-34

Osteoarthritis of the glenohumeral joint—Axillary view

Axillary view of the left shoulder shows OA of the glenohumeral joint. Note the severe loss of joint space and posterior erosion of the glenoid fossa (arrow).

DIFFERENTIAL DIAGNOSIS

AC joint arthritis (osteophytes and narrowing of AC joint on radiographs; bone edema and synovitis on MRI)

Adhesive capsulitis (frozen shoulder) (no abnormalities seen on radiographs)

Bone neoplasm (benign, malignant, or metastatic) (lytic lesion seen on AP view)

Calcific tendinitis (calcium in tendons of rotator cuff on radiographs; homogeneous abnormally low signal intensity within the tendons on MRI)

Cervical spondylosis and/or radiculopathy (narrowing of disk spaces and foramen seen on cervical radiographs)

CPPD crystal deposition disease (same radiographic findings as osteoarthritis; calcifications in the joint possible)

Impingement syndrome (subacromial spur on radiographs; tendinosis or subacromial/subdeltoid edema on MRI)

Neuropathic shoulder (radiographic findings similar to osteoarthritis but sometimes more severe)

Osteonecrosis (subchondral lucency in the humeral head, flattening of the humeral head)

Proximal biceps tendinitis (no abnormalities on radiographs)

Proximal humeral fracture (disruption of the cortex of the proximal humerus)

Rheumatoid arthritis (marginal bony erosion, symmetric joint space narrowing, periarticular osteopenia on radiographs)

Rotator cuff tear (acromial spur, proximal migration of the humeral head on radiographs; full-thickness tearing with or without tendon retraction and muscle atrophy on MRI and arthrogram)

Septic conditions (glenohumeral sepsis, subacromial septic bursitis, AC sepsis) (intra-articular effusion, fluid, or edema signal on MRI)

Seronegative arthropathies (marginal bony erosion, symmetric joint space narrowing, periarticular osteopenia on radiographs)

SECTION 4 ■ SHOULDER

OSTEONECROSIS

ICD-9 Codes

715.21
Osteoarthrosis, localized, secondary, shoulder region

716.81
Other unspecified arthropathy, shoulder region

733.4
Aseptic necrosis of bone

SYNONYMS

Aseptic necrosis
Avascular necrosis of the humeral head
AVN

DEFINITION

Osteonecrosis (ON) of the humeral head is a relatively uncommon condition, but it is the second most common site for ON, after the femoral head. Its clinical course varies but always includes necrosis, or death, of the subchondral bone. The area of the humeral head in contact with the glenoid at 90° of abduction, the superocentral humeral head, is most commonly involved. Known risk factors or etiologies include steroid use, sickle cell disease, trauma, Gaucher's disease, caisson disease, alcoholism, and prior radiation treatment.

With progressive ON, the area of necrosis eventually fractures and is followed by collapse of the humeral head. As the disease progresses, the glenoid is affected with subsequent loss of articular cartilage and progressive arthritic changes. Not all patients progress to end-stage degenerative joint disease.

HISTORY AND PHYSICAL FINDINGS

Not all patients are symptomatic. Some patients are only diagnosed after ON of the femoral head is found and being treated. In patients with early ON, pain is often the most common symptom. Function may be limited but often only because of pain. In the later stages, pain is still the most common symptom; however, as the joint progressively degenerates, loss of motion and function become more common. Bilateral involvement is common.

Physical examination of a patient with early-stage disease may be unremarkable, except for pain with active motion. With advanced disease, findings on physical examination are similar to those in a patient with osteoarthritis, specifically loss of active and passive range of motion. There is no specific clinical test to diagnose ON of the humeral head.

IMAGING STUDIES

Required for diagnosis

A five-view shoulder series consisting of AP (in the plane of the scapula) in neutral, internal, and external rotation; transscapular; and axillary views are needed to make the diagnosis. ON of the humeral head is classified radiographically in stages. Stage I is a preradiographic stage in which radiographs are negative. However, a bone scan may reveal either increased or decreased uptake in the humeral head, and an MRI scan will show characteristic abnormalities on T1-weighted images, including decreased marrow signal intensity. Stage II is characterized by osteoporosis, osteosclerosis, or both on radiographs. A subchondral osteolytic lesion may also be present. Stage III is characterized by a crescent sign (subchondral radiolucent line) that represents a fracture of the subchondral bone with loss of congruity. Stage IV consists of extensive collapse of the subchondral bone, severe articular incongruity, and progressive degenerative changes. In stage V disease, joint space narrowing and pathologic changes of the glenoid are seen in addition to stage IV changes.

Required for comprehensive evaluation

If osteonecrosis is suspected but radiographs are normal, MRI or bone scan can establish the diagnosis, but MRI is preferred because it has greater sensitivity and specificity than a bone scan. MRI is also useful in determining the location and degree of possible subchondral collapse.

Special considerations

None

Pitfalls

Normal radiographs do not rule out ON, especially early in the course of the disease. MRI should be obtained in patients with known risk factors.

SECTION 4 ■ SHOULDER

IMAGE DESCRIPTIONS

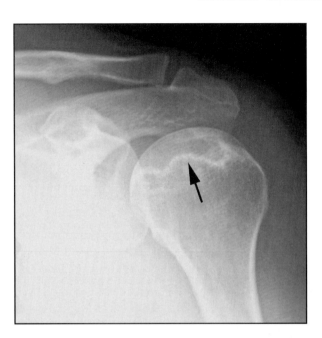

Figure 4-35

Osteonecrosis of the humeral head—AP view

AP view of the right shoulder in a patient with stage II osteonecrosis of the humeral head shows subchondral osteoporosis and sclerosis (black arrow).

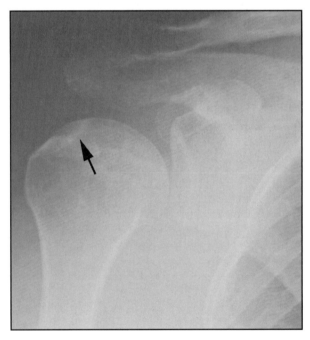

Figure 4-36

Osteonecrosis of the humeral head—AP view

AP view of the shoulder shows the typical area of involvement of ON in the superior aspect of the humeral head (black arrow).

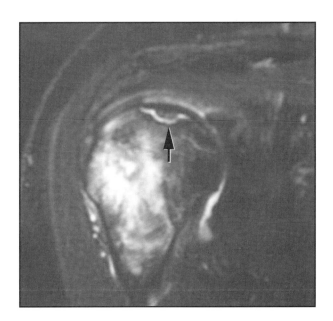

Figure 4-37

Osteonecrosis of the humeral head— Oblique coronal MRI

Oblique coronal fat-suppressed T2-weighted MRI scan of the right shoulder in a patient with osteonecrosis of the humeral head shows involvement of the superior humeral head (black arrow) with surrounding edema in the rest of the humeral head.

DIFFERENTIAL DIAGNOSIS

AC joint arthritis (osteophytes and narrowing of the AC joint on plain radiographs; bone edema and synovitis on MRI)

Adhesive capsulitis (frozen shoulder) (no radiographic abnormalities)

Bone neoplasm (benign, malignant, or metastatic) (visible on MRI)

Cervical spondylosis and/or radiculopathy (narrowing of disk spaces and foramen on cervical radiographs)

Glenohumeral osteoarthritis (primary or secondary) (osteophyte formation, asymmetric narrowing of glenohumeral joint space, subchondral sclerosis, subchondral cysts)

Proximal humeral fracture (disruption of the cortex of the proximal humerus)

Rheumatoid arthritis (marginal bony erosion, symmetric joint space narrowing, periarticular osteopenia)

Septic conditions (glenohumeral sepsis, subacromial septic bursitis, AC sepsis) (presence of intra-articular effusion or edema signal in the affected regions on MRI)

RHEUMATOID ARTHRITIS

ICD-9 Codes

714.0
Rheumatoid arthritis

716.91
Arthropathy, unspecified,
shoulder region

SYNONYMS

Arthritis (monoarticular, pauciarticular, polyarticular)
Inflammatory arthritis
RA
Rheumatism
Rheumatoid factor–positive arthropathy
Seropositive arthritis

DEFINITION

Rheumatoid arthritis (RA) is the prototypic inflammatory arthritis. It is a systemic disease and has a variety of clinical manifestations. The age of onset and number of joints affected varies. Shoulder involvement, often bilateral, is relatively common and may include the glenohumeral joint, acromioclavicular (AC) joint, and occasionally the sternoclavicular (SC) joint. The rheumatoid pannus is the inflamed synovial tissue responsible for erosion of the articular cartilage and also leads to characteristic periarticular erosions. The soft tissues are often thin and atrophic in patients with RA, and concomitant rotator cuff tears are common.

HISTORY AND PHYSICAL FINDINGS

Patients with RA typically have a long history of pain, but loss of motion is less common than in osteoarthritis (OA). It is important to review with patients the history of other joint involvement and drug therapy because many patients are on cytotoxic and immunosuppressive medications. Findings on the physical examination vary, depending on the stage of the disease process. In early-stage RA, patients may have preserved but painful active range of motion. As the disease progresses, the joints may become stiff and more painful, with losses of active and passive range of motion. The overall appearance of the shoulder girdle will often appear atrophic. Any weaknesses of the shoulder girdle, specifically the rotator cuff muscles, should be documented. Lag signs, the hallmarks of tendon rupture, are important to document as well. The AC and SC joints can be a source of pain and must be examined.

IMAGING STUDIES

Required for diagnosis

A standard five-view radiographic series should be obtained, including AP (in the plane of the scapula) in neutral, external rotation, and internal rotation; transscapular; and axillary views. RA in the shoulder joint has a classic appearance: symmetric and global joint space narrowing, periarticular osteopenia, and erosive changes of the humeral head and glenoid. The typical medial erosion of the glenoid is best seen on the axillary view.

One classification system divides the radiologic patterns of glenohumeral RA into four groups: (1) the wet form, which is characterized by periarticular erosions; (2) the dry form, which is similar to OA, with subchondral sclerosis and osteophyte formation; (3) the resorptive form, which is associated with significant bone loss but minimal bone reaction; and (4) the end-stage form, in which there is significant bone loss with structural changes of the joint. Often the inferior glenoid has an articulation with the proximal humeral shaft.

Required for comprehensive evaluation

Because of associated soft-tissue deficiencies (eg, rotator cuff pathology), MRI or ultrasound is very useful in the evaluation of patients with RA. In addition to identifying rotator cuff tears, an MRI scan will show any associated muscle atrophy and the extent of rheumatoid pannus penetration into the associated soft tissues. CT is less commonly used but may provide additional information when severe bony deficiency is present or loose bodies are suspected.

Special considerations

None

Pitfalls

RA can be easily confused with other inflammatory arthritides. It also must be distinguished from cuff tear arthropathy, which has distinct radiographic features.

SECTION 4 ■ SHOULDER

IMAGE DESCRIPTIONS

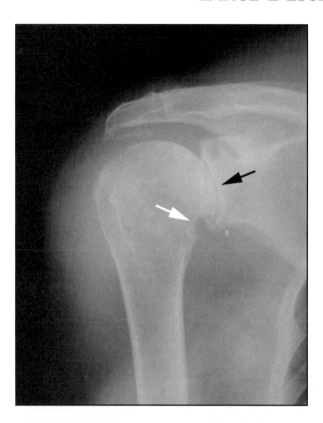

Figure 4-38

Rheumatoid arthritis (shoulder)— AP view

AP view of the right shoulder shows the characteristic findings of RA, specifically loss of joint space in the absence of osteophytes (black arrow). Note the erosive changes, with periarticular erosion of the medial humeral neck (white arrow).

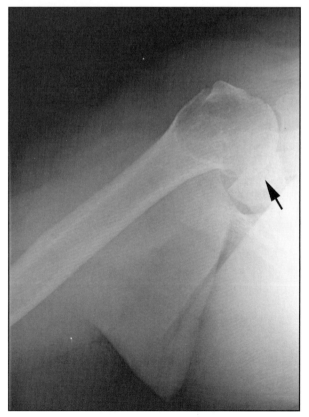

Figure 4-39

Rheumatoid arthritis (shoulder)— Axillary view

Axillary view of the right shoulder shows the characteristic findings of RA, specifically the loss of joint space and medialization of the humeral head as it erodes into the glenoid fossa (black arrow). Note the concentric erosion of the center of the glenoid, in contrast to the eccentric posterior erosion common in OA.

DIFFERENTIAL DIAGNOSIS

Adhesive capsulitis (frozen shoulder) (no radiographic abnormalities)

AC joint arthritis (osteophytes and narrowing of AC joint on radiographs; bone edema and synovitis on MRI)

Bone neoplasm (benign, malignant, or metastatic) (bone resorption [lytic lesions] or new bone formation [blastic lesions])

Calcific tendinitis (calcium in tendons of rotator cuff on radiographs; low signal intensity within the tendons on MRI)

Cervical spondylosis and/or radiculopathy (narrowing of disk spaces and foramen seen on cervical radiographs)

Glenohumeral osteoarthritis (primary or secondary) (osteophyte formation, asymmetric narrowing of the glenohumeral joint space, subchondral sclerosis, subchondral cysts on radiographs)

Impingement syndrome (acromial spur on radiographs; tendinosis or subacromial/subdeltoid edema on MRI)

Neuropathic shoulder (severe lytic changes of the glenohumeral joint with complete bony destruction)

Osteonecrosis (subchondral lucency of the humeral head)

Rotator cuff tear (acromial spur, proximal migration of the humeral head on radiographs; full-thickness tearing with or without tendon retraction and muscle atrophy on MRI)

Rotator cuff tear arthropathy (erosive changes of the inferior acromion and superolateral humeral head with acetabularization of the acromion)

Septic conditions (glenohumeral sepsis, subacromial septic bursitis, AC sepsis) (presence of intra-articular effusion or edema in the affected regions on MRI)

Rotator Cuff Tear Arthropathy

ICD-9 Codes

712.12
Chondrocalcinosis due to calcium diphosphate crystals, upper arm

712.91
Unspecified crystal arthropathy, shoulder region

716.61
Unspecified monoarthritis, shoulder region

Synonyms

Cuff tear arthropathy
Milwaukee shoulder

Definition

Rotator cuff arthropathy is a less common form of glenohumeral arthritis and is distinctly different from other arthritides of the glenohumeral joint. It is characterized by a massive rotator cuff tear and erosive arthritis of the glenohumeral joint. The humeral head migrates upward and abuts against the undersurface of the acromion, resulting in erosive changes (referred to as acetabularization). While the exact etiology is unclear, both mechanical and nutritional factors play a role in its pathogenesis, and there is evidence to support the theory that it is a crystal-induced (basic calcium phosphate) disease.

History and Physical Findings

Patients typically report pain and decreased function; they may also have a history of failed rotator cuff surgery. Recurrent, large sterile effusions (hygromas) are a common finding. Physical examination typically reveals atrophy of the rotator cuff muscles, significant loss of active and passive range of motion, soft-tissue contractures, and fixed subluxations. Palpable and audible crepitus usually accompanies any motion. External rotation is profoundly weak given the absence of the rotator cuff muscles, and lag signs indicating rotator cuff deficiencies are frequent.

Imaging Studies

Required for diagnosis

A standard five-view series, including AP (in the plane of the scapula) in neutral, internal, and external rotation; transscapular; and axillary views are required to make the diagnosis. Classic findings include superior migration, collapse of the humeral head, and erosive changes of the glenoid and acromion resulting in acetabularization. Sclerosis of the greater tuberosity and inferior acromion are common as well.

In later stages, erosion of the coracoid and distal clavicle may be seen on radiographs. Coracoid erosion can be best seen on a West Point lateral view. Anterior or posterior subluxation is often noted on axillary lateral views.

Required for comprehensive evaluation

When the humeral head is seen to articulate with the undersurface of the acromion on a radiograph, the diagnosis of rotator cuff tear can be made with certainty; MRI is not needed. However, if on physical examination, a cystic mass is found in the region of the AC joint, MRI can be helpful to show a communication between the glenohumeral and AC joints—a common finding in cuff tear arthropathy.

CT is rarely used and is indicated only for assessing bony deficiencies such as erosion of the glenoid in preparation for surgery.

Special considerations

None

Pitfalls

The severe erosive changes of rotator cuff arthropathy can be confused with septic or inflammatory arthritis, and these diagnoses should be considered.

IMAGE DESCRIPTIONS

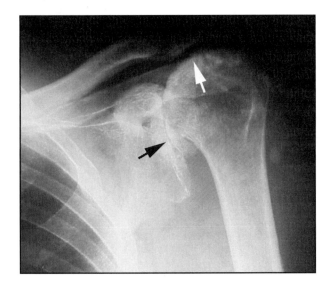

Figure 4-40

Rotator cuff arthropathy—AP view

AP view of the left shoulder in a patient with rotator cuff arthropathy shows the loss of joint space (black arrow) and superior migration of the humeral head relative to the glenoid (white arrow).

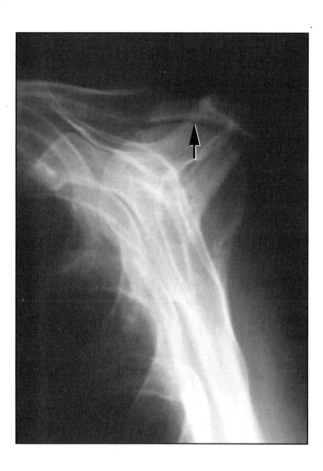

Figure 4-41

Rotator cuff arthropathy— Transscapular view

Transscapular view in a patient with rotator cuff arthropathy shows complete loss of the acromiohumeral interval (space between the acromion and humeral head) (arrow), resulting from complete absence of the rotator cuff.

DIFFERENTIAL DIAGNOSIS

Adhesive capsulitis (frozen shoulder) (no radiographic abnormality)

Bone neoplasm (benign, malignant, or metastatic) (lytic lesion in the humeral head on radiographs and MRI)

Calcific tendinitis (calcium in tendons of the rotator cuff on radiographs; low signal intensity within the tendons on MRI)

Cervical spondylosis and/or radiculopathy (narrowing of disk spaces and foramen seen on cervical radiographs)

Glenohumeral osteoarthritis (primary or secondary) (no superior migration of the humeral head)

Neuropathic arthropathy (marked deformity, resorption of the humeral head)

Osteonecrosis (subchondral lucency of the humeral head)

Rheumatoid arthritis (marginal bony erosion, symmetric joint space narrowing, periarticular osteopenia on radiographs)

Septic conditions (glenohumeral sepsis, subacromial septic bursitis, AC sepsis) (intra-articular effusion or edema in the affected regions on MRI)

CALCIFIC TENDINITIS

SYNONYMS
Calcifying tendinitis
Hydroxyapatite deposition disease (HADD)

ICD-9 Code
726.11
Calcifying tendinitis of
shoulder

DEFINITION
Calcific tendinitis is an idiopathic condition in which the tendons of the rotator cuff, more often the supraspinatus or less commonly the infraspinatus, undergo a process of calcium deposition and subsequent resorption. The disease process tends to affect women more frequently than men, typically in the fourth or fifth decade of life.

The disease is progressive but usually self-limiting. While its etiology remains unknown, calcific tendinitis most likely represents a degenerative condition that results in subsequent calcification. The process is thought to occur in three stages: precalcific, calcific, and postcalcific. The calcific stage consists of two phases: the formative and resorptive phases. The formative phase is marked by calcium deposition within the tendon(s) of the rotator cuff. The resorptive phase is typically the most inflammatory, and therefore the most painful. During this phase, the calcium is often thick and looks and feels like toothpaste. The resorptive phase is followed by the formation of granulation tissue, which occurs as part of a repair response. Eventually, the involved area undergoes fibrosis and tendon reconstitution.

HISTORY AND PHYSICAL FINDINGS
Patients typically report anterosuperior shoulder pain that is focused near the proximal humerus or deltoid region. The pain is of varying intensity, depending on the stage or phase of the disease. Acute episodes may be particularly intense, especially in the resorptive phase. As the disease progresses to the postcalcific stage, pain tends to diminish and eventually resolve.

Physical examination reveals findings similar to those associated with impingement syndrome or rotator cuff pathology. Atrophy, deformity, or swelling are rarely seen. Classic signs of impingement are common, such as pain with overhead positioning of the arm or with internal rotation. A painful arc is often present and occurs as patients report discomfort when they actively lower their arm from 120° to 70° of elevation. In general, range of motion is preserved unless limited by secondary contracture. The neurovascular examination is typically normal.

SECTION 4 ■ SHOULDER

IMAGING STUDIES

Required for diagnosis

A standard five-view series, including AP (in the scapular plane) in neutral, external rotation, and internal rotation; transscapular; and axillary views, is needed to make the diagnosis. The internal and external rotation AP views are particularly necessary because calcium deposits may be obscured by surrounding normal bone. The three AP views will typically show mineralization within the tendons of the rotator cuff. The neutral and external rotation views are particularly useful for visualizing calcium deposits within the supraspinatus tendon. The AP internal rotation or transscapular view is best for showing calcification of the infraspinatus and teres minor tendons. The axillary view demonstrates calcification in the subscapularis tendon. Mineralization may appear with varying degrees of density or opacity on radiographs. Usually, the deposited mineral has an amorphous appearance and no trabecular formation, thereby differentiating this condition from heterotopic ossification.

Required for comprehensive evaluation

Calcific tendinitis is not well seen and is nonspecific on MRI; therefore, conventional radiographs may be needed for correlation.

Special considerations

None

Pitfalls

MRI may demonstrate swelling and edema in the tendon with calcific tendinitis, mimicking tendinosis or rotator cuff tear. The indication for ultrasound in evaluation of calcific tendinitis is limited. It may be helpful in situations in which a rotator cuff tear should be ruled out. Actual visualization of calcium deposits in rotator cuff tendons has been described using this technique.

IMAGE DESCRIPTIONS

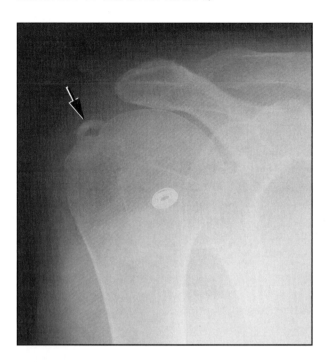

Figure 4-42

Calcific tendinitis—AP external rotation view

AP external rotation view of the right shoulder shows homogeneous curvilinear calcification, consistent with calcific tendinitis of the supraspinatus tendon into the greater tuberosity (arrow). This is a typical location.

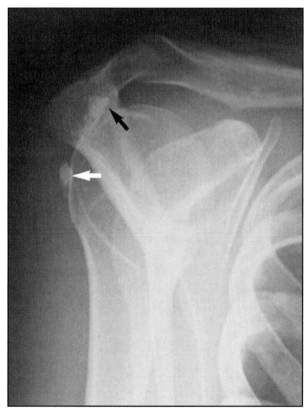

Figure 4-43

Calcific tendinitis— Transscapular view

Transscapular lateral view of the right shoulder shows calcium deposits within the supraspinatus tendon (black arrow). Note an additional deposit posterior within the infraspinatus tendon (white arrow). The information provided in these images underscores the importance of the three orthogonal views, as well as rotational views, to identify this condition.

SECTION 4 ■ SHOULDER

Differential Diagnosis

AC joint arthritis (osteophytes and narrowing of the AC joint on radiographs; bone edema and synovitis on MRI)

Adhesive capsulitis (frozen shoulder) (no radiographic abnormalities)

Cervical spondylosis and/or radiculopathy (narrowing of disk spaces and foramen seen on cervical radiographs)

Glenohumeral osteoarthritis (primary or secondary) (osteophyte formation, asymmetric narrowing of the glenohumeral joint space, subchondral sclerosis, subchondral cysts on radiographs)

Impingement syndrome (acromial spur on radiographs; tendinosis or subacromial/subdeltoid edema on MRI)

Proximal biceps tendinitis (no abnormalities on radiographs)

Proximal humeral fracture (disruption of the cortex of the proximal humerus)

Pulmonary disease (lesion seen on apical view of the chest)

Rheumatoid arthritis (marginal bony erosion, symmetric joint space narrowing, periarticular osteopenia on radiographs)

Rotator cuff tear (acromial spur, proximal migration of the humeral head on radiographs; full-thickness tearing with or without tendon retraction and muscle atrophy on MRI)

Septic conditions (glenohumeral sepsis, subacromial septic bursitis, AC sepsis) (intra-articular effusion, increased fluid or edema signal intensity in the affected regions on MRI)

SLAP (superior labrum anterior and posterior) lesion (tear in the superior labrum; best seen on MR arthrogram)

IMPINGEMENT SYNDROME

SYNONYMS
Rotator cuff disease
Rotator cuff tendinitis
Subacromial bursitis
Subacromial impingement
Subdeltoid subacromial bursitis

ICD-9 Code

726.10
Rotator cuff syndrome NOS

DEFINITION
Inflammation of the subacromial bursa and underlying rotator cuff tendons is a common cause of shoulder pain in middle-aged and elderly patients. The thickened bursa and supraspinatus tendon "impinge" against the undersurface of the coracoacromial arch when the arm is abducted and flexed forward. Anatomic considerations predisposing the development of an impingement syndrome include a prominent acromion and acromioclavicular (AC) joint; a hook-shaped acromion and degenerative spurs on the acromion or lateral aspect of the clavicle may create mechanical impingement on the bursa and rotator cuff. These changes lead to bursitis, tendinitis, and the development of shoulder pain. Occasionally, impingement syndrome may result from associated trauma such as fractures or dislocations of the glenohumeral joint.

HISTORY AND PHYSICAL FINDINGS
The classic history of impingement syndrome consists of shoulder pain, frequently of insidious onset, that is typically focused around the proximal humerus or deltoid region and radiates to the elbow. Anterior shoulder pain may also be seen. The symptoms are typically made worse with overhead activities, repetitive lifting, or reaching behind the back. In young patients, symptoms are associated with throwing or other overhead sports. Patients frequently describe symptoms at night and may have difficulty finding a comfortable position to sleep.

Physical examination should include thorough inspection of the cervical spine and both shoulder girdles. Comparison to the unaffected side is paramount, keeping in mind, however, that some patients may have bilateral involvement. The presence of previous scars or incisions, skin changes, gross deformity, swelling, ecchymosis, erythema, and atrophy should be noted. All anatomic structures, including the clavicle, scapula (spine, coracoid process, and acromion), proximal humerus, sternoclavicular (SC) joint, and AC joint, should be palpated to identify tenderness or crepitus. Typical findings include tenderness over the proximal humerus and pain with passive elevation of the arm (Neer impingement sign) or passive elevation to 90° followed by internal rotation (Hawkins impingement sign). Occasionally, associated tenderness may also be elicited at the AC joint. Active and passive range of motion of the shoulder must be documented, as should strength of the rotator cuff and distal arm, forearm, and hand musculature. A thorough neurovascular examination is necessary as well, including assessment of associated symptoms in the cervical spine and possible radiculopathy.

IMAGING STUDIES

Required for diagnosis

Five standard views, including three AP (neutral, external rotation, and internal rotation), an axillary, and a supraspinatus outlet view, are needed to establish the diagnosis. Subacromial spurs, if large, may occasionally be identified on the AP views. The axillary view visualizes the acromion in the axial plane and documents the location of the humeral head relative to the glenoid. In the supraspinatus outlet view, which is a modified transscapular view, the supraspinatus outlet is visualized, which helps identify acromial morphology, the presence of degenerative changes, and the space available for the rotator cuff. This view is obtained with the x-ray beam angled at a 10° caudal tilt from medial to lateral in the scapular plane. Another useful view to visualize a subacromial spur is an AP view with the x-ray beam angled 30° caudally.

Required for comprehensive evaluation

Additional imaging studies may be considered in patients in whom initial nonsurgical management has failed and a rotator cuff tear is suspected. The presence of antecedent trauma, muscular atrophy, or anatomic deformity also may warrant more advanced studies. Ultrasound, MRI, or arthrography is used in certain circumstances as described below.

Ultrasound previously was an unreliable diagnostic tool for the evaluation of rotator cuff pathology. However, in some centers with skilled radiologists, ultrasound has become a valuable noninvasive means to evaluate the rotator cuff. In patients with impingement syndrome, ultrasound may provide some useful information in evaluating underlying bursitis, edema, and the presence or absence of rotator cuff tears. However, it is not required to diagnose impingement syndrome and should not be considered as an initial diagnostic tool unless nonsurgical treatment has failed.

MRI provides information on the condition of the subacromial and subdeltoid bursae, acromial morphology, the AC joint, and the presence of cysts and muscle atrophy. It is particularly helpful in patients who are believed to have a concomitant rotator cuff tear, or after trauma, where it is helpful in identifying minimally displaced fractures not seen on radiographs. However, MRI should be considered a confirmatory test; it is not required to establish impingement syndrome, which is a clinical diagnosis.

Arthrography of the glenohumeral joint is most helpful in confirming or excluding the presence of a rotator cuff tear in association with impingement syndrome but is not required to diagnose impingement syndrome. Since the advent of MRI, however, arthrography has had limited application, as it is invasive, requires radiation exposure, and provides limited information on the condition of soft tissues beyond plain radiography. Occasionally, arthrography may be combined with either CT or MRI to improve the ability to detect bony or soft-tissue pathology.

Special considerations
None

Pitfalls
None

IMAGE DESCRIPTIONS

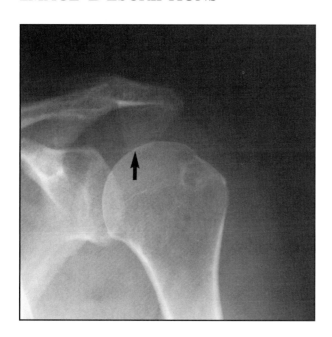

Figure 4-44

Impingement syndrome (subacromial spur)— 30° caudal tilt view

This 30° caudal tilt view of the shoulder shows a large subacromial spur (arrow).

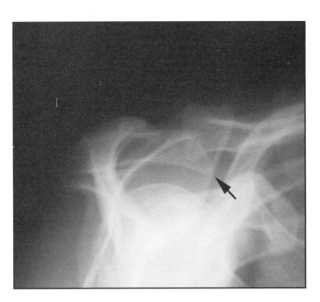

Figure 4-45

Impingement syndrome (hook-shaped acromion)—Transscapular view

Transscapular view of the shoulder shows a hook-shaped acromion (arrow), a finding often seen in association with impingement syndrome, with or without a rotator cuff tear.

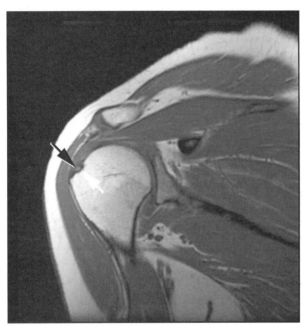

Figure 4-46

Supraspinatus tendinosis—Oblique coronal MRI

Oblique coronal T1-weighted MRI scan of the right shoulder shows swelling and intermediate signal intensity at the insertion of the supraspinatus tendon onto the greater tuberosity (black arrow). Note the cyst located at the insertion point onto the humeral head (white arrow). No full-thickness tearing is seen.

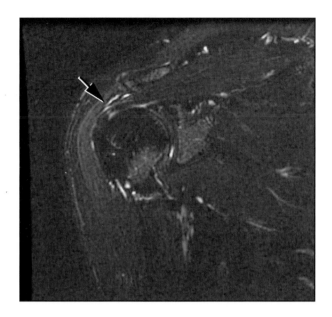

Figure 4-47

Supraspinatus tendinosis— Oblique coronal MRI

Oblique coronal T2-weighted MRI scan of the same shoulder shown in Figure 4-46 demonstrates abnormal signal intensity within the substance of the supraspinatus tendon. A normal tendon will demonstrate a homogeneous, low-intensity signal on T2-weighted images. Here, abnormally high signal intensity (arrow) is noted medial to the tendon insertion onto the greater tuberosity, indicating tendinosis. No full-thickness tearing is seen.

DIFFERENTIAL DIAGNOSIS

AC joint arthritis (osteophytes and narrowing of AC joint on radiographs; bone edema and synovitis on MRI)

Adhesive capsulitis (frozen shoulder) (no radiographic abnormalities)

Bone neoplasm (benign, malignant, or metastatic) (extensive bony erosion or proliferation distorting the normal anatomy of the shoulder)

Calcific tendinitis (calcium in the tendons of the rotator cuff on radiographs; homogeneous hypointense signal within the tendons on MRI)

Cervical spondylosis and/or radiculopathy (narrowing of disk spaces and foramen on cervical radiographs)

Glenohumeral osteoarthritis (primary or secondary) (osteophyte formation, asymmetric narrowing of the glenohumeral joint space, subchondral sclerosis, subchondral cysts)

Rheumatoid arthritis (marginal bony erosion, symmetric joint space narrowing, periarticular osteopenia)

Rotator cuff tear (acromial spur, proximal migration of the humeral head on radiographs; full-thickness tearing with or without tendon retraction and muscle atrophy on MRI and arthrogram)

Superior labrum anterior and posterior (SLAP) tear (tear in the superior labrum; best seen on MR arthrogram)

SECTION 4 ■ SHOULDER

ROTATOR CUFF TEAR

ICD-9 Codes

727.61
Complete rupture of rotator cuff

840.3
Sprains and strains of shoulder and upper arm, infraspinatus

840.4
Sprains and strains of shoulder and upper arm, rotator cuff

840.5
Sprains and strains of shoulder and upper arm, subscapularis

840.6
Sprains and strains of shoulder and upper arm, supraspinatus

SYNONYMS

Infraspinatus tear
Subscapularis tear
Supraspinatus tear
Teres minor tear

DEFINITION

A rotator cuff tear is defined as a disruption of the tendinous portion of the rotator cuff, typically at or near its bony insertion on the proximal humerus; theoretically, it may involve any of the four rotator cuff tendons (infraspinatus, subscapularis, supraspinatus, teres minor). Of these, the supraspinatus tendon is torn most frequently. The acromion and acromioclavicular (AC) joint may be involved as well. Variable acromial morphology and degenerative spurs on the acromion or lateral aspect of the clavicle may create a mechanical impingement on the bursa and rotator cuff; these factors are thought to accelerate tendon degeneration and tear formation.

Rotator cuff tears most commonly occur with aging or in conjunction with impingement syndrome in middle-aged and elderly patients. They rarely are seen in younger patients, but when they occur, it is most often in association with frequent overhead use such as that seen in throwers or other overhead athletes. Traumatic rotator cuff tears are rare in young patients. However, traumatic tears do occur in older patients, particularly following a traumatic glenohumeral dislocation.

HISTORY AND PHYSICAL FINDINGS

Patients typically report pain around the proximal aspect of the humerus or deltoid region. Anterior shoulder pain is also common. The symptoms are often made worse with overhead activities, repetitive lifting, or reaching behind the back. Patients frequently report symptoms at night and may have difficulty finding a comfortable position to sleep. Symptoms are typically worse at night.

As in impingement syndrome, the physical examination begins with full inspection of the cervical spine and both shoulder girdles to identify any atrophy. Particular emphasis should be placed on an assessment of the rotator cuff musculature. All four tendons should be isolated and evaluated to assess integrity and strength. The presence of lag signs, which result from a discrepancy between active and passive rotation of the glenohumeral joint, indicates a relatively large rotator cuff tear and should not be missed. Limited active motion may indicate pain inhibition or true weakness, but differentiating them is often difficult, if not impossible. The use of diagnostic injections of a local anesthetic into the subacromial space (impingement test) can be helpful in making the diagnosis.

Imaging Studies

Required for diagnosis

A five-view series of the shoulder consisting of AP (in the scapular plane), internal rotation, external rotation; transscapular; and axillary views is needed to make the diagnosis. The transscapular view typically shows a curved or hook-shaped acromial morphology and sclerosis of the greater tuberosity at the supraspinatus insertion. In more advanced disease and in the presence of massive rotator cuff tears, the AP view will show that the distance between the top of the humeral head and the acromion (acromiohumeral interval) is decreased to less than 7 mm.

Required for comprehensive evaluation

Advanced imaging studies should be considered if initial nonsurgical management fails or if the patient has limited active range of motion or lag signs. Other conditions in which advanced imaging is appropriate include advanced atrophy of the supraspinatus or infraspinatus fossae or in patients who have symptoms following trauma.

MRI or shoulder arthrography can be used to document a suspected rotator cuff tear. With MRI, typical findings include a discontinuity in the normal course of the tendon adjacent to its insertion. In severe cases, tendon retraction, edema, fatty infiltration, and atrophy of the associated muscles may also be seen. The axial view MRI is particularly helpful in diagnosing subscapularis tendon tears. In cases of subscapularis tears, biceps tendon dislocation from its groove is common and may be a clue to this condition.

Arthrography of the glenohumeral joint is most helpful in confirming or excluding the presence of a rotator cuff tear in association with impingement syndrome. Since the advent of MRI, arthrography is used less often, as it is invasive, requires exposure to radiation, and provides limited information on the soft tissues beyond plain radiography.

Ultrasound may occasionally be used to image rotator cuff tears, particularly full-thickness tears; in many instances, the amount of tendon retraction in both AP and medial-lateral dimensions can be determined.

Special considerations

In the presence of a fracture or bone contusion of the humeral head, MRI may show reactive edema that simulates a rotator cuff tear. Follow-up MRI in 2 to 3 months can clarify the clinical picture.

Occasionally, the use of arthrography may be combined with either CT or MRI to enhance the ability to detect bony or soft-tissue pathology. Glenohumeral contrast (MR arthrogram) may occasionally be required in cases of prior surgery where scarring makes routine imaging difficult. MR arthrogram or CT with air contrast can be used to evaluate tears of the glenoid labrum.

Pitfalls

Occasionally, granulation tissue may fill in a rotator cuff tear, making it difficult to diagnose on arthrography or MRI. Supraspinatus muscle atrophy can also be caused by entrapment of the suprascapular nerve. If MRI or arthrogram does not show a tear, this diagnosis should be considered. Regarding ultrasound, its value depends on the skill of the technician, and few radiology centers in the United States have extensive experience with its application.

IMAGE DESCRIPTIONS

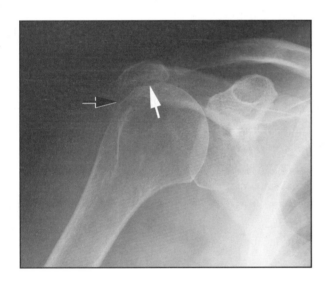

Figure 4-48

Rotator cuff tear—AP view

AP view of the shoulder shows the characteristic findings of rotator cuff tear. Note the sclerosis of the greater tuberosity (black arrow), indicating mechanical impaction between the acromion and the humeral head. Also note the decreased acromiohumeral interval (white arrow), which is consistent with proximal humeral migration and a large to massive rotator cuff tear.

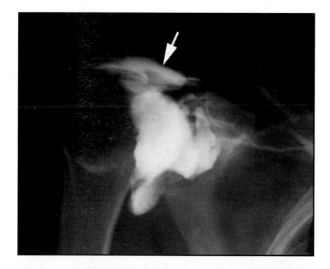

SECTION 4 ■ SHOULDER

Figure 4-49

Rotator cuff tear—AP arthrogram

AP arthrogram of the right shoulder in a patient with rotator cuff tear shows extension of the contrast medium into the subacromial space (arrow), indicating a full-thickness rotator cuff tear.

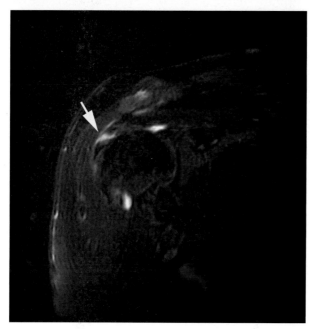

Figure 4-50

Rotator cuff tear (supraspinatus)— Oblique coronal MRI

Oblique coronal fat-suppressed T2-weighted MRI scan shows a focal full-thickness tear in the supraspinatus tendon (arrow).

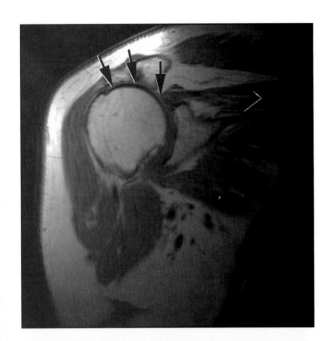

Figure 4-51

Rotator cuff tear (supraspinatus)—Oblique coronal MRI

Oblique coronal T1-weighted MRI scan shows a massive full-thickness tear of the supraspinatus tendon (black arrows) with muscle retraction, fatty infiltration (arrowhead), and atrophy. Note the high-riding humerus closely approximating the acromion.

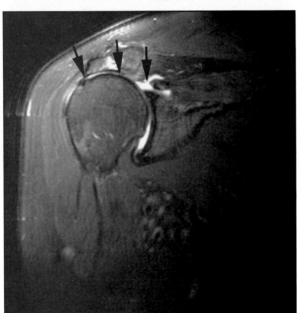

Figure 4-52

Rotator cuff tear (supraspinatus)—Oblique coronal MRI

Oblique coronal T2-weighted MRI scan shows the same patient as in Figure 4-51. The arrows point to the massive full-thickness tear of the supraspinatus tendon.

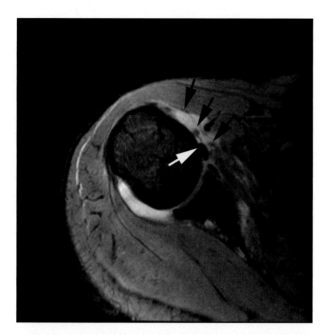

Figure 4-53

Rotator cuff tear (subscapularis)— Axial MRI

Axial gradient echo MRI scan shows a full-thickness tear of the subscapularis tendon (black arrows) with associated biceps tendon dislocation (white arrow).

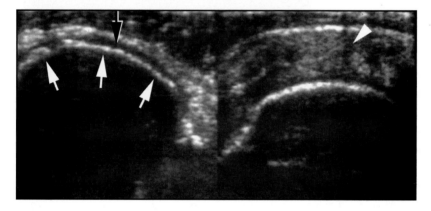

Figure 4-54

Rotator cuff tear— Ultrasound

Transverse bilateral view of the shoulders shows a massive rotator cuff tear of the right shoulder (black arrow). The supraspinatus tendon cannot be seen. Note also that the humeral head on the right is riding high (white arrows) as well. By comparison, the left supraspinatus tendon is normal (arrowhead).

(Courtesy of Fredrick Matsen III, MD.)

DIFFERENTIAL DIAGNOSIS

Acromioclavicular arthritis (osteophytes and narrowing of the AC joint on plain radiographs; bone edema and synovitis on MRI)

Adhesive capsulitis (frozen shoulder) (no radiographic abnormalities)

Calcific tendinitis (presence of calcium in the tendons of the rotator cuff on plain radiographs; homogeneous area of abnormally low signal intensity within the tendons on T2-weighted MRI)

Cervical spondylosis and/or radiculopathy (narrowing of disk spaces and foramen seen on cervical radiographs)

Glenohumeral osteoarthritis (primary or secondary) (osteophyte formation, asymmetric narrowing of the glenohumeral joint space, subchondral sclerosis, subchondral cysts)

Impingement syndrome (acromial spur on plain radiographs; tendinosis or subacromial/subdeltoid edema on MRI)

Rheumatoid arthritis (marginal bony erosion, symmetric joint space narrowing, periarticular osteopenia)

Superior labrum anterior and posterior (SLAP) tear (tear in the superior labrum; best seen on MR arthrogram)

RUPTURE OF THE BICEPS TENDON

SYNONYM
Proximal biceps tendon tear

ICD-9 Code

727.62
Rupture of tendon of biceps
(long head), nontraumatic

DEFINITION
A tear of the proximal biceps tendon is defined as a disruption of the long head of the biceps at or near its origin on the supraglenoid tubercle of the scapula. Rupture can occur at any point within the glenohumeral joint or within the intertubercular groove of the proximal humerus. It most often occurs as part of a spectrum of impingement syndrome and usually is associated with tears of the rotator cuff. A tear of the proximal biceps tendon is distinct from a distal biceps tendon rupture, which occurs at the insertion of the biceps tendon onto the bicipital tuberosity of the radius at the elbow.

HISTORY AND PHYSICAL FINDINGS
The history of a proximal biceps rupture is typically similar to that of impingement syndrome or rotator cuff tear. The condition often develops insidiously, although an episode of significant trauma sometimes precedes more acute tears. The pain associated with such tears may be located more anteriorly than with impingement syndrome; however, pain may also be referred and more generalized. Occasionally, patients report cramping or aching pain distally in the arm, particularly with activities requiring biceps function such as elbow flexion and forearm supination.

The classic physical finding is the presence of a soft-tissue mass in the mid to distal upper arm, proximal to the elbow. This "Popeye" sign, although diagnostic, is not always present and is not required to make the diagnosis. In the setting of an acute or an acute on chronic rupture, ecchymosis or swelling may be noted proximally near the intertubercular groove. With active flexion of the elbow or supination of the forearm, movement of the distal mass may be noted. Once completely ruptured, the tendon origin often becomes less painful. Typically, there is little functional impairment from a rupture of the long head of the biceps, and it seldom needs to be repaired. However, in circumstances of incomplete rupture or isolated biceps tendon degeneration, local tenderness on palpation and/or positive Speed's or Yergason's tests may be present. Motor weakness and impingement signs consistent with impingement syndrome and rotator cuff pathology may be seen as well.

SECTION 4 ■ SHOULDER

Imaging Studies

Required for diagnosis

Diagnostic imaging should begin with the standard shoulder series of five views: AP (in the plane of the scapula) in neutral, external rotation, and internal rotation; transscapular; and axillary. However, no specific radiographic findings are consistent exclusively with biceps tendon tears. Features such as a high-riding humerus, acromial sclerosis, acromial spurs, and tuberosity prominence may be present.

Required for comprehensive evaluation

The diagnosis of a complete rupture of the long head of the biceps is easily made by physical examination. Additional imaging studies are seldom needed. Biceps tendon tears are almost always associated with tears of the rotator cuff. If shoulder pain persists after a biceps tendon rupture, imaging of the rotator cuff and biceps tendon is indicated.

MRI is the most useful diagnostic imaging study for evaluating the proximal biceps tendon. In addition to demonstrating associated subacromial bursitis, inflammation, and rotator cuff pathology, MRI can visualize the proximal biceps tendon. In particular, axial sequences will demonstrate the presence of the long head of the tendon within the tubercular groove. If the tendon has migrated distally after rupture, it may be poorly visualized or absent. Occasionally, the tendon will appear thinned or flattened, and T2-weighted images will show abnormally high signal intensity in the midsubstance, consistent with tendinosis. The tendon may also be seen anteriorly on the oblique coronal sequences, coursing from its origin at the superior aspect of the glenoid, over the humeral head, and into the tubercular groove. Finally, a distal soft-tissue mass with signal intensity similar to that of the surrounding muscle may be seen, although edema may also be present, in addition to the retracted tendon.

Special considerations

Plain arthrography is not recommended for the diagnosis of proximal biceps tears. However, intra-articular contrast medium injected prior to MRI (MR arthrography) can increase the sensitivity of MRI in diagnosing biceps pathology.

Pitfalls

Ultrasound for the diagnosis of biceps pathology is difficult, and few centers in the United States are experienced in its use.

IMAGE DESCRIPTION

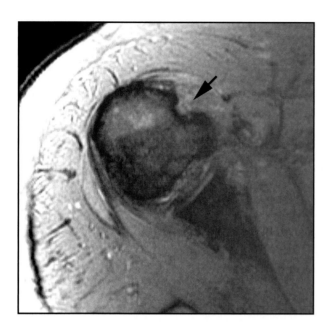

Figure 4-55

Rupture of the proximal biceps tendon—Axial MRI

Axial gradient echo MRI scan of the shoulder shows absence of the biceps tendon in the intertubercular groove (arrow), consistent with a tear.

DIFFERENTIAL DIAGNOSIS

Acromioclavicular arthritis (osteophytes and narrowing of the AC joint on radiographs; bone edema and synovitis on MRI)

Calcific tendinitis (presence of calcium in the tendons of the rotator cuff on radiographs; homogeneous, abnormally low signal intensity within the tendons on MRI)

Glenohumeral osteoarthritis (primary or secondary) (osteophyte formation, asymmetric narrowing of the glenohumeral joint space, subchondral sclerosis, subchondral cysts)

Impingement syndrome (acromial spur on radiographs; tendinosis or subacromial/subdeltoid edema on MRI)

Proximal humeral fracture (disruption of the cortex of the proximal humerus)

Rheumatoid arthritis (marginal bony erosion, symmetric joint space narrowing, periarticular osteopenia)

Rotator cuff tear (acromial spur, proximal migration of the humeral head on radiographs; full-thickness tearing with or without tendon retraction and muscle atrophy on MRI)

Superior labrum anterior and posterior (SLAP) tear (tear in the superior labrum; best seen on MR arthrogram)

RUPTURE OF THE DELTOID AND PECTORALIS MAJOR

ICD-9 Codes

727.6
Rupture of tendon, nontraumatic

840.8
Sprains and strains of shoulder and upper arm, other specified sites

840.9
Sprains and strains of shoulder and upper arm, unspecified site

SYNONYMS
None

DEFINITION
The deltoid and pectoralis major muscles provide most of the power to the arm. The pectoralis major is a large, triangular-shaped muscle that arises from the clavicle, sternum, and ribs and inserts along the bicipital groove of the humerus. Rupture of this muscle is relatively rare and follows extreme muscle tension. Weight lifters are at increased risk, especially when bench pressing weights. Another reported mechanism is an attempt to break a fall. Direct trauma can also result in a tear. The deltoid muscle arises from the outer aspect of the spine of the scapula, the acromion, and the lateral end of the clavicle. It covers the rotator cuff and inserts into the upper end of the humerus. Rupture of the deltoid muscle is very rare. Most cases are iatrogenic in which the deltoid has been detached at surgery and fails to heal after reattachment.

HISTORY AND PHYSICAL FINDINGS
The history of any deltoid or pectoralis major injury most often involves trauma. Patients may report a sudden jerk or pull during exercise or other activity, followed by sudden pain and/or swelling localized to the specific anatomic region. The mechanism of injury may be suggestive of the muscle or tendon involved. For instance, sudden pain or weakness during forceful internal rotation or adduction of the arm may suggest an injury to the pectoralis major, whereas a direct blow to the proximal and lateral aspects of the arm may result in a deltoid injury. Direct trauma can lead to muscle contusion or hematoma as opposed to muscle strain or tendon injury.

Physical examination typically reveals obvious ecchymosis and marked swelling in the upper arm and anterior chest. Local tenderness is also common. The integrity of the pectoralis major can be seen as a normal contour at the proximal aspect of the axilla. When this tendon is completely ruptured, there may be a palpable defect in the area, as well as weakness with resisted adduction of the flexed arm. The tendon is normally palpable at its insertion point on the proximal humerus; its absence suggests disruption of the musculotendinous unit.

The deltoid is also directly subcutaneous and easily examined. It is most often injured by a direct blow, resulting in contusion and potentially hematoma. The tendon origin or insertion is rarely disrupted, although if it occurs, it will likely be associated with violent trauma and concomitant injury. Local swelling and ecchymosis in the area are common on physical examination. Weakness or discomfort with active abduction of the arm may be present as well.

IMAGING STUDIES

Required for diagnosis
A standard five-view series (AP in neutral, internal rotation, and external rotation; transscapular; and axillary views) or, in the setting of acute trauma, a three-view series (AP, transscapular, and axillary views) can be obtained to make the diagnosis. In general, a fracture must be ruled out first, as any direct or indirect injury to the shoulder girdle could potentially produce a fracture. In particular, bony avulsion fractures should be identified, as they may suggest more significant underlying musculotendinous injury.

Required for comprehensive evaluation
When radiographs are negative or inconclusive, additional diagnostic imaging is indicated. MRI is the most helpful for these injuries. T2-weighted images should be scrutinized for swelling, either subcutaneous or intramuscular. Coronal images may be helpful for localizing the deltoid insertion on the proximal humerus; axial images are better for visualizing the pectoralis insertion. If the tendon is disrupted, edema will typically appear as increased signal intensity on T2-weighted images. When there is concern about either of these muscles or tendons, the MRI should contain the entire muscle and tendon groups, as a routine shoulder MRI may not include them entirely.

Special considerations
None

Pitfalls
Arthrography and ultrasound are not typically helpful, although ultrasound may occasionally be used for locating an intramuscular hematoma.

SECTION 4 ■ SHOULDER

IMAGE DESCRIPTION

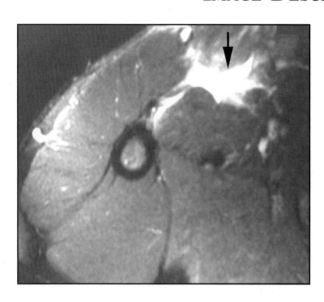

Figure 4-56

Rupture of the pectoralis major tendon—Axial MRI

Fat-suppressed axial T2-weighted MRI scan of the right shoulder shows an acute rupture of the pectoralis major tendon. Note the location of the rupture at the musculotendinous junction, with retraction of the muscle belly medially (black arrow).

DIFFERENTIAL DIAGNOSIS

Cervical spondylosis and/or radiculopathy (narrowing of disk spaces and foramen on cervical radiographs)

Impingement syndrome (acromial spur on radiographs; tendinosis or subacromial/subdeltoid edema on MRI)

Proximal biceps tendinitis (no abnormalities on radiographs)

Proximal humeral fracture (disruption of the cortex of the proximal humerus)

Rotator cuff tear (acromial spur, proximal migration of the humeral head on radiographs; full-thickness tear, with or without tendon retraction, and muscle atrophy on MRI)

Superior Glenoid Labrum Tears

Synonyms

Biceps anchor tear

SLAP lesion

Definition

SLAP is the acronym for a superior labrum anterior to posterior tear or lesion. This condition is defined as a tear involving the superior glenoid labrum that affects, in varying degrees, the proximal biceps anchor. Labral tears in this region range in severity from only degeneration or fraying of a portion of the biceps to frank disruption of the biceps anchor and gross instability. These lesions may occur in association with concomitant intra-articular or extra-articular pathology or in isolation.

History and Physical Findings

The classic history for a SLAP lesion can be hard to define and has resulted in much debate in the literature. It appears that these lesions may develop either acutely, following sudden trauma, or chronically, as a degenerative condition. Typically, traumatic events occur in throwers who may feel a sudden twinge or pop at some point during throwing, or in individuals who fall on an abducted, flexed arm, resulting in an axial load through the glenohumeral joint. When these lesions are seen chronically, it is typically in throwers or other overhead athletes; chronic lesions may also be associated with either rotator cuff tears or subacromial impingement syndrome. Occasionally, SLAP lesions are also seen in laborers whose occupation involves repetitive motion. The location and character of the pain is often similar to that of impingement; however, the symptoms may more typically be activity related, especially activities such as throwing or lifting.

Physical examination findings can also be difficult to define and, like the history, have been the topic of great debate. Examination findings consistent with subacromial impingement or rotator cuff pathology may be positive. In addition, numerous tests have been purported to aid in the diagnosis of the lesion, including the active compression test; biceps load test, modified load and shift, Speed's test, and Yergason's test. However, no test is universally accepted, and the diagnosis is most often made in the setting of the history and physical examination, combined with findings at the time of arthroscopy.

ICD-9 Code

840.7
Superior glenoid labrum lesion

Section 4 ■ Shoulder

IMAGING STUDIES

Required for diagnosis

The five-view shoulder series consisting of AP (in the scapular plane) in neutral, internal rotation, and external rotation; transscapular; and axillary views are needed to make the diagnosis. If radiographs fail to conclusively identify the lesion, other associated pathology should be considered. Impingement syndrome with subacromial spur formation and acromioclavicular joint arthritis are often confused with SLAP lesions, and both have characteristic radiographic findings.

Required for comprehensive evaluation

Advanced imaging studies are indicated when initial nonsurgical management of a suspected impingement syndrome has failed, or if a patient has objective findings potentially consistent with a SLAP lesion.

Special considerations

MRI with intra-articular contrast can aid in diagnosis. Contrast medium is usually recommended because it enhances visualization of pathology compared with standard MRI. However, distinguishing normal labral anatomy (which is variable) from that which is truly pathologic can be difficult. In general, the contrast medium, which clearly tracks beneath the superior labrum and passes onto the superior glenoid rim, will identify detachment of the superior labrum. Thin-cut CT scans with air contrast are also useful in visualizing SLAP lesions.

Pitfalls

Plain arthrography and ultrasound have not been shown to be helpful in the diagnosis of SLAP lesions.

IMAGE DESCRIPTION

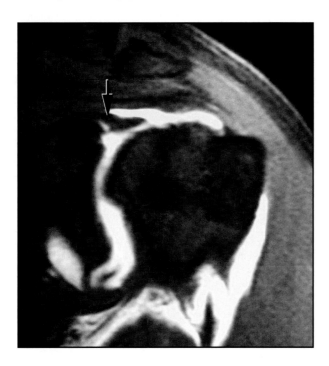

Figure 4-57

SLAP lesion—Oblique coronal MR arthrogram

Oblique coronal T2-weighted MR arthrogram of the left shoulder shows tracking of contrast material medial to the labral attachment (arrow), consistent with a SLAP lesion.

DIFFERENTIAL DIAGNOSIS

Acromioclavicular arthritis (osteophytes and narrowing of the AC joint on radiographs; bone edema and synovitis on MRI)

Calcific tendinitis (calcium in the tendons of the rotator cuff on radiographs; homogeneous low signal intensity within the tendons on MRI)

Cervical spondylosis and/or radiculopathy (narrowing of disk spaces and foramen seen on cervical radiographs)

Glenohumeral instability (history of frank dislocation, bony lesion anterior to the glenoid, anterior capsular tear on MRI)

Glenohumeral osteoarthritis (primary or secondary) (osteophyte formation, asymmetric narrowing of the glenohumeral joint space, subchondral sclerosis, subchondral cysts on radiographs)

Impingement syndrome (acromial spur on radiographs; tendinosis or subacromial/subdeltoid edema on MRI)

Proximal biceps tendinitis (no abnormalities on radiographs)

Rotator cuff tear (acromial spur, proximal migration of the humeral head on radiographs; full-thickness tearing with or without tendon retraction and muscle atrophy on MRI)

ELBOW AND FOREARM

Section Editor
Theodore Blaine, MD

Imaging the Elbow—An Overview

Anatomy

The elbow joint consists of three bones (humerus, radius, and ulna) and three joints (humeroulnar [ulnotrochlear], proximal radioulnar, and humeroradial [radiocapitellar]). The elbow can flex 150°, from 0° (in which the elbow is straight) to 150° of flexion. Viewing the elbow from the front, the forearm long axis deviates 15° outward from the arm, the so-called "carrying angle." The forearm can rotate from up to 90° of supination to up to 90° of pronation. A strong annular ligament holds the radial head in place against the radial notch of the ulna. Two ligaments, the radial collateral and ulnar collateral ligaments, hold the elbow in reduction. The principal elbow flexors are the brachialis, biceps, and brachioradialis. The biceps is the prime supinator of the forearm, whereas the triceps is the prime elbow extensor.

Elbow Fractures in Children and Ossification Centers

Fractures about the elbow joint and forearm are common fractures in children, accounting for 10% to 15% of all children's fractures about the elbow and about 50% of all children's fractures of the forearm. The multiple ossification centers about the child's elbow make interpreting elbow injuries quite difficult in the young child. Secondary centers of ossification usually appear in the following sequence: (1) capitellum at 1 year; (2) radial head at 3 to 6 years; (3) medial epicondyle at 4 years; (4) trochlea at 8 to 9 years; (5) lateral epicondyle at 9 to 10 years; and (6) olecranon at 8 to 10 years.

Standard Imaging Views

Radiographs

AP and lateral views are adequate to evaluate most conditions about the elbow and forearm. Oblique views may be added to further evaluate fractures, if needed. In children, comparison views of the opposite (normal) elbow are often helpful to differentiate an abnormal radiographic appearance because the ossification centers can easily be confused with fractures. Two "lines" are helpful in identifying abnormalities about the elbow. On a lateral view, a line drawn along the anterior cortex of the distal humerus should normally intersect the midportion of the capitellum. Likewise, a line bisecting the proximal radius normally will pass through the midsection of the capitellum, regardless of the degree of elbow flexion.

On a lateral view, the presence of a fat pad sign is a useful indicator of an underlying fracture in the joint. Normally, a small anterior fat pad can be seen but a posterior fat pad usually is not visible. Fat, blood, and marrow are released in intra-articular fractures, causing an elevation of both anterior and posterior fat pads. In adults, the presence of both fat pads often indicates a radial head fracture, whereas in children, a supracondylar fracture should be suspected in this instance. A special view—the radial head view—is helpful in evaluating suspected fractures of the radial head.

Computed tomography

CT combined with contrast medium is useful for detecting osteochondral loose bodies within the joint. Subtle chondral and osteochondral fractures also can be diagnosed with CT. The extent of heterotopic bone formation around the elbow also can be well assessed with CT.

Magnetic resonance imaging

MRI is helpful in diagnosing soft-tissue injuries such as a rupture of the distal biceps tendon and a triceps tendon tear. Tears of the collateral ligaments and joint effusions also can be seen on MRI scans. Osteochondritis dissecans can be evaluated with either MRI or CT.

EMERGENCIES

Three conditions about the elbow constitute emergencies: (1) dislocation, (2) compartment syndrome, and (3) sepsis about the elbow joint. Prolonged dislocation can increase the risk of neurovascular damage and compartment syndrome. Fractures about the elbow place the forearm at risk for a compartment syndrome. Pain that is out of proportion to physical findings and pain that occurs with passive extension of the fingers should prompt referral to a specialist. Pulses may be normal in the presence of a compartment syndrome and therefore cannot be used as a guide to the presence or absence of compartment syndrome. A delay in diagnosis of a septic joint leads to cartilage destruction and a stiff, painful joint.

NORMAL VARIANTS

A number of findings on imaging studies can appear to be a result of trauma or another type of problem when, in fact, they are simply normal variants of anatomy. In the elbow, three bear mentioning. First is the supracondylar process, a bony, hook-shaped process that can occur on the medial aspect of the distal humerus. It may be the source of median nerve entrapment symptoms. The second is the trochlea, which can have several ossification centers that look fragmented and be confused with fractures. Third is the radial tuberosity, which may look like a lytic lesion if the x-ray beam strikes it head on.

IMAGING TIPS

1. Always order two views of the elbow—AP and lateral.

2. In children, order comparison views of the contralateral elbow if there is any question about the diagnosis.

3. Look for the fat pad signs on the lateral view. In adults, a positive fat pad sign may indicate a radial head fracture. In children, a positive fat pad sign may suggest a supracondylar fracture. If there is any question about the diagnosis, an oblique view and radial head view can sometimes detect a radial head fracture.

4. Remember the lines that can help identify abnormalities. A line bisecting the proximal radius should pass through the capitellum, regardless of the degree of elbow flexion; if not, the radial head is dislocated. A line drawn along the anterior humerus should pass through the midportion of the capitellum. If not, suspect a displaced supracondylar fracture.

5. On a lateral view, the normal appearance of the elbow resembles a hockey stick (ie, the distal humerus is angled anteriorly about 40°). Loss of this angle indicates a supracondylar fracture.

6. With a possible dislocation of the radial head, order a radiograph as if you are looking for an ulnar fracture. Likewise, if a fracture of the ulna is present, look for a dislocation of the radial head.

7. In children, the medial epicondyle ossification center appears around age 4 and the trochlea around age 8. In children younger than 8 years who have a history of elbow trauma and have radiographs that show what looks like a trochlea but no medial epicondyle, suspect an avulsion of the medial epicondyle that has displaced into the trochlea's position.

BOTH-BONE FRACTURES

SYNONYM
Diaphyseal fractures of radius and ulna

DEFINITION
Both-bone forearm fractures are shaft fractures of both the radius and ulna. These fractures are common in children but relatively uncommon in adults. Adult both-bone fractures are usually high-energy injuries, with a high incidence of open fractures and associated neurologic injuries.

HISTORY AND PHYSICAL FINDINGS
Patients present with obvious deformity of the forearm, as well as pain and swelling at the fracture site. Assessment of the forearm compartments is necessary, as compartment syndrome can occur. Temporary stabilization with a well-padded forearm splint is acceptable; however, the perfusion and neurologic function of the fingers must be assessed frequently within the first 24 hours. Adult both-bone fractures require surgical stabilization, and early specialty involvement is necessary.

IMAGING STUDIES

Required for diagnosis
AP and lateral radiographs of the forearm, including the elbow and wrist joints, will allow adequate visualization of the fracture pattern and associated injuries.

Required for comprehensive evaluation
None

Special considerations
None

Pitfalls
Forearm compartment syndrome is possible secondary to vascular compromise and swelling. If the patient reports pain out of proportion to physical findings, and if physical examination reveals severe pain with passive extension of the finger, pallor, paresthesias or pulselessness, immediate specialty evaluation is required. An untreated compartment syndrome can lead to permanent neurologic deficit in a matter of hours.

ICD-9 Codes

813.23
Fracture of the radius with ulna

813.33
Fracture of the radius and ulna, ulna (alone)

SECTION 5 ■ ELBOW AND FOREARM

SECTION 5 ■ ELBOW AND FOREARM

IMAGE DESCRIPTIONS

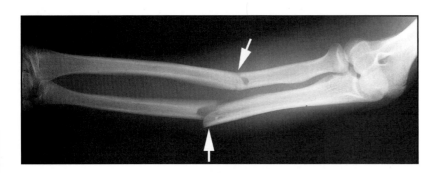

Figure 5-1

Both-bone fracture—AP view

AP view of the forearm in a patient with a both-bone fracture shows that both fractures have occurred at the same level (arrows), which is typical with this injury. There is also angulation at the fracture site. Note also that both the wrist and elbow joints are included in the image.

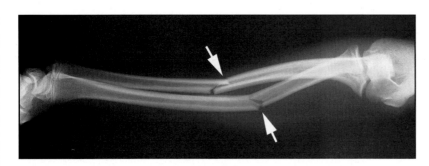

Figure 5-2

Both-bone fracture— Lateral view

Lateral view of the forearm in a patient with a both-bone fracture shows that both fractures have occurred at the same level (arrows), which is typical with this injury. There is also angulation at the fracture site. Note also that both the wrist and elbow joints are included in the image.

DIFFERENTIAL DIAGNOSIS

Galeazzi fracture (fracture of the distal radius with distal radioulnar joint dislocation)

Isolated shaft fracture (fracture of one forearm bone only)

Monteggia fracture (fracture of the proximal ulna with radial head dislocation)

ELBOW DISLOCATION

SYNONYMS
Radiocapitellar dislocation (nursemaid's elbow)
Radiohumeral dislocation
Ulnohumeral dislocation

ICD-9 Codes
832.00
Closed dislocation, of elbow,
unspecified

DEFINITION
Elbow dislocations are common, with an annual incidence of 6 per 100,000 persons, second in frequency only to shoulder dislocations. The elbow is a modified hinge joint that is stabilized by osseous and ligamentous structures. The osseous architecture, including the trochlea, olecranon fossa, coronoid process, and coronoid fossa, is the main contributor to anterior-posterior stability. However, varus-valgus stability is maintained primarily by ligamentous structures. Normal elbow range of motion is 0° to 150° of flexion and 80° of supination and pronation. Minimum functional range of motion is considered to be 30° to 130° of flexion and 50° of supination and pronation.

Elbow dislocations are typically classified based on the relationship of the ulna to the distal humerus. Posterolateral dislocations are the most common, with the highest incidence between the second and third decades of life, and account for more than 90% of elbow dislocations. These injuries are frequently associated with sports activities. Neurologic and vascular injuries can occur; therefore, a careful and well-documented vascular and neurologic exam is necessary. Radial head and/or coronoid process fractures occur in approximately 5% of these injuries.

HISTORY AND PHYSICAL FINDINGS
Patients present with obvious deformity, pain, and swelling at the elbow and require closed reduction with IV sedation or regional anesthesia. Careful neurologic evaluation and documentation are necessary before and after reduction. Following reduction, AP and lateral radiographs must be obtained to confirm anatomic reduction and to assess the presence of associated fractures. Once reduction is verified radiographically, careful assessment and documentation of the stable range of motion is necessary to set limits for rehabilitation. Patients should be placed in a splint at 90° of flexion and referred to a specialist within 5 days of injury. Optimal outcomes are most frequently achieved by beginning range of motion within 13 days of injury; prolonged immobilization has been associated with poor outcomes.

IMAGING STUDIES

Required for diagnosis

AP and lateral radiographs of the elbow should be sufficient for the initial evaluation and should be repeated to confirm reduction.

Required for comprehensive evaluation

MRI may be required for more complete evaluation of a potential ligamentous injury (medial or lateral collateral ligament) once the immediate injury has been addressed and stable reduction achieved.

Special considerations

Isolated dislocations of the radial head are uncommon in adults but are very common in children. These injuries have been called "nursemaid's elbow," as the mechanism of injury involves forceful traction and pronation of the elbow, such as when a nursemaid pulls forcefully on a child's arm. These injuries should be expected in any child with pain and loss of motion of the elbow. Often the radiographs are normal in this condition. Evaluation of location of the radial head with respect to the capitellum, as well as comparison to the opposite normal elbow, is useful when the clinical diagnosis is uncertain. Reduction is easily performed by a skilled physician by supination and flexion of the elbow, occasionally with force directly on the radial head.

Pitfalls

Fractures of the coronoid process or radial head may be associated with elbow dislocations. These injuries should always be suspected when an elbow dislocation occurs. Blocks to motion from fracture fragments following reduction should be assessed and treated (see Fracture of the Coronoid Process and Fracture of the Radial Head).

IMAGE DESCRIPTIONS

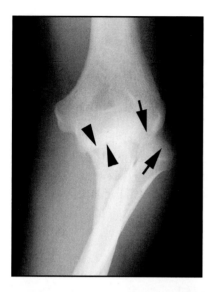

Figure 5-3

Elbow dislocation—AP view

AP view of the elbow in a patient with a posterolateral dislocation shows incongruity of the radiocapitellar (black arrows) and ulnotrochlear articulations (arrowheads), indicating dislocation. No fracture is apparent.

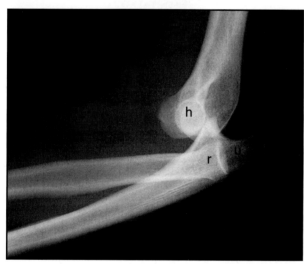

Figure 5-4

Elbow dislocation—Lateral view

Lateral view of the elbow and forearm in a patient with a posterolateral dislocation shows lack of articulation of the radius (r) and ulna (u) with the humerus (h), indicating dislocation. No fracture is apparent.

DIFFERENTIAL DIAGNOSIS

Coronoid process fracture (commonly associated with elbow dislocations; CT occasionally required to make the diagnosis)

Distal humerus fracture (cortical disruption of the distal humerus at the elbow; intra-articular or extra-articular fracture possible)

Monteggia fracture (proximal ulna fracture with radial head dislocation)

Olecranon fracture (cortical disruption of the proximal ulna at the elbow; intra-articular or extra-articular fracture possible)

Radial head fracture (cortical disruption of the radial head, positive fat pad sign on lateral radiograph)

FRACTURE OF THE CORONOID PROCESS

SYNONYM

Elbow fracture-dislocation

DEFINITION

Fractures of the coronoid process are uncommon, but they occur frequently in association with elbow dislocations. A small chip or avulsion fracture of the coronoid on a lateral radiograph of the elbow is highly suggestive of an associated elbow dislocation. Fractures that involve more than 50% of the coronoid process may be associated with persistent elbow instability. Surgical fixation may be required in such cases to restore elbow stability.

HISTORY AND PHYSICAL FINDINGS

Patients typically present with pain, swelling, and ecchymosis about the elbow and may report a history of elbow dislocation. A careful neurovascular examination of the entire extremity is necessary. Application of a well-padded splint with the elbow in 90° of flexion is appropriate. However, if the elbow is stable, the patient should resume early range of motion to prevent excessive elbow stiffness. If an elbow dislocation has occurred or elbow instability is suspected, careful documentation of the stable range of motion is necessary to guide the rehabilitation process. These patients require specialty consultation within 5 days of the injury so that appropriate treatment and rehabilitation can begin.

IMAGING STUDIES

Required for diagnosis
AP, lateral, and oblique views of the elbow are required for diagnosis. The coronoid process may be obscured by the radial head on the lateral view, which is the primary view for diagnosis.

Required for comprehensive evaluation
If a small fragment is suspected, especially if elbow motion is blocked, CT may be necessary because small fragments may not be apparent on radiographs. If ligamentous disruption has occurred with an associated elbow dislocation, MRI may provide additional information, but it is not required in the acute setting.

Special considerations

Small displaced coronoid fragments can block elbow motion and lead to permanent elbow stiffness if not addressed urgently. Range of motion of the elbow should be assessed immediately. If pain limits the examination, an intra-articular injection of lidocaine can allow more accurate assessment of any mechanical block to elbow motion.

Pitfalls

Coronoid fractures are most often seen in association with elbow dislocations. When a coronoid fracture is identified, therefore, a careful history, physical examination, and radiographic evaluation are required to identify elbow dislocations.

IMAGE DESCRIPTIONS

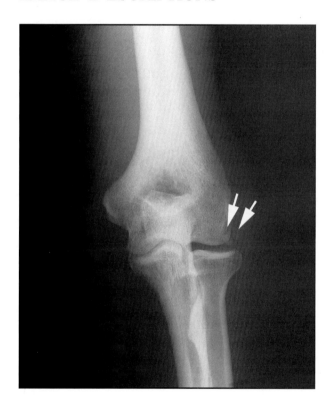

Figure 5-5

Fracture of the coronoid process—AP view

AP view of the elbow reveals that the ulnohumeral and radiohumeral joints are reduced to anatomic alignment. The major coronoid fragment cannot be seen on this view, but smaller comminuted fragments (arrows) are seen laterally.

SECTION 5 ■ ELBOW AND FOREARM

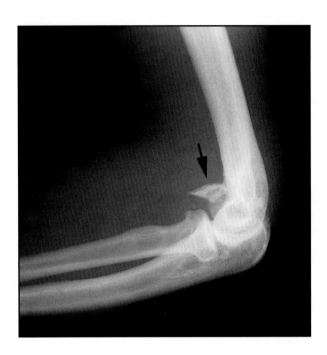

Figure 5-6

Fracture of the coronoid process—Lateral view

Lateral view of the elbow in a patient with a displaced coronoid fracture reveals that the ulnohumeral and radiohumeral joints are reduced to anatomic alignment. Note the large displaced coronoid fragment anterior to the humerus (arrow).

DIFFERENTIAL DIAGNOSIS

Elbow dislocation (incongruity of the distal humerus and the ulna or radius and capitellum)

Monteggia fracture (fracture of the proximal ulna with dislocation of the radial head)

Osteochondral loose body (ossified body in the elbow joint without a fracture)

FRACTURE OF THE DISTAL HUMERUS

SYNONYMS
Intercondylar fracture
Supracondylar fracture
T condylar fracture
Transcondylar fracture
Y condylar fracture

DEFINITION
Traditionally, the distal humerus is described as being composed of a medial and lateral condyle separated by the trochlea. From this anatomic description, fractures of the distal humerus are classified as supracondylar, intercondylar, and transcondylar. Recently the term medial column has been substituted for medial condyle and lateral column for lateral condyle. The traditional classification is used here. Most fractures of the distal humerus are unstable and are best treated surgically with some form of fixation.

Intercondylar fractures are the most common fractures of the distal humerus in adults, accounting for up to 60% of all distal humerus fractures. However, compared with the overall incidence of fractures, intercondylar fractures are rare, accounting for less than 1% of all fractures. The mechanism of injury is usually a fall onto the posterior part of the elbow, driving the ulna into the trochlea and thereby splitting apart the condyles.

Transcondylar fractures occur primarily in elderly patients with osteoporotic bone. The fracture line passes just proximal to the articular surface, extending through the coronoid and olecranon fossa. These fractures are less common, accounting for less than 10% of all distal humerus fractures.

Supracondylar fractures occur above the condyles of the distal humerus and do not have intra-articular extension. These fractures are more common in children and result from a fall on an outstretched hand.

HISTORY AND PHYSICAL FINDINGS
The typical mechanism of injury includes a fall on an outstretched hand, a direct blow to the elbow, or trauma from a motor vehicle accident. Patients report pain, swelling, and limited motion. Physical examination will reveal deformity, ecchymosis, and tenderness to palpation. Any movement of the elbow joint is painful and guarded. A neurovascular examination may reveal injuries to the radial or median or ulnar nerves, as well as arterial injury. Monitoring the forearm for compartment syndrome is essential.

ICD-9 Codes

812.41
Closed fracture of humerus, supracondylar fracture

812.44
Closed fracture of humerus, condyle(s) unspecified

812.51
Open fracture of humerus, supracondylar fracture

SECTION 5 ■ ELBOW AND FOREARM

IMAGING STUDIES

Required for diagnosis
AP, lateral, and oblique views are usually sufficient to define the extent and characteristics of the fracture.

Required for comprehensive evaluation
CT is useful for the specialist to plan surgical reconstruction.

Special considerations
None

Pitfalls
Failure to monitor for compartment syndrome in these patients could have devastating results.

IMAGE DESCRIPTIONS

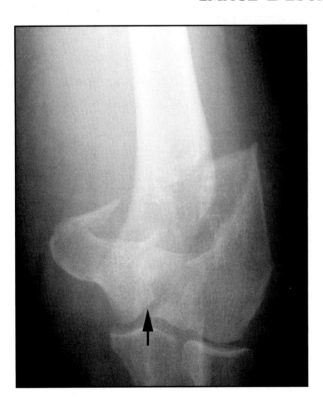

Figure 5-7

Intercondylar fracture of the distal humerus—AP view

AP view of the elbow in a patient with an intercondylar fracture shows that the fracture line extends into the trochlea at the articular surface of the distal humerus (arrow).

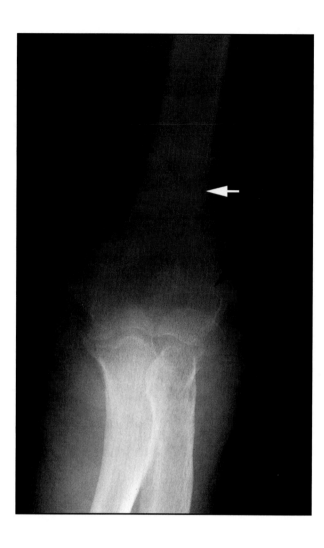

Figure 5-8

Transcondylar fracture of the distal humerus—AP view

AP view of the elbow in a patient with an extra-articular fracture shows that the fracture line is located just above the articular surface (transcondylar) (black arrow). Note the osteopenic appearance of the humerus (white arrow).

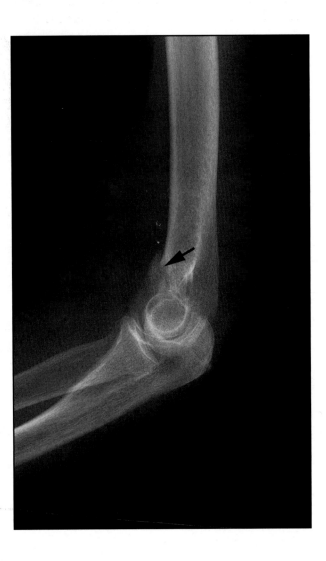

Figure 5-9

Transcondylar fracture of the distal humerus—Lateral view

Lateral view of the elbow in a patient with an extra-articular fracture of the distal humerus shows the fracture line just above the articular surface (arrow). This patient lacks the characteristic fat pad or sail sign.

DIFFERENTIAL DIAGNOSIS

Elbow dislocation (incongruity of the distal humerus and ulna)

Fracture of the olecranon (apparent on radiographs)

Fracture of the radial head (apparent on radiographs)

FRACTURE OF THE OLECRANON

SYNONYM
Proximal ulnar fracture

DEFINITION
Fractures of the olecranon occur as a result of either direct or indirect trauma. The subcutaneous location of the olecranon renders it susceptible to direct trauma in which the olecranon is impacted against the distal humerus, often resulting in comminuted fractures with depression of the articular surface. With indirect trauma, the mechanism is a forceful contraction of the triceps muscle during a fall on an outstretched hand, which usually produces a transverse or short oblique fracture.

HISTORY AND PHYSICAL FINDINGS
Patients present with pain and swelling about the elbow. The most common causes of injury include motor vehicle accidents, falls, and assaults. As these are frequently high-energy injuries, the incidence of associated injuries, including long bone fractures, abdominal injury, pulmonary contusion, and vascular compromise, is as high as 20%. Nondisplaced fractures can be treated nonsurgically, but displaced fractures require surgical intervention and anatomic reduction to reconstruct the articular surface of the olecranon and the extensor mechanism of the elbow. After a careful neurovascular examination; documentation of radial, ulnar, and median nerve function; and careful assessment of skin and distal pulses, a well-padded splint should be applied with the elbow in 30° to 60° of elbow flexion.

IMAGING STUDIES

Required for diagnosis
AP and lateral views of the elbow are necessary for the diagnosis of this injury.

Required for comprehensive evaluation
CT may be useful in cases of severe comminution, but it is rarely required.

Special considerations
Open fractures occur in up to one third of olecranon fractures. These fractures require emergent débridement and fixation, and immediate specialty consultation should be obtained.

SECTION 5 ■ ELBOW AND FOREARM

Pitfalls

Radiographs should be assessed carefully to rule out concomitant elbow subluxation or dislocation, which may occur if the ligaments have been disrupted. Radiohumeral or ulnohumeral dislocations can occur, and if these injuries are suspected, prompt specialty consultation is required.

IMAGE DESCRIPTIONS

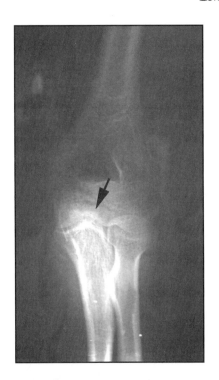

Figure 5-10

Fracture of the olecranon—AP view

AP view of the elbow shows a displaced comminuted olecranon fracture (arrow). Fractures of the olecranon are sometimes difficult to see on the AP view.

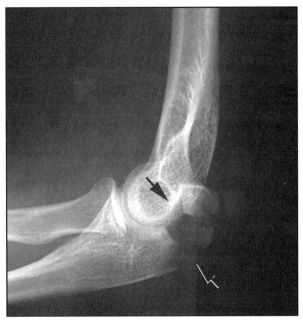

Figure 5-11

Fracture of the olecranon— Lateral view

Lateral view of the elbow shows a displaced comminuted olecranon fracture (arrows). The lateral view is the best view to see fractures of the olecranon. The pull of the triceps muscle tends to displace the proximal fragment.

DIFFERENTIAL DIAGNOSIS

Fracture of the distal humerus (radiographs will show fracture)

Fracture of the radial head (evident on radiographs)

Monteggia fracture (radiographs will show fracture of the proximal ulna with dislocation of the radial head)

FRACTURE OF THE RADIAL HEAD

ICD-9 Code

813.05
    Closed fracture of radial head

813.15
    Open fracture of radial head

SECTION 5 ■ ELBOW AND FOREARM

SYNONYM

Proximal radius fracture

DEFINITION

Radial head fractures are intra-articular fractures of the radius at the elbow that usually occur as a result of a fall on an outstretched hand. Radial head and olecranon fractures account for more than 50% of fractures about the elbow.

HISTORY AND PHYSICAL FINDINGS

Patients present with limited active range of motion and well-localized tenderness directly over the radial head, which can be easily palpated just distal to the lateral epicondyle. Passive pronation and supination of the forearm is very painful and may be limited by a mechanical block. Medial collateral ligament competence should be tested, especially in patients with associated elbow dislocations. A careful neurovascular examination is also important. Occasionally, sterile aspiration of the elbow hemarthrosis and injection of lidocaine will decrease acute pain enough to allow evaluation of passive range of motion. This assessment will help identify a mechanical block to motion.

Nondisplaced fractures can be treated nonsurgically with early range of motion. Displaced and comminuted fractures require surgical intervention for fixation, removal, or replacement, depending on the amount of comminution, the stability of the elbow, and the presence of concomitant injuries. The elbow should be placed in a sling for comfort. Prompt specialty referral is required. Immobilization for longer than 2 weeks has been associated with elbow stiffness and loss of motion; therefore, timeliness of referral is critical.

IMAGING STUDIES

Required for diagnosis
Radiographic evaluation consists of AP, lateral, and oblique views of the elbow.

Required for comprehensive evaluation

A special radial head view also may be indicated when complete assessment from standard views is not adequate. The radial head view is obtained with the forearm resting on its ulnar side, the elbow joint flexed to 90° and the thumb pointing upward. The central x-ray beam is then directed toward the radial head at a 45-degree angle. In cases of comminuted fractures, CT may provide additional information. Additionally, MRI may be helpful when concomitant ligamentous injury (medial collateral ligament or lateral collateral ligament) or occult fracture is suspected.

Special considerations

Nondisplaced radial head fractures are extremely common and are often missed on initial evaluation. If pain is present over the radial head and an intra-articular effusion is present clinically or radiographically, a radial head fracture should be suspected until proven otherwise.

Pitfalls

Mechanical blocks to motion may occur from displaced radial head fragments. A mechanical block to motion can lead to permanent elbow stiffness and must be identified. Both flexion-extension and pronation-supination should be evaluated. Occasionally, sterile aspiration of the elbow hemarthrosis with injection of lidocaine will decrease acute pain enough to allow evaluation of passive range of motion.

Examination of the radioulnar joint is critical to assess for pain. A combined radial head fracture and distal radioulnar joint injury is referred to as an Essex-Lopresti injury, an injury that occurs in less than 5% of radial head fractures. If not identified, an Essex-Loprestri injury may result in significant morbidity secondary to potential proximal migration of the radius following radial head excision.

IMAGE DESCRIPTIONS

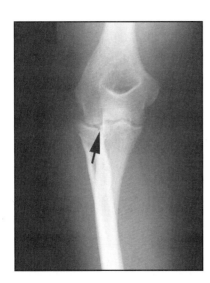

Figure 5-12

Fracture of the radial head—AP view

AP view of the elbow shows a radial head fracture that extends to the articular surface (arrow).

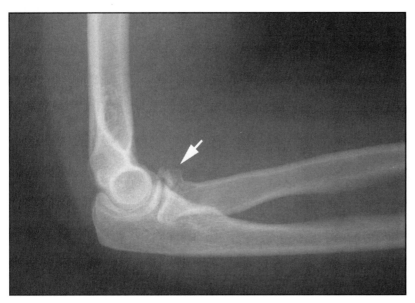

Figure 5-13

Fracture of the radial head—Lateral view

Lateral view of the elbow shows a radial head fracture that is slightly rotated (arrow).

DIFFERENTIAL DIAGNOSIS

Elbow dislocation (incongruity of the distal humerus and the ulna or radius and capitellum)

Coronoid process fracture (displaced coronoid process fractures can be mistaken for radial head fractures; CT is occasionally required to make the diagnosis)

Lateral epicondylitis (no fracture seen on radiographs)

Monteggia fracture (proximal ulna fracture with radial head dislocation)

Radiohumeral arthritis (joint space narrowing, no fracture seen on radiographs)

GALEAZZI FRACTURE

SYNONYMS

Distal radial shaft fracture with distal radioulnar joint dissociation

Piedmont fracture

Reversed Monteggia fracture

DEFINITION

Galeazzi fractures, also referred to as Piedmont fractures, are diaphyseal fractures of the radius at the junction of the middle and distal thirds with dislocation of the distal radioulnar joint (DRUJ). There may be a fracture of the ulnar styloid as well.

HISTORY AND PHYSICAL FINDINGS

Patients have pain and swelling at the distal forearm and wrist and forearm rotation can be very painful. A well-documented neurovascular examination is essential, and adequate radiographic evaluation of the forearm, elbow, and wrist is necessary. After radiographic evaluation, a well-padded forearm splint will comfortably immobilize the injury. These fractures require surgical reduction and stabilization to restore forearm anatomy and function.

IMAGING STUDIES

Required for diagnosis

AP and lateral radiographs of the forearm and wrist are needed to confirm the diagnosis, along with AP and lateral radiographs of the elbow to identify any associated injuries.

Required for comprehensive evaluation

None

Special considerations

Once the radius has been repaired, surgical attention needs to be directed at the distal radioulnar joint. The lateral radiographs of the wrist should be obtained in neutral rotation or in supination because the normal, uninjured distal radioulnar joint will not appear reduced with the wrist in pronation. A cross-sectional imaging study such as CT is often required to evaluate for distal radioulnar joint dislocation, as radiographs can be misleading.

ICD-9 Codes

813.40
Fracture of radius and ulna, distal end unspecified

833.01
Closed dislocation of wrist, unspecified

SECTION 5 ■ ELBOW AND FOREARM

Pitfalls

Unrecognized Galeazzi fractures can lead to permanent distal radioulnar joint dysfunction and chronic wrist pain. Therefore, complete physical and radiographic evaluation of the wrist is necessary when fractures of the distal radial shaft are identified.

IMAGING DESCRIPTIONS

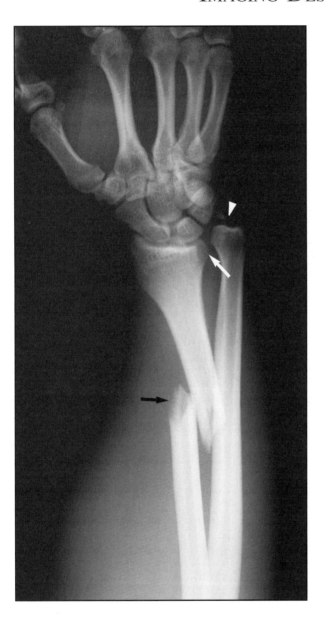

Figure 5-14

Galeazzi fracture—AP view

AP view of a forearm and wrist in a 15-year-old boy shows a fracture of the distal third of the radius (black arrow) and a dislocation of the distal radioulnar joint (white arrow). Note also the fracture of the ulnar styloid (arrowhead) and the positive ulnar variance (the ulna is longer than the radius).

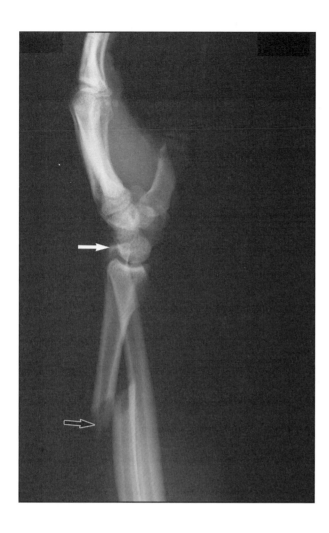

Figure 5-15

Galeazzi fracture—Lateral view

Lateral view of the patient shown in Figure 5-14 shows that the distal radial fracture fragment is displaced dorsally (black arrow). This view also shows the positive ulnar variance (white arrow).

DIFFERENTIAL DIAGNOSIS

Distal radioulnar dislocation (no fracture seen on radiographs)

Distal radius fracture (metaphyseal Colles, fracture; more common and occurs distal to the radial diaphysis)

Isolated radial shaft fracture (no distal radioulnar joint injury, appears reduced on lateral radiographs)

ISOLATED SHAFT FRACTURES

ICD-9 Codes

813.21
Closed fracture of radius and ulna, radial shaft alone

813.22
Closed fracture of radius and ulna, ulnar shaft alone

813.31
Open fracture of radius and ulna, radial shaft alone

813.32
Open fracture of radius and ulna, ulnar shaft alone

SYNONYMS
Nightstick fracture
Radial shaft fracture
Ulnar shaft fracture

DEFINITION
Isolated ulnar shaft fractures, also known as nightstick fractures, usually occur from direct trauma to the subcutaneous border of the ulna and are more common than isolated fractures of the radius. Isolated radial shaft fractures must be scrutinized more carefully because the anatomic radial bow may cause loss of forearm rotation.

HISTORY AND PHYSICAL FINDINGS
Patients typically have pain, swelling, and ecchymosis over the ulnar or radial aspect of the forearm. As with all other fractures, a careful neurovascular evaluation and assessment of skin integrity overlying the fracture are necessary. These injuries are safely treated acutely with a forearm splint, and most nondisplaced ulnar fractures can be treated nonsurgically and will heal without difficulty. The exception is an isolated fracture of the radius with significant displacement because nonanatomic alignment of the radius may obstruct forearm rotation.

IMAGING STUDIES

Required for diagnosis
AP and lateral radiographs of the forearm are necessary to establish the diagnosis. AP and lateral views of the wrist and elbow joints are also necessary when associated dislocations (Monteggia or Galeazzi) are suspected.

Required for comprehensive evaluation
None

Special considerations
None

Pitfalls

The proximal and distal articulations (radiohumeral joint, distal radioulnar joint) must be examined to rule out associated dislocations, as seen in Monteggia and Galeazzi fractures. Failure to obtain AP and lateral radiographs of both the elbow and the wrist can result in missing these associated injuries. Cross-sectional imaging such as CT may be necessary to evaluate for subtle radioulnar joint dislocation, as radiographs can be misleading.

IMAGE DESCRIPTIONS

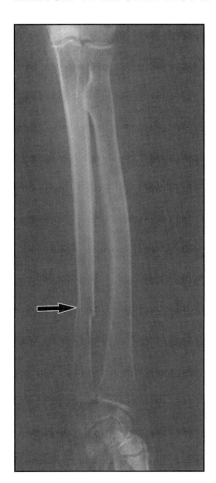

Figure 5-16

Fracture of the ulna—PA view

PA view of the forearm shows an isolated fracture of the ulna (arrow) at the junction of the middle and distal thirds with only minimal displacement. This fracture is sometimes called a nightstick fracture, as it results from a direct blow to the ulna.

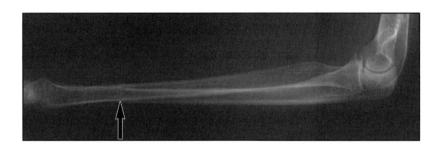

Figure 5-17

Fracture of the ulna— Lateral view

Lateral view of the forearm shows the same fracture as in Figure 5-16 and demonstrates that the fracture ends are in good alignment (arrow).

DIFFERENTIAL DIAGNOSIS

Both-bone forearm fractures (cortical disruption with or without displacement of both the radius and ulna, usually at the same or adjacent level)

Galeazzi fracture (fracture of the distal radius with distal radioulnar joint dislocation)

Monteggia fracture (fracture of the proximal ulna with radial head dislocation)

MONTEGGIA FRACTURE

SYNONYM
Proximal ulnar shaft fracture with associated radial head dislocation

DEFINITION
Monteggia fractures are fractures of the ulnar shaft, typically the proximal ulna, with an associated dislocation of the radial head. These injuries are more common in children, but they also occur in adults. Adult Monteggia injuries are usually caused by high-energy trauma, including falls from heights and motor vehicle accidents.

HISTORY AND PHYSICAL FINDINGS
Patients present with pain along the ulnar border of the forearm and at the elbow. Physical examination requires a thorough neurovascular evaluation with documentation of radial, ulnar, and median nerve function. Of these, the radial nerve is most frequently injured. AP and lateral radiographs of the elbow, forearm, and wrist are necessary to assess the fracture pattern and look for any associated injuries. Management includes reduction of the radial head, splinting with the elbow at 90° of flexion, and prompt specialty referral. Definitive treatment requires surgical intervention for anatomic reduction of the ulnar fracture and radial head dislocation.

IMAGING STUDIES

Required for diagnosis
AP and lateral radiographs of the elbow, forearm, and wrist are necessary to assess the fracture pattern and identify any associated injuries.

Required for comprehensive evaluation
None

Special considerations
None

Pitfalls
Unrecognized Monteggia fractures can lead to permanent elbow joint dysfunction and chronic wrist pain. Therefore, complete physical and radiographic evaluation of the elbow is necessary when fractures of the proximal ulnar shaft are identified. An AP view of the wrist must be included.

ICD-9 Codes

813.03
Monteggia fracture, closed

813.13
Monteggia fracture, open

SECTION 5 ■ ELBOW AND FOREARM

IMAGE DESCRIPTION

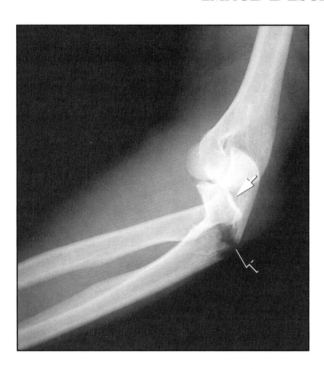

Figure 5-18

*Monteggia fracture (elbow)—
Lateral view*

Lateral view of the elbow shows a displaced fracture of the ulna (black arrow) and posterior dislocation of the radial head (white arrow), consistent with a Monteggia fracture.

DIFFERENTIAL DIAGNOSIS

Coronoid process fracture (commonly associated with elbow dislocations; CT occasionally required to make the diagnosis)

Distal humerus fracture (cortical disruption of the distal humerus at the elbow; fracture may be intra-articular or extra-articular)

Elbow dislocation (incongruity of the distal humerus and the ulna or radius and capitellum without fracture of the ulna)

Olecranon fracture (cortical disruption of the proximal ulna at the elbow; fracture may be intra-articular or extra-articular)

Radial head fracture (cortical disruption of the radial head)

Heterotopic Ossification

Synonyms
Ectopic bone
Heterotopic bone
HO
Myositis ossificans

ICD-9 Code

728.10
Muscular calcification and
ossification, unspecified

Definition
Heterotopic ossification (HO) is defined as bone formation that
occurs in the soft tissues. These formations may present as an
extension from native bone or may form de novo within muscle
(myositis ossificans). The rapid and abundant bone formation of HO
distinguishes these formations from the osteophytes of osteoarthritic
joints. Direct trauma to the muscle usually precedes myositis
ossificans.

History and Physical Findings
Patients who have experienced elbow trauma such as a dislocation,
surgery for a fracture-dislocation of the elbow, or distal biceps
repair are at risk for developing HO. Traumatic brain injury and
third-degree burns are also risk factors for the development of HO.

Radioulnar synostosis is a type of HO in which a bridge of bone
fuses the radius to the ulna. This condition is most often seen with
fracture of the radius, ulna, or both. The formation can also occur
secondary to soft-tissue injuries. A congenital form of radioulnar
synostosis also exists.

Patients with HO about the elbow may be completely
asymptomatic except for the bone mass. Of reported symptoms,
pain and loss of motion are the most common. With radioulnar
synostosis, limited forearm rotation and pain are common.

Imaging Studies

Required for diagnosis
AP and lateral views are used for evaluation of HO. Radiographs
can reveal bone extending posteriorly from the olecranon, which
would limit extension, or ectopic bone that creates a bridge from
the humerus to the ulna. In the latter case, little if any motion is
possible. If limited forearm rotation is the primary symptom,
radiographs of the elbow and forearm should be obtained. With
radioulnar synostosis, bone bridging the ulna and radius is present.

SECTION 5 ■ ELBOW AND FOREARM

Required for comprehensive evaluation
In situations in which surgery is being considered, CT with sagittal reconstructions can be extremely helpful in visualizing the location and extent of bone formation.

Special considerations
None

Pitfalls
None

IMAGE DESCRIPTIONS

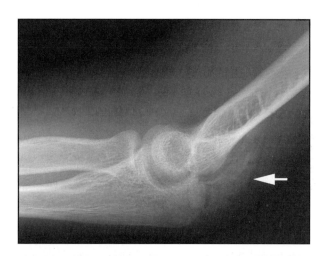

Figure 5-19

Heterotopic ossification (elbow)— Lateral view

Lateral view of the elbow demonstrates heterotopic ossification extending posteriorly (arrow).

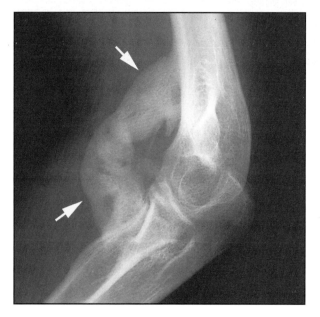

Figure 5-20

Heterotopic ossification (elbow)— Lateral view

Lateral view of the elbow demonstrates heterotopic ossification in the anterior soft tissues, creating a bony bridge (arrows) that extends from the distal humerus to the ulna and radius.

DIFFERENTIAL DIAGNOSIS

Osteoarthritis (osteophytes, joint space narrowing, cystic erosions, subchondral sclerosis)

Osteochondral loose bodies (multiple small, discrete, usually round bodies of bone or cartilage present within the elbow joint)

Posttraumatic arthritis (radiographic features similar to osteoarthritis, history of prior trauma)

Soft-tissue contracture (no additional bone formation seen on any imaging study)

Tumor (productive or destructive osseous changes with associated soft-tissue mass)

SECTION 5 ■ ELBOW AND FOREARM

OLECRANON BURSITIS

ICD-9 Code
726.33
Olecranon bursitis

SYNONYM
Coal miner's bursitis

DEFINITION
Olecranon bursitis, or inflammation of the olecranon bursa, is confined to the bursa overlying the olecranon process and does not involve the elbow joint. The condition has several etiologies, including overuse, inflammation, infection, and trauma. Alcoholism and diabetes mellitus have been found to be predisposing factors. In addition, a history of hemodialysis and the use of anticoagulants have been shown to be risk factors.

HISTORY AND PHYSICAL FINDINGS
A careful history should be taken, including questioning about the risk factors named above. Rheumatoid arthritis or gout can present with olecranon bursitis. When the bursitis is caused by overuse, onset is usually insidious and painless. Acute bursitis is sometimes seen with direct-impact injuries. The condition is painful in the presence of infection. Septic bursitis should be suspected in patients with a history of fever, erythema, and tenderness, although these findings are not specific. A more specific finding is elevated skin temperature over the septic bursa relative to that of the contralateral arm. When the condition is symptomatic, the patient usually experiences bursal pain when the elbow is flexed more than 90°. This helps to distinguish olecranon bursitis from a septic joint, where the entire arc of motion is painful. The bursa itself is most often completely filled with fluid. Bogginess may indicate rheumatoid arthritis.

IMAGING STUDIES

Required for diagnosis
AP and lateral views of the elbow should be obtained to rule out a foreign body or underlying arthropathy. Increased soft-tissue density of varying degrees may be seen in the area of the bursa. Olecranon spurs have been implicated in olecranon bursitis, but their presence is not always causal.

Required for comprehensive evaluation

Ultrasound or MRI can be used to assess the extent of disease and to determine whether the mass is cystic or solid. Olecranon bursitis is confined to the bursa overlying the olecranon process and does not involve the elbow joint, but it may be associated with intra-articular involvement in patients with rheumatoid arthritis. The presence of a "fat pad" sign or other intra-articular findings (eg, erosions) suggests an associated intra-articular process.

Special considerations

Distinguishing between septic and aseptic bursitis can sometimes be difficult. Preexisting cellulitis can become bursitis. The organism most commonly associated with septic bursitis is *Staphylococcus aureus*. Aspiration of the bursa with culture and Gram stain is necessary to confirm the diagnosis.

Pitfalls

None

IMAGE DESCRIPTION

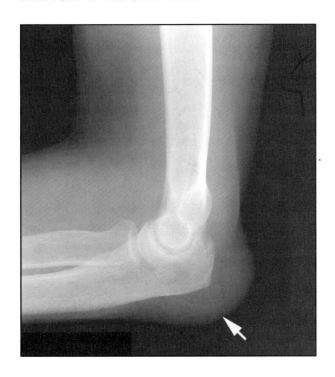

Figure 5-21

Olecranon bursitis—Lateral view

Lateral view of an elbow with gout and olecranon bursitis shows soft-tissue swelling posterior to the olecranon (arrow), where the bursa is filled with fluid.

Differential Diagnosis

Cellulitis (soft-tissue edema and swelling may be seen on radiographs)

Infectious arthritis (radiographs may demonstrate a fat pad sign indicating an elbow joint effusion; minimal radiographic changes except with long-standing disease, where severe joint destruction may be present)

Rheumatoid arthritis (characteristic intra-articular findings, including effusion osteopenia, periarticular erosions, erosions, bony destruction in severe disease, rheumatoid nodules)

Soft-tissue tumor (solid rather than cystic characteristics)

OSTEOARTHRITIS

SYNONYMS
Degenerative joint disease
Radiohumeral osteoarthritis
Ulnohumeral osteoarthritis
Wear-and-tear osteoarthritis

ICD-9 Code
715.12
Localized primary
osteoarthrosis, forearm

DEFINITION
Primary osteoarthritis of the elbow is relatively uncommon. The condition occurs five times as often in men as in women and is most commonly seen in men with a history of overuse of the arm, such as carpenters, weightlifters, and throwing athletes. Peak onset is during the fifth and sixth decades of life, with a mean age of presentation of 55 years.

HISTORY AND PHYSICAL FINDINGS
A thorough history, including the patient's work history, is helpful in diagnosing this condition. Patients usually report pain when the arm is fully extended. A classic report is that of being unable to carry an object such as a briefcase because of pain. In more advanced stages, pain is present throughout the arc of motion. A flexion contracture of about 20° to 30° is common. The most reproducible finding on examination is pain with forced extension.

IMAGING STUDIES

Required for diagnosis
AP and lateral views of the elbow are sufficient to make the diagnosis. Radiographs will show osteophytes of the coronoid and olecranon processes and their respective fossae, and the ulnohumeral and radiohumeral joint spaces will be reduced. The olecranon and coronoid fossae will be narrowed because of osteophytic encroachment. There can be adjacent subchondral sclerosis. Loose bodies may also be present.

Required for comprehensive evaluation
CT is helpful in the identification and location of loose bodies if mechanical symptoms such as elbow locking or catching are present.

Special considerations
None

Pitfalls
None

IMAGE DESCRIPTIONS

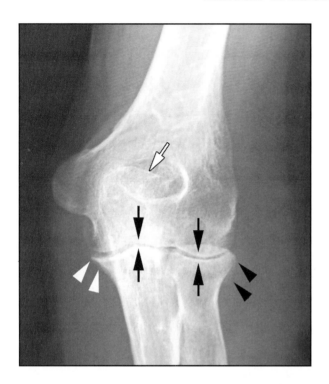

Figure 5-22

Osteoarthritis of the elbow— AP view

AP view of an elbow with osteoarthritis demonstrates decreased ulnohumeral and radiohumeral joint space (black arrows). The olecranon fossa is not well visualized because of osteophytic encroachment (white arrow), and osteophytes are present around the radial head (black arrowheads) and coronoid process (white arrowheads).

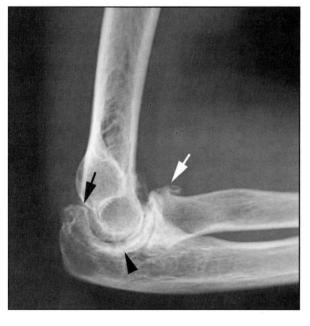

Figure 5-23

Osteoarthritis of the elbow— Lateral view

Lateral radiograph of the same elbow shown in Figure 5-22 demonstrates osteophytes on the olecranon process, filling the olecranon fossa of the distal humerus (black arrow). Osteophytes on the radial head (white arrow) are well visualized on this view. Note the subchondral sclerosis in the greater sigmoid notch of the olecranon (arrowhead).

DIFFERENTIAL DIAGNOSIS

Lateral epicondylitis (normal radiographs)

Neuropathic joint (extreme changes of osteoarthritis)

Posttraumatic arthritis (radiographic features similar to osteoarthritis, history of prior trauma)

Radial head fracture (apparent on radiographs)

Rheumatoid arthritis (osteopenia, periarticular erosions, cystic erosions, bony destruction in severe disease)

Ulnar nerve entrapment (normal radiographs)

OSTEOCHONDRAL LOOSE BODIES

ICD-9 Code

718.12
Loose body in joint, upper arm

SYNONYMS

Degenerative joint disease
Osteoarthritis
Osteochondromatosis
Synovial chondromatosis

DEFINITION

Osteochondral loose bodies within the elbow may be congenital or acquired. Acquired loose bodies include degenerative ossicles, synovial chondromatosis (osteochondromatosis), and fragments from old articular fractures.

HISTORY AND PHYSICAL FINDINGS

Most patients report loss of motion and a sense of catching or locking of the elbow. Not all patients will report pain, however, and in those who do, the intensity of pain varies. Limited motion will be apparent on physical examination. Crepitus may also be observed.

IMAGING STUDIES

Required for diagnosis

AP and lateral views are required for diagnosis. Small bodies may be masked by the normal osseous architecture, so cross-sectional imaging will be needed if loose bodies are suspected and not seen on radiographs.

Required for comprehensive evaluation

Radiographs may not detect loose bodies that have not yet ossified. Suspected loose bodies usually can be visualized on CT arthrogram.

Special considerations

None

Pitfalls

Accessory ossicles in the elbow, which are often incidental findings on radiographs, may be confused with intra-articular loose bodies. Accessory ossicles may originate from just distal to the medial epicondyle, at the tip of the olecranon process, or within the olecranon fossa. In infants or children with small bony components, acute fractures of the medial or lateral condyle may also be confused with loose bodies. Loose bodies are rare in children, however, so radiographic findings that resemble loose bodies but that occur in the context of trauma should be considered fractures until proven otherwise.

IMAGE DESCRIPTIONS

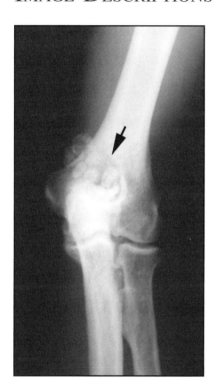

Figure 5-24

Osteochondral loose bodies (elbow)— AP view

AP view demonstrates multiple loose bodies within the olecranon fossa of the distal humerus (arrow).

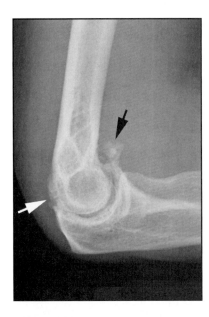

Figure 5-25

Osteochondral loose bodies (elbow)—Lateral view

Lateral view of the elbow with osteoarthritis demonstrates a large coronoid osteophyte anteriorly (black arrow) and multiple loose bodies filling the olecranon fossa posteriorly (white arrow).

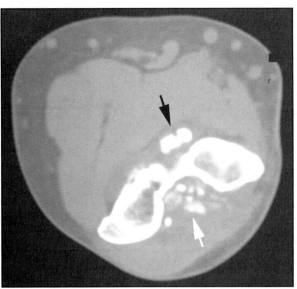

Figure 5-26

Osteochondral loose bodies (elbow)—Axial CT

Axial CT scan of the same elbow shown in Figure 5-25 demonstrates loose bodies posteriorly, in the olecranon fossa (white arrow), and anteriorly, in the coronoid fossa (black arrow).

DIFFERENTIAL DIAGNOSIS

Fracture (cortical disruption of the radius, humerus, or ulna; fragments without sclerotic margins in the setting of trauma)

Osteoarthritis (osteophytes, joint space narrowing, cystic erosions, subchondral sclerosis)

RHEUMATOID ARTHRITIS

SYNONYMS
Inflammatory arthritis
RA
Seropositive arthritis

ICD-9 Code

714.0
Rheumatoid arthritis

DEFINITION
Rheumatoid arthritis (RA), the most common form of arthritis of the elbow, is an inflammatory arthritis usually characterized by the presence of rheumatoid factor in the blood (seropositive arthritis). This is distinguished from other inflammatory arthropathies where no rheumatoid factor is present (seronegative arthritis). The etiology of RA is not completely understood, but a genetic link has been established. In RA, an autoimmune process produces inflammation that can cause both osseous and soft-tissue destruction that can lead to arthritis of the joint and instability.

HISTORY AND PHYSICAL FINDINGS
RA may affect one, several, or all joints. RA should be suspected and appropriate laboratory studies performed when a patient has a family history of RA or presents with symmetric symptoms in multiple joints. In patients with symptoms about the elbow, pain and limited motion secondary to synovitis will be present, and the patient will usually hold the elbow in a flexed position.

Physical examination typically reveals symmetric swelling of the joint. Depending on the stage of the disease, the synovitis may extend both proximally and distally from the joint, manifesting as a boggy, mobile, subcutaneous mass. Olecranon bursitis may also be present. As the disease progresses, extension of the elbow may become limited. The joints of the hand and wrist are most commonly involved and are the site of characteristic deformities. Soft-tissue extra-articular manifestations may also be present in the form of rheumatoid nodules, subcutaneous masses that usually occur on the extensor surface of the arms (near the elbow) and areas under mechanical pressure.

IMAGING STUDIES

Required for diagnosis

AP and lateral views of the elbow are recommended for initial evaluation of suspected RA. Characteristic radiographic findings include periarticular osteopenia and joint space narrowing. Erosions of the bone are often present; periarticular erosions caused by invasion by the rheumatoid pannus are characteristic of RA. The osteophytes seen in osteoarthritis are absent with RA.

Required for comprehensive evaluation

MRI with intravenous contrast (gadolinium) can be useful to show the extent of the disease and disease activity.

Special considerations

None

Pitfalls

None

IMAGE DESCRIPTIONS

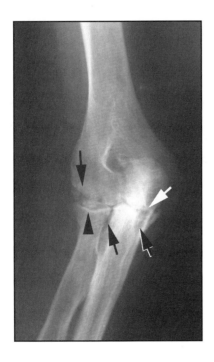

Figure 5-27

Rheumatoid arthritis (elbow)—AP view

AP view demonstrates radiographic findings characteristic of rheumatoid arthritis: periarticular erosions (black arrows) and complete loss of ulnohumeral (white arrow) and radiohumeral (arrowhead) joint space. Note the absence of osteophyte formation.

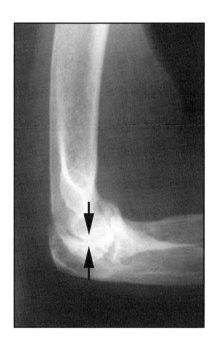

Figure 5-28

Rheumatoid arthritis (elbow)—Lateral view

Lateral view of the elbow of a patient with rheumatoid arthritis demonstrates complete loss of the joint space (arrows) without osteophyte formation.

DIFFERENTIAL DIAGNOSIS

Infectious arthritis (minimal radiographic changes except with long-standing disease, where severe joint destruction may be present; usually only one elbow, not both)

Osteoarthritis (osteophytes, joint space narrowing, cysts, subchondral sclerosis)

Posttraumatic arthritis (radiographic features similar to osteoarthritis, history of prior trauma)

LATERAL EPICONDYLITIS

ICD-9 Code

726.32
Lateral epicondylitis

SYNONYMS

Common extensor tear
Common extensor tenosynovitis
Extensor carpi radialis brevis tear
Lateral epicondylosis
Tennis elbow

DEFINITION

Lateral epicondylitis, commonly called tennis elbow, is an overuse injury of the common extensor origin at the lateral epicondyle of the elbow. Pathology studies have demonstrated that the extensor carpi radialis brevis tendon is usually involved. Improper technique or overuse in sports or work activities involving the elbow has been implicated as a causative factor. Treatment includes rest, ice, nonsteroidal anti-inflammatory drugs, counterforce bracing, and cessation of activities. Injection of lidocaine and steroids is effective in recalcitrant cases. Treatment is followed by a physical therapy regime with the goal of maintaining motion and strength. Additionally, adjusting work-related activities or training in proper sports techniques is essential. In racquet sports players, proper fitting of racquets has been shown to be beneficial as well.

HISTORY AND PHYSICAL FINDINGS

Patients most commonly present in the fourth decade of life, usually reporting an insidious onset of pain with particular activities. A history of playing tennis or other racquet sports is common. Painting, weaving, and raking are also associated with the condition.

Tenderness just anterior and distal to the lateral epicondyle is the most common physical finding. Provocative testing involves resisted wrist extension and forearm supination, which will reproduce the discomfort at the elbow.

IMAGING STUDIES

Required for diagnosis
The diagnosis of lateral epicondylitis is largely made based on clinical evaluation. However, AP and lateral views of the elbow, which are usually normal in patients with lateral epicondylitis, are required to rule out other causes of pain. Calcification of the common extensor origin may be seen occasionally.

Required for comprehensive evaluation

In cases of revision surgery or profound extensor weakness where complete common extensor rupture is suspected, MRI may provide additional information. On MRI, the soft tissues surrounding the epicondyle may show tendinosis or tear at the origin of the extensor carpi radialis brevis muscle. In some cases, cervical degenerative joint disease manifests as elbow pain. If pain is present in the neck in combination with elbow pain, or if neurologic symptoms such as weakness, numbness, or tingling are present, AP, lateral, and oblique views of the cervical spine should be obtained. MRI of the cervical spine may be necessary for more comprehensive evaluation.

Special considerations

None

Pitfalls

Entrapment of the radial nerve as it passes through the supinator muscle (radial tunnel syndrome) may be confused with tennis elbow.

IMAGE DESCRIPTIONS

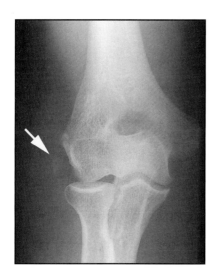

Figure 5-29

Lateral epicondylitis—AP view

AP view of the elbow of a patient with lateral epicondylitis demonstrates calcification within the soft tissues at the common extensor origin (arrow).

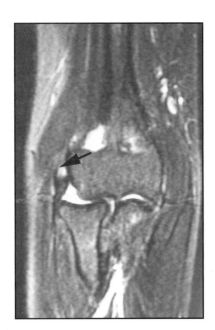

Figure 5-30

Lateral epicondylitis—Coronal MRI

Coronal fat-suppressed T2-weighted MRI scan of the elbow of a patient with lateral epicondylitis shows disruption of the fibers of the common extensor origin at the lateral epicondyle (arrow).

DIFFERENTIAL DIAGNOSIS

Cervical osteoarthritis (osteophytes, disk space narrowing, subchondral sclerosis of the cervical spine)

Radial nerve entrapment (no radiographic abnormality)

Radiocapitellar arthritis (osteophytes, joint space narrowing, cystic erosions, subchondral sclerosis of the radiocapitellar joint)

Medial Epicondylitis

Synonyms

Common flexor tendon tear
Common flexor tenosynovitis
Golfer's elbow
Handball player's elbow
Medial epicondylosis

ICD-9 Code

726.31
Medial epicondylitis

Definition

Medial epicondylitis, or golfer's elbow, is less common than lateral epicondylitis (tennis elbow). The incidence in men is twice that in women. Medial epicondylitis may be work related in approximately 50% of patients (common activities are bricklaying, typing, and hammering) and sports related in as many as 20% of patients (sports commonly associated are tennis, rowing, handball, and baseball). Because of the proximity of the ulnar nerve to the medial epicondyle, ulnar neuropathy may be present in 50% of patients. The pathology involves microtears of the flexor-pronator muscle group, with the flexor carpi radialis and pronator teres most commonly involved. Nonsurgical management, including nonsteroidal anti-inflammatory drugs, rest, bracing, and physical therapy, often is not as successful for medial epicondylitis as for lateral epicondylitis. Surgical consultation should be considered if the condition does not improve after 10 to 12 weeks of therapy.

History and Physical Findings

Patients present with a history of medial elbow pain that is characteristically worse with forceful pronation. Physical examination will reveal tenderness immediately anterior and distal to the medial epicondyle. Resisted pronation of the forearm or resisted wrist flexion will elicit the tenderness. In throwing athletes, medial collateral ligament (MCL) insufficiency should be considered as part of the differential diagnosis, and prompt specialty referral should be considered if the diagnosis is in question. Ulnar neuropathy may be diagnosed by a positive Tinel's sign at the cubital tunnel, decreased strength in the area innervated by the ulnar nerve, or decreased sensation in the ring and little fingers.

IMAGING STUDIES

Required for diagnosis

AP, lateral, and oblique views of the elbow should be obtained to rule out other intra-articular causes of elbow pain. Calcification at the medial epicondyle may be seen in some patients with medial epicondylitis.

Required for comprehensive evaluation

MRI may demonstrate edema of the flexor-pronator origin at the medial epicondyle but is not necessary for the diagnosis. However, MRI may be useful in patients with chronic (longer than 1 year) tennis elbow, in patients who have had previous surgery for medial epicondylitis, and in patients with suspected MCL insufficiency.

Special considerations

None

Pitfalls

None

IMAGE DESCRIPTION

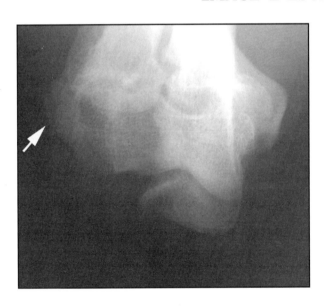

Figure 5-31

Medial epicondylitis— Cubital tunnel view

Cubital tunnel view of the elbow shows calcification medial to the medial epicondyle (arrow), consistent with medial epicondylitis.

DIFFERENTIAL DIAGNOSIS

MCL insufficiency (no abnormal radiographic findings; MRI may show edema or disruption of the MCL fibers)

Ulnar neuropathy (no abnormal radiographic findings; MRI may show edema or enlargement or subluxation of the ulnar nerve)

Ulnohumeral osteoarthritis (posteromedial olecranon osteophytes, joint space narrowing, cystic lesions, subchondral sclerosis of the ulnohumeral joint)

SECTION 5 ■ ELBOW AND FOREARM

RUPTURE OF THE DISTAL BICEPS TENDON

ICD-9 Codes

727.69
Rupture of tendon, nontraumatic (other)

881.21
Open wound of elbow, forearm, and wrist, with tendon involvement (scapular region)

SYNONYMS

Avulsion

Distal biceps tendon tear

DEFINITION

The biceps muscle is the strongest supinator of the forearm and assists the brachialis in elbow flexion. Rupture of the distal biceps tendon occurs most commonly in the dominant arm of men in the fourth to sixth decades of life. Almost all reported cases of complete biceps tendon ruptures have occurred in men. The mechanism of injury is usually an identifiable traumatic event in which an unexpected extension force is applied to an arm flexed 90°. The tendon typically avulses from the radial tuberosity.

Partial ruptures are uncommon. Complete ruptures have arbitrarily been classified as acute or chronic, with a chronic rupture being defined as one of more than 3 to 4 weeks' duration. Surgical intervention with anatomic repair of the tendon to the radial tuberosity is necessary to restore strength and endurance in supination and flexion.

HISTORY AND PHYSICAL FINDINGS

Patients typically report a sudden, painful tearing sensation in the antecubital fossa and a weakness in flexion that is profound immediately after the injury but tends to diminish over time. Examination reveals tenderness, ecchymosis, and a palpable defect in the antecubital fossa. If the biceps tendon cannot be palpated in the antecubital fossa and the biceps muscle belly has migrated, complete rupture is indicated. If the biceps tendon is palpable, a partial rupture of the tendon must be considered. Weakness in supination as well as some weakness in flexion can usually be demonstrated.

When acute ruptures are diagnosed early, they can be easily reattached to the radial tuberosity with predictably good results. However, repairs of chronic ruptures have variable results, are difficult to reattach to the radial tuberosity, and occasionally require interpositional grafting. Therefore, prompt referral to an orthopaedic specialist is required when a distal biceps tendon rupture is suspected. Unlike ruptures of the proximal biceps tendon, which usually do not require surgical treatment because there is little functional deficit, ruptures of the distal biceps tendon should be repaired surgically. Unrepaired distal biceps tendon ruptures can be quite disabling.

IMAGING STUDIES

Required for diagnosis

AP, lateral, and oblique views of the elbow are required and in rare cases will demonstrate a fleck of bone avulsed from the radial tuberosity of the radius. MRI or ultrasound of the elbow is required, however, to definitively diagnose a ruptured biceps tendon.

Required for comprehensive evaluation

None

Special considerations

None

Pitfalls

None

IMAGE DESCRIPTIONS

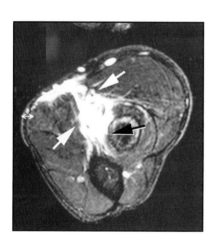

Figure 5-32

Distal biceps tendon rupture—Axial MRI

Axial fat-suppressed T2-weighted MRI scan demonstrates that the distal biceps tendon attachment to the bicipital tuberosity is missing (black arrow). Edema is present within the soft tissues in the area where the normal biceps tendon should be (white arrows).

SECTION 5 ■ ELBOW AND FOREARM

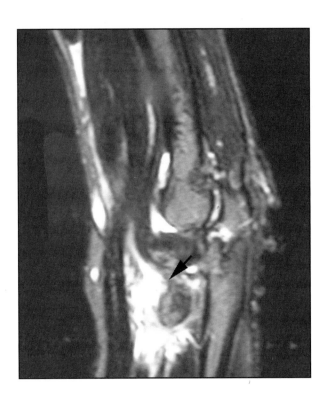

Figure 5-33

Distal biceps tendon rupture—Sagittal MRI

Sagittal fat-suppressed T2-weighted MRI scan shows edema in the region of the tear near the radial tuberosity (arrow).

DIFFERENTIAL DIAGNOSIS

Elbow dislocation (incongruity of the distal humerus and the ulna or radius and capitellum)

Fracture of the radial head (cortical disruption of the radial head, positive "fat pad" sign on lateral radiographs)

Median nerve entrapment (normal MRI; abnormal nerve conduction may be present)

HAND AND WRIST

Section Editor

Thomas R. Johnson, MD

Contributors

James F. Schwarten, MD

Curtis Settergren, MD, MS

IMAGING THE HAND AND WRIST—AN OVERVIEW

ANATOMY

The wrist joint consists of two joints—the radiocarpal and radioulnar joints. The articular surface of the radius slopes, on average, 18° toward the ulna when viewed from the front or back of the wrist. When viewed from the side, the articular surface of the radius tilts down an average of 15°. The distal radius and ulna articulate at the ulnar notch of the radius. The length of the ulna relative to the radius is referred to as ulnar variance. Positive ulnar variance means that the ulna is longer than the radius, whereas negative ulnar variance means the opposite. When the distal ulna is the same length as the distal radius, the term is ulnar neutral.

The carpus consists of two rows of small carpal bones, a proximal and distal carpal row linked together through the scaphoid. Gilula has described three arcs drawn along the proximal and distal carpal rows that help to evaluate carpal bone alignment on PA views of the wrist (see p. 373). A useful mnemonic device to remember the carpal bones is SLTP for the proximal row and TTCH for the distal carpal row—Show (Scaphoid) Larry (Lunate) The (Triquetrum) Phone (Pisiform) To (Trapezium) Try (Trapezoid) Calling (Capitate) Home (Hamate).

The hand is composed of five metacarpal bones and 14 phalanges. The thumb has only two phalanges (a proximal and distal phalanx), while the fingers each have three phalanges (a proximal, middle and distal phalanx). The phalanges and metacarpals are held together by paired collateral ligaments, the radial and ulnar collateral ligaments. A tear of the ulnar collateral ligament of the thumb metacarpophalangeal (MCP) joint is referred to as a gamekeeper's thumb or a skier's thumb.

The epiphyses of the metacarpals (index through little) are located distally just before the metacarpal heads. In the thumb metacarpal, the epiphysis is located proximally at the base of the metacarpal. The epiphyses of the phalanges are all located at the proximal base of the phalanx.

OSSIFICATION CENTERS

At birth, all carpal bones are cartilaginous. Ossification centers about the hand and wrist appear, on average, in the following sequence: (1) capitate and hamate and radial epiphysis at year 1; (2) triquetrum at year 3; (3) trapezium and lunate at year 5; (4) scaphoid at year 6; (5) trapezoid and ulnar styloid at year 7; (6) pisiform at year 10; and (7) thumb sesamoids at year 12.

Standard Imaging Views

Radiographs

PA and lateral views are adequate to diagnose most conditions about the hand and wrist. A 45° PA oblique view is often added to complete the so-called standard hand series. For the standard PA view, the shoulder is abducted 90°, the elbow flexed 90°, and the forearm held in neutral. Ulnar deviation PA and oblique views of the wrist are useful to visualize the scaphoid bone in its long axis, as well as the scaphoid, trapezium, and trapezoid joints. Scapholunate dissociation may also be visualized by this view. A clenched fist view is helpful to see a scapholunate dissociation. A Robert view best demonstrates carpometacarpal (CMC) arthritis of the thumb.

Computed tomography

CT in the long axis of the scaphoid will reveal scaphoid fractures and nonunions of the scaphoid. Distal radioulnar dislocations are also nicely visualized. Fractures of the hook of the hamate are often better seen on CT than on radiographs. In the setting of one carpal fracture, CT often reveals others that are not apparent on radiographs.

Magnetic resonance imaging

MRI is valuable in the diagnosis of osteonecrosis of the lunate (Kienböck's disease) and scaphoid after fractures. Occult fractures are well visualized with this modality, as are soft-tissue masses. For suspected occult fractures of the wrist, MRI is the modality of choice. Ligamentous injuries and triangular fibrocartilage complex (TFCC) tears also can be easily seen with MRI.

Bone scans

Bone scans are still useful in diagnosing occult fractures of the scaphoid and other carpal bones; however, the use of this modality remains controversial, particularly given the availability of MRI and CT.

Emergencies

None

Normal Variants

A number of findings on imaging studies can appear to be a result of trauma or another type of problem when, in fact, they are simply a normal variant of anatomy. In the hand, three bear mentioning. The first is congenital fusions, also called carpal coalitions. Fusion of the lunotriquetral joint is most common, followed by fusion of the capitate-hamate and the trapezium and trapezoid. The second is the presence of accessory ossicles/sesamoids. Two sesamoids are always present at the base of the thumb MCP joint; one occurs at the base of the little finger MCP joint in 8 of 10 individuals; and one occurs at the proximal interphalangeal joint of the thumb in 7 of 10 individuals. Infrequently, sesamoids are seen at the MCP joints of the index, middle, or ring fingers. Not uncommonly, however, these are mistaken for fractures or avulsions. The third normal variant is the so-called congenital bipartite scaphoid. Whether this condition actually exists remains controversial. Recent evidence suggests that it may indeed be a fracture rather than a congenital condition.

IMAGING TIPS

1. Always order PA and lateral views of the fingers, hand, or wrist. Fractures easily can be missed when only a PA view is obtained. Likewise, a dislocated lunate can be missed on a PA view but is relatively easy to see on a lateral view.

2. When looking at PA views of the wrist, check for the continuity of the three lines (Gilula's lines) that define the proximal and distal carpal rows. Lack of continuity of one or more of these lines indicates a dislocation or fracture-dislocation of one or more of the carpal bones.

3. When assessing fractures of the distal radius, look for the slope of the distal radius (15° to 20°) on the PA view, the volar tilt of the distal radius (10° to 20°) on the lateral view, and the length of the ulna relative to the radius (ulnar variance) on PA views.

4. When concerned about a possible tear of the ulnar collateral ligament of the MCP joint of the thumb (gamekeeper's or skier's thumb), order an abduction (radial deviation) stress view of the MCP joint.

5. When looking at lateral views of the wrist, the capitate, lunate, and radius should be aligned. If they are not colinear, a lunate or perilunate dislocation may be present.

6. On a PA view of the wrist, the space between the carpal bones should be the same (approximately 2 mm). If the space between the scaphoid and lunate bones is twice as wide as the spaces between the other carpal bones, a scapholunate dissociation is likely present. A clenched fist PA view will often accentuate this separation. If doubt arises as to whether the degree of separation is normal, a PA comparison view of the opposite wrist is helpful.

7. Increased space between the scaphoid and lunate has been likened to a set of teeth with a wide gap between the front teeth. Names of a famous British actor, Terry-Thomas, and numerous famous Americans have been affixed to this sign.

8. If a fracture of the scaphoid is suspected clinically but not seen on radiographs, MRI or CT of the scaphoid is helpful to make the diagnosis. Bone scans also can be ordered.

9. Persistent tenderness at the base of the palm on the radial side of the hand suggests the possibility of a fracture of the hook of the hamate (often seen in golfers). Radiographs seldom show this fracture; therefore, CT is helpful to make the diagnosis. A carpal tunnel view will show the base of the hamate, but patients with this fracture usually are in too much pain for a good carpal tunnel view to be obtained.

10. Dislocations or fracture-dislocations of the carpometacarpal (CMC) joint at the base of the little finger (fifth metacarpal) are frequently missed. PA and lateral views may look normal. If a fracture-dislocation is suspected clinically, oblique views in pronation and supination should be obtained. The fracture is usually an avulsion off the dorsum of the hamate.

11. Avulsion fractures at the volar base of the middle phalanx, the dorsum of the distal phalanx, the volar base of the distal phalanx, and the ulnar side of the base of the thumb proximal phalanx are all significant injuries that frequently require surgical treatment.

12. Soft-tissue masses in the hand may be due to underlying bony abnormalities; therefore, PA and lateral views are required.

13. Carpal fractures in children are rare, but when in doubt, order comparison views of the opposite, uninjured extremity.

SECTION 6 ■ HAND AND WRIST

Avulsion of the Flexor Digitorum Profundus Tendon Insertion

Synonym
Jersey finger

ICD-9 Code

816.02
Fracture of distal phalanx or phalanges, closed

Definition
The name "jersey finger" comes from a common mechanism of injury in football in which a player grabs an opponent's jersey, causing an avulsion at the insertion of the flexor digitorum profundus (FDP) of the ring finger. The fragment usually is small, but occasionally a large fragment is involved. Large fragments will "hang up" on the distal flexor pulleys, preventing the FDP from retracting back into the hand. A small fragment may retract more proximally, making it more difficult to retrieve and repair.

History and Physical Findings
The history includes sudden onset of pain and inability to flex the distal interphalangeal (DIP) joint of the ring finger following an incident during football play, as described above. Physical examination will reveal tenderness and swelling along the flexor surface of the ring finger and sometimes into the palm. The patient will be unable to bend the DIP joint.

Imaging Studies

Required for diagnosis
AP and lateral radiographs of the finger will show the avulsed fragment unless it is small and has retracted into the palm. The vincula that connect to the flexor tendon often prevent the tendon from retracting into the palm.

Required for comprehensive evaluation
If there is any doubt as to the diagnosis, MRI will show whether the flexor tendon has been avulsed and, if so, where the end of the tendon is located in the finger.

Special considerations
None

Pitfalls
The lack of a bone fragment may lull the unwary practitioner into thinking the tendon is intact. Clinical testing for function of the FDP should eliminate this confusion.

IMAGE DESCRIPTION

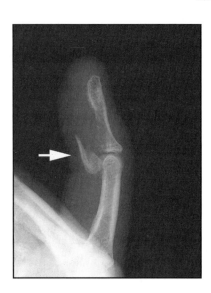

Figure 6-1

Avulsion fracture of the flexor digitorum profundus tendon insertion—Lateral view

Lateral view of a finger shows a large fragment off of the volar aspect of the distal phalanx (arrow). Note that the fragment is translated about 3 mm proximally and is tipped away, or volarly, from the distal phalanx.

DIFFERENTIAL DIAGNOSIS

Nerve injury or paralysis (anterior interosseous nerve syndrome paralysis; no active flexion at the DIP joint of the index finger)

Rupture of the flexor tendon at the wrist (usually seen in rheumatoid arthritis; carpal tunnel view may show a bony spike)

BOUTONNIÈRE DEFORMITY

SYNONYM
Buttonhole deformity

ICD-9 Code

736.21
Boutonnière deformity

DEFINITION

Disruption of the central slip of the extensor tendon at the middle phalanx of the proximal interphalangeal (PIP) joint with volar subluxation of the lateral bands results in the so-called boutonnière deformity. The name is derived from the position the index finger assumes when pinning a boutonnière onto the lapel of a gentleman's jacket. The position is one of flexion at the PIP joint and hyperextension at the distal interphalangeal (DIP) joint. As the lateral band slips below the axis of rotation, active extension of the PIP joint becomes impossible, creating a situation of paradoxical flexion at the PIP joint. The harder the person tries to extend the PIP joint, the more the joint flexes and the DIP joint extends. This situation creates the typical posture of a finger with a boutonnière deformity. Rheumatoid arthritis and connective tissue diseases can also affect the central slip of the extensor tendon and result in the boutonnière deformity.

HISTORY AND PHYSICAL FINDINGS

A central slip injury may occur secondary to blunt trauma with acute forced flexion of the PIP joint or a direct blow to the area of the insertion. A volar dislocation of the PIP joint may also result in avulsion of the central slip, with subsequent development of a boutonnière deformity. A wound with laceration of the central slip may also result in this deformity. This condition is often missed and should be suspected in patients with a jammed or sprained finger with a 15° to 20° loss of active extension at the PIP joint when the wrist and metacarpophalangeal joint are fully flexed. Examination of the finger shows that the PIP joint is flexed 30° or more and the joint cannot be actively extended. During the first few weeks after injury, the joint can be passively extended. Later, a flexion contracture develops, resulting in loss of both active and passive extension.

IMAGING STUDIES

Required for diagnosis

Fractures are not typically associated with a routine boutonnière deformity, but PA and lateral views of the finger will rule out an associated fracture. A lateral view will also show the flexion deformity of the PIP joint and the extension deformity of the DIP joint.

Required for comprehensive evaluation

None

Special considerations

None

Pitfalls

With closed injuries, this condition is often missed acutely and may not be recognized for 2 to 3 weeks following the injury.

IMAGE DESCRIPTIONS

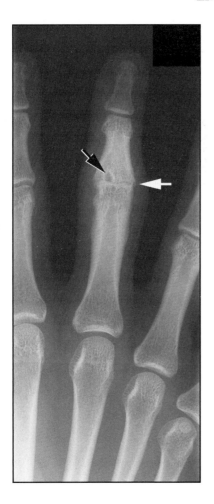

Figure 6-2

Boutonnière deformity—PA view

PA view of the middle finger shows an incidental cyst or erosion in the base of the middle phalanx (black arrow). Because of the flexion contracture of the PIP joint, the joint space is not visualized (white arrow).

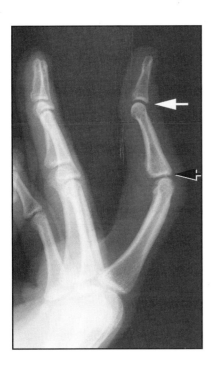

Figure 6-3

Boutonnière deformity—Lateral view

Lateral view of the middle finger shows a flexion deformity of the PIP joint (black arrow) and an extension deformity of the DIP joint (white arrow), characteristic of a boutonnière deformity. Some irregularity and narrowing of the joint space of the PIP joint also can be seen.

DIFFERENTIAL DIAGNOSIS

Finger sprain (no flexion deformity of the PIP joint)

Septic joint (positive results of joint aspirate, erythema)

SECTION 6 ■ HAND AND WRIST

CARPOMETACARPAL DISLOCATIONS

ICD-9 Codes

814.00
Fracture of carpal bone(s), unspecified, closed

833.04
Fracture of wrist, carpometacarpal joint, closed

SYNONYMS
None

DEFINITION
The metacarpals of the index and middle fingers form a strong, stable articulation with the trapezoid and capitate bones, producing little motion. Conversely, on the ulnar side of the hand, the metacarpals of the ring and little (fifth) fingers are more mobile, with up to 20° of flexion and extension. Strong ligamentous attachments between these bones, along with tendon insertions, make these joints quite stable; therefore, pure dislocations are rare. Most injuries at these joints are dorsal fracture-dislocations.

The carpometacarpal (CMC) joint of the little finger is the most frequently injured. Dislocations of the fourth and fifth metacarpals often occur together, along with a fracture of the dorsal half of the articular surface of the hamate. Dorsally displaced injuries of the fifth metacarpal are unstable because of the pull of the extensor carpi ulnaris tendon. Palmar (volar) dislocations are less common and are usually stable following closed reduction. Neurapraxia of the ulnar nerve may accompany dislocations of the lateral metacarpals.

HISTORY AND PHYSICAL FINDINGS
A typical mechanism of injury involves direct trauma to the hand, such as a blow to the dorsum of the metacarpal head, which causes the base of the metacarpal to be forced dorsally. Physical examination reveals swelling, direct tenderness, and a flexion deformity of the metacarpal. A rotational malalignment also may be seen.

IMAGING STUDIES

Required for diagnosis
PA and lateral views should be obtained, but this injury may be easily missed with these views alone. A 30° pronated oblique view will better visualize the fifth CMC joint in an attempt to identify a dislocation.

Required for comprehensive evaluation
If there is any doubt after viewing the radiographs, CT should be ordered because it better visualizes the small carpal bone fractures that often accompany these dislocations.

Special considerations
None

Pitfalls
Fracture-dislocations of the CMC joints are easily missed on radiographs. Careful evaluation of the lateral view may reveal increased flexion of the fifth metacarpal, suggesting the possibility of a CMC dislocation.

IMAGE DESCRIPTIONS

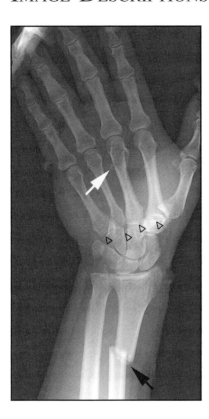

Figure 6-4

Dislocation of the CMC joints—PA view

PA view of a left wrist and distal forearm shows an obvious fracture of the shaft of the radius (black arrow). A fracture of the neck of the middle finger metacarpal (white arrow) can be seen as well. Less obvious is that the CMC joints of the index, middle, ring, and little fingers are dislocated (arrowheads). These dislocations would be seen best on a lateral view.

SECTION 6 ■ HAND AND WRIST

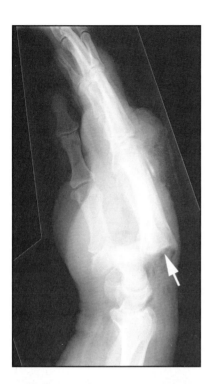

Figure 6-5

Dislocation of the CMC joints—
Lateral view

Lateral view of the same wrist shown in Figure 6-4 shows a dorsal dislocation of the CMC joints of the index through little fingers (arrow).

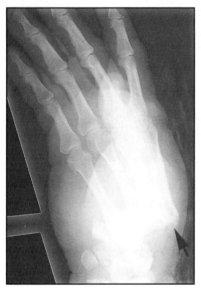

Figure 6-6

Dislocation of the CMC joints—
Oblique view

Oblique view shows dislocation of the CMC joints of the index through ring fingers (arrow). The dislocation at the little finger cannot be seen on this view.

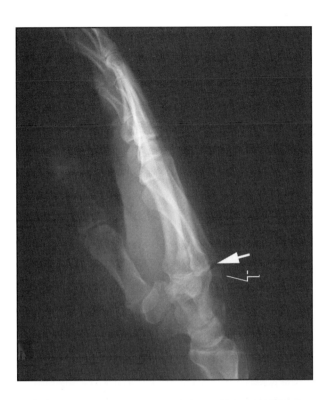

Figure 6-7

Fracture of the hamate with dislocation of the base of the fourth and fifth metacarpals—Lateral view

In this lateral view, the displaced fragment of the hamate (black arrow) can be seen with the dorsally displaced base of the fourth and fifth metacarpals (white arrow).

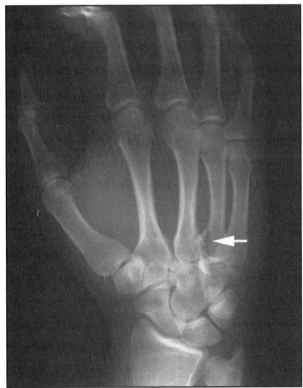

Figure 6-8

Fracture of the hamate with dislocation of the base of the fourth and fifth metacarpals—Oblique view

In this oblique view of the same hand shown in Figure 6-7, the metaphyseal fracture in the base of the fourth metacarpal can be seen (arrow).

SECTION 6 ■ HAND AND WRIST

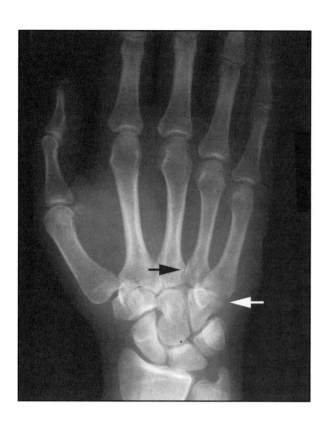

Figure 6-9

Fracture of the hamate with dislocation of the base of the fourth and fifth metacarpals— PA view

This PA view of the same hand shown in Figures 6-7 and 6-8 demonstrates the subtle signs that may be missed with these types of fractures. A faint fracture line can be seen at the base of the fourth metacarpal (black arrow). Note also that the base of the fifth metacarpal appears to overlap the hamate (white arrow).

DIFFERENTIAL DIAGNOSIS

Fracture of the metacarpal (easily seen on radiographs)

Rupture of wrist flexor or extensor tendons (defect on palpation of tendons)

Dislocation of the Finger

Synonyms

None

Definition

The stability of the metacarpophalangeal (MCP) and interphalangeal (IP) joints depends primarily on the ligamentous structures surrounding the joint. The stability of the IP joints depends on two strong lateral collateral ligaments, which connect with a volar plate complex to form a ligament box complex. The weakest part of this system is on the dorsal side, so it is not surprising that dorsal dislocations of the proximal interphalangeal (PIP) joint are the most common ligamentous injury in the hand. Pure dislocations of the distal interphalangeal (DIP) joint are uncommon; when they occur, these injuries are often open and warrant careful evaluation of tendon function. Volar dislocations disrupt the central slip extensor mechanism and may be irreducible because of a buttonhole entrapment of the condyles by the central slip and the lateral band of the extensor mechanism (boutonnière deformity). Dorsal dislocations of the PIP joint may be unstable if a volar avulsion fracture of the base of the middle phalanx is greater than 20% of the articular surface.

The MCP joints have additional ligamentous support in the form of the deep transverse metacarpal ligament, which connects the volar plates of the adjacent MCP joints. MCP dislocations may be dorsal or volar. A dorsal dislocation, in which the proximal phalanx is dorsal and the metacarpal head volar, is the most common. The MCP joint of the index finger is most often involved. Dorsal dislocations of this joint may be irreducible by closed means because the volar plate attached to the base of the proximal phalanx becomes trapped between the joint surfaces. This dislocation is also called a "complex dorsal dislocation." A complex dorsal dislocation may not appear as badly distorted as a pure dorsal dislocation. Three clinical and radiographic signs are strong clues that a complex dislocation has occurred: (1) the joint appears only slightly hyperextended; (2) there is puckering of the palmar skin at the joint; and (3) the presence of a sesamoid that appears trapped in the joint is pathognomonic of a complex dislocation.

ICD-9 Codes

834.01
Dislocation of metacarpophalangeal joint, closed

834.11
Dislocation of metacarpophalangeal joint, open

HISTORY AND PHYSICAL FINDINGS

Patients will report a history of significant trauma. Physical examination reveals pain, swelling, and deformity in the affected finger. Active flexion and extension will be limited and painful on examination. Following reduction, stability must be carefully evaluated. The most common residual problem with injured joints is limited motion and stiffness, not instability.

IMAGING STUDIES

Required for diagnosis

PA and lateral views should be adequate to identify most dislocations. The addition of an oblique view may be helpful to evaluate a fracture-dislocation. Postreduction PA and lateral views should be obtained to evaluate the adequacy of the reduction.

Required for comprehensive evaluation

None

Special considerations

None

Pitfalls

Failure to carefully evaluate the lateral view may miss a subluxation of the DIP or PIP joint.

IMAGE DESCRIPTIONS

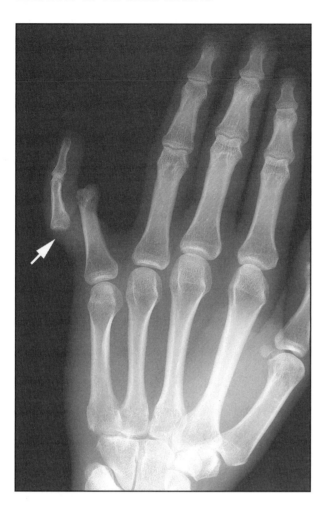

Figure 6-10

Dislocation of the PIP joint— PA view

PA view of the left hand shows an obvious and complete dislocation of the PIP joint of the little finger (arrow). No other views are needed to make this diagnosis. A lateral view would be helpful to exclude a fracture.

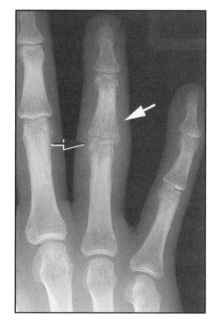

Figure 6-11

Dislocation of the PIP joint— PA view

PA view of a ring finger shows slightly narrowed joint spaces (black arrow) and obvious soft-tissue swelling (white arrow). Without a lateral view, this fracture-dislocation can easily be missed.

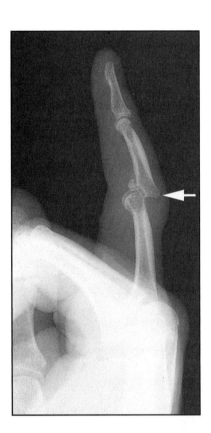

Figure 6-12

Fracture-dislocation of the PIP joint—Lateral view

Lateral view of the finger shown in Figure 6-11 shows a dorsal fracture-dislocation of the PIP joint (arrow). This image illustrates the importance of obtaining two views; this dislocation cannot be seen on the PA view.

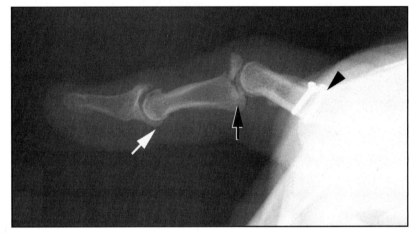

Figure 6-13

Fracture-dislocation of the PIP joint— Lateral view

Lateral view of a volar fracture-dislocation of the PIP joint (black arrow) also shows degenerative changes about the DIP joint (white arrow). Two screws are seen in the proximal phalanx (arrowhead), indicating an old fracture.

DIFFERENTIAL DIAGNOSIS
Finger sprain (normal radiographs)

DISTAL RADIOULNAR JOINT DISORDERS

SYNONYMS

Distal radioulnar arthritis
Distal radioulnar dislocation
Distal radioulnar subluxation
Triangular fibrocartilage complex tears
Ulnar impaction syndrome

ICD-9 Codes

716.94
Arthropathy, unspecified;
hand

833.11
Dislocation of radioulnar
(joint), distal

DEFINITION

The distal radioulnar joint is stabilized by a complex anatomic soft-tissue arrangement that allows rotation of the radius about the ulna and permits flexion and extension and radial and ulnar deviation of the wrist. The primary stabilizer of the distal radioulnar joint is the triangular fibrocartilage complex (TFCC). This complex is made up of the dorsal and the palmar (volar) ligaments, which run from the radius to the ulna; the triangular fibrocartilage, a soft-tissue articular disk that lies between these ligaments; and the sheath about the extensor carpi ulnaris. Although ulnar-sided wrist pain is sometimes caused by TFCC injuries, central tears, which are common, are often asymptomatic. Peripheral tears, especially when associated with subluxation or dislocation of the distal radioulnar joint, often require surgical repair. For a complete dislocation to occur, several of the stabilizing structures must be torn, including the dorsal and palmar radioulnar ligaments, the distal interosseous membrane, and the pronator quadratus muscle. Dislocations may occur either palmarly or, more commonly, dorsally.

Several types of fractures occur at the distal radioulnar joint. Fracture of the radial head with injury to the interosseous membrane (the Essex-Lopresti fracture) may be associated with injury to the TFCC and distal radioulnar instability. Fractures of the ulnar styloid may be associated with instability of the distal radioulnar joint. Fractures of the distal third of the radial shaft, which are often associated with distal radioulnar joint disruption, are called Galeazzi fractures.

HISTORY AND PHYSICAL FINDINGS

The history typically includes a fall on a pronated wrist. Another mechanism of injury is a direct blow to the top of the wrist over the radius. On presentation, the forearm is often rotated inward, and may be locked in this position, and the ulna is prominent dorsally. In actuality, the carpus and radius are dislocated palmarly, and the ulna is fixed in position, giving the appearance of the ulna being prominent dorsally. In contrast, palmar dislocations occur from a fall on a supinated wrist and forearm (ie, the wrist and forearm are rotated outward).

IMAGING STUDIES

Required for diagnosis

PA and lateral views of the wrist in neutral rotation should be ordered initially. The lateral view will often show a dislocation or subluxation. The PA view may show a separation of the distal radioulnar joint. A clenched fist, or grip, view will often accentuate the separation.

Required for comprehensive evaluation

CT is useful for evaluating the distal radioulnar joint. Comparison scans of the opposite wrist are helpful in diagnosing subluxation or dislocation of the joint. If tears of the TFCC are suspected and no subluxation or dislocation is obvious, MRI is useful in making the diagnosis.

Special considerations

Arthroscopy of the wrist is being used increasingly as a diagnostic tool for suspected TFCC tears.

Pitfalls

Positioning of the wrist for the lateral view is critical because small variations in positioning may lead to false-positive diagnoses. Central tears of the TFCC are common in older individuals and may not be the cause of ulnar-sided wrist pain.

IMAGE DESCRIPTIONS

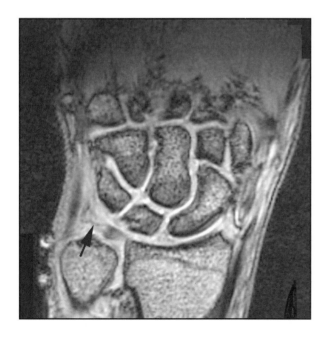

Figure 6-14

TFCC disruption—Coronal MRI

Coronal gradient echo MRI scan of a left wrist shows disruption of the TFCC (arrow).

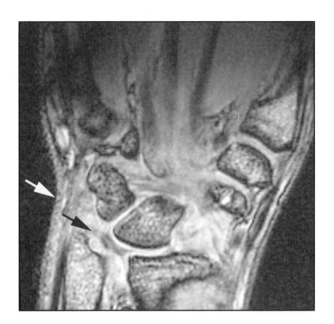

Figure 6-15

TFCC disruption—Coronal MRI

Coronal gradient echo MRI scan of the same wrist as in Figure 6-14 shows disruption of the TFCC (black arrow), along with the area of maximum tenderness on palpation (white arrow).

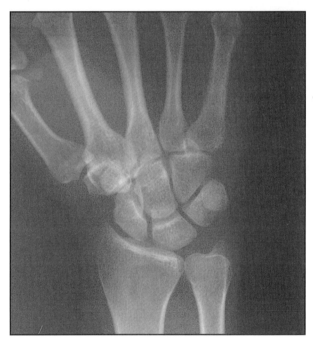

Figure 6-16

Ulnar subluxation (normal comparison view)—PA view

PA view of a right wrist with dorsal subluxation of the ulna appears normal.

SECTION 6 ■ HAND AND WRIST

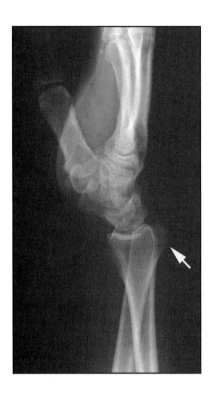

Figure 6-17

Ulnar subluxation—Lateral view

Lateral view of the same wrist as in Figure 6-16 shows a dorsal dislocation of the ulna (arrow) with the wrist in pronation. In actuality, the ulna is fixed and the carpus and radius are dislocated palmarly, making the ulna appear to be dislocated dorsally.

DIFFERENTIAL DIAGNOSIS

Distal radioulnar joint arthritis (narrowing and sclerosis on AP view of wrist)

Extensor carpi ulnaris tendinitis (calcification about the tendon may be seen on radiographs)

Pisotriquetral arthritis (tenderness on compression over the pisiform; sclerosis seen between the pisiform and triquetrum on pisiform view)

Subluxation of the extensor carpi ulnaris (ulnar deviation of the wrist causes the tendon to slip out of its groove; lateral radiographs are normal)

Triquetral impingement ligament tear (TILT) syndrome (localized tenderness over the triquetrum; lateral radiographs are normal)

Ulnar impaction syndrome (positive ulnar variance; cyst in lunate or triquetrum)

FRACTURE OF THE CAPITATE

SYNONYMS

None

ICD-9 Code

814.07
Fracture of the capitate bone
(os magnum), closed

DEFINITION

Fractures of the capitate sometimes occur as isolated injuries to the body or neck of the capitate, but they are more commonly accompanied by other carpal fractures and dislocations. These fractures are quite rare, representing as few as 1% to 3% of all carpal bone fractures. The waist of the capitate is the most common site for a fracture. Because the proximal pole of the capitate is covered with hyaline cartilage and has a limited blood supply, nonunion is common with fractures through the waist of the capitate. A fracture of the waist of the scaphoid associated with a fracture of the neck of the capitate with rotation of the proximal fragment is known as scaphocapitate syndrome.

HISTORY AND PHYSICAL FINDINGS

Fractures of the capitate result from a direct blow to the dorsum of the palmarly (volarly) flexed wrist or, more commonly, a fall on an outstretched hand with the wrist in dorsiflexion. Diagnosis requires a high degree of suspicion, which should occur when a scaphoid fracture is present. On physical examination, swelling and tenderness are noted over the dorsum of the wrist.

IMAGING STUDIES

Required for diagnosis

PA views will reveal a fracture through the waist of the capitate. Lateral views will show any displacement, such as would be present with scaphocapitate syndrome.

Required for comprehensive evaluation

CT or tomography should be ordered if radiographs are inconclusive. These studies also are helpful to plan optimal surgical treatment if necessary. MRI can be useful for demonstrating occult capitate fractures.

Special considerations

None

SECTION 6 ■ HAND AND WRIST

Pitfalls

Initial radiographs may be normal. Also, with capitate fractures, associated injury to the scaphoid may be present and should be recognized.

IMAGE DESCRIPTIONS

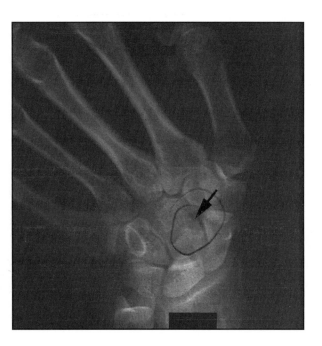

Figure 6-18

Fracture of the capitate—PA view

PA view of a wrist in ulnar deviation shows a fracture through the waist of the capitate (arrow).

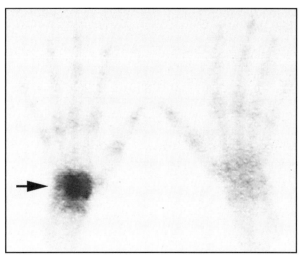

Figure 6-19

Fracture of the capitate—Bone scan

Bone scan shows increased uptake in the midcarpal region of a left wrist (arrow) compared with normal uptake in the right wrist. Note the lack of specificity.

DIFFERENTIAL DIAGNOSIS

Carpal boss (positive carpal boss view; may have associated ganglion cyst)

Hand sprain (normal radiographs and CT scans)

FRACTURE OF THE DISTAL RADIUS

SYNONYMS

Barton's fracture
Chauffeur's (Hutchinson's) fracture
Colles' fracture
Die-punch fracture
Reverse (volar) Barton's fracture
Smith's fracture

DEFINITION

Fractures of the distal radius are the most frequently occurring
fractures in adults, accounting for up to 15% of all fractures seen in
the emergency department. Women older than 60 years are
particularly at risk. With the most common mechanism for these
injuries, a fall on the outstretched hand, the type of injury sustained
is related to the age of the patient. In children age 5 to 10 years,
distal radial metaphyseal fractures are common, whereas
adolescents tend to sustain distal radial epiphyseal fractures.
Patients age 15 to 40 years are more likely to sustain a fracture of
the scaphoid, whereas patients older than 40 years are likely to
incur fractures of the distal radius and ulna. Both types of fracture
may be intra-articular or extra-articular.

Several eponyms continue to be used to describe various types
of distal radius fractures. The most common is the Colles' fracture,
in which the distal radius fragment is tilted upward, or dorsally
(apex volar). An intra-articular component may or may not be
present. The ulnar styloid may be fractured as well. Smith's fracture
is the opposite of the Colles' fracture: the distal fragment is tilted
downward, or volarly (apex dorsal). A Barton's fracture is an intra-
articular fracture of the dorsal lip of the radius with a subluxation
of the carpus. A reverse, or volar, Barton's fracture is an intra-
articular fracture of the volar lip with subluxation of the carpus. A
chauffeur's, or Hutchinson's, fracture is an intra-articular fracture of
the radial styloid. The term chauffeur's fracture comes from a
common mechanism of injury in the early 1900s: a car would
backfire while a person was cranking the engine, causing the
starting crank to strike the person's wrist. A die-punch fracture is a
depressed fracture of the articular surface of the radius opposite the
lunate or scaphoid.

No absolute guidelines exist as to which distal radius fractures
are stable; that is, which fractures, once anatomically reduced, will
stay reduced. However, the presence of any of the following
characteristics would suggest that the fracture is unstable: dorsal
angulation of 20° or more, extensive intra-articular involvement,

ICD-9 Codes

813.41
Colles' fracture

813.42
Other fractures of distal end
of radius (alone), closed

813.44
Fracture of radius with ulna,
lower end, closed

813.54
Fracture of radius with ulna,
lower end, open

SECTION 6 ■ HAND AND WRIST

dorsal comminution, or shortening of 5 mm or more. Although anatomic reduction of distal radius fractures is ideal, less-than-perfect alignment can provide acceptable function, as shown in the figure below.

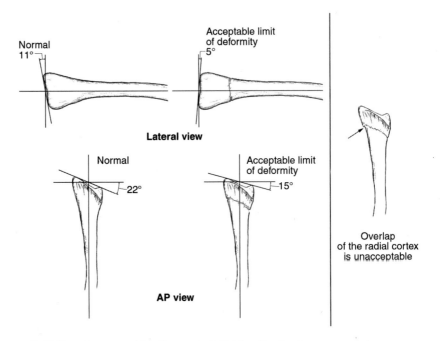

Guidelines for acceptable alignment of distal radius fractures.
Reproduced from Greene WB (ed): Essentials of Musculoskeletal Care, ed 2. Rosemont, IL, American Academy of Orthopaedic Surgeons, 2001, p 251.

HISTORY AND PHYSICAL FINDINGS

Patients will usually report a history of a fall on an outstretched hand or, less often, a direct blow to the wrist, as well as acute onset of pain, swelling, and deformity. Any wrist motion is painful. Physical examination reveals swelling, deformity, and discoloration. Sensation testing may show decreased sensation in the median nerve distribution. Examination of the elbow may reveal swelling and tenderness. Any distal radius fracture that appears unstable should be evaluated by a specialist.

IMAGING STUDIES

Required for diagnosis

PA and lateral views of the wrist should be ordered initially. If tenderness is present about the elbow, AP and lateral views of the elbow should be obtained as well. Although these two views will usually show the fracture, oblique views are helpful to check for intra-articular involvement.

Required for comprehensive evaluation
CT should be obtained to evaluate comminuted intra-articular fractures. The degree of displacement is often underappreciated on radiographs.

Special considerations
The treating surgeon may want to perform fluoroscopic examination with the patient under anesthesia if the exact nature of the fracture is unclear.

Pitfalls
Radiographs often fail to show the true degree of displacement of intra-articular fractures.

IMAGE DESCRIPTIONS

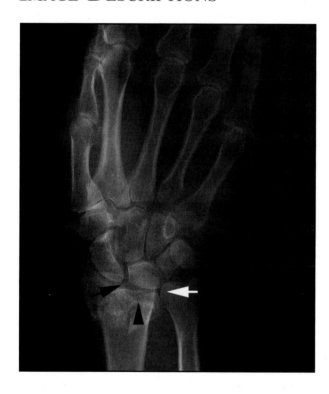

Figure 6-20

Fracture of the distal radius (Colles')—PA view

PA view of the wrist shows a Colles' fracture of the distal radius. Note the loss of ulnar inclination (black arrow), the shortening of the radius (white arrow), and the intra-articular extension of the fracture (arrowhead).

SECTION 6 ■ HAND AND WRIST

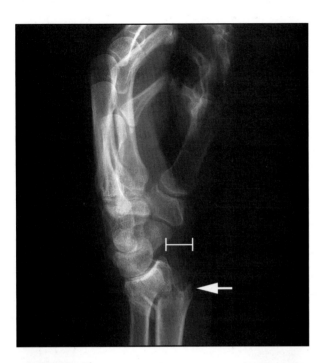

Figure 6-21

Fracture of the distal radius (Colles')—Lateral view

Lateral view of the same wrist shown in Figure 6-20 demonstrates that the radius is translated dorsally about 50% of the metaphyseal diameter (lines) and is dorsally angulated (apex volar) about 30° (arrow).

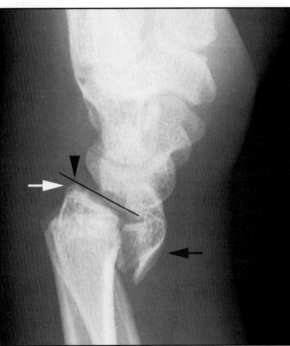

Figure 6-22

Fracture of the distal radius (reverse Barton's)—Lateral view

Lateral view of the wrist shows a volar, or reverse, Barton's fracture. Note the volarly displaced distal radius fragment (black arrow). The dorsal half of the articular surface shows increased volar angulation (white arrow, line), suggesting that the fracture runs through the metaphysis dorsally, creating a three-part fracture. Note that the carpus is subluxated volarly (arrowhead, line) along with the volar radial fragment.

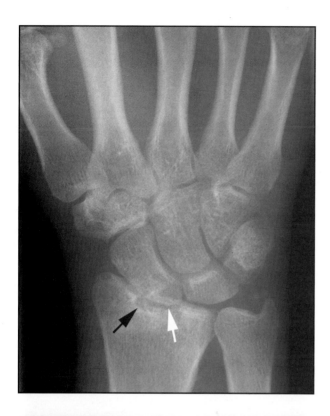

Figure 6-23

Fracture of the distal radius (die-punch)—PA view

PA view of a wrist with a die-punch fracture (black arrow) shows that the scaphoid fossa is depressed, with apparent loss of joint space. The lucency in the proximal pole of the scaphoid adjacent to the attachment to the scapholunate ligament (white arrow) is an incidental finding of little significance.

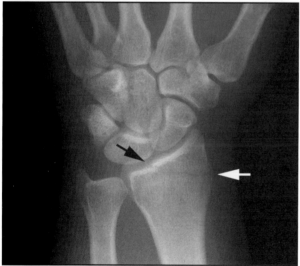

Figure 6-24

Fracture of the distal radius (chauffeur's)—PA view

PA view of a left wrist shows a large, nondisplaced radial styloid fracture (chauffeur's, or Hutchinson's, fracture) extending from the lunate fossa (black arrow) to the radial cortex (white arrow).

DIFFERENTIAL DIAGNOSIS

de Quervain's disease (normal radiographs, positive Finkelstein's test)

Fracture of the scaphoid (fracture apparent on radiographs)

Radiocarpal arthritis (joint space narrowing seen on radiographs)

Scapholunate dissociation (widening of the scapholunate interval)

Fracture of the Hamate

Synonyms

Fracture of the body of the hamate
Fracture of the hamular process
Fracture of the hook of the hamate

ICD-9 Code

814.08
Fracture of the hamate
(unciform) bone, closed

Definition

Fractures of the hamate occur in two locations: the body of the hamate and the hook (hamular process) of the hamate. Fractures through the body often occur with dislocations of the fourth and fifth metacarpals. Fractures through the hook of the hamate are most commonly found in players of racquet sports, golf, and baseball.

History and Physical Findings

Ulnar-sided wrist pain that occurs after the patient participates in a racquet sport or plays golf should raise suspicion of a fracture of the hook of the hamate. Pressure over the hook of the hamate and over the dorsal ulnar aspect of the wrist will elicit pain, and swelling may be observed. Resisted flexion of the little finger with the wrist in ulnar deviation increases the pain. Numbness along the ulnar nerve distribution (little finger and ulnar half of the ring finger) may be present. Occasionally, ruptures of the flexor tendons to the ulnar fingers may occur.

Imaging Studies

Required for diagnosis

PA and lateral views of the wrist will show a fracture of the body of the hamate but rarely will reveal a fracture of the hook of the hamate. A carpal tunnel view is useful in diagnosing a fracture of the hook of the hamate.

Required for comprehensive evaluation

If radiographs are normal and a fracture of the hamate is suspected, CT, which is excellent for visualization of the hamate, should be ordered.

Special considerations

None

Section 6 ■ Hand and Wrist

Pitfalls

Fractures of the hook of the hamate are easily missed. A high index of suspicion is needed to obtain the correct diagnosis. When diagnosed early, these fractures can heal with cast immobilization. When diagnosed late, excision of the hook of the hamate is often required.

IMAGE DESCRIPTION

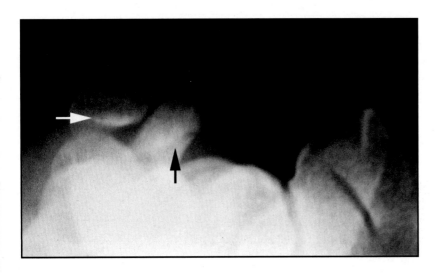

Figure 6-25

Fracture of the hamate (hook)— Carpal tunnel view

This carpal tunnel view of the wrist demonstrates an oblique fracture through the hook of the hamate (black arrow). The pisiform bone (white arrow) can be seen to the left of the hamate.

DIFFERENTIAL DIAGNOSIS

Flexor carpi ulnaris tendinitis (pain with wrist flexion against resistance, may see calcification on radiographs)

Pisotriquetral arthritis (signs of arthritis on lateral view)

Ulnar hammer syndrome or thrombosis of the ulnar artery (positive Allen's test)

FRACTURE OF THE METACARPALS

SYNONYM
Boxer's fracture

DEFINITION
Fractures of the metacarpals and phalanges constitute 10% of all fractures. The finger metacarpals are diminutive long bones, with their weakest point behind the metacarpal head at the neck. A fracture of the metacarpal neck, usually of the fourth or fifth metacarpal, is called a boxer's fracture and is the most common type of metacarpal fracture. With this fracture, there is comminution of the volar cortex, creating a relative instability that results in the metacarpal head being angulated toward the palm.

Angulation of more than 15° in the index and middle fingers interferes with function and requires reduction. Greater degrees of angulation are tolerated in the fourth and fifth metacarpals without loss of function because these metacarpals normally have increased mobility. As much as 60° of angulation in a boxer's fracture may be tolerated without significant impairment of function.

Fractures of the metacarpal head are uncommon and are usually intra-articular. When they occur, the metacarpal of the index finger is most frequently involved. Metacarpal shaft fractures may be transverse, spiral and oblique, and comminuted. Transverse fractures tend to angulate dorsally at the apex as a result of the pull of the interosseous muscles. Spiral and comminuted fractures tend to shorten and rotate.

HISTORY AND PHYSICAL FINDINGS
Patients typically report a history of direct trauma or a fall on an outstretched hand. Physical examination will reveal pain, swelling, ecchymosis, and perhaps malrotation or shortening of the finger. To identify malrotation, ask the patient to flex the fingers and then check for any overlap of the fingers. If the metacarpophalangeal (MCP) joint is swollen, a fracture of the metacarpal head must be ruled out.

IMAGING STUDIES

Required for diagnosis
PA, lateral, and oblique views should be taken of all suspected hand fractures because the fracture may be seen on only one of the views.

ICD-9 Codes

815.02
Fracture of the base of other metacarpal bone(s), closed

815.03
Fracture of the shaft of metacarpal bone(s), closed

815.09
Multiple fractures of metacarpal bones, closed

815.12
Fracture of the base of other metacarpal bone(s), open

815.14
Fracture of the neck of metacarpal bone(s), open

815.19
Multiple fractures of metacarpal bones, open

See also "F" codes under phalanges

SECTION 6 ■ HAND AND WRIST

Required for comprehensive evaluation

Fractures of the metacarpal head may require special views because they are sometimes hard to visualize on standard views. The Brewerton view can be used to evaluate ligament avulsions and fractures off the head. This view is obtained by placing the dorsum of the fingers flat against the x-ray plate and flexing the MCP joint 65°. The central x-ray beam is angled from a point 15° to the ulnar side of the hand. A skyline view is useful to evaluate for metacarpal head fractures after a closed fist injury. In this view, the back of the patient's hand is placed against the x-ray cassette and the MCP joints are fully flexed. The central x-ray beam is directed perpendicular to the cassette. In this way, the profiles of the metacarpal head and the articular fracture can be seen. CT of the metacarpal is useful in planning treatment options.

Special considerations

None

Pitfalls

Fractures of the metacarpal head and fracture-dislocations at the base of the metacarpal are easily missed on radiographs. A high index of suspicion based on clinical examination will guide the clinician to order additional views.

IMAGE DESCRIPTIONS

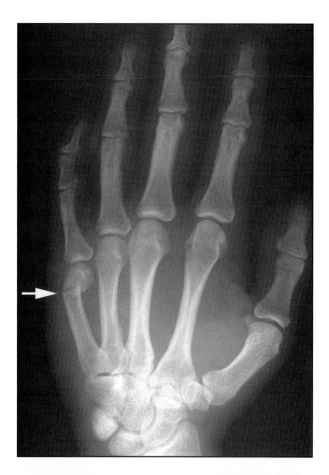

Figure 6-26

Boxer's fracture—PA view

PA view of the left hand shows an angulated fracture of the neck of the fifth metacarpal (boxer's fracture) (arrow). The degree of angulation shown here is well tolerated without loss of function.

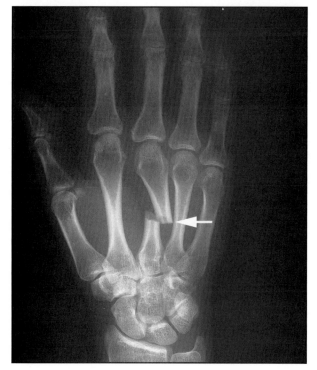

Figure 6-27

Metacarpal fracture—PA view

PA view of a right hand shows a displaced transverse fracture of the middle metacarpal (arrow). Treatment is likely to consist of closed reduction and casting.

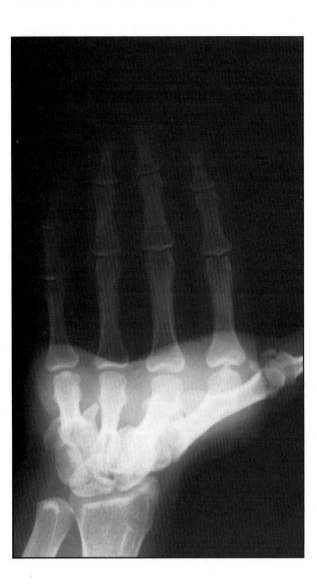

Figure 6-28

Metacarpal fracture (normal comparison view)— Brewerton view

Brewerton view of a right hand shows the metacarpal head and collateral recesses and is helpful in detecting collateral ligament avulsions and fractures off the metatarsal head. In this case, no fractures can be seen.

DIFFERENTIAL DIAGNOSIS

Cellulitis of the hand (erythema and fever; normal bony architecture)

Contusion of the hand (normal radiographs)

Gout (elevated serum uric acid; may see soft-tissue calcification)

FRACTURE OF THE PHALANGES

SYNONYMS
Finger fractures
Fractures of the digits

DEFINITION
Fractures of the phalanges account for 8% to 10% of all fractures, most commonly occurring in individuals younger than 40 years. Kelsey found the cost to society of phalangeal injuries, both in terms of medical costs as well as lost time and wages, to be enormous. More than 850,000 phalangeal fractures occur annually, with days lost from work exceeding 700,000.

The proximal and middle phalanges can be divided anatomically into four distinct areas: the base, the shaft, the neck, and the condyles. Fractures can occur through any of these regions. The distal phalanx is most commonly affected; these fractures comprise 50% of all phalangeal fractures. Distal phalangeal fractures have a surprisingly high rate of associated complications, including cold sensitivity, loss of motion in the distal interphalangeal joint, decreased sensation, and nail deformities. Distal phalangeal fractures may involve the tuft, the shaft, or the joints. With any phalangeal fracture, the nail plate can be injured, resulting in nail plate deformities.

A large percentage of phalangeal fractures can be treated nonsurgically. The radiographic appearance of these fractures helps identify whether the fracture is nondisplaced, minimally displaced, or impacted. Fractures that generally require specialty evaluation include oblique and spiral fractures, markedly displaced or comminuted fractures, and displaced intra-articular fractures.

HISTORY AND PHYSICAL FINDINGS
Patients report a history of direct trauma to the hand and fingers, specifically pain and swelling in the affected fingers. Physical examination reveals tenderness to palpation, swelling, and deformity if the fracture is displaced. Careful assessment for rotational malalignment is critical. The best way to evaluate for malalignment is to ask the patient to flex the fingers. When the fingers are extended, a phalangeal fracture may appear to be nondisplaced; however, when flexed, the affected finger may appear to overlap the adjacent finger, indicating a rotational malalignment. Examination of neurovascular status and tendon function is also important, particularly with open injuries.

ICD-9 Codes

816.01
Fracture of middle or proximal phalanx or phalanges, closed

816.02
Fracture of distal phalanx or phalanges, closed

816.11
Fracture of middle or proximal phalanx or phalanges, open

816.12
Fracture of distal phalanx or phalanges, open

SECTION 6 ■ HAND AND WRIST

IMAGING STUDIES

Required for diagnosis

PA, lateral, and oblique views should be obtained to establish the diagnosis. Of these, the oblique view often is the only view to show the fracture; it is also helpful in adequately assessing angulation, displacement, and rotation.

Required for comprehensive evaluation

CT can be helpful in evaluating potential displaced intra-articular fractures. MRI is seldom indicated.

Special considerations

None

Pitfalls

Rotational malalignment may not be recognized from plain radiographs, so the clinical evaluation testing for malalignment is essential.

IMAGE DESCRIPTIONS

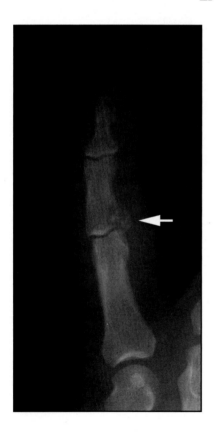

Figure 6-29

Fracture of the phalanx (intra-articular)— PA view

PA view of the little finger shows an intra-articular fracture of the middle phalanx (arrow). The radial collateral ligament is attached to this small bone fragment. The joint is reduced into its normal position.

SECTION 6 ■ HAND AND WRIST

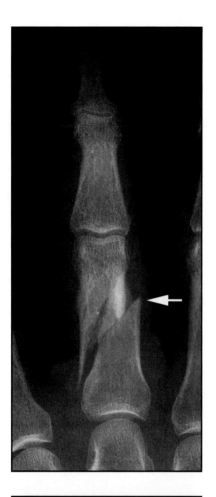

Figure 6-30

Fracture of the proximal phalanx—PA view

PA view of a middle finger shows an oblique fracture of the shaft of the proximal phalanx (arrow). Note that shortening has occurred, but it is impossible to tell from this view whether rotational malalignment exists. This type of fracture tends to be unstable and likely needs some type of surgical fixation.

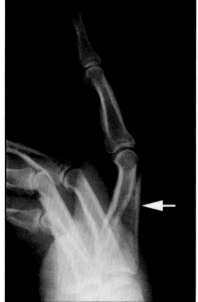

Figure 6-31

Fracture of the proximal phalanx—Lateral view

Lateral view of the same finger shown in Figure 6-30 shows a displaced fracture of the proximal phalanx (arrow). The fracture has shortened and angulated with the apex palmarly (volarly).

SECTION 6 ■ HAND AND WRIST

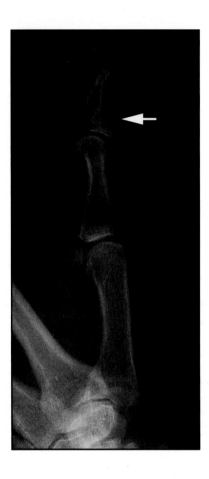

Figure 6-32

Fracture of the distal phalanx—
Lateral view

Lateral view of the distal phalanx of the thumb shows a transverse fracture through the shaft (arrow). The distal fragment is displaced palmarly (volarly), about half the width of the phalanx. This fracture should be considered stable because the flexor and extensor tendons insert onto the base of the distal phalanx. In this case, the nail is at risk for nail deformity because of likely injury to the nail matrix.

DIFFERENTIAL DIAGNOSIS

Cellulitis (soft-tissue swelling possible on radiographs, but no fracture)

Dislocation (lack of normal joint alignment on radiographs)

Gout (soft-tissue swelling possible on radiographs, but no fracture)

Septic joint (soft-tissue swelling possible on radiographs, but no fracture)

FRACTURE OF THE PISIFORM

SYNONYMS
None

ICD-9 Code

814.04
Fracture of the pisiform,
closed

DEFINITION
Fractures involving the body of the pisiform are quite rare,
accounting for only 1% of all carpal fractures. When they occur,
these fractures are commonly associated with other fractures of the
upper extremity. Arthritis of the pisotriquetral joint may develop as
a long-term sequela.

HISTORY AND PHYSICAL FINDINGS
Pisiform fractures are typically caused by acute trauma sustained
either in a fall or from a direct blow from the butt end of a golf
club, baseball bat, or tennis racquet. Tenderness is elicited directly
with palpation over the pisiform on the ulnar side of the wrist.
Numbness in the little and ring fingers may occur from bleeding of
the fracture into Guyon's canal.

IMAGING STUDIES

Required for diagnosis
PA and lateral views should be ordered, but they are not good for
visualizing these fractures. If these views appear normal and a
fracture of the pisiform is suspected, a carpal tunnel view and an
oblique view with the wrist in supination can help make the
diagnosis.

Required for comprehensive evaluation
If the views described above are normal despite the high index of
suspicion for a pisiform fracture, CT should be ordered as it will
reveal the fracture.

Special considerations
None

Pitfalls
None

IMAGE DESCRIPTION

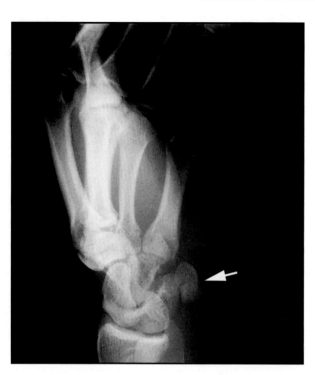

Figure 6-33

Fracture of the pisiform—Oblique view

Oblique view (also called pisiform or Norgaard view) of the left wrist with the wrist in supination shows a nondisplaced fracture through the body of the pisiform (arrow).

DIFFERENTIAL DIAGNOSIS

Flexor carpi ulnaris tendinitis (normal radiographs, calcification around the tendon possible)

Pisotriquetral arthritis (joint space narrowing seen on pisiform view)

Triangular fibrocartilage complex (TFCC) tear (tear seen on MRI)

Ulnar artery thrombosis (positive Allen's test; ultrasound will show clot)

FRACTURE OF THE SCAPHOID

SYNONYMS
None

ICD-9 Code

814.01
Fracture of the navicular
(scaphoid) of wrist, closed

DEFINITION
Fractures of the scaphoid account for 80% of all carpal bone fractures. Of all fractures about the wrist, only fractures of the distal radius occur more frequently. The mechanism of injury is a fall on the extended and radially deviated wrist. The proximal pole of the scaphoid is covered by cartilage and has no independent blood supply. The main blood supply to the scaphoid enters through the waist and distal pole. Therefore, fractures in the proximal pole of the scaphoid are slower to heal and have a higher incidence of nonunion and osteonecrosis than do fractures in the more distal portions of the scaphoid.

HISTORY AND PHYSICAL FINDINGS
Fractures of the scaphoid are typically caused by a fall on an outstretched hand or by axial loading with the wrist in extension. Patients usually report diffuse radial-sided wrist pain and have tenderness in the anatomic snuffbox area. Some isolated scaphoid fractures have few symptoms, and the patient may not seek treatment in a timely manner, increasing the chances of delayed healing or nonunion.

IMAGING STUDIES

Required for diagnosis
PA, lateral, and scaphoid views should be obtained initially. If the fracture is not evident on the initial views, the wrist and thumb should be immobilized and radiographs should be repeated 2 to 3 weeks later, when bone resorption at the fracture site may make the fracture line more evident.

Required for comprehensive evaluation
If the repeat radiographs are normal but suspicion of a scaphoid fracture remains high based on the clinical examination, MRI of the wrist should be obtained.

Special considerations
None

Pitfalls
Initial radiographs of the wrist may be normal in the presence of an occult scaphoid fracture.

IMAGE DESCRIPTIONS

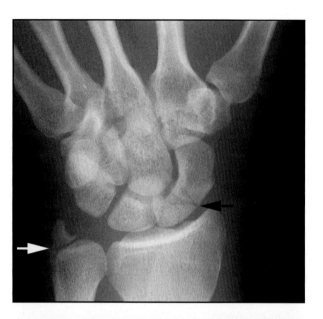

Figure 6-34

Fracture of the scaphoid—PA view

PA view of a left wrist shows a fracture at the junction of the proximal and middle thirds of the scaphoid (black arrow) and a fracture of the ulnar styloid (white arrow).

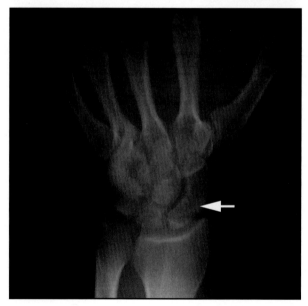

Figure 6-35

Fracture of the scaphoid— Scaphoid view

In this scaphoid view of the left wrist, the fracture in the middle third of the bone (arrow) is visualized. Note that this view causes the scaphoid to appear elongated.

Differential Diagnosis

Carpometacarpal arthritis (older age group; positive stress test; radiographs show arthritis at the carpometacarpal joint)

de Quervain's disease (positive Finkelstein's test, negative radiographs)

Flexor carpi radialis tendinitis (localized tenderness over the flexor tendon; calcification may be seen about the tendon on radiographs)

Radioscaphoid arthritis (easily seen on PA views)

Section 6 ■ Hand and Wrist

FRACTURE OF THE THUMB METACARPAL

ICD-9 Codes

815.01
Fracture of base of thumb [first] metacarpal, closed

815.03
Fracture of shaft of metacarpal bone(s), closed

815.11
Fracture of base of thumb [first] metacarpal, open

815.13
Fracture of shaft of metacarpal bone(s), open

SYNONYMS

Bennett's fracture
Rolando's fracture

DEFINITION

Thumb metacarpal fractures differ from fractures of the finger metacarpals in that neither the metacarpal head nor the shaft of the thumb is commonly affected. Rather, most thumb metacarpal fractures occur at the base and may be intra-articular (called Bennett's or Rolando's fractures) or extra-articular.

Bennett's fracture is an intra-articular fracture that usually occurs after a direct axial load is applied to the flexed metacarpal. The fracture line separates the large portion of the metacarpal dorsally from the smaller, triangular-shaped fragment volarly. This triangular bone fragment remains attached to the trapezium through the strong anterior oblique ligament. The larger fragment is displaced proximally and radially by the pull of the adductor pollicis and the abductor pollicis longus, resulting in dislocation of the metacarpal shaft. Approximately one third of thumb metacarpal fractures are Bennett's fractures.

The classic Rolando's fracture is a comminuted three-part fracture in which the fracture pattern has a T- or Y-shaped intra-articular component. The term Rolando's fracture is now used for any comminuted intra-articular fracture of the base of the thumb metacarpal. This fracture pattern is much less common than the Bennett's type and has a poorer prognosis.

A third type of fracture is a transverse or oblique extra-articular fracture at the base of the thumb metacarpal. This fracture is often confused with a Bennett's fracture, but whereas Bennett's fractures tend to be unstable, many of these are stable and can be treated with closed reduction and casting.

HISTORY AND PHYSICAL FINDINGS

A typical history is of a direct longitudinal blow to the thumb with the thumb metacarpal flexed. This may occur from a fall on the thumb or from an object such as a baseball striking the tip of the thumb with the metacarpal flexed. Swelling and deformity at the base of the thumb are evident. Any active or passive motion of the thumb is painful and limited.

IMAGING STUDIES

Required for diagnosis
PA and lateral views will easily demonstrate the fracture. Other views are seldom needed.

Required for comprehensive evaluation
CT can be useful in planning treatment for a comminuted Rolando's fracture.

Special considerations
None

Pitfalls
Bennett's fracture is really a fracture-subluxation, and the tendency for this fracture to subluxate over time may not be appreciated. Careful scrutiny of a lateral view and repeat lateral views will easily reveal this subluxation.

IMAGE DESCRIPTIONS

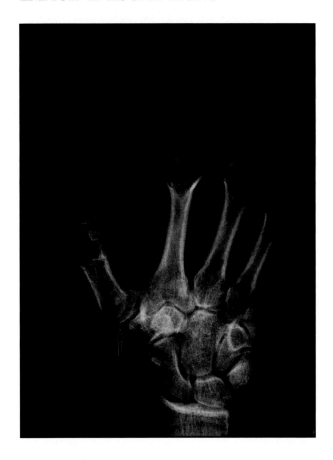

Figure 6-36

Rolando's fracture—PA view

PA view of the hand and wrist shows a fracture at the base of the left thumb metacarpal (arrow). On this view, it appears as if it may be a Bennett's fracture with only two parts, but the oblique view (Figure 6-37) shows three fracture parts.

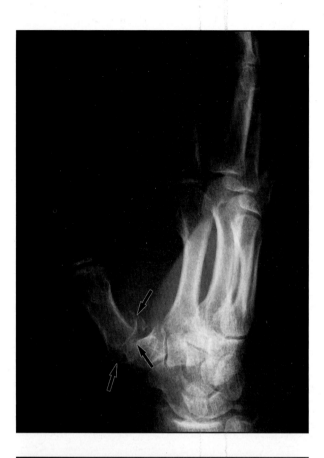

Figure 6-37

Rolando's fracture—Oblique view

Oblique view of the hand and wrist shows a three-part fracture at the base of the left thumb metacarpal (arrows). This fracture is displaced and considered unstable; therefore, surgical treatment is indicated.

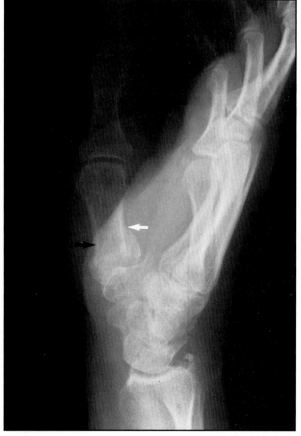

Figure 6-38

Bennett's fracture—AP view

AP view of the hand and wrist shows a healed fracture at the base of the thumb metacarpal (black arrow). Note the callus formation (white arrow). From this view, the Bennett's fracture cannot be seen.

SECTION 6 ■ HAND AND WRIST

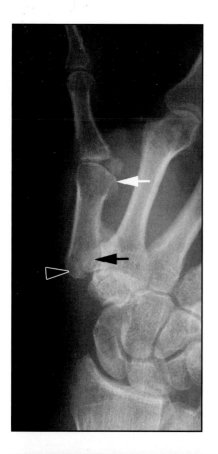

Figure 6-39

Bennett's fracture—Lateral view

Lateral view of the hand shown in Figure 6-38 shows a healed Bennett's fracture (black arrow), proximal migration of the distal thumb metacarpal (arrowhead), and an adducted position of the thumb metacarpal (white arrow).

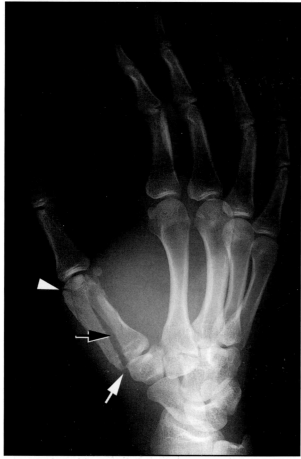

Figure 6-40

Fracture of the metacarpal (thumb)—Oblique view

Oblique view of the right hand shows a longitudinal fracture of the thumb metacarpal (black arrow). The fracture extends into the carpometacarpal (CMC) (white arrow) and metacarpophalangeal (arrowhead) joints.

SECTION 6 ■ HAND AND WRIST

DIFFERENTIAL DIAGNOSIS

CMC arthritis (no history of acute trauma)

CMC dislocation or subluxation (radiographs will show the difference)

Fracture of the Triquetrum

Synonym
Dorsal chip fracture

ICD-9 Code

814.03
Fracture of triquetral
(cuneiform) bone of wrist,
closed

Definition
Fractures of the triquetrum are the second most common carpal bone fracture, after fractures of the scaphoid. Isolated triquetral fractures are uncommon; these fractures are usually associated with other carpal fractures or dislocations. Triquetral fractures are most commonly produced by impaction, avulsion, or shear forces that occur when the ulnar styloid impacts the triquetrum with the wrist in dorsiflexion and ulnar deviation. Two types of triquetral fractures occur: dorsal cortical fractures and fractures of the body of the triquetrum. With dorsal cortical fractures, which are the more common, impaction is believed to be the mechanism of injury, and a longer than normal ulnar styloid is often present. Closed management is sufficient for most dorsal cortical fractures. Fractures of the body of the triquetrum are much less common and are usually associated with other carpal injuries. Most triquetral fractures will heal with casting alone. When nonunion occurs, it is usually asymptomatic.

History and Physical Findings
Localized swelling and tenderness over the dorsal ulnar aspect of the wrist are typical.

Imaging Studies

Required for diagnosis
PA, lateral, and oblique views will be adequate to diagnose most triquetral fractures. The lateral and oblique views will demonstrate a dorsal cortical fracture, and the PA view often shows a fracture of the body of the triquetrum.

Required for comprehensive evaluation
CT or bone scans should be ordered if radiographs are normal and a fracture is suspected based on clinical examination.

Special considerations
None

Pitfalls

Fractures of the triquetrum may occur as part of a perilunate fracture-dislocation pattern. Associated fractures and ligamentous injuries should therefore be suspected.

IMAGE DESCRIPTIONS

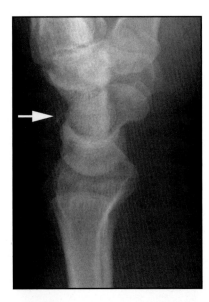

Figure 6-41

Fracture of the triquetrum (cortical)— Lateral view

Lateral view of a wrist demonstrates a small osseous density just dorsal to the wrist (arrow), which is a cortical fragment from the dorsum of the triquetrum. Note that the carpal alignment is normal.

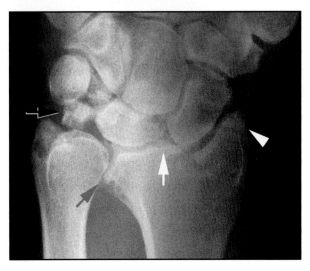

Figure 6-42

Fracture of the triquetrum (body)—PA view

PA view of a left wrist shows a comminuted fracture of the body of the triquetrum (black arrow). In addition, a fracture of the radial styloid is present (white arrowhead), as well as an injury to the scapholunate joint (white arrow). Arthritic changes are also present at the distal radioulnar joint (gray arrow).

DIFFERENTIAL DIAGNOSIS

None

Lunotriquetral Instability

Synonyms

Lunotriquetral dissociation
Lunotriquetral sprain

Definition

Lunotriquetral instability, a disruption of the anatomy or motion dynamics between the lunate and triquetrum, leads to a spectrum of wrist conditions. This disruption occurs as a result of ulnar-sided wrist trauma. The exact mechanism is not known, but it is hypothesized to be the result of an extreme wrist dorsiflexion, radial deviation, and intercarpal pronation. With complete disruption of the ligaments between the lunate and triquetrum, the scaphoid and lunate flex in a pattern referred to as VISI (volar intercalated segment instability). The ligaments between the lunate and triquetrum are subject to attritional and degenerative changes, and ligamentous defects are increasingly common after age 40 years. Cadaver studies have demonstrated a 55% occurrence of lunotriquetral tears, suggesting that these tears are a normal part of aging and may not be the cause of a patient's wrist pain.

History and Physical Findings

With acute injuries, patients report a history of significant trauma resulting in ulnar-sided wrist pain, swelling, decreased grip strength, and focal tenderness over the injured joint. With chronic sprains, patients will usually report a painful "click" or "pop" with ulnar deviation. Frequently, the patient has no recollection of an injury. Three clinical tests have been described as helpful in making this diagnosis: the shear test, the shuck sign, and the ballottement maneuver. These require a great deal of skill and experience to perform and interpret. The diagnosis of ulnar-sided wrist pain remains very difficult and often requires specialty referral.

Imaging Studies

Required for diagnosis

PA and lateral views will show the VISI pattern in advanced cases. On the PA view, a step-off can be seen between the lunate and triquetrum, and the triquetrum can be seen to have migrated proximally. Variations in anatomy, which are more common in women, may lead to an incorrect diagnosis of lunotriquetral instability. Comparison views of the opposite wrist are helpful.

ICD-9 Codes

718.83
Other joint derangement, not elsewhere classified; forearm

736.09
Acquired deformities of forearm, excluding fingers; other

833.03
Dislocation of wrist, midcarpal (joint), closed

842.01
Sprains and strains of wrist and hand, carpal (joint)

Section 6 ■ Hand and Wrist

Required for comprehensive evaluation
Wrist arthrography, high-resolution MRI, or MR arthrography can demonstrate a tear of the lunotriquetral ligaments. However, there is no consensus at this time on which is the preferred modality. Cineradiography can demonstrate abnormal motion between the lunate and triquetrum.

Special considerations
None

Pitfalls
In patients older than 40 years, attritional tears occur normally and may not be the cause of wrist pain.

IMAGE DESCRIPTION

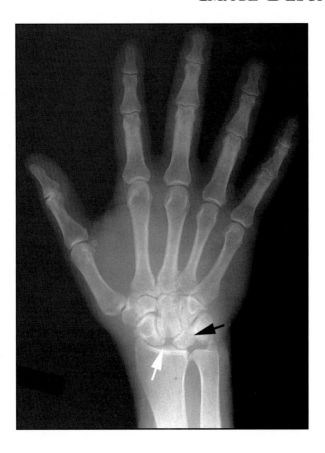

Figure 6-43

Lunotriquetral instability—PA view

PA view of the hand and wrist shows disruption of the lunotriquetral ligament with overlap of the lunotriquetral bones and tilting of the lunate (black arrow). Note also the widening of the scapholunate interval (white arrow), consistent with scapholunate dissociation.

DIFFERENTIAL DIAGNOSIS

Disruption of the distal radioulnar joint (dorsal subluxation of ulna on CT)

Fracture of the triquetrum (fracture seen on radiographs)

Midcarpal instability (demonstrated on cineradiography)

Subluxation of the extensor carpi ulnaris (clinical examination)

Triangular fibrocartilage complex (TFCC) tears (positive arthrogram)

Ulnar impaction syndrome (positive ulnar variance, appearance of the lunate on MRI)

SECTION 6 ■ HAND AND WRIST

MALLET FINGER

SECTION 6 ■ HAND AND WRIST

ICD-9 Codes

736.1
Mallet finger

816.02
Fracture of the distal phalanx
or phalanges, closed

SYNONYMS

Baseball finger
Extensor avulsion fracture of the distal phalanx

DEFINITION

When the insertion of the extensor tendon is avulsed from the distal phalanx, the unopposed flexor digitorum profundus tendon flexes the distal interphalangeal (DIP) joint. The finger assumes a bent position like the head of a mallet, hence the term "mallet" deformity. With some of these injuries, the tendon may avulse a fragment of the distal phalanx. If a large fragment is broken off, the joint may become unstable, causing the distal phalanx to subluxate palmarly (volarly).

HISTORY AND PHYSICAL FINDINGS

The most common mechanism of injury is a blow to the end of the finger that acutely flexes the DIP joint, such as a ball hitting the end of the finger. Occasionally, these injuries result from minor trauma, such as stubbing the end of the finger when reaching for something or when reaching into a pocket. Pain and swelling may be absent, depending on the extent of injury. The patient will report the inability to extend the finger at the DIP joint. Shortly after the injury, tenderness to palpation is noted over the top of the DIP joint.

IMAGING STUDIES

Required for diagnosis
PA and lateral views of the finger are sufficient to diagnose this injury. If bone is avulsed with the tendon, it should be noted what percentage of the joint is involved and whether the distal phalanx is subluxated. On the lateral view, a line drawn through the intramedullary canal of the distal phalanx will intersect the midportion of the condyle of the middle phalanx if the joint is reduced.

Required for comprehensive evaluation
None

Special considerations
None

Pitfalls

A subluxation of the DIP joint can easily be missed on the PA view, so a lateral view must always be obtained.

IMAGE DESCRIPTIONS

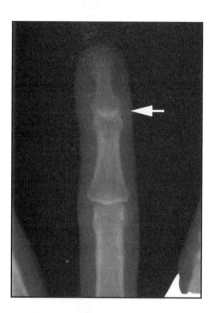

Figure 6-44

Mallet finger—PA view

PA view of a middle finger with a bony mallet deformity shows narrowing of the joint space (arrow), even though the fracture cannot be appreciated on this view.

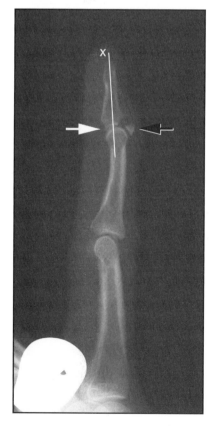

Figure 6-45

Mallet finger—Lateral view

Lateral view of the middle finger in Figure 6-44 shows a bone fragment avulsed from the distal phalanx (black arrow). The fracture is intra-articular and involves approximately 40% of the joint space. Note that the joint remains reduced (white arrow), as shown by the fact that line X intersects the midportion of the condyle of the proximal middle phalanx.

SECTION 6 ■ HAND AND WRIST

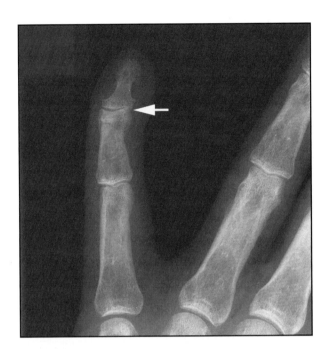

Figure 6-46

Mallet finger—PA view

PA view of a little finger shows a mallet deformity caused by rupture of the extensor tendon without an associated fracture. Note that the finger also shows signs of osteoarthritis (arrow).

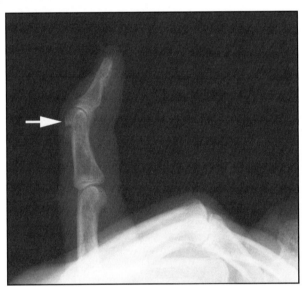

Figure 6-47

Mallet finger—Lateral view

On the lateral view, the dorsal osteophyte coming off the middle phalanx can be appreciated (arrow).

DIFFERENTIAL DIAGNOSIS

Flexion contracture (no history of acute trauma; no fracture visible on radiographs)

PERILUNATE INSTABILITY AND DISLOCATION

ICD-9 Codes

718.83
Other joint derangement, not elsewhere classified; forearm

736.09
Acquired deformities of forearm, excluding fingers; other

833.02
Dislocation of radiocarpal (joint), closed

833.03
Dislocation of midcarpal (joint), closed

842.01
Sprains and strains of carpal (joint)

SYNONYMS

Carpal instability
Carpal instability combined-perilunate dislocation
"Lesser arc" disruption or dislocation
Perilunate dislocation

DEFINITION

Most wrist injuries occur with the wrist under extreme load in extension and radial or ulnar deviation. Several factors determine whether the carpal bones or ligaments will fail, including the age of the patient, the position of the wrist at impact, and the magnitude of the force at impact. The pattern of injury represents a spectrum from simple ligament tears with lesser energy dissipation to complete dislocations from higher impact injuries. Mayfield described four stages of progressive perilunate instability depending on the amount of energy imparted into the system. In stage 1, the scapholunate ligaments are torn, resulting in scapholunate dissociation. In stages 2 and 3, the forces continue in an ulnar direction, separating the lunate from the adjacent carpal bones and resulting in a dorsal perilunate dislocation. In stage 4, the lunate is forced palmarly, resulting in a lunate dislocation—the most severe degree of instability.

Fractures of adjacent carpal bones frequently occur in combination with ligament injuries and follow a specific pattern of energy dissipation referred to as the "greater arc," which involves fractures of the scaphoid and capitate. "Lesser arc" injuries pass through soft tissue only, as shown in the figure below. Gilula

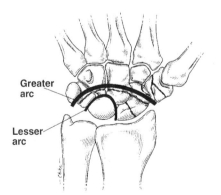

Greater arc

Lesser arc

Palmar view of a right hand showing the pathways of ligamentous and bone injury about the wrist. The lesser arc injuries represent the ligamentous disruptions described by Mayfield and associates. Greater arc injuries are those that occur through the carpal bones.

Reproduced with permission from Kozin SH, Murphy MS, Cooney WP: Perilunate dislocations, in Cooney WP, Linscheid RL, Dobyns JH (eds): The Wrist: Diagnosis and Operative Treatment. St. Louis, MO, Mosby, 1998.

has described three carpal arcs, as shown in the figure below, on neutral PA or AP views of the wrist, which help define normal carpal anatomy. Arc I outlines the proximal margins or convex surfaces of the scaphoid, lunate, and triquetrum. Arc II outlines the distal margins or concave surfaces of these three bones. Arc III outlines the proximal or convex surfaces of the capitate and hamate. These arcs should be concentric in the normal wrist. Loss of parallelism and/or broken arcs with a step-off or overlaps indicate ligament disruption and carpal malalignment. The distance between the carpal bones normally is 2 mm; a space of more than 4 mm suggests ligamentous disruption. A space between the scaphoid and lunate of more than 3 to 4 mm is considered abnormal and is referred to as the "Terry-Thomas sign," referring to the widened space between the front teeth in this celebrity. Likewise, any overlap of the carpal bones indicates ligamentous injury.

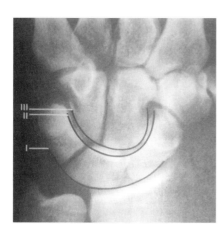

Carpal arcs described by Gilula.
Reproduced from Blazar PE, Lawton JN: Diagnosis of acute carpal ligament injuries, in Trumble TE (ed); Carpal Fracture-Dislocations. Rosemont, IL, American Academy of Orthopaedic Surgeons, 2002, pp 19-26.

HISTORY AND PHYSICAL FINDINGS

These injuries are usually the result of high-energy trauma to the extended wrist and hand. Severe pain and swelling are typical with high-impact injuries. Decreased sensation may occur in the median nerve distribution with perilunate or lunate dislocations. Patients often mistake stage 1 injuries for simple sprains and may delay seeking treatment.

IMAGING STUDIES

Required for diagnosis

PA, lateral, PA in ulnar deviation (scaphoid view), and 45° pronated oblique views should be obtained in suspected carpal injuries. Note that careful evaluation of these studies is mandatory, particularly with severe injuries, because it is reported that up to 20% of initial radiographs are misread.

SECTION 6 ■ HAND AND WRIST

Required for comprehensive evaluation

If these views do not confirm a suspected carpal instability, a PA clenched fist view is helpful in demonstrating scapholunate instability. MRI has a limited role in evaluating carpal instabilities.

Special considerations

Wrist arthrography, MRI, and MR arthrography can show ligament tears if further workup is needed.

Pitfalls

Lunate dislocations are frequently missed. The PA view may look normal, but a lateral view must be obtained and studied carefully. The dislocated lunate is always visible on the lateral view.

IMAGE DESCRIPTIONS

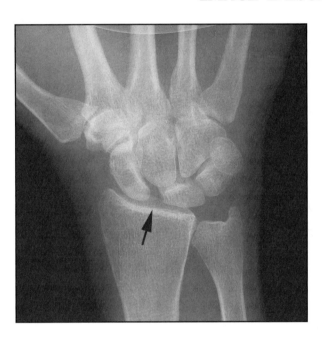

Figure 6-48

Scapholunate dissociation—PA view

PA view of a right wrist shows the separation between the scaphoid and lunate (Terry-Thomas sign) (arrow).

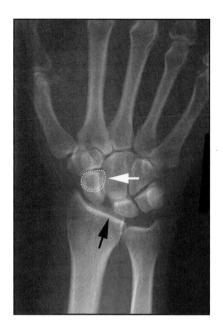

Figure 6-49

Scapholunate dissociation—PA view

PA view of a right wrist shows the increased space between the scaphoid and lunate (black arrow). Note also the scaphoid ring sign, indicating that the scaphoid is rotated into a more vertical position (white arrow, dotted ring).

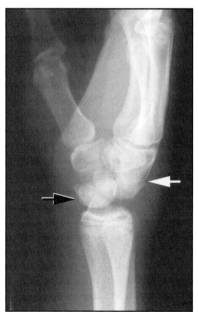

Figure 6-50

Perilunate dislocation—Lateral view

Lateral view of a dorsal perilunate dislocation shows that the lunate remains in line with the radius (black arrow), but the capitate is not colinear with the lunate but rather sits dorsal to the lunate (white arrow).

SECTION 6 ■ HAND AND WRIST

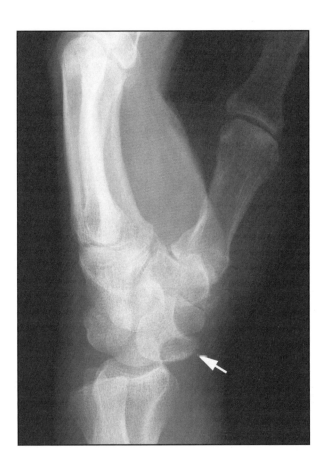

Figure 6-51

Lunate dislocation—Lateral view

Lateral view of a wrist shows a lunate dislocation in which the lunate is not colinear with the radius but rather is dislocated and faces downward (arrow). This is the most extreme form of instability.

DIFFERENTIAL DIAGNOSIS

Fracture of carpal bone (seen on radiograph, MRI, or bone scan)

Kienböck's disease (seen on radiograph or MRI)

Occult ganglion (seen on MRI)

Triangular fibrocartilage complex (TFCC) tear (seen on arthroscopy, arthrography, MRI, or MR arthrography)

Wrist sprain (normal radiographs)

ULNAR COLLATERAL LIGAMENT INJURY OF THE THUMB

SYNONYMS
Gamekeeper's thumb
Skier's thumb

ICD-9 Code

842.12
Sprains and strains of the metacarpophalangeal (joint)

DEFINITION
The metacarpophalangeal (MCP) joint of the thumb depends on a pair of strong proper and accessory collateral ligaments for its stability. The ulnar collateral ligament (UCL) is especially susceptible to injury, occurring at least 10 times more often than radial collateral ligament tears. A force that directs the proximal phalanx of the thumb radially (away from the palm) will result in a UCL tear. The ligament most often tears at its distal insertion onto the proximal phalanx.

Stener has described a pathology in which the UCL folds back and becomes trapped proximally behind the aponeurosis of the adductor pollicis tendon when the thumb spontaneously relocates after injury. The aponeurosis prevents the torn end of the ligament from reattaching to its normal insertion. This injury is called the Stener lesion. Surgery is almost always required for repair of this lesion. Occasionally, a fleck of bone attached to the lateral collateral ligament will be pulled off the base of the proximal phalanx. The Stener lesion is rarely present in skeletally immature patients with open epiphyses.

HISTORY AND PHYSICAL FINDINGS
Patients commonly report a fall on an outstretched hand and thumb, often while holding a ski pole with the strap securely around the wrist. Pain and swelling along the inside of the thumb in the first web space are typical, as is diminished pinch strength. Examination of the thumb reveals focal tenderness and swelling over the ulnar aspect of the MCP joint, and the thumb distal to the MCP joint may appear pronated and radially deviated after a severe injury. Stress testing may reveal laxity on the affected side. Ecchymosis may not appear immediately after the injury.

IMAGING STUDIES

Required for diagnosis
PA and lateral radiographs of the thumb will show an avulsion fracture off the base of the proximal phalanx. The radiographs will appear normal, however, if the injury is purely ligamentous.

Required for comprehensive evaluation

A stress PA radiograph of the MCP joint will show a complete tear. To obtain this view, the thumb must be forced into radial deviation while the radiograph is taken. With complete tears, the proximal phalanx may form an angle of 45° or more with the thumb metacarpal.

Special considerations

Stress views may require administration of a local anesthetic block to the thumb to eliminate pain and adequately stress the thumb. MRI can demonstrate tears and the degree of retraction of the UCL.

Pitfalls

Without a stress view or MRI, a complete tear of the UCL may be missed. Failure to treat a complete tear will lead to chronic loss of pinch strength.

IMAGE DESCRIPTIONS

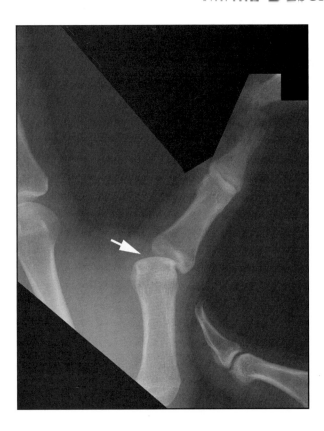

Figure 6-52

Ulnar collateral ligament injury— Stress view

Stress view of the MCP joint of the thumb shows how the joint space opens up on the inside (ulnar) of the thumb (white arrow). A Stener lesion is likely present, and surgery will be needed to repair the ligament. When the UCL is intact, this space will open only slightly with stress.

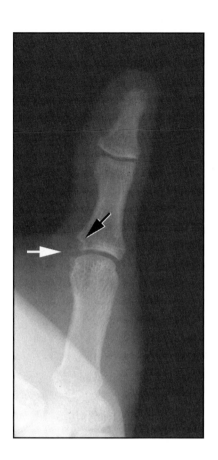

Figure 6-53

Ulnar collateral ligament injury—PA view

PA view of the left thumb shows erosion at the base of the proximal phalanx on the ulnar side (black arrow). Note that an avulsed fragment is attached to the UCL (white arrow), but this fragment will heal with immobilization alone.

DIFFERENTIAL DIAGNOSIS

Fracture of the base of the proximal phalanx or metacarpal head (apparent on radiographs)

Radial collateral ligament tear (tenderness on the outside of the thumb at the MCP joint)

Volar plate injury (tenderness is volar at the MCP joint; possible hyperextension of the thumb)

ULNAR IMPACTION SYNDROME

ICD-9 Code

718.83
Other joint derangement, not elsewhere classified, forearm

SECTION 6 ■ HAND AND WRIST

SYNONYM
Ulnocarpal abutment

DEFINITION
In ulnar impaction syndrome, the ulnar head abuts against the triangular fibrocartilage complex (TFCC) and the ulnar carpus, especially the ulnar side of the lunate. Over time, the TFCC degenerates and chondromalacia and cystic changes develop in the lunate. This condition has become recognized as one of the more common causes of ulnar-sided wrist pain. Ulnar impaction syndrome may be caused by any of a variety of conditions: an abnormally long ulna relative to the radius (positive ulnar variance); a long ulnar styloid; malunion of a radial fracture with shortening of the radius; premature closure of the distal radial epiphysis; or excision of the radial head causing the radius to shift proximally, making the ulna appear longer than the radius. In rare cases, when the TFCC is abnormally thick, ulnar impaction syndrome may occur when the ulnar length is normal (normal ulnar variance) or even shorter than normal (negative ulnar variance). Typical radiographic findings are positive ulnar variance and cystic changes in the lunate.

HISTORY AND PHYSICAL FINDINGS
A history of a fracture of the radius may be present, although often patients will report no history of trauma. Patients commonly report ulnar-sided wrist pain, especially with ulnar deviation of the wrist. Some patients may report a clicking sensation along the ulnar side of the wrist. Tenderness on palpation over the lunate may be present.

IMAGING STUDIES

Required for diagnosis
PA and lateral views will show the positive ulnar variance and any cystic changes in the lunate or triquetrum.

Required for comprehensive evaluation
A PA clenched fist view will often show the ulna impacting against the TFCC and ulnar carpus. MRI will show changes in the ulnar aspect of the lunate or the radial aspect of the triquetrum, as well as damage to the TFCC, lunotriquetral ligament, and cartilage.

Special considerations
None

Pitfalls
None

IMAGE DESCRIPTIONS

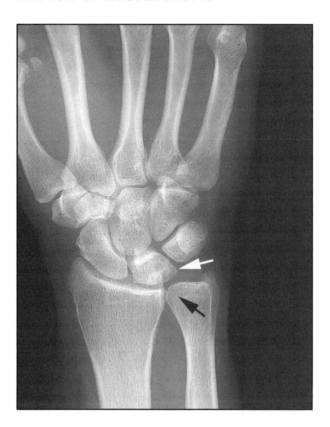

Figure 6-54

*Ulnar impaction syndrome—
PA clenched fist view*

PA clenched fist view of a right wrist shows a positive ulnar variance (black arrow). Cystic changes can be seen in the lunate, opposite the ulna (white arrow).

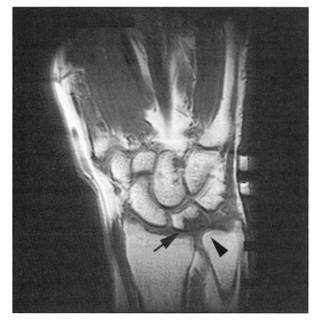

Figure 6-55

Ulnar impaction syndrome—MRI

T1-weighted MRI scan of a right wrist shows low signal intensity within the ulnar and proximal aspects of the lunate (arrow) with positive ulnar variance (arrowhead), consistent with ulnocarpal impaction.

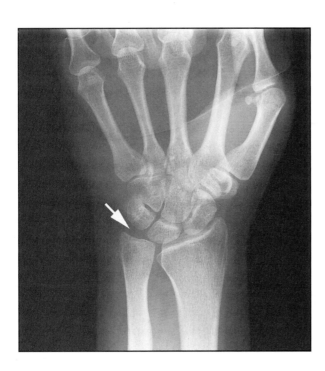

Figure 6-56

Ulnar impaction syndrome— PA clenched fist view

In this PA clenched fist view of a left wrist, the ulna can be seen to abut against the lunate (arrow).

DIFFERENTIAL DIAGNOSIS

Extensor carpi ulnaris tendinitis (normal radiographs; localized tenderness over the extensor carpi ulnaris)

Lunotriquetral ligament tear (tear seen on MRI or wrist arthrogram without positive ulnar variance or bone changes)

Pisotriquetral arthritis (lateral pisiform view shows osteoarthritic changes)

Triangular fibrocartilage complex (TFCC) tear (tear is seen on MRI or wrist arthrogram without positive ulnar variance or bone changes)

CARPOMETACARPAL ARTHRITIS OF THE THUMB

SYNONYMS
Basal joint arthritis
CMC arthritis

DEFINITION
The carpometacarpal (CMC) joint of the thumb is the second most common site of osteoarthritis in the hand, second only to the distal interphalangeal joints. The incidence in postmenopausal women ranges from 16% to 25%, which is two to three times higher than in men. Bilateral involvement is common. Patients with CMC arthritis, however, are not at increased risk for osteoarthritis in other joints of the hand.

The CMC joint of the thumb has a characteristic shape; each side of the joint is shaped like a saddle. The arrangement of the joint surfaces allows for increased range of motion not only in flexion and extension but also in side-to-side motion. A certain amount of incongruity is present between these surfaces that allows for the increased motion. This incongruity, however, may be responsible for or contribute to the development of osteoarthritis of this joint.

Large forces are transmitted across the CMC joint. The joint reaction force across the CMC joint is 10 times higher than that of the tip pinch force of the thumb, which is why even a simple pinching motion can be very painful in patients with CMC arthritis. The cause of thumb CMC arthritis is unknown, but the large forces transmitted across this joint probably play a role. The stability of this joint also depends on six ligaments along with the saddle-shaped architecture of the joint itself. Ligamentous laxity commonly is seen in patients with CMC arthritis. It is not clear whether this laxity is a cause or the result of the arthritis.

HISTORY AND PHYSICAL FINDINGS
Pain at the base of the thumb in women older than 30 years suggests a diagnosis of CMC arthritis or synovitis. Hand weakness is common, especially during activities involving pinching. The pain is relieved by rest and by nonsteroidal anti-inflammatory drugs. Intra-articular steroid injections provide several months of pain relief. Swelling over the base of the thumb is common. Loss of thumb motion occurs years after the onset of symptoms. The thumb draws into the palm, and patients have trouble getting the thumb around objects such as a drinking glass. The decrease in motion usually is accompanied by a decrease in pain. Carpal tunnel

ICD-9 Codes
715.14
Osteoarthrosis of the hand, localized, primary

715.24
Osteoarthrosis of the hand, localized, secondary

715.94
Osteoarthrosis of the hand, unspecified whether generalized or localized

SECTION 6 ■ HAND AND WRIST

syndrome often accompanies CMC arthritis with the characteristic intermittent numbness in the thumb, index, middle, and ring fingers.

A Watson's stress test is very useful to diagnose CMC arthritis. With the palm facing up and the back of the hand resting on the table, the thumb is pushed down toward the table with the MCP and interphalangeal joints extended. Pain elicited with this maneuver is specific for CMC arthritis. Grinding the thumb metacarpal against the trapezium also causes pain. Tenderness is common over the volar and radial aspects of the joint in the region of the base of the thumb metacarpal.

IMAGING STUDIES

Required for diagnosis

PA and lateral views of the thumb, along with a Robert view, will clearly demonstrate CMC arthritis. With the Robert view, the forearm and hand are fully pronated, which provides a clear view of the thumb metacarpotrapezium joint.

Required for comprehensive evaluation

MRI and CT are not needed to make this diagnosis.

Special considerations

None

Pitfalls

None

IMAGE DESCRIPTIONS

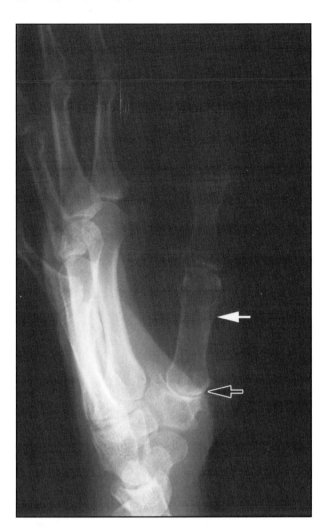

Figure 6-57

CMC arthritis of the thumb— Robert view

Robert view of the left hand of a 61-year-old woman shows that the joint space between the trapezium and thumb metacarpal is obliterated (black arrow). Note also the thumb metacarpal is in an adducted position (white arrow).

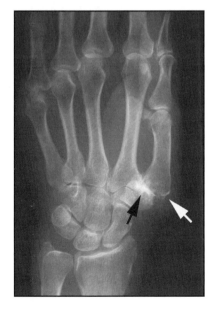

Figure 6-58

CMC arthritis of the thumb—Oblique view

Oblique view of the CMC joint in profile shows joint space narrowing (black arrow) and clear formation of marginal osteophytes (white arrow).

SECTION 6 ■ HAND AND WRIST

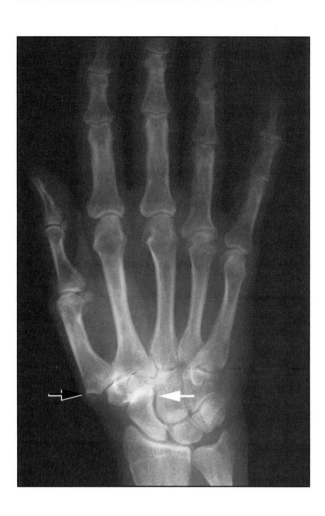

Figure 6-59

Pantrapezial arthritis—PA view

PA view of the right hand of a 71-year-old woman shows CMC arthritis (black arrow). Note also the development of arthritis between the trapezium and scaphoid (white arrow). This is referred to as pantrapezial arthritis.

DIFFERENTIAL DIAGNOSIS

de Quervain's disease (normal radiographs, tenderness over the first extensor compartment)

Neuritis of the sensory branch of the radial nerve (positive Tinel's sign over the radial side of the wrist; normal radiographs)

Scaphoid-trapezium-trapezoid (STT) arthritis (CMC joint appears normal on plain radiographs)

Scapholunate advanced collapse (SLAC) wrist (radioscaphoid arthritis apparent on radiographs)

GOUT

SYNONYMS
None

ICD-9 Code
274.0
Gouty arthropathy

DEFINITION
Gout is a metabolic condition in which monosodium urate crystals cause synovial inflammation in the joints, most commonly in the feet and hands. The metatarsophalangeal joint of the great toe is involved at least 75% of the time. In addition to the hands and feet, the knees and elbows can be involved. Deposits of sodium urate, called tophi, may accumulate in the soft tissues about the joints, as well as in the olecranon bursa and the earlobe.

Gout occurs predominantly in middle-aged and elderly men, but postmenopausal women also can be affected. Hyperuricemia, which is almost always present with gout, may be idiopathic or result from chronic renal disease or myeloproliferative disorders. An elevated serum uric acid level confirms the diagnosis, as does visualizing urate crystals in synovial fluid using a polarizing microscope. Certain diuretics may also increase the serum uric acid level. Radiographic changes are slow to develop, occurring months to years after the onset of the disease.

HISTORY AND PHYSICAL FINDINGS
The typical patient is a middle-aged man with acute onset of a swollen, red, painful joint. Gout may be precipitated by stress, such as following surgery, or after excessive alcohol intake. A family history of gout may be present. An acute episode of gout is very painful. Any joint of the hand or wrist can be affected. Joint aspirate that is positive for monosodium urate crystals gives a definitive diagnosis.

SECTION 6 ■ HAND AND WRIST

IMAGING STUDIES

Required for diagnosis

PA and lateral views are adequate to show the characteristic radiographic features of gout, which include well-defined erosions with sclerotic margins and overhanging edges. CT and MRI are usually not necessary for diagnosis.

Required for comprehensive evaluation

None

Special considerations

None

Pitfalls

None

IMAGE DESCRIPTIONS

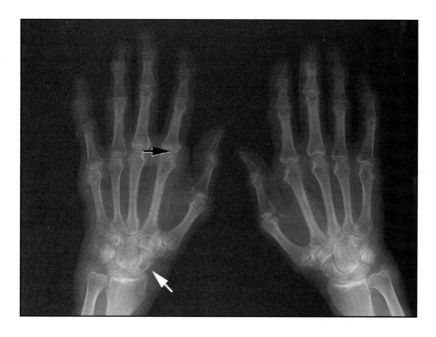

Figure 6-60

Gout (hand)—PA view

PA view of the wrists and hands of a 55-year-old man shows a periarticular erosion with an overhanging edge at the base of the proximal phalanx and the radial aspect of the metacarpal head of the left index finger (black arrow). Note also the large cystic lesion in the scaphoid (white arrow). Scattered soft-tissue masses compatible with tophi are seen elsewhere. Microscopic examination revealed sodium urate crystals.

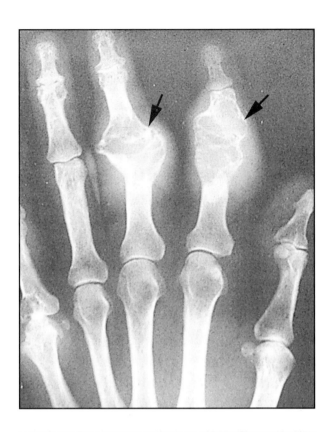

Figure 6-61

Gout (hand)—PA view

PA view of the left hand of a 66-year-old man shows advanced tophaceous gout involving the proximal interphalangeal joints of the index and middle fingers (arrows).

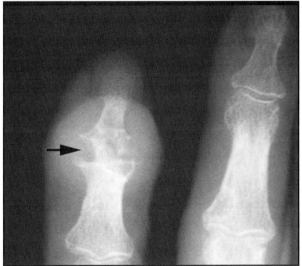

Figure 6-62

Gout (hand)—PA view

PA view of the right index finger of a 60-year-old man shows advanced tophaceous gout with soft-tissue swelling and a large erosion with an overhanging edge (arrow). The bone density appears normal.

DIFFERENTIAL DIAGNOSIS

CPPD crystal deposition disease (intra-articular calcification, location in wrist radiocarpal joint)

Psoriatic arthritis (characteristic skin lesions, peripheral erosions)

Rheumatoid arthritis (multiple joint involvement [except the distal interphalangeal joint], osteopenia, symmetric soft-tissue swelling)

PSORIATIC ARTHRITIS

ICD-9 Code

696.0
Psoriatic arthropathy

SYNONYM

Seronegative spondyloarthropathy

DEFINITION

Psoriatic arthritis is one of a group of four conditions called seronegative spondyloarthropathies. The others are ankylosing spondylitis, Reiter's syndrome, and enteropathic arthropathies associated with inflammatory bowel disease. The age of onset is similar to that in rheumatoid arthritis—young adulthood to middle age. However, psoriasis in childhood has been reported.

Inflammatory arthritis develops in up to 6% of patients with psoriasis. The characteristic scaly erythematous skin rash usually precedes the onset of the arthritis, although in 20% of patients, the articular manifestations appear first. The more severe the skin changes, the more likely the arthritic changes are to develop. Flares of the skin changes, however, do not necessarily correlate with flares of the arthritis. Fingernail changes, including pitting, thickening, ridging, splintering, and separation, are a better predictor of the development of arthritis, especially of the nearby distal interphalangeal (DIP) joints. Joint involvement, however, varies considerably.

Bony erosion accompanied by adjacent bony proliferation typifies psoriatic arthritis. In advanced stages, the phalanges assume a pencil-in-cup deformity characterized by narrowing of the proximal phalanx and cupping of the distal phalanx. The term "opera glass hand" has been used to describe the extreme form of psoriatic arthritis—arthritis mutilans characterized by collapse of the fingers. Although osteolysis of the phalanges is common, spontaneous fusions, especially of the DIP joints, can also occur. Wrist involvement is common. Extra-articular manifestations such as tenosynovitis and tendon ruptures are rare.

HISTORY AND PHYSICAL FINDINGS

In the hand, the site of articular involvement varies from a single joint to several joints. Swelling of the joint or of the entire finger (the so-called sausage digit) may occur. The rheumatoid factor is usually negative, whereas the HLA-B27 antigen is often positive.

IMAGING STUDIES

Required for diagnosis

PA, lateral, and oblique radiographs will reveal most of the changes of psoriatic arthritis.

Required for comprehensive evaluation

Early in the course of the disease, a bone scan or MRI can be useful in detecting early arthritis.

Special considerations

None

Pitfalls

None

IMAGE DESCRIPTION

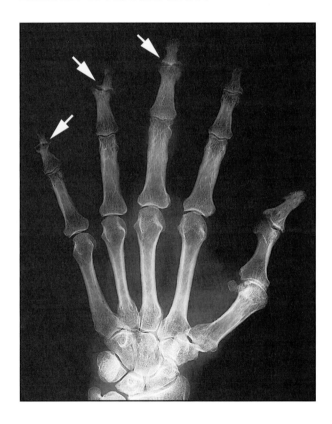

Figure 6-63

Psoriatic arthritis—PA view

PA view of the left hand of a 45-year-old woman with psoriatic arthritis shows the destruction of the DIP joints of the middle, ring, and little fingers (arrows), consistent with the early articular changes in psoriasis. The erosions start at the margins and work toward the middle of the joint. Clinically, the patient's fingernails showed characteristic pitting, splitting, and ridging.

DIFFERENTIAL DIAGNOSIS

Ankylosing spondylitis (spine and sacroiliac joint involvement)

Arthritis of inflammatory bowel disease (lower gastrointestinal symptoms)

Erosive osteoarthritis (older women, symmetric erosions that begin centrally)

Reiter's syndrome (conjunctivitis and urethritis)

RHEUMATOID ARTHRITIS

SYNONYMS
Polyarthritis of unknown etiology
RA

ICD-9 Code
714.0
Rheumatoid arthritis

DEFINITION
Rheumatoid arthritis (RA) is a chronic systemic inflammatory disease of unknown etiology that affects the synovial joints and the synovium surrounding tendons. Synovial inflammation can cause articular destruction and tendon rupture. Women are three times more likely to be affected than men, and the onset of disease ranges from adolescence through the fourth decade of life. Chronic inflammatory synovial disease can also affect children, resulting in a condition called juvenile chronic arthritis (JCA). The term JCA encompasses four or five different childhood diseases that have in common juvenile arthritis.

Anti-gamma-globulin antibodies called rheumatoid factors are found in roughly 80% of patients with RA. These factors are thought to play a role in the release of enzymes that cause joint destruction. Extra-articular manifestations include nodules along the olecranon border of the elbow, swelling about the extensor and flexor tendons, and pulmonary nodules and pleural effusion. With persistent extensor synovitis, the extensor tendons may rupture. Persistent synovitis about the flexor tendons leads to carpal tunnel syndrome and potential flexor tendon rupture.

HISTORY AND PHYSICAL FINDINGS
Morning stiffness, joint pain, and swelling in several joints are typical symptoms. Early involvement of the metacarpophalangeal (MCP) and proximal interphalangeal (PIP) joints is common, as is swelling over the distal radioulnar and ulnocarpal joints. Over time, the fingers at the MCP joints and the wrist tend to drift ulnarly. Two types of deformities develop in the fingers: (1) a swan-neck deformity characterized by hyperextension of the PIP joint and hyperflexion of the distal interphalangeal (DIP) joint; and (2) a boutonnière deformity characterized by hyperflexion of the PIP joint and hyperextension of the DIP joint.

IMAGING STUDIES

Required for diagnosis

PA and lateral radiographs typically show bony erosions that begin at the articular margins and ultimately involve the entire joint surface. The bone also appears osteopenic. Subchondral cysts are common, but calcifications are not. In addition, the wrist tends to shift or translocate ulnarly and palmarly (volarly), slipping off the radius. The tip of the ulna then tends to appear shaped like the tip of a pencil.

Required for comprehensive evaluation

MRI is seldom indicated but can be helpful if the degree of synovial or tendon involvement is in question.

Special considerations

None

Pitfalls

None

IMAGE DESCRIPTIONS

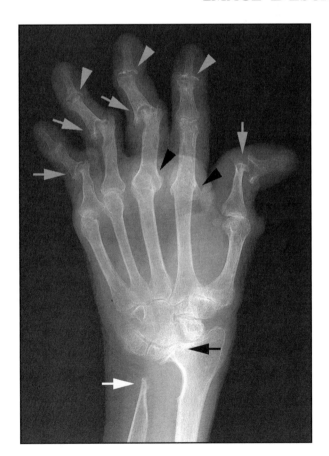

Figure 6-64

Rheumatoid arthritis—PA view

PA view of the left hand of a 42-year-old woman with RA shows that the carpus is translocated ulnarly (black arrow) with the lunate slipped off the radius. Note the pencil shape to the ulna (white arrow). The MCP joints of the index and middle fingers are dislocated (black arrowheads), and there is marked destruction of the interphalangeal joint of the thumb and the PIP joints of the middle, ring, and little fingers (gray arrows). The DIP joints also show advanced arthritic changes (gray arrowheads).

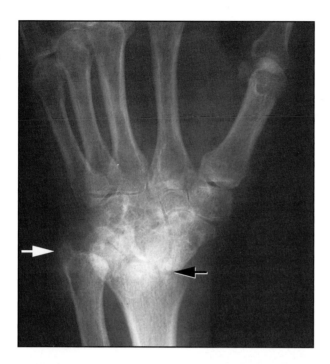

Figure 6-65

Rheumatoid arthritis—PA view

PA view of the left wrist of a 53-year-old woman with RA shows marked radiocarpal destruction (black arrow). The ulna appears long (positive ulnar variance) (white arrow). The MCP joints of the thumb and ring and little fingers appear unaffected.

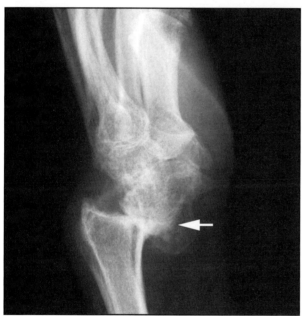

Figure 6-66

Rheumatoid arthritis—Lateral view

Lateral view of the wrist shown in Figure 6-65 shows marked palmar (volar) subluxation of the carpus on the radius (arrow). Lateral views are essential to appreciate this deformity.

SECTION 6 ■ HAND AND WRIST

DIFFERENTIAL DIAGNOSIS

CPPD crystal deposition disease (calcification of cartilage)

Osteoarthritis (negative rheumatoid factor, normal bone density)

Psoriatic arthritis (more changes to the DIP joint)

Scleroderma (skin changes, calcifications)

Systemic lupus erythematosus (erosions usually not apparent)

SCAPHOLUNATE ADVANCED COLLAPSE WRIST

SYNONYMS

Degenerative arthritis of the wrist
Radiocarpal arthritis
Radioscaphoid arthritis
SLAC wrist

DEFINITION

Up to 70% of patients with wrist arthritis will demonstrate the scapholunate advanced collapse (SLAC) pattern on plain radiographs. This pattern is characterized by a tear between the scaphoid and lunate bones, resulting in rotation of the scaphoid bone into a vertical position. This rotation, referred to as rotary subluxation of the scaphoid, is the most common etiology of SLAC wrist. Another common cause is calcium pyrophosphate dihydrate (CPPD) crystal deposition disease. Advanced Kienböck's disease may also progress to SLAC wrist. A similar pattern of collapse can be seen in long-standing nonunions of the scaphoid, sometimes called SNAC (scaphoid nonunion advanced collapse) wrist.

SLAC wrist involves arthritis between the scaphoid and radius and the capitate and lunate. Once the scaphoid flexes or rotates into a vertical position, arthritis develops between the radial styloid and scaphoid because of an incongruous fit. The radioscaphoid joint then wears out and collapses, which renders the capitolunate joint unable to bear the increased loads. The latter joint then disintegrates.

HISTORY AND PHYSICAL FINDINGS

A history of trauma is typical, and the patient often recalls an injury to the wrist, but radiographs obtained at the time of the injury are normal. Radiographs obtained months or even years after the initial injury, however, often reveal nonunion of a scaphoid fracture or scapholunate dissociation.

Pain over the top and radial aspect of the wrist is the most common presenting symptom. Swelling of the wrist after activity is usual. Loss of motion and grip strength is also typical. Management with a wrist splint and over-the-counter nonsteroidal anti-inflammatory drugs is helpful in partially alleviating these symptoms. For some patients, restricting activities that involve the wrist may be helpful in relieving pain.

Physical examination will show limited flexion and extension and radial and ulnar deviation. Grip strength in the hand with the affected wrist will be significantly decreased compared with that of the opposite uninjured side. Swelling over the dorsum of the wrist may be visible, while palpation on the radial side of this area will reveal tenderness. Applying pressure over the scaphoid tuberosity while the patient moves the wrist from radial to ulnar deviation (Watson's scaphoid shift test) produces pain.

IMAGING STUDIES

Required for diagnosis

PA and lateral radiographs of the wrist are the only imaging studies needed to establish the diagnosis. The PA view will show narrowing of the joint space between the radius and scaphoid, as well as between the capitate and lunate in advanced cases. The space between the lunate and radius is preserved. Increased separation between the scaphoid and lunate (Terry-Thomas sign) is easily seen. A circle can be drawn over the scaphoid, the aptly named ring sign, demonstrating the horizontal rotation of the scaphoid. The lateral view will show the horizontal position of the scaphoid and sometimes a dorsal rotation of the lunate (dorsal intercalated segmental instability, or DISI deformity) is seen.

Required for comprehensive evaluation
None

Special considerations
None

Pitfalls
None

IMAGE DESCRIPTIONS

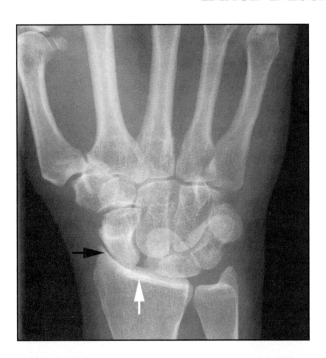

Figure 6-67

SLAC wrist—PA view

PA view of the right hand of a 35-year-old woman shows an early SLAC wrist. Note the narrowing of the joint space between the radius and scaphoid bones (black arrow). Also note the increased space between the scaphoid and lunate (white arrow).

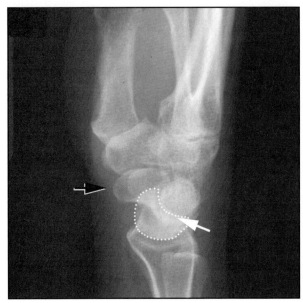

Figure 6-68

SLAC wrist—Lateral view

Lateral view of the wrist in Figure 6-67 shows the horizontal orientation of the scaphoid (black arrow) plus the rotation of the lunate (white arrow) so that its cup is pointing up (DISI). In time, if left untreated, the capitolunate joint will wear out and appear narrow on a PA view.

DIFFERENTIAL DIAGNOSIS

Carpal tunnel syndrome (sensory abnormalities in the median nerve distribution)

de Quervain's disease (positive Finkelstein's test; radiographs will be normal)

Fracture of the distal radius (easily seen on PA view)

Fracture of the scaphoid (easily seen on PA view)

KIENBÖCK'S DISEASE

SYNONYMS

Aseptic necrosis of the lunate
Avascular necrosis of the lunate

DEFINITION

Kienböck's disease is characterized by sclerosis of the lunate and, in late stages, collapse of the bone as a result of osteonecrosis. The condition is twice as common in men as in women, most commonly affecting men between the ages of 30 and 50. Heavy laborers are more prone to osteonecrosis of the lunate, and the dominant hand is more often involved.

The precise etiology is unkown, but several theories such as acute trauma and uneven load across the radiocarpal joint have been proposed. Patients with Kienböck's disease are more likely to have a short ulna relative to the radius (negative ulnar variance). In a normal wrist, the radiocarpal joint supports approximately 80% of the load. In a wrist with negative ulnar variance, the radiocarpal joint supports roughly 95% of the load. Repeated injuries or repetitive loading is believed by many to be the cause of Kienböck's disease. Venous congestion also appears to play a significant role in the development of osteonecrosis.

Lichtman described four stages of Kienböck's disease, based on PA radiographs of the wrist. In stage 1, radiographs appear normal. In stage 2, there is increased radiodensity in the lunate, but the bone retains its normal shape. Stage 3A is characterized by collapse of the lunate, but the relationship between the scaphoid and lunate remains normal, while in stage 3B, advanced collapse of the lunate with rotary subluxation (flexion) of the scaphoid is characteristic. Stage 4 is considered end stage and is marked by extensive arthritis in the area of the radius, scaphoid, and lunate.

HISTORY AND PHYSICAL FINDINGS

Early in the course of Kienböck's disease, patients will note the gradual onset of mild dorsal wrist pain and swelling. Later, loss of motion accompanies more severe wrist pain. On physical examination, tenderness is noted with pressure over the central portion of the back of the wrist. Loss of wrist flexion and extension is accompanied by a decrease in grip strength. Swelling can be seen over the back of the wrist.

SECTION 6 ■ HAND AND WRIST

IMAGING STUDIES

Required for diagnosis

In most instances, PA and lateral radiographs are sufficient to establish the diagnosis. However, at the onset of symptoms, radiographs appear normal (stage 1). Therefore, if Kienböck's disease is suspected at this stage, MRI should be ordered. A T1-weighted image will show decreased signal intensity within the lunate. Note that MRI is not needed to establish stage 2, 3, or 4 disease.

Required for comprehensive evaluation

Bone scans have been used in the past as a screening test but are not specific. CT has also been used, but MRI has become the imaging study of choice for stage 1 disease.

Special considerations

None

Pitfalls

A normal radiograph of the wrist in a patient with wrist pain does not rule out Kienböck's disease. If the patient exhibits tenderness over the mid-dorsum of the wrist, MRI should be considered.

IMAGE DESCRIPTIONS

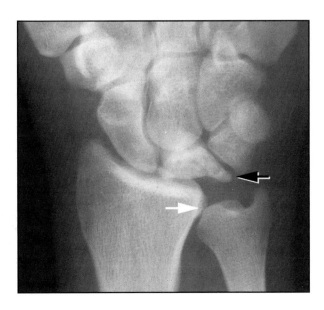

Figure 6-69

Kienböck's disease (stage 3A)— PA view

PA view of the right wrist in a 30-year-old male laborer shows sclerosis and collapse of the lunate (black arrow), but the relationship with the scaphoid is maintained. These findings are characteristic of stage 3A Kienböck's disease. The scaphoid is not rotated, and the carpal height is normal. Note also the short ulna relative to the radius (negative ulnar variance) (white arrow).

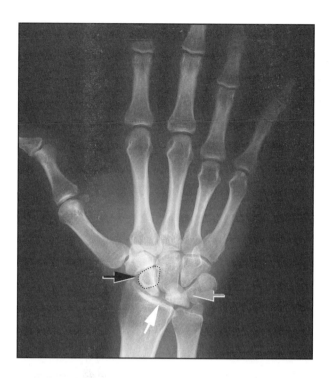

Figure 6-70

*Kienböck's disease (stage 3B)—
PA view*

PA view of a right wrist shows that the lunate appears dense with signs of collapse (gray arrow), characteristic of stage 3B Kienböck's disease. Note the separation between the scaphoid and the lunate (white arrow). Also note that the scaphoid is rotated, indicated by a cortical ring sign (black arrow).

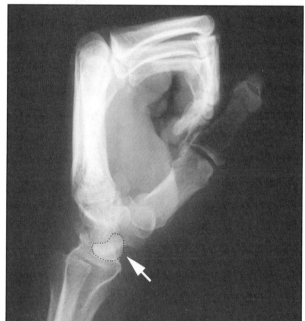

Figure 6-71

Kienböck's disease—Lateral view

Lateral view of a right wrist shows a dense lunate that is also rotated into extension. The distal articular surface of the lunate is rotated dorsally (arrow), which is sometimes referred to as dorsal intercalated segmental instability (DISI) or dorsiflexion instability.

SECTION 6 ■ HAND AND WRIST

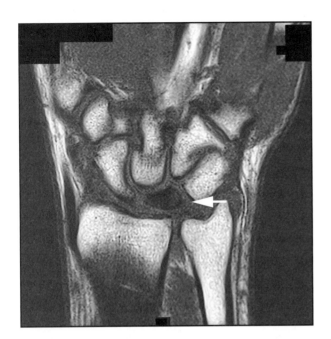

Figure 6-72

Kienböck's disease—Coronal MRI

Coronal T1-weighted MRI scan shows decreased signal intensity in the avascular lunate (arrow) because dead bone has replaced the normal fatty marrow. The other carpal bones show high signal intensity typical of normal fatty bone marrow.

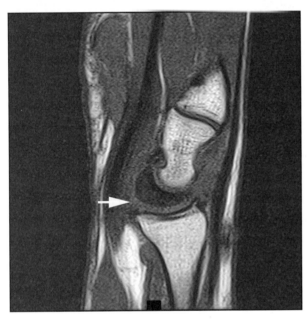

Figure 6-73

Kienböck's disease—Sagittal MRI

Sagittal T1-weighted MRI scan shows decreased signal intensity in the lunate (arrow). Note also how the distal articular surface of the lunate is rotated dorsally (DISI).

DIFFERENTIAL DIAGNOSIS

Deep capsular ganglion (lunate appears normal on MRI)

Intraosseous ganglion (round, lucent appearance in the lunate)

Scapholunate dissociation (increased space between the lunate and scaphoid)

Ulnar impaction syndrome (long ulna/positive ulnar variance)

Osteonecrosis of the Scaphoid

Synonyms
Aseptic necrosis
Avascular necrosis

ICD-9 Code
733.4
Aseptic necrosis of bone

Definition
Fractures through the waist of the scaphoid are most commonly the result of a fall on an outstretched hand. The mechanism of forced dorsiflexion creates the fracture. The blood supply to the scaphoid enters the waist and distal pole. The proximal pole, however, is intra-articular and covered with hyaline cartilage; its blood supply is very limited. Fractures that occur through the waist or more proximally severely interfere with this blood supply. For this reason, fractures of the proximal pole of the scaphoid have a high incidence (between 20% and 40%) of nonunion and eventual osteonecrosis.

History and Physical Findings
Patients often report progressive pain, somewhat more to the radial aspect than to the ulnar aspect of the wrist. Some localized swelling is possible, but most often there is tenderness in the anatomic snuffbox and dorsal radial aspect of the wrist. Loss of wrist motion is also a frequent finding. The patient may or may not recall the inciting event; often, several months will have transpired before radiographs show evidence of osteonecrosis.

Imaging Studies

Required for diagnosis
PA, lateral, and oblique radiographs will demonstrate osteonecrosis but only after at least 4 weeks after the injury. The proximal pole appears more white, or radiodense, than the surrounding tissues. This increased density is the result of mineral resorption in the surrounding bones, not in the proximal pole, and is not always specific for osteonecrosis.

Required for comprehensive evaluation
MRI can detect osteonecrosis earlier than radiographs but is nonspecific for osteonecrosis. Abnormal signal intensity in the proximal pole may be related to hyperemia and granulation tissue. No imaging test is specific for scaphoid osteonecrosis. Ultimately, the diagnosis is made by biopsy of the scaphoid.

Special considerations
None

Pitfalls
None

IMAGE DESCRIPTION

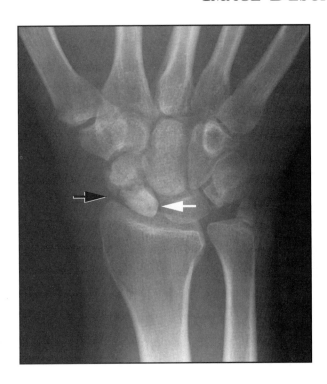

Figure 6-74

Osteonecrosis (wrist)—PA view

PA view of a wrist shows an obvious scaphoid nonunion (black arrow), as well as increased density (whiteness) of the proximal pole (white arrow), suggestive of but not definitive for osteonecrosis.

DIFFERENTIAL DIAGNOSIS

Carpometacarpal arthritis of the thumb (radiographs show the difference)

de Quervain's disease (positive Finkelstein's test, localized tenderness over the first extensor compartment)

Flexor carpi ulnaris tenosynovitis (tenderness over the flexor carpi ulnaris)

GANGLIONS

SYNONYMS

Flexor sheath ganglion
Mucoid cyst
Retinacular ganglion
Synovial cyst

ICD-9 Codes

727.41
Ganglion of joint

727.42
Ganglion of tendon sheath

DEFINITION

Ganglions are cysts composed of mucinous material with a fibrous lining that can originate from the synovial joints of the wrist or from tendon sheaths. They are the most common soft-tissue tumors of the hand and will transilluminate when a penlight is held against the overlying skin. Ganglions may develop insidiously or over a matter of days. They can vary in size depending on activity and may resolve spontaneously. The diagnosis is usually obvious based on the specific location of a visible and palpable mass.

The dorsal wrist ganglion arises from the scapholunate joint and is the most common ganglion, accounting for up to 70% of all ganglions about the hand and wrist. The palmar (volar) wrist ganglion is located along the radial aspect of the palmar surface of the wrist. The flexor sheath ganglion is located on the flexor surface at the base of the fingers. Ganglions that arise just in front of the fingernail over the distal interphalangeal (DIP) joint are called mucoid cysts. A ganglion seen over a bony prominence at the base of the second and third metacarpals is called a carpal boss.

Women in the second, third, and fourth decades are most likely to be affected. Infrequently, ganglions can be seen in children. The etiology of ganglions remains unknown, but a history of wrist trauma preceding the development of a ganglion is not uncommon. Even if untreated, ganglions do not cause osteoarthritis of joints to which they are connected. Malignancy has never been reported in a ganglion.

HISTORY AND PHYSICAL FINDINGS

Patients with ganglions seek treatment for two main reasons: the unsightly cosmetic appearance of the mass and pain. The mass typically is soft and cystic but may be so firm that it is mistaken for a bony mass. Usually, it is not tender on palpation. Decreased sensation or loss of motor function may occur if the mass is adjacent to a peripheral nerve, such as the motor branch of the ulnar nerve or the superficial branch of the radial nerve. Ganglions within the carpal tunnel or Guyon's canal may cause neurologic symptoms as a result of pressure on the median or ulnar nerves. A mucoid cyst may cause furrowing of the fingernail as a result of pressure on the germinal matrix.

IMAGING STUDIES

Required for diagnosis

PA and lateral radiographs are useful to identify any underlying carpal abnormalities such as radiocarpal arthritis or carpometacarpal arthritis. Lateral views of the DIP joint in patients with a mucoid cyst will reveal osteoarthritis with a typical dorsal bone spur off the middle or distal phalanx.

Required for comprehensive evaluation

Radiographs using soft-tissue penetration techniques may outline a soft-tissue mass, but the real value of radiography is in its ability to identify associated bone pathology. A special oblique view of the wrist, the carpal boss view, is helpful in visualizing a carpal boss, which consists of osteophytes or an ossicle at the base of the index and middle metacarpals and the distal edge of the trapezoid and capitate bones.

MRI usually is not needed to make the diagnosis of a ganglion. However, if an occult ganglion is suspected as a cause of wrist pain, MRI is the imaging modality of choice. MRI may also demonstrate internal derangement associated with a ganglion. Diagnostic ultrasound is being increasingly used to evaluate soft-tissue masses of the hand and wrist but requires an experienced technician to obtain images. It has the advantage of low cost.

Special considerations

None

Pitfalls

Ganglions may occur over an arthritic joint. Failure to obtain a radiograph of the wrist will result in a missed diagnosis.

IMAGE DESCRIPTIONS

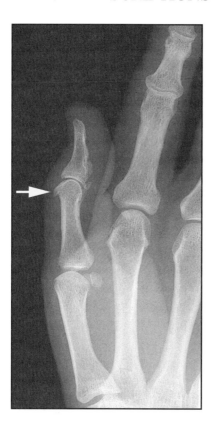

Figure 6-75

Mucoid cyst—Lateral view

Lateral view of the DIP joint of a 60-year-old woman with a mucoid cyst shows a dorsal osteophyte (arrow). This patient's fingernail showed the typical furrowing secondary to pressure from the cyst.

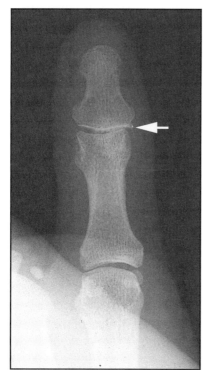

Figure 6-76

Mucoid cyst—PA view

PA view of the same patient in Figure 6-75 shows joint space narrowing (arrow).

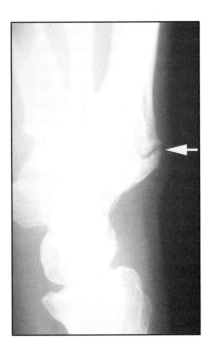

Figure 6-77

Carpal boss—Lateral view

Slightly oblique lateral view of a 35-year-old man with a symptomatic carpal boss and an overlying ganglion shows that the ganglion arises over this arthritic joint (arrow).

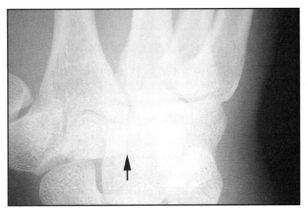

Figure 6-78

Carpal boss—PA view

PA view of the same patient as in Figure 6-77 shows that the carpal boss is not visualized on this view (arrow).

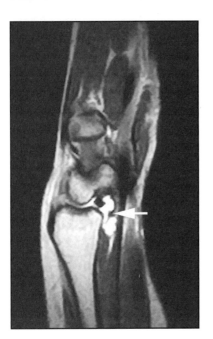

Figure 6-79

Ganglion (wrist)—Sagittal MRI

Sagittal T2-weighted MRI scan of a wrist of a 26-year-old woman with volar wrist pain shows a multilobulated volar ganglion (arrow).

DIFFERENTIAL DIAGNOSIS

Aneurysm or pseudoaneurysm (pulsating mass but easily confused with a volar radial ganglion, which may transmit pulsations)

Epidermal inclusion cyst (history of penetrating trauma)

Giant cell tumor (tendon sheath) (atypical location along side of phalanx)

Hemangioma (red-blue discoloration)

Lipoma (does not transilluminate, atypical location)

Ruptured tendon (history of trauma and loss of function)

SCLERODERMA

SYNONYM

Progressive systemic sclerosis

DEFINITION

Scleroderma is a generalized connective tissue disorder that affects the skin, subcutaneous tissue, musculoskeletal system, kidneys, heart, and often the hands. Women between the ages of 20 and 30 years are at highest risk. There are two forms of scleroderma: (1) a localized form that affects only the skin and (2) a generalized or diffuse form. The hands are commonly involved in the diffuse form, with severe contractures of the proximal interphalangeal (PIP) joints and painful subcutaneous calcifications. Patients with the diffuse form commonly have a group of symptoms referred to as CREST syndrome: Calcinosis, Raynaud's phenomenon, Esophageal abnormalities, Sclerodactyly, and Telangiectasia. Results of laboratory tests for rheumatoid factor and antinuclear antibodies are positive in at least one third of patients. Radiographs show subcutaneous calcifications, calcifications about the joints, degenerative changes about the interphalangeal joints, and narrowing of the distal phalanges.

HISTORY AND PHYSICAL FINDINGS

Tightness of the skin about the face and hands is characteristic in the diffuse form of scleroderma. Early in the course of the disease, Raynaud's phenomenon affects the fingers, characterized by decreased circulation to the fingers that can lead to painful ulcerations and even gangrene of the fingertips. With progression of the disease, progressive flexion contractures develop in the PIP joints and extension contractures develop in the metacarpophalangeal joints. Contracture of the first web space is also common. Calcification can develop in the subcutaneous tissues, creating hard, tender plaques in the hands and fingers.

IMAGING STUDIES

Required for diagnosis
PA, lateral, and oblique views of the hands will show the typical changes in the soft tissues and bones.

Required for comprehensive evaluation
No additional studies are needed.

Special considerations

None

Pitfalls

Scleroderma may be confused with other conditions that cause subcutaneous calcifications, as listed in the Differential Diagnosis below.

IMAGE DESCRIPTION

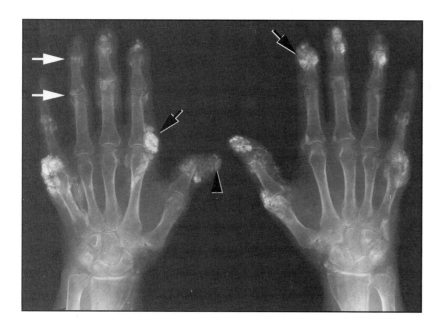

Figure 6-80

Scleroderma—PA view

PA view of the hands of a 42-year-old woman shows the subcutaneous and periarticular calcifications (black arrows) common in scleroderma. Note that most of the PIP and DIP joints show destructive changes (white arrows). Significant resorption of the distal phalanx of the left thumb is present as well (arrowhead).

DIFFERENTIAL DIAGNOSIS

Gout (elevated uric acid, periarticular erosions)

Polymyositis/dermatomyositis (abnormal serum enzymes and positive muscle biopsy)

Systemic lupus erythematosus (usually no subcutaneous calcification)

HIP AND THIGH

Section Editor
Joseph M. Erpelding, MD

Contributors
Paul J. Herzwurm, MD
Albert D. Olszewski, MD

IMAGING THE HIP AND THIGH— AN OVERVIEW

ANATOMY

The pelvis comprises two iliopubic bones connected anteriorly at the symphysis pubis and posteriorly to the sacrum at the sacroiliac joints. The iliopubic bone forms the acetabulum, which connects to the femur at the hip joint.

The shape of the pelvic ring can vary considerably among individuals and also differs by sex, but the normal configuration of the acetabulum and proximal femur is more uniform. For example, because the hip flexes much farther than it extends, the acetabulum extends farther posteriorly than anteriorly. This is further facilitated by a femoral anteversion at the hip joint. Finally, to allow the hip to function as a ball-and-socket joint, the proximal femur is usually angled about 135° at the junction of the femoral shaft with the neck, which allows for a greater range of motion. The normal ranges of motion at the hip, which vary somewhat with age but generally are symmetric, include flexion to 115°, extension to 20°, internal rotation to 30°, external rotation to 45°, abduction to 45°, and adduction to 30°. The symphysis and sacroiliac joints have very little or no functional motion, except during childbirth. One function of the pelvis is to allow locomotion. The pelvis also provides structural protection and support for the visceral organs, which is important to remember when dealing with certain types of pelvic injuries.

The pelvis and femur have anatomic landmarks that are easily visualized on images and serve as sites of origin or attachment for a variety of muscles and ligaments. Some of the most apparent include the anterior superior iliac spine (ASIS), the origin of the sartorius; the anterior inferior iliac spine (AIIS), the origin of a portion of the rectus femoris; the posterior superior iliac spine (PSIS), the site of insertion of part of the lumbodorsal fascia and origin of the gluteus maximus; and the cotyloid notch of the acetabulum and the fovea of the femoral head, the origin and attachment of the ligamentum teres. The proximal femur has the greater and lesser trochanters, which serve as attachments for the hip abductors (gluteus medius and minimus) and hip flexors (iliopsoas), respectively. The femoral shaft has an anterior bow that ranges from 10° to 20° (seen on the lateral view). These anatomic landmarks and others such as the teardrop, sourcil, and medial clear space are used to distinguish normal from abnormal when viewing images of the hip, pelvis, and thigh.

OSSIFICATION CENTERS

Centers of ossification in the hip and pelvis form, on average, at the following ages: (1) femoral head at 4 months; (2) greater trochanter at 5 to 7 years; (3) lesser trochanter at 11 to 12 years; (4) acetabulum at 10 to 13 years; (5) ischial spine at 13 to 15 years; (6) iliac spine at 13 to 15 years; (7) tubercle of ischium at 13 to 15 years; (8) tubercle of ilium at 13 to 15 years; (9) tubercle of pubis at 18 to 20 years; and (10) iliac crest at puberty.

STANDARD IMAGING VIEWS

Radiographs

The hip joint is typically primarily viewed on the AP view of the hip or pelvis, with a frog-lateral or cross-table lateral of the proximal femur viewed secondarily. A lateral view of the acetabulum is rarely helpful, except in very specific circumstances. A modified lateral view is sometimes used to assess the degree of deficiency of the anterior acetabulum in patients with evidence of dyplasia of the hip.

If an injury to the pelvic ring is suspected, and in instances of high-energy trauma, an AP view of the pelvis is obtained first. If an injury to the acetabulum is suggested on the initial radiograph, then iliac and obturator oblique (Judet) views should be obtained to identify the character of the injury to the acetabulum (transverse, or anterior or posterior wall or column). If disruption of the pelvic ring is suggested on the initial AP radiograph, then a Ferguson view of the sacrum (AP 30° cephalad) or an inlet view (AP 40° to 60° caudad) with an outlet view (AP 40° cephalad) is frequently helpful in identifying the nature of the disruption.

To evaluate most conditions of the femur, AP and lateral views of the femur, including the proximal femur, are adequate.

Computed tomography

Imaging of acetabular fractures includes thin-cut CT with three-dimensional reformation, with the latter reserved for complex injury patterns. CT is useful in assessing pelvic fractures, especially those involving the sacrum and sacroiliac joints. CT is also helpful in defining the degree of stability of pelvic ring disruptions. Loose bodies in the hip joint following dislocations or fracture-dislocations can be seen on CT scans.

SECTION 7 ■ HIP AND THIGH

Magnetic resonance imaging

If radiographs are negative for suspected fractures, MRI is a useful diagnostic tool because it can identify fractures before they are evident on radiographs. MRI will also confirm the presence of stress fractures. MR arthrography can identify tears of the labrum, as well as osteochondral defects. MRI is also a sensitive tool for detecting osteonecrosis of the hip. Bone scans have been used to image conditions such as osteomyelitis, stress fractures, and osteonecrosis, but MRI has largely supplanted bone scans for these conditions.

EMERGENCIES

Three conditions of the hip constitute emergencies: septic hip joint, hip joint dislocation, and unstable pelvic ring injuries. These conditions warrant immediate referral to a specialist. Radiographs of a septic hip frequently are normal. MRI will show the fluid, but a definitive diagnosis depends on aspiration under fluoroscopy with Gram stain and culture of the joint fluid. Hip dislocations should be apparent on AP views of the hip and pelvis with clinical correlation (with a posterior dislocation, the hip will be in flexion and adduction and internally rotated). However, a cross-table lateral view should be added to assess for associated injuries. Following reduction, CT is needed if an intra-articular fragment is suspected. Unstable pelvic ring disruptions usually will be apparent on an AP view of the pelvis. These are associated with a high rate of neurovascular and urinary tract injuries.

NORMAL VARIANTS

1. Herniation pits are ring-shaped radiolucencies with well-marginated sclerotic borders that can be seen in the superolateral aspect of the femoral neck. They are thought to be caused by herniation of synovium into cortical bone. They may be mistaken for tumors.
2. Ward's triangle is a triangular radiolucent area in the femoral neck caused by thin, loosely arranged trabeculae. This is a normal finding.
3. Fovea capitis femoris is the central defect in the femoral capital epiphysis through which passes the ligamentum teres. This may vary considerably in size and can be mistaken for osteochondritis dissecans, a fracture, or osteonecrosis.
4. An AP view of the pelvis superimposes the acetabulum on the femoral head. This may give rise to the appearance of a large lytic lesion in the femoral head.
5. Hypertrophic changes in the femoral neck may simulate a fracture. Also, skin folds overlying the femoral neck may be misinterpreted as a fracture.

6. An accessory ossification center of the greater trochanter may mimic a calcific tendinitis.

7. Notches may be seen in various locations in the superior aspect of the acetabulum. On MRI, fluid may be seen filling the notches. These are a normal variant of anatomy and of no clinical significance.

8. In adolescents, notching of the inferior and superior aspects of the femoral neck can be seen much like the notching seen in the upper humerus. This notching usually disappears at skeletal maturity.

9. Os acetabuli marginalis superior is a persistent ossification center at the superior lateral edge of the acetabulum that may be mistaken for a fracture or for an area of calcification.

IMAGING TIPS

1. A fracture of the transverse process of L5 is often associated with fractures of the sacrum or disruption of the sacroiliac joints.

2. Groin pain in the elderly in the presence of normal radiographs should raise suspicion of a stress fracture of the hip or pubic rami. MRI will show these fractures.

3. Fractures of the acetabulum are best visualized on Judet views, but CT is usually added to better define the complexity of the fracture pattern.

4. Most hip dislocations are posterior and are often associated with a fracture of the posterior acetabular rim.

SECTION 7 ■ HIP AND THIGH

LABRAL TEAR

SYNONYM
Internal derangement of the hip

ICD-9 Code

718.85
Other derangement of the pelvic region and thigh, not elsewhere classified

DEFINITION
The acetabular labrum is a fibrocartilaginous rim-like structure that encircles the bony margin of the acetabulum, much like the glenoid labrum in the shoulder. It serves to deepen the socket of the hip and functions to seal the hip joint, aiding the fluid film lubrication mechanism. Labral tears may result from hip dislocations or subluxations as a natural consequence of aging or from minor injuries such as twisting or falling. Most tears occur in the anterior superior aspect of the labrum. Recently, tears of the acetabular labrum have been recognized as a cause of groin pain, especially in athletes. In fact, labral tears may be the cause of groin pain in one out of five athletes. Attention has focused on athletes, but these injuries can occur in nonathletes of either sex and in all age groups.

HISTORY AND PHYSICAL FINDINGS
Patients may or may not report a history of trauma. In some cases, a twisting injury is reported, typically resulting in groin pain; pain in the buttock or greater trochanteric region is reported less often. Patients may report a catching, clicking, or locking of the hip. On physical examination certain provocative maneuvers will reproduce symptoms. Flexing, adducting, and internally rotating the hip will reproduce pain with an anterior superior tear. Range of motion usually is normal, but the patient may experience pain at the extremes of motion

IMAGING STUDIES

Required for diagnosis
AP and lateral views of the hip are not adequate to diagnose this condition but should be ordered initially to rule out associated pathology such as osteoarthritis and dysplasia.

Required for comprehensive evaluation
MRI alone is not adequate or reliable to diagnose a labral tear. However, MR arthrography is much more accurate in making this diagnosis.

Special considerations
When in doubt, hip arthroscopy, typically done by a specialist, is being used increasingly to make this diagnosis.

Pitfalls

Many clinicians are not aware of this diagnosis as a cause of hip pain. It may be confused with iliopsoas pathology.

IMAGE DESCRIPTION

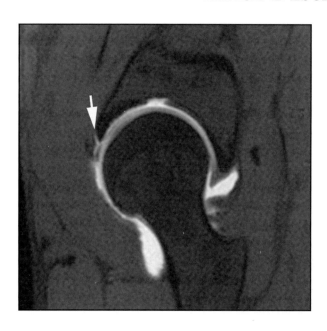

Figure 7-1

Labral tear— Sagittal MR arthrogram

Sagittal T1-weighted, fat-suppressed MR arthrogram of the hip following intra-articular injection of dilute gadolinium shows contrast extending through the base of the anterior superior labrum (arrow), consistent with a tear.

DIFFERENTIAL DIAGNOSIS

Fracture (apparent on radiographs)

Iliopsoas bursitis (MR arthrography should show the difference)

Infection (joint effusion on MRI, positive culture on joint aspirate)

Osteoarthritis (joint space narrowing on radiographs)

Sciatica (nerve root impingement apparent on MRI)

ANTERIOR PELVIC RING INJURIES

SYNONYMS
Bucking horse injury
Ischium fracture
Obturator foramen fracture
Pelvic fracture
Straddle injury
Symphysis pubis disruption

ICD-9 Codes
808.2
Fracture of the pelvis; pubis, closed

808.42
Fracture of the ischium, closed

808.43
Multiple pelvic fractures

DEFINITION
Anterior pelvic ring injuries occur as a consequence of trauma. The most common fractures involve the superior or inferior pubic rami, located between the symphysis pubis and acetabulum. Single ramus fractures are the most common, typically occurring in elderly patients as a result of a fall. Double fractures involving both the superior and inferior rami also can occur as a result of a fall, but these are more commonly associated with other high-energy pelvic fractures.

The mechanism of injury in young patients often is a motorcycle or motor vehicle accident or a fall from a height. These high-energy injuries are usually associated with a second break in the pelvic ring, such as an unstable acetabular fracture or injury to the sacroiliac joint. In contrast to the more stable low-energy injuries, high-energy injuries with potential instability have associated problems, including potential hemodynamic instability, inability to ambulate, and multiple foci of pain. With both types of injuries, hospitalization is nearly always required. For patients with older, low-energy injuries, pain control and gait training are indicated, whereas in patients with high-energy injuries, assessment for associated problems is critical, and surgical treatment is frequently required.

HISTORY AND PHYSICAL FINDINGS
Patients typically report pain directly over the area of injury, and they cannot ambulate. Pain also is elicited with direct palpation or lateral compression of the pelvis. Most patients with low-energy injuries can walk if aided by a cane, crutch, or walker. Laboratory studies are not necessary for patients with single ramus fractures; however, serial hematocrit levels may need to be obtained for patients with unstable pelvic ring injuries, particularly if the anterior pelvic ring is involved. Patients with high-energy injuries can have occult vascular injury with significant blood loss.

SECTION 7 ■ HIP AND THIGH

IMAGING STUDIES

Required for diagnosis

An AP radiograph of the pelvis is sufficient to establish the diagnosis in cases where the fracture pattern is stable. These same fractures, however, can be difficult to detect on the AP view alone, in which case core additional views are needed.

An AP view of the pelvis that appears normal does not rule out fracture of the pubic rami; however, a high index of suspicion is needed based on mechanism of injury and physical examination. If radiographs show more than 1 cm of widening at the symphysis pubis, a second injury to the pelvic ring should be suspected. If the radiograph shows 2 cm or more of widening, then there is a second break to the pelvic ring in virtually all circumstances. CT may best allow for diagnosis in this instance.

Required for comprehensive evaluation

Nondisplaced fractures or insufficiency fractures in elderly patients can be difficult to detect on the AP view alone. In patients who have sustained a high-energy injury, injuries in other parts of the pelvic ring may be difficult to detect. In these instances, a pelvic outlet view (AP 40° cephalad) not only highlights the superior pubic rami and the symphysis pubis but it also helps identify the fracture pattern and other injuries in the anterior aspect of the pelvis. If the patient reports pain in the posterior aspect of the pelvis, a Ferguson view (AP 30° cephalad) better visualizes fractures of the sacrum or sacroiliac joint. Finally, the pelvic inlet view (AP 40° to 60° caudad) is sometimes the only view that actually demonstrates superior pubic rami fractures.

MRI is the imaging modality of choice if the index of suspicion for fracture is high but radiographs are normal. MRI will not only identify a stress fracture but will also identify a potential pathologic fracture. If symptoms (such as anterior and posterior pain) suggest an unstable fracture pattern but radiographs are not definitive, then CT typically provides definitive diagnosis for the purpose of planning treatment. Low-energy injuries that are difficult to confirm on plain radiographs should be assessed with MRI, whereas high-energy injuries with a potentially unstable pelvic ring disruption and involvement of both aspects of the pelvis should be definitively diagnosed with CT.

Special considerations
None

Pitfalls
None

IMAGE DESCRIPTION

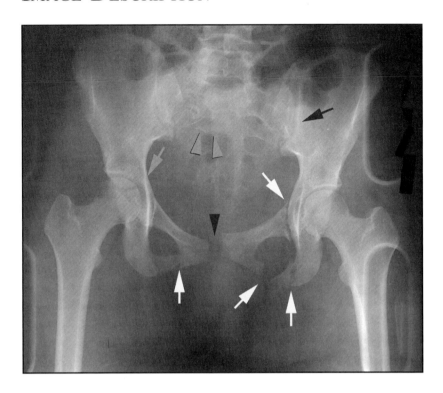

Figure 7-2

Multiple fractures of the pelvis—AP view

AP view of the pelvis in an adult patient shows multiple interruptions of the pelvic ring, including widening of the left sacroiliac joint (black arrow); multiple rami fractures (white arrows), including a segmental ischial ramus fracture on the left; a pubic ramus fracture on the left side; an ischial ramus fracture on the right side; disruption of the symphysis pubis (black arrowhead); and a nondisplaced transverse fracture of the right acetabulum (gray arrow). Note the disruption of the sacral foramina on this view (gray arrowheads), which often is the only notable finding on a radiograph suggesting an injury to the sacrum.

DIFFERENTIAL DIAGNOSIS

Inflammation of the pubic symphysis (irregularity with sclerosis about the symphysis pubis on radiographs)

Ischium fracture (isolated fractures exceedingly rare; more commonly associated with acetabular fractures and a second break in the obturator foramen complex, ie, fracture of the pubic rami)

Metastatic disease (lytic lesion on radiographs, MRI evidence of associated pathologic fracture)

Osteoarthritis of the hip (joint space narrowing apparent on radiographs)

DISLOCATION OF THE HIP

ICD-9 Codes

835.01
Dislocation of hip, closed,
posterior

835.02
Dislocation of hip, closed,
obturator

835.03
Dislocation of hip, closed,
other anterior dislocation

SYNONYMS
None

DEFINITION

Hip dislocation is characterized as a disruption of the relationship between the femoral head and the acetabulum. Because the hip joint is inherently stable, high-energy trauma such as a collision between a pedestrian and motor vehicle, a motor vehicle accident, or a fall from a height is necessary to dislocate the hip. The femoral head can be dislocated posteriorly, anteriorly, or inferiorly (obturator), depending on the position of the leg and the direction of the force. Posterior dislocations account for approximately 90% of injuries; anterior dislocations account for about 10%. Obturator dislocations are quite rare.

About half of patients with hip dislocations have associated musculoskeletal injuries. Injuries to the posterior acetabular wall are common, as are ipsilateral knee injuries, which occur in roughly 25% of patients with hip dislocations. Ipsilateral femur fractures are also common. The vascular supply of the femoral head depends on the vessels about the femoral neck, especially the posterior aspect. Dislocations may either tear these vessels or occlude them, which can result in eventual osteonecrosis. A delay of 12 hours in reducing a hip dislocation results in osteonecrosis of the femoral head in up to 50% of patients. Sciatic nerve injuries, especially the peroneal portion of the sciatic nerve, can occur in up to 20% of patients with posterior dislocations; therefore, neurologic examination is necessary prior to treatment.

HISTORY AND PHYSICAL FINDINGS

Severe pain about the hip and the inability to ambulate after some type of high-energy injury are common presenting symptoms. Patients may report numbness in the affected extremity. Because associated injuries are common, detailed vascular, neurologic, and musculoskeletal examinations are mandatory, including evaluation of the integrity of the knee joint ligaments. Patients with hip dislocations have a characteristic appearance, depending on the direction of the dislocation. With an anterior dislocation, the leg will be in a shortened, externally rotated, and abducted position. With the more common posterior hip dislocation, the leg will appear shortened, flexed, and internally rotated. With the rare obturator dislocation, the leg will appear relatively lengthened, abducted, and in slight neutral or internal rotation.

IMAGING STUDIES

Required for diagnosis

An AP view of the pelvis should be ordered first and typically is sufficient to confirm the diagnosis and identify the direction of the dislocation.

Required for comprehensive evaluation

Following closed reduction of the dislocation, iliac and obturator oblique (Judet) views will show the condition of the anterior and posterior acetabular walls in the pelvic columns if an associated acetabular fracture is suspected. CT is indicated after the reduction to evaluate the congruency of the reduction and to identify any intra-articular bony fragments.

Special considerations

Because the amount of time that passes prior to reduction is related to the incidence of osteonecrosis, timely reduction (less than 6 hours) is paramount once the diagnosis is established. Therefore, the hip should be reduced first, before proceeding with CT.

Pitfalls

Ipsilateral femoral shaft fractures commonly occur with hip dislocations. The obvious deformity with this fracture may tempt some practitioners to simply order an AP radiograph of the femur, without an AP view of the pelvis, in which case a hip dislocation may be missed.

SECTION 7 ■ HIP AND THIGH

IMAGE DESCRIPTION

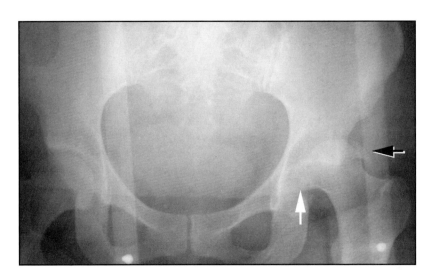

Figure 7-3

Hip dislocation— AP view

AP view of the pelvis shows a dislocation of the left femoral head (white arrow) with an associated marginal acetabular fracture. Note evidence of the latter by the presence of a bone fragment lateral to the ilium and superior to the femoral head (black arrow). This patient most likely has a posterior dislocation, given that the left femoral head appears to be smaller than the right. Because the left femoral head is closer to the film, it is less magnified; the closer an object is to the film, the less divergent the x-ray beams.

DIFFERENTIAL DIAGNOSIS

Acetabular fracture (apparent on radiographs and further evaluated with CT and Judet views)

Displaced femoral neck fracture (apparent on AP view of the pelvis)

Pelvic fracture (apparent on radiograph or CT of the pelvis)

Fracture of the Acetabulum

Synonym
Pelvic fracture

ICD-9 Code

808.0
Fracture of the acetabulum,
closed

Definition
Acetabular fractures involve the portion of the pelvis that articulates with the femoral head and are usually caused by a force transmitted to the acetabulum by the femoral head. The femoral head is driven into the acetabulum, causing the fracture. Most acetabular fractures involve high-energy injuries such as motor vehicle and motorcycle accidents or falls from heights. The fracture pattern is determined by the position of the leg at the time of impact. These fractures can occur at the anterior wall, the posterior wall, the roof segment, or in any combination of these locations. Fractures of the posterior wall are most common. Associated injuries are common and can involve not only the musculoskeletal system (eg, femoral head fracture, pelvic ring fracture, hip dislocation, or degloving injury to the soft tissue) but also the urinary tract and the vascular and neurologic systems. The incidence of osteoarthritis following fractures of the acetabulum is as high as 20%, and the incidence of osteonecrosis is 7.5%.

History and Physical Findings
A history of a motorcycle accident or a motor vehicle accident is common. The patient may report that the knee struck the dashboard on impact; this mechanism causes a posterior dislocation of the hip and fracture of the acetabulum—a so-called dashboard injury. A history of a fall from a height is also common. Because sciatic nerve paralyses are present in up to 20% of patients with a posterior wall fracture, a careful neurologic examination is needed to detect any sensory or motor deficits in the lower extremities.

Imaging Studies

Required for diagnosis
An AP radiograph of the pelvis is needed to establish a diagnosis of a bony injury to the acetabulum. Both 45° iliac and obturator oblique (Judet) views can be added to confirm the diagnosis and determine if other imaging studies are needed.

Section 7 ■ Hip and Thigh

Required for comprehensive evaluation

In most instances, CT also should be obtained. CT with 1- to 2-mm cuts will identify loose fragments within the joint, the articular surface geometry, and the number of fracture lines.

Special considerations

Emergency angiography may be needed if unexplained bleeding occurs in a patient with acetabular fracture, as the mortality rate in patients with pelvic and hemodynamic instability is as high as 45%. A retrograde urethrogram may also be indicated to assess for an associated urinary tract injury.

Pitfalls

Plain radiographs underestimate the severity of the fracture. A CT scan should eliminate this possibility.

IMAGE DESCRIPTIONS

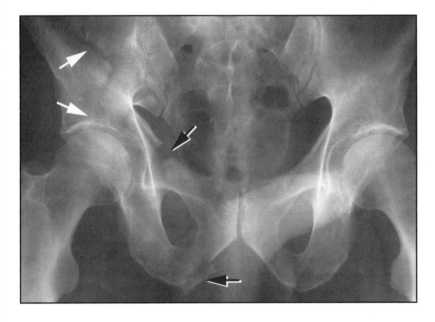

Figure 7-4

Fracture of the acetabulum—AP view

AP view of an adult with multiple fractures on the right side of the pelvis shows inferior and superior rami fractures (black arrows). Note also a fracture of the ilium that extends down to the superior dome of the acetabulum (white arrows). Definitive assessment of the acetabular fracture is likely with the addition of Judet views.

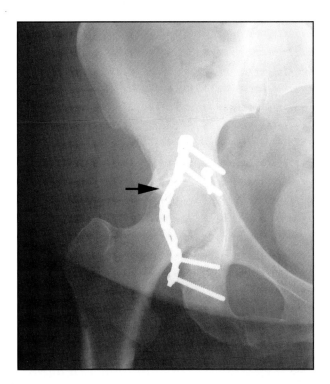

Figure 7-5

*Fracture of the acetabulum—
AP view*

Postoperative AP view of the pelvis in which
plate and screw fixation has been applied to
the posterior wall of this acetabular fracture
(arrow). Loss of cartilage space, consistent
with posttraumatic osteoarthritis, is evident.

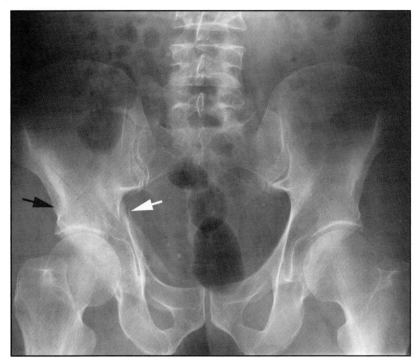

Figure 7-6

*Fracture of the
acetabulum—AP view*

AP view of the pelvis shows
a subtle fracture on the
lateral aspect of the
acetabulum (black arrow).
Note, however, that this
fracture is not easily seen on
this view, but it does show
apparent involvement of the
anterior column and/or
medial wall of the
acetabulum (white arrow).
The fracture also extends
into the right ilium.

SECTION 7 ■ HIP AND THIGH

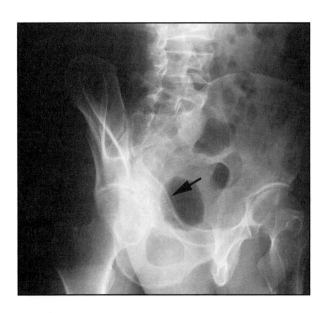

Figure 7-7

Fracture of the acetabulum extending into the ilium—Judet view

Judet view of the pelvis shows the degree of displacement of the medial wall with this fracture (arrow); it also appears to involve both columns. Note how well the anterior column is visualized and how there is a disruption in the normal continuity of the iliopectineal line.

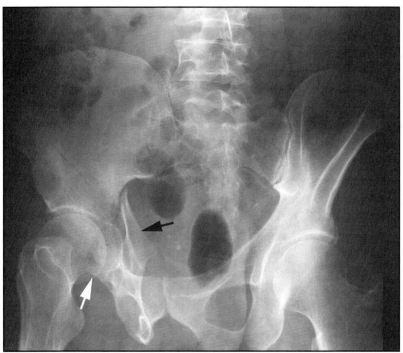

Figure 7-8

Fracture of the acetabulum extending into the ilium— Opposite Judet view

Opposite Judet view of the pelvis of the same patient shown in Figure 7-7 better illustrates the medial wall and the posterior aspect of the acetabulum (black arrow). Note also an associated transverse fracture involving the posterior aspect of the acetabulum, exiting the lower quadrant of the posterior wall (white arrow).

DIFFERENTIAL DIAGNOSIS

Fracture of the femoral head (may appear on AP radiograph, will appear on CT scan)

Fracture of the pelvic ring (apparent on AP view of the pelvis)

FRACTURE OF THE COCCYX

SYNONYMS

Coccydynia

Tailbone fracture

ICD-9 Code

806.6
Fracture of sacrum and coccyx, closed

DEFINITION

The coccyx is a triangular-shaped bony structure located at the end of the spine and made up of three to five bony segments (vertebrae). The coccyx corresponds to the tail in animals, hence the term "tailbone." Roughly two thirds of people have a coccyx that curves down and slightly forward with an intercoccygeal angle (the angle between the first and last segment of the coccyx) of 50°; in the other third, the coccyx points straight forward. In a minority of patients, the coccyx will show a deviation to one side or the other when viewed from the front. This variation makes it difficult to diagnose an acute fracture on radiographs. Most coccygeal fractures occur in women, probably because of the female pelvic anatomy. The female pelvis is broader, so the coccyx is more vulnerable.

HISTORY AND PHYSICAL FINDINGS

A typical history is of a fall with the buttocks striking a hard surface. A history of direct trauma to the coccyx from contact sports is also possible. "Tubing" fractures of the coccyx occur in people who ride the rapids sitting on a rubber inner tube. A fall on the buttocks during snowboarding is another mechanism of injury. Coccygeal fractures also have been reported during childbirth. The patient reports severe pain in the upper crease of the buttocks that is aggravated by sitting. Straining to move the bowels is painful. Physical examination reveals local tenderness on palpation of the coccyx. On rectal examination, palpation of the coccyx is painful, and frank motion of the coccyx may be noted.

IMAGING STUDIES

Required for diagnosis

A 10° caudal angulated AP view of the coccyx and a lateral view with the legs flexed at the hip should be taken initially. Lateral views can also be taken with the patient standing and then sitting to identify any change in the position of the coccyx.

Required for comprehensive evaluation
If the original radiographs are normal and pain persists despite an adequate trial of nonsurgical treatment (at least 4 weeks), CT can be ordered as it may reveal a fracture. Bone scan is also sensitive for these fractures and can be obtained at the time of injury.

Special considerations
None

Pitfalls
The coccyx has many shapes, and a normal coccyx may be misdiagnosed as a fracture.

IMAGE DESCRIPTION

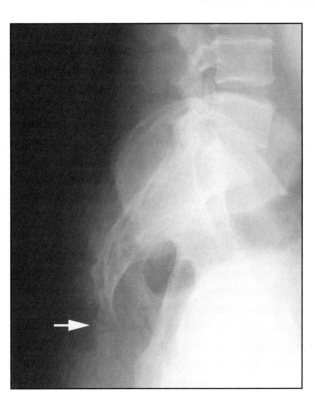

Figure 7-9

Fracture of the coccyx—Lateral view

Lateral view of the sacrococcygeal aspect of the pelvis in an adult shows an oblique fracture line about the last coccygeal segment (arrow). The fracture is apparent on this radiograph, but in many cases these fractures cannot be seen on a lateral view. In these cases, bone scan or CT is needed if there is a high level of suspicion for coccygeal fracture based on the physical examination and the mechanism of injury.

DIFFERENTIAL DIAGNOSIS

Metastatic disease (lytic lesion seen on radiograph; MRI will show the metastasis)

Perirectal abscess (radiographs normal; diagnosis made by clinical examination)

Rectal carcinoma (radiographs normal; palpated on rectal examination or seen on colonoscopy)

Sacral fracture (seen on radiographs or CT)

FRACTURE OF THE FEMORAL NECK

SYNONYMS

Hip fracture
Intracapsular hip fracture
Subcapital femur fracture

ICD-9 Code

820.00
Fracture of the femoral neck, intracapsular section, unspecified

DEFINITION

The hip joint consists of the acetabulum and the femoral head, which is connected to the shaft by way of the femoral neck and intertrochanteric region. Historically, fractures of the femoral head, femoral neck, intertrochanteric region, and subtrochanteric region have been combined under the broad category "hip fractures." The blood supply to the femoral head is supplied primarily by the lateral epiphyseal artery, which courses along the posterior surface of the femoral neck. Displaced femoral neck fractures interrupt this blood supply, accounting for the high incidence (up to 35%) of osteonecrosis of the femoral head. However, osteonecrosis also occurs with nondisplaced or impacted femoral neck fractures, occurring in up to 15% of patients. This anatomic arrangement also explains the high incidence of nonunion in one third of patients with femoral neck fractures who have had internal fixation of the fracture. Women older than 50 years are at increased risk for femoral neck fracture and overall are three to four times more likely than men to sustain this injury. Younger adults are more likely to sustain femoral neck fractures than intertrochanteric fractures. Femoral neck fractures are associated with increased mortality (approximately 15% in men and 8% in women) during the first month after the injury.

HISTORY AND PHYSICAL FINDINGS

A fall from a standing position is the most common mechanism of injury. Less commonly, with an insufficiency fracture of the femoral neck, groin pain may precede the fall. In a small group of patients, usually younger patients, there is a history of a high-energy injury such as a fall from a height or a motor vehicle accident in which the knee strikes the dashboard. Rarely, a young running athlete with long-standing groin pain may report the sudden inability to bear weight as a result of a displaced stress fracture of the femoral neck. Physical examination reveals that the patient cannot bear weight and has a shortened, externally rotated limb. Usually, there are no associated neurologic or vascular injuries. Patients with nondisplaced fractures have no visible deformity on physical examination and can usually ambulate with some type of aid such as a cane or crutch. However, these patients may report groin and buttocks pain with both active and passive motion at the hip, especially in internal and external rotation.

IMAGING STUDIES

Required for diagnosis
AP and lateral views of the hip will show displaced and impacted fractures of the femoral neck. However, nondisplaced fractures or stress fractures can be difficult to detect on radiographs.

Required for comprehensive evaluation
If clinical suspicion is high and radiographs appear normal, MRI of the hip should be obtained, as it will show the fracture line with surrounding marrow edema if a fracture is present.

Special considerations
None

Pitfalls
Stress fractures of the hip are not easily seen. If an undetected stress fracture or nondisplaced fracture is suspected, the patient should be advised to avoid weight bearing to minimize potential displacement and the high risk of osteonecrosis. A radiologist should be consulted regarding the best modality available locally for proper diagnosis.

IMAGE DESCRIPTIONS

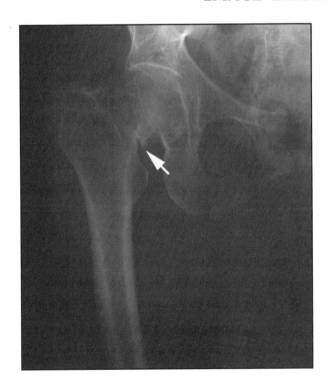

Figure 7-10

Fracture of the femoral neck— AP view

AP view shows a cortical step-off in the medial femoral neck (arrow) with foreshortening of the femoral neck.

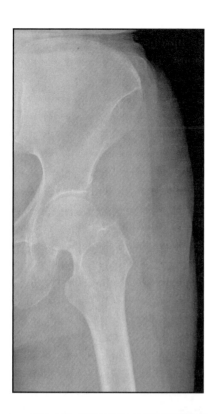

Figure 7-11

Fracture of the femoral neck, subtle—AP view

AP view of the left femur does not reveal a fracture.

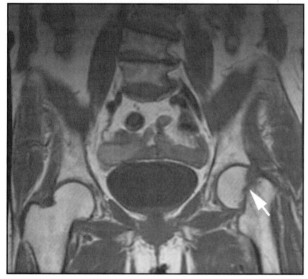

Figure 7-12

Fracture of the femoral neck, subtle—MRI

A T1-weighted MRI of the same patient shown in Figure 7-11 shows the low signal intensity fracture line across the left femoral neck (arrow).

DIFFERENTIAL DIAGNOSIS

Acetabular fracture (seen on radiographs; CT may be needed)

Intertrochanteric fracture (readily seen on AP radiograph)

Metastatic disease (lytic lesion seen in the region of the fracture)

Pubic ramus fracture (seen on AP view of the pelvis)

FRACTURE OF THE FEMORAL SHAFT

ICD-9 Code

821.0
Fracture of shaft or
unspecified part of the femur,
closed

SYNONYMS

Fracture of the femoral diaphysis
Fracture of the femur

DEFINITION

The femoral shaft begins 5 cm below the lesser trochanter and ends
at the junction of the diaphysis and metaphysis distally. As with all
femoral fractures, those that occur in the shaft are usually the result
of significant trauma and are most commonly seen in young adults.
However, osteopenic fractures of the femoral shaft are being seen
with increased frequency in patients older than 90 years. Open
fractures are not unusual (approximately 20%) and require special
treatment. Associated injuries involving multiple organ systems are
common. Forty percent of patients with femoral shaft fractures have
associated injuries, including head, chest, and abdominal injuries.
Causes of femoral shaft fractures include falls, motor vehicle
accidents (including collisions between motor vehicles and
pedestrians), and gunshot injuries. The femoral shaft is surrounded
by muscle on all sides and has excellent vascular supply and
therefore great healing potential.

HISTORY AND PHYSICAL FINDINGS

A history of a fall in an older individual is typical for a femoral
shaft fracture. In younger individuals, a high-energy injury such as
a motor vehicle accident, a motor vehicle–pedestrian collision, or a
gunshot wound is more typical. Sports-related femoral shaft
fractures are uncommon, with the exception of competitive skiers
who sustain a high-energy type of fracture. The diagnosis is usually
quite obvious on physical examination, with swelling and deformity
readily apparent. Anterior and lateral angulation of the thigh and a
large hematoma are common on initial evaluation. Swelling of the
knee may indicate an associated fracture about the knee. Vascular
and neurologic injuries and closed fractures are not common but
may be present with gunshot wounds. Any difference in the pulses
at the wrist or ankle will require further evaluation.

IMAGING STUDIES

Required for diagnosis

AP and lateral views are almost always adequate to diagnose a
femoral shaft fracture.

Required for comprehensive evaluation

AP views of the pelvis are also essential because concurrent femoral neck fractures are present in up to 10% of patients with femoral shaft fractures. AP and lateral views of the knee joint also should be obtained because of the potential for associated fractures in this area. Because of considerable deformity associated with femoral shaft fractures, true AP and lateral views are sometimes difficult to obtain. Therefore, two orthogonal views (two views at 90° from each other) without rotation of the limb are usually adequate to plan treatment.

Special considerations

If peripheral pulses are absent or if the limb appears ischemic, Doppler ultrasound of the wrist and ankle can be obtained. If blood flow at the ankle is less than 90% of that at the wrist, angiography should be strongly considered.

Pitfalls

Failure to recognize an associated hip fracture, especially a femoral neck fracture, can have devastating results.

IMAGE DESCRIPTIONS

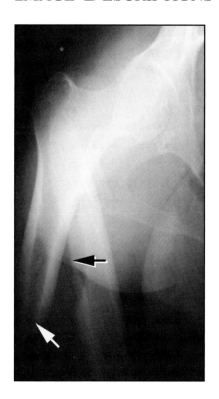

Figure 7-13

Fracture of the femoral shaft—AP view

AP view of an adult patient with a femoral shaft fracture shows a spiral fracture pattern (black arrow) with the apex of the deformity lateral (white arrow).

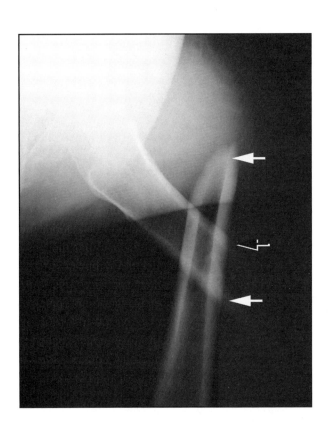

Figure 7-14

Fracture of the femoral shaft—
Frog-lateral view

Frog-lateral view of the same patient shown in Figure 7-13 shows that the apex of the deformity is lateral (black arrow). Note also the degree of displacement present (white arrows), indicating that this patient is not in any form of traction or splinting.

DIFFERENTIAL DIAGNOSIS

Hematoma of the thigh (may be seen on soft-tissue views, but MRI most likely needed to visualize)

Subtrochanteric fracture (seen on radiographs that include the hip)

Supracondylar fracture (seen on radiographs that include the knee)

FRACTURES OF THE SACROILIAC JOINT AND SACRUM

SYNONYMS
Pelvic fracture
Spine fracture

ICD-9 Code
806.6
Fracture of the sacrum and coccyx, closed

DEFINITION
The sacroiliac joint consists of the sacrum and ilium on each side. Each side is stabilized by very strong ligaments, both anteriorly and especially posteriorly, with the latter considered the primary stabilizers of the joint. Injuries of the sacroiliac joint result from high-energy trauma and typically occur with other injuries to the pelvis. Fractures of the sacrum involve that portion of the spine below the fifth lumbar vertebra and above the coccyx. Up to 30% of patients with pelvic ring injuries will have concomitant fractures of the sacrum. Isolated sacral fractures are rare (less than 10%), but when they occur are typically transverse and the result of a fall from a height. The mortality rate with fractures of the sacrum and pelvic ring is as high as 20%, with hemorrhage the leading cause of death. Associated neurologic and genitourinary injuries occur in more than one third of patients with sacral fractures.

HISTORY AND PHYSICAL FINDINGS
A high-energy injury such as a motor vehicle accident is typical of an acute fracture. Patients with a history of osteoporosis, steroid use, or radiation therapy to the pelvis are prone to insufficiency fractures of the sacrum. Physical examination reveals pain and ecchymosis over the posterior aspect of the pelvis. The sacroiliac joint is not only tender to palpation but also to lateral compression of the pelvis. Sacral fractures are tender to direct palpation and on palpation during rectal examination. With sacral injuries, urinary retention and decreased anal sphincter tone are possible. Other neurologic deficits may include sensory and motor loss in the lower extremity.

SECTION 7 ■ HIP AND THIGH

IMAGING STUDIES

Required for diagnosis

A 30° cephalad AP view of the pelvis is the initial study of choice for suspected sacroiliac joint injuries or sacral fractures. A lateral view of the sacrum should be obtained as well. If a rare transverse fracture of the sacrum is suspected given the mechanism of injury (fall onto the buttocks) and suspicious on the initial AP view, a lateral view of the pelvis with the hips flexed may show the degree of fracture displacement. Isolated fractures of the sacrum are difficult to detect on radiographs. Only 30% of these fractures appear on radiographs.

Required for comprehensive evaluation

CT provides excellent visualization of the sacrum and sacroiliac joint. CT allows evaluation of potential disruption of the sacroiliac joint or subtle vertical fractures of the sacrum and is valuable in deciding whether surgical treatment is necessary. MRI is indicated for patients with acute sacral fractures accompanied by neurologic deficits. MRI is also useful in elderly patients with suspected insufficiency fractures of the sacrum.

Special considerations

If significant arterial bleeding is detected, embolization of the bleeding arteries is 90% effective when done early but less than 20% effective if the patient's hemodynamic status has not been stabilized. Cystometry and sphincter electromyography may be indicated if bowel and bladder dysfunction are suspected on clinical examination.

Pitfalls

Sacral fractures in the elderly are frequently missed because they are not recognized as a source of low back pain.

IMAGE DESCRIPTIONS

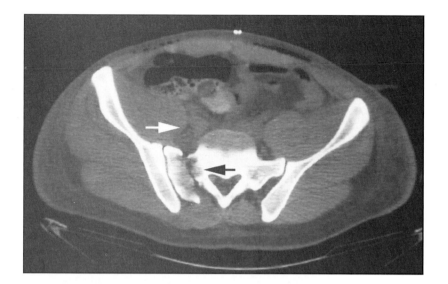

Figure 7-15

Fracture of the sacrum—Axial CT

Axial CT scan of the pelvis shows a minimally displaced vertical fracture through the right side of the sacrum (black arrow). Note the hematoma anterior to the fracture (white arrow).

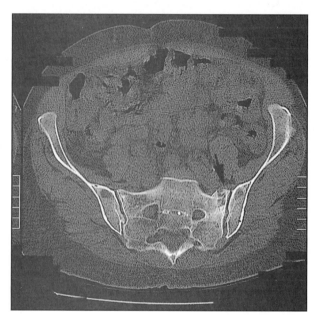

Figure 7-16

Fracture of the sacrum— Axial CT

Axial CT scan of a sacral insufficiency fracture shows compression of the sacrum in an area adjacent to the sacroiliac joint (arrow).

DIFFERENTIAL DIAGNOSIS

Coccyx fracture (seen on lateral radiograph or CT)

Iliac wing fracture (seen on AP view of the pelvis)

Metastatic disease (lytic or blastic lesion seen on MRI)

Spinal stenosis (seen on MRI)

Intertrochanteric Fracture

ICD-9 Code

820.21
Fracture of neck of femur, intertrochanteric section, closed

Synonym
Hip fracture

Definition
The intertrochanteric region of the hip extends from the extracapsular region of the femoral neck to just below the lesser trochanter. Fractures in this area usually result from a fall involving a direct blow to the greater trochanter. Intertrochanteric fractures occur between the greater and lesser trochanter and may have two, three, or four parts. This fracture occurs through an area of cancellous bone that has an excellent blood supply because of the many muscles that originate and insert on the trochanters. Therefore, in contrast to a femoral neck fracture, osteonecrosis following an intertrochanteric fracture is quite rare. Intertrochanteric fractures typically occur in older individuals. More than 90% of hip fractures occur in individuals older than 65 years, and 40% to 50% of these will be intertrochanteric fractures. Women are two to three times more likely to sustain a hip fracture than men.

History and Physical Findings
A history of slipping and falling at home or an episode of syncope preceding a fall is common. When an insufficiency fracture of the hip has occurred, the patient may experience pain first and then fall after the onset of the pain. Physical examination will reveal that the affected limb is usually shortened and externally rotated and that the patient is unable to bear weight on the leg. Ecchymosis over the posterior aspect of the greater trochanter may be present. Neurologic and vascular injuries are rare. However, careful examination of the opposite hip and upper extremities is indicated to ensure there are no other associated fractures.

Imaging Studies

Required for diagnosis
An AP view of the pelvis and a cross-table lateral view of the affected limb will show the fracture in almost all cases. The cross-table lateral view is particularly important to obtain in these fractures because the stability of an intertrochanteric fracture is based on the condition of the posteromedial cortex in the direction of the fracture line, which is visualized on this view.

Required for comprehensive evaluation

If the history and physical examination are consistent with a hip fracture but radiographs are normal, MRI is indicated. MRI will show the fracture line and surrounding marrow edema with a high degree of sensitivity and specificity. Also, MRI will readily visualize a pathologic fracture.

Special considerations

None

Pitfalls

Failure to image the opposite hip and upper extremities may result in missing associated fractures, which are not uncommon in these patients.

IMAGE DESCRIPTIONS

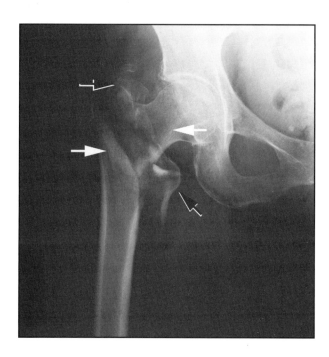

Figure 7-17

Intertrochanteric fracture—AP view

AP view of a right hip shows a four-part unstable intertrochanteric fracture. Note that both the greater and lesser trochanters (black arrows) are separated from the shaft and the femoral head and neck (white arrows).

SECTION 7 ■ HIP AND THIGH

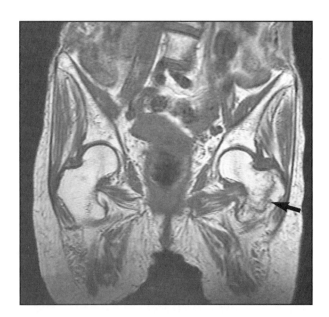

Figure 7-18

Intertrochanteric fracture— Coronal MRI

Coronal T1-weighted MRI scan of a patient with pain in the left hip shows low signal intensity in the intertrochanteric region of the left hip (arrow), consistent with a nondisplaced intertrochanteric hip fracture.

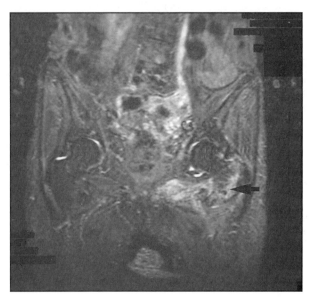

Figure 7-19

Intertrochanteric fracture—MRI

Inversion-recovery image of the pelvis in the patient shown in Figure 7-18 shows edema along the fracture line in the intertrochanteric region of the left hip (black arrow).

DIFFERENTIAL DIAGNOSIS

Acetabular fracture (may be seen on radiographs, CT may be necessary)

Femoral neck fracture (can be seen on AP view)

Metastatic disease (lytic lesion seen on radiographs)

PELVIC RING INSTABILITY

SYNONYMS
Osteitis condensans ilii
Osteitis pubis
Sacroiliitis

ICD-9 Codes

720.2
Sacroiliitis, not elsewhere classified

733.5
Osteitis condensans

DEFINITION
Pelvic instability is a painful condition caused by pathologic changes to the joints of the pelvic ring. The pelvic ring consists of three joints: two sacroiliac joints posteriorly and the symphysis pubis anteriorly. Instability in these joints often occurs as the result of repetitive microtrauma, degenerative osteoarthritis, inflammatory arthritis, and iatrogenic causes.

Sacroiliitis is a common inflammatory condition of the sacroiliac joint that is often an underdiagnosed source of low back and posterior buttock pain. It can be caused by many arthritides and is frequently associated with seronegative spondyloarthropathies such as ankylosing spondylitis. It is bilateral in nature.

Osteitis condensans ilii is an unusual cause of pelvic instability that occurs in up to 2% of multiparous women following pregnancy. Excessive stress across the sacroiliac joints is thought to stretch or disrupt the adjacent ligamentous structures. This condition is painful but usually considered self-limiting.

Osteitis pubis is an uncommon type of instability, usually resulting from excessive stress and strain across the symphysis pubis from repetitive vigorous activities. It also can be associated with pregnancy.

HISTORY AND PHYSICAL FINDINGS
Patients with pelvic instability typically report pain about the sacroiliac joint of insidious onset that may radiate into the posterior buttock and thigh. Less common is localized pubic pain. The pain may be described as dull, sharp, or aching. Sitting or twisting the trunk of the body exacerbates the pain, whereas lying or standing relieves it. Preexisting conditions such as ankylosing spondylitis are usually present.

Physical examination reveals localized tenderness on palpation of the sacroiliac joint posteriorly or the symphysis pubis anteriorly. Provocative testing that can cause rotation or shear across the sacroiliac joint can reproduce the pain. Pain typically does not radiate to the lower extremities on a straight leg raising test.

SECTION 7 ■ HIP AND THIGH

IMAGING STUDIES

Required for diagnosis

An AP view of the sacroiliac joints (Ferguson view) may be normal or show subtle sclerosis and widening of the sacroiliac joints in the early stages. As the instability progresses, increased sclerosis is typically found adjacent to these joints. The sclerosis always involves the inferior sacroiliac joint, which distinguishes it from degenerative changes that may only affect more central areas. In later stages of sacroiliitis, the sclerosis becomes more prominent and the joints become narrow. The end stage of sacroiliitis is characterized by ankylosis of the sacroiliac joint, and radiographs show that the joint is obliterated. An AP view of the pelvis is diagnostic for osteitis pubis or osteitis condensans ilii. Osteitis pubis presents with sclerosis, irregularity, and widening of the symphysis pubis. Bilateral, triangle-shaped sclerosis can be seen adjacent to the sacroiliac joint on the iliac side in cases of osteitis condensans ilii. There is no evidence of narrowing or obliteration of the sacroiliac joint.

Required for comprehensive evaluation

A pelvic inlet (30° caudad tilt) view provides a true AP view of the sacrum and is ordered to further delineate any mild abnormality seen on the AP view. Oblique views of the pelvis and arthrography are unnecessary. Technetium Tc 99m bone scan may show increased uptake at or about the sacroiliac joint or symphysis pubis, but it lacks specificity and adds very little additional information. CT or MRI is helpful in ruling out other pathology such as infection, tumor, or stress fractures. CT can identify fusion of the sacroiliac joint or destruction of the adjacent bone. T2-weighted and post–gadolinium-contrast MR images may reveal increased signal intensity in the sacroiliac joint or symphysis pubis, consistent with inflammation.

Special considerations

Unilateral sacroiliitis may require aspiration under fluoroscopy to rule out sepsis, especially if intravenous drug use is suspected or noted.

Pitfalls

These conditions can be confused with infection.

IMAGE DESCRIPTIONS

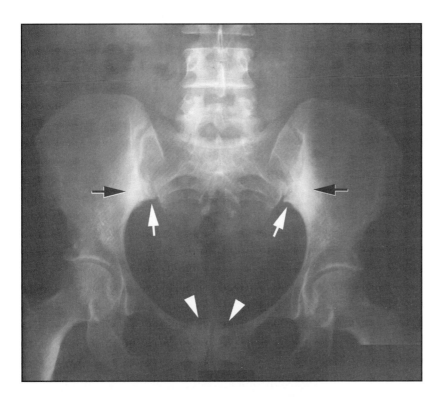

Figure 7-20

Osteitis condensans ilii—AP view

AP view of the pelvis of a multiparous woman shows a bilateral, triangular-shaped sclerosis on the iliac side of the sacroiliac joints (black arrows). The sacroiliac joint architecture is preserved (white arrows), but the increased sclerosis about the symphysis pubis is characteristic of osteitis pubis (arrowheads).

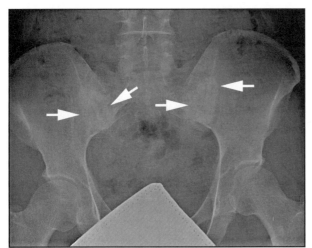

Figure 7-21

Sacroiliitis—AP view

AP view of the pelvis shows extensive sclerosis and narrowing of the sacroiliac joints (arrows) in this patient with ankylosing spondylitis.

SECTION 7 ■ HIP AND THIGH

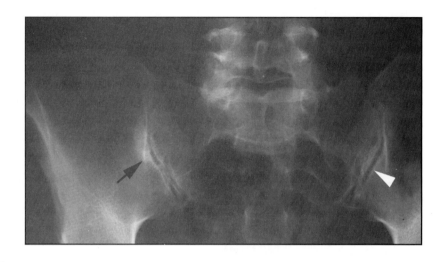

Figure 7-22

Degenerative change of sacroiliac joint— AP view

AP view of the pelvis shows iliac sclerosis at the middle aspect of the right sacroiliac joint (black arrow). The left sacroiliac joint appears normal (arrowhead). Lack of involvement of the inferior sacroiliac joint excludes sacroiliitis.

DIFFERENTIAL DIAGNOSIS

Iatrogenic etiology (history of aggressive posterior iliac crest bone graft harvest)

Infection (acute onset, fever, elevated white blood cell count, elevated erythrocyte sedimentation rate, unilateral)

Osteoarthritis (degenerative findings on radiographs, usually asymptomatic)

Rheumatoid arthritis (bilateral, positive serologic tests, multiple joint involvement)

Seronegative spondyloarthropathy (bilateral involvement, osteoarthritis in spine, associated symptoms)

Stress fracture (history of increased vigorous activities, evident on MRI)

Traumatic fracture (history of significant direct trauma, radiographic findings)

Tumor (night pain, evident on MRI)

STRESS FRACTURES OF THE HIP AND PELVIS

SYNONYMS

Fatigue fracture

Insufficiency fracture

ICD-9 Code

733.95

Stress fracture of other bone

DEFINITION

Stress fractures occur in two situations: (1) when normal bone is subjected to abnormal stress and repeatedly loaded beyond its ability to heal (fatigue fracture); and (2) when normal stress is applied to abnormal bone such as osteoporotic or osteopenic bone, resulting in microfractures in the trabecular and cortical bone that with continuous stress eventually fracture completely (insufficiency fracture). Fatigue fractures most commonly occur in individuals involved in a vigorous training program or in athletes involved in running activities. Marathon runners, track athletes, and military recruits in basic training are in the highest risk groups. Insufficiency fractures typically occur in frail elderly individuals who have weakened bone from osteoporosis or osteomalacia.

Stress fractures about the hip commonly occur at the femoral neck, the pubic rami, and the symphysis pubis, but they rarely occur at the sacrum. Stress fractures can occur in patients of all ages and in both sexes; however, they are infrequent among blacks. Female runners with amenorrhea or oligomenorrhea are at increased risk. The morbidity associated with stress fractures can be significant.

HISTORY AND PHYSICAL FINDINGS

Patients with fatigue fractures usually report engaging in a new and vigorous activity within a couple of weeks of the development of symptoms. Symptoms usually include a gradual, increasingly dull, aching pain in the groin and anterolateral thigh that may radiate to the medial aspect of the knee. Stress fractures of the pelvic ring are associated with inguinal pain or pubic pain but rarely with sacroiliac or buttock pain. Early on, the symptoms occur during activity and are relieved by rest. As a stress fracture progresses, symptoms may occur during activities of daily living. In time, the pain becomes constant and prevents weight bearing on the affected extremity. On physical examination, localized tenderness about the groin, pubic region, and anterolateral thigh or sacral region is noted. Pain is also elicited at the limits of range of motion. Internal rotation of the hip may be limited as in figure-of-four testing. In advanced stages, an antalgic gait is usually observed.

SECTION 7 ■ HIP AND THIGH

IMAGING STUDIES

Required for diagnosis

AP views of the hip and pelvis and a frog-lateral view of the affected hip are the appropriate initial imaging studies. Even though radiographs are often normal in the early stages of a stress fracture, radiographic evidence of increased sclerosis about the femoral neck, pubic rami, or sacrum may actually precede the onset of symptoms by 2 to 3 weeks. Radiographs are considered positive when increased sclerosis within the femoral neck is evident. Sclerosis represents osteal or periosteal callus formation and may be readily apparent in the femoral neck or pubic rami.

Required for comprehensive evaluation

For many years, a bone scan was considered the gold standard in identifying stress fractures. Now, however, if radiographs are normal, MRI of the hip and pelvis should be obtained. MRI is more specific than a bone scan in detecting stress fractures of the femoral neck and pelvis and can rule out other possible diagnoses simultaneously. Therefore, if radiographs are normal and if a stress fracture is suspected, MRI is the next study to obtain.

Special considerations

None

Pitfalls

A normal radiograph within the first 4 to 6 weeks of onset of symptoms does not rule out a stress fracture. Radiographic changes may not be seen for several months on radiographs. Therefore, with a high index of suspicion for stress fracture and a compatible history, MRI should be ordered early.

IMAGE DESCRIPTIONS

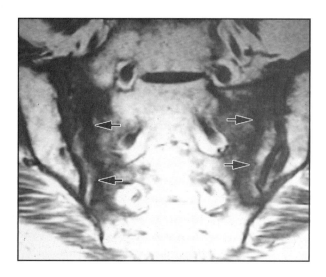

Figure 7-23

Stress fracture of the sacrum— Coronal MRI

Coronal T1-weighted MRI scan of the sacrum shows bilateral low signal intensity black lines medial and parallel to the sacroiliac joints (black arrows). These black lines represent bilateral sacral stress fractures.

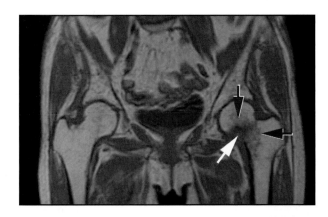

Figure 7-24

Stress fracture of the medial femoral neck—Coronal MRI

Coronal T1-weighted MRI scan of the hips reveals a low signal intensity linear stress fracture along the medial left femoral neck (white arrow) surrounded by low signal intensity reactive edema (black arrows).

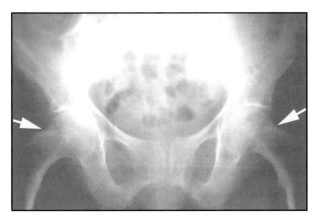

Figure 7-25

Stress fractures of the femoral necks—AP view

Subtle linear cortical lucencies are seen in the lateral femoral necks (arrows) of this patient with osteomalacia.

DIFFERENTIAL DIAGNOSIS

Hip strain (normal radiographs, MRI positive for muscle involvement)

Infection (fluid in the joint on MRI, positive culture of joint aspirate)

Osteoarthritis (joint space narrowing evident on radiographs)

Osteonecrosis (collapse or early changes evident on radiographs)

Traumatic fracture (evidence of fracture on radiographs immediately at the onset of symptoms)

Trochanteric bursitis (normal radiographs; pain relief by anesthetic injection)

Tumor (lytic lesion seen on radiograph)

SECTION 7 ■ HIP AND THIGH

SUBTROCHANTERIC FRACTURE

SYNONYMS
Fracture of the femur
Hip fracture

DEFINITION
Subtrochanteric fractures occur below the level of the lesser
trochanter and 5 cm distal to this point (or the isthmus of the
diaphysis of the femoral shaft) and account for up to 30% of all hip
fractures. This area of the femur is composed of cortical bone that
is subjected to high biomechanical stresses. Subtrochanteric
fractures occur in two distinct groups with different mechanisms of
injury for each group. In elderly (average age 75 years) patients,
the fracture results from low-energy trauma such as from a fall. In
younger (average age 40 years) patients, the fracture is caused by
high-energy injuries accompanied by significant soft-tissue injuries
of the chest and abdomen. In high-energy injuries, fractures of the
patella and tibia on the same limb are common, as are fractures of
the pelvis and spine.

HISTORY AND PHYSICAL FINDINGS
Patients in the younger age group commonly have a history of a
motor vehicle accident, a motor vehicle-pedestrian accident, or a
fall from a height. Penetrating injuries such as from a gunshot
wound are the cause in up to 10% of subtrochanteric fractures.
Severe pain is typical. On physical examination the leg is swollen,
shortened, and externally rotated. The vascular and neurologic
examinations usually are normal in closed injuries. The hemoglobin
and hematocrit levels need close monitoring as patients can lose
four or more units of blood into the thigh, resulting in hypovolemia
and hypotension.

IMAGING STUDIES

Required for diagnosis
AP and lateral views are usually sufficient to establish the diagnosis
and delineate the fracture pattern.

Required for comprehensive evaluation
An AP pelvis radiograph should be obtained, along with AP and
lateral views of the entire femur including the hip and the knee to
rule out a fracture about the knee.

Special considerations

Because of the considerable deformity and pain associated with this fracture, it is often difficult to obtain true AP and lateral views. Two orthogonal views (two views at 90° from each other) can be obtained instead to provide imaging in two planes. In gunshot wounds, if no peripheral pulses are palpated in the lower extremity, immediate referral to a specialist is indicated, and Doppler arterial pressures at the ankle and wrist should be measured. If the Doppler pressure at the ankle is less than 90% of the pressure at the wrist, arteriography should be considered to rule out a vascular injury.

Pitfalls

Failure to include the knee and hip joints on radiographs may miss associated fractures often seen in conjunction with subtrochanteric fractures.

IMAGE DESCRIPTIONS

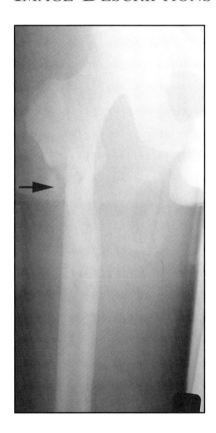

Figure 7-26

Subtrochanteric fracture—AP view

AP view of the right hip and femur shows an oblique comminuted subtrochanteric fracture (arrow).

SECTION 7 ■ HIP AND THIGH

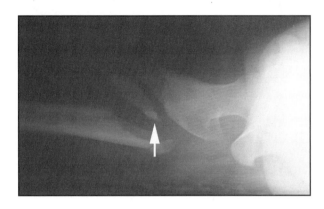

Figure 7-27

Subtrochanteric fracture—
Cross-table lateral view

Cross-table lateral view of the same patient shown in Figure 7-26 shows the comminuted subtrochanteric fracture, which is distracted and posteriorly displaced.

DIFFERENTIAL DIAGNOSIS

Fracture of the femoral shaft (seen on AP view more distally in the femur)

Intertrochanteric fracture (seen on AP view more proximally in the femur)

Metastatic disease (fracture through a lytic lesion)

Congenital and Developmental Abnormalities of the Hip Joint

Synonyms

Acetabular dysplasia
Congenital subluxation or dislocation
Coxa breva
Coxa magna
Coxa valga
Coxa vara
Developmental dysplasia
Legg-Calvé-Perthes disease
Slipped capital femoral epiphysis

Definition

Congenital dislocations most commonly occur at the hip joint, with approximately 1 in 1,000 neonates affected. Dislocations occur in girls eight to ten times more frequently than in boys; bilateral dislocation occurs in one quarter of patients who have a dislocation. The progressive loss of cartilage around the hip joint can be a consequence of the abnormal shape of the acetabulum (acetabular dysplasia) or the femur (excessive valgus or varus), or it can be the end result of Legg-Calvé-Perthes disease or slipped capital femoral epiphysis. Another consequence of these abnormalities is that joint reaction forces are altered sufficiently to cause activity-related pain that usually is a precursor to secondary osteoarthritis. Occasionally the joint is incongruent or aspherical as a consequence of the original condition, resulting in accelerated joint space narrowing.

If symptoms develop in early adulthood, timely intervention may delay or halt the progression of secondary osteoarthritis. Identifying these potential conditions, then, is critical for early diagnosis and treatment. To allow for early diagnosis, both the normal and abnormal configurations of the hip joint must be understood.

If the secondary osteoarthritis is caused by a slipped capital femoral epiphysis, the slip is usually seen on the AP view (Herndon hump), and the previous slip of the epiphysis is best seen on the lateral view.

The consequences of Legg-Calvé-Perthes disease with secondary osteoarthritis may include a large femoral head (coxa magna) or short femoral neck (coxa breva) and, in extreme cases, lateral subluxation of the femoral head after reconstitution and healing of the osteonecrosis. Adult onset osteonecrosis with secondary osteoarthritis is described in Osteonecrosis and Transient Osteoporosis.

ICD-9 Codes

715.25
Osteoarthrosis, hip and thigh, secondary

718.4
Contracture of joint

732.1
Juvenile osteochondrosis of hip and pelvis

732.2
Nontraumatic slipped upper femoral epiphysis

736.31
Coxa valga (acquired)

736.32
Coxa vara (acquired)

754.3
Congenital dislocation of hip

820.01
Transcervical fracture of neck of femur, epiphysis (separation) (upper), closed

Section 7 ■ Hip and Thigh

HISTORY AND PHYSICAL FINDINGS

The history and physical examination usually reveal the potential causes of secondary osteoarthritis (eg, trauma, slipped capital femoral epiphysis, Legg-Calvé-Perthes disease). Symptoms are similar to those of osteoarthritis, including loss of motion, pain with extremes of motion, abnormal gait, limb-length discrepancy, and pain that typically becomes worse with high-demand activities.

Altered joint reaction forces may be associated with a limp and can be further accentuated as a result of a limb-length discrepancy. Slipped capital femoral epiphysis is more commonly associated with external rotation contracture, and the late sequelae of Legg-Calvé-Perthes disease are more typically associated with decreased abduction, especially if persistent lateral subluxation of the femoral head is apparent on the subsequent radiographs.

IMAGING STUDIES

Required for diagnosis

An AP view of the pelvis (with gonadal shielding in children and young adults) is standard to establish the diagnosis because it frequently will identify congenital or developmental abnormalities of the hip joint with secondary osteoarthritis. The acetabular index, which is the angle created with one line vertical from the center of the femoral head and the other from the center of the head to the margin of the acetabulum, is about 30° on the AP view. An angle of less than 20° suggests acetabular dysplasia. Cross-table lateral or groin lateral views may suggest an associated increase in anteversion, which typically is about 25° or 30° anterior. With increased anteversion, more of the relatively uncovered femoral head is exposed anteriorly. AP views also may show a significant variation in the neck-shaft angle. Normally, the angle ranges from 120° to 140° (typically, 130°), with a relative varus (less than 120°) or valgus (greater than 140°) configuration.

Required for comprehensive evaluation

A low AP view of the hip (to include the proximal 8 to 10 inches of the femur) and a lateral view (frog-lateral or cross-table lateral) are added for comprehensive evaluation. For patients who have loss of joint motion, a cross-table lateral is more comfortable for the patient and easier to obtain than the frog-lateral view.

Special considerations

Shielding of the gonads in children and young adults is suggested.

Pitfalls

The pain may be attributed to the patient's hip problem when a spine condition may be the problem.

IMAGE DESCRIPTIONS

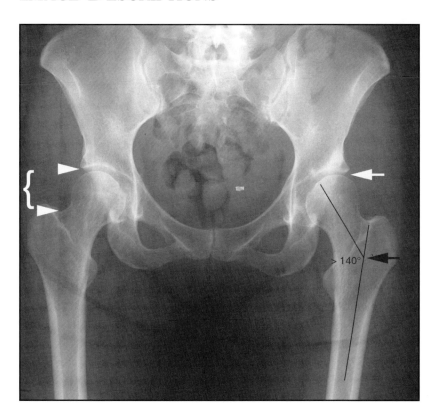

Figure 7-28

Coxa valga of the hip—AP view

AP view of an adult patient with a valgus alignment at the hip joint shows a neck-shaft angle that exceeds 140° (black arrow). Note also the increased portion of the articular aspect of the femoral head that is uncovered (white arrow). This attribute becomes even more important if the superior aspect of the weight-bearing surface of the acetabulum is smaller than normal. In this patient, the trochanteric acetabular distance (the distance from a line drawn parallel to the superior aspect of the weight-bearing surface of the dome to a line parallel to the superior aspect of the tip of the greater trochanter) exceeds 2.5 cm (arrowheads). Normally, the trochanteric acetabular distance in adults averages about 2.2 cm.

SECTION 7 ■ HIP AND THIGH

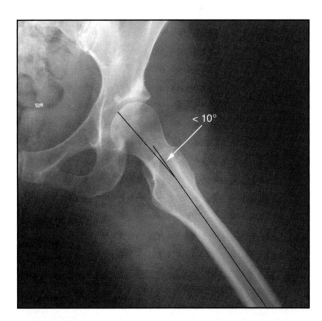

Figure 7-29

Coxa valga of the hip— Frog-lateral view

Frog-lateral view of the same patient shown in Figure 7-28 shows a relative absence of anteversion (arrow). In this patient, the neck-shaft angle is slightly retroverted. The consequence of these developmental findings is an increased risk of degenerative changes as a result of altered joint reaction forces in the hip.

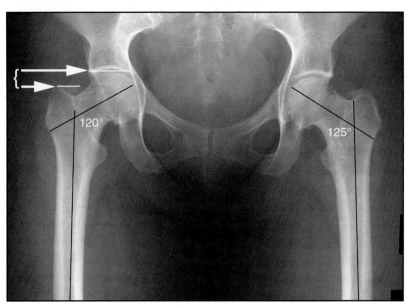

Figure 7-30

Coxa vara of the hip—AP view

AP view of the pelvis in an adult patient with coxa vara of the hip joint shows a neck-shaft angle of less than 125° and a decreased trochanteric acetabular distance (white arrows). This configuration contributes to the potential for abnormal joint reaction forces, with an increased risk of a medial osteoarthritis developing at the hip joint. In this patient, the loss of the medial joint space and/or early arthrokatadysis or medial migration of the femoral heads can be seen, as can early development of osteophytes at the acetabulum and femoral head.

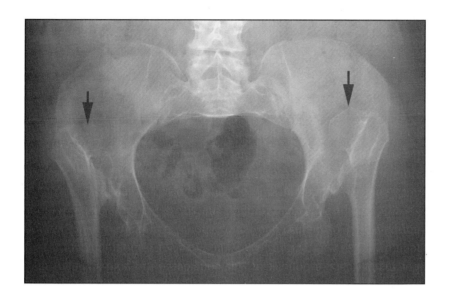

Figure 7-31

Developmental dysplasia of the hip—AP view

AP view of the pelvis of an adult with long-standing dislocation of the hips bilaterally shows that the femoral heads are relatively small and underdeveloped (arrows) and the acetabulum is not readily apparent, perhaps having never truly formed. With a deformity this severe, the patient's legs are likely shortened by 3 to 4 inches.

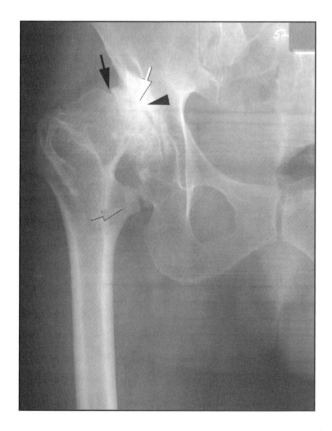

Figure 7-32

Developmental dysplasia of the hip—AP view

AP view of an adult patient shows severe subluxation of the femoral head relative to the normal position of the severely dysplastic acetabulum (black arrow). This view also shows loss of joint space (white arrow) and sclerosis (arrowhead), consistent with long-standing changes of the abnormal articular region of the hip. Note the high position of the lesser trochanter relative to the inferior margin of the ischium, which is in the more normal relative position of the lesser trochanter (gray arrow). This abnormal positioning confirms a long-standing shortening of the limb.

SECTION 7 ■ HIP AND THIGH

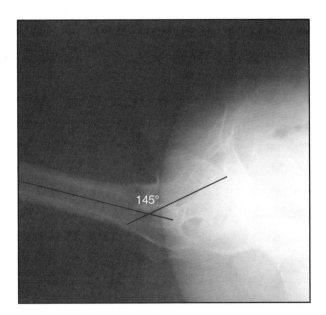

Figure 7-33

Developmental dysplasia of the hip—Lateral view

Lateral view of the patient shown in Figure 7-32 shows an increase in the angle of anteversion (145°) of the femoral head relative to the femoral shaft.

DIFFERENTIAL DIAGNOSIS

Midlumbar disk disease (pain, weakness, and numbness in a dermatomal pattern; nerve root impingement apparent on MRI)

Primary osteoarthritis (no abnormal measurements of the hip region)

Septic joint (abnormal laboratory and/or aspiration data)

INFLAMMATORY ARTHROPATHY

SYNONYMS

Ankylosing spondylitis
Erosive osteoarthritis
Psoriatic arthritis
Reiter's syndrome
Rheumatoid arthritis

DEFINITION

Inflammatory arthropathy of the hip is seen in a group of systemic disorders that have in common a progressive uniform loss of cartilage about the hip joint. This group of systemic disorders includes rheumatoid arthritis, perhaps the most commonly recognized, and juvenile rheumatoid arthritis; erosive osteoarthritis; ankylosing spondylitis; psoriatic arthritis; and enteropathic arthropathies (Crohn's disease, ulcerative colitis, and patients with a history of gastric bypass surgery). These conditions may be the most difficult to accurately diagnose in the hip and can occur in any age group. Of these conditions, rheumatoid arthritis is the most common and/or most widely recognized. However, other conditions as noted can produce similar radiographic abnormalities. Frequently, medial and/or axial femoral head migration is seen. The end stage is known as arthrokatadysis.

Extra-articular manifestations are common with these conditions, including central and marginal erosions and associated reactive synovitis with relative osteopenia, an absence of marginal osteophytes, and an absence of reactive subchondral sclerosis. Multiple joints are usually involved, often bilaterally. Some of these conditions commonly affect the hip (eg, rheumatoid arthritis, Reiter's syndrome, ankylosing spondylitis) and some rarely do (erosive osteoarthritis and psoriatic arthritis).

HISTORY AND PHYSICAL FINDINGS

Stiffness, especially in the morning, or with start-up related activities and aching in the groin region are common presenting symptoms. Up to 15% of patients may have trochanteric buttock or thigh- and/or knee-related symptoms, but referred pain to the medial aspect of the knee is rarely seen. These patients initially may respond to anti-inflammatory drugs and limited activities. For a patient who has symptoms in multiple joints, a comprehensive history, physical examination, and serologic or laboratory evaluation should be considered. Medical treatment and observation can potentially slow or stop disease progression in many cases.

ICD-9 Codes

274.0
Gouty arthropathy

696.0
Psoriatic arthropathy

710.0
Systemic lupus erythematosus

713.0
Arthropathy associated with other endocrine and metabolic disorders

713.1
Arthropathy associated with gastrointestinal conditions other than infections

714.0
Rheumatoid arthritis

714.30
Polyarticular juvenile rheumatoid arthritis, chronic or unspecified

720.0
Ankylosing spondylitis

SECTION 7 ■ HIP AND THIGH

IMAGING STUDIES

Required for diagnosis

An AP view of the pelvis is standard to establish the diagnosis. Gonadal shielding is recommended for children and young adults.

Required for comprehensive evaluation

A low AP view of the hip (to include the proximal 8 to 10 inches of the femur) and a lateral view (frog-lateral or cross-table lateral) are added for comprehensive evaluation. For a patient with loss of joint motion as a result of this condition, a cross-table lateral is kinder to the patient and easier to obtain than a frog-lateral view.

Special considerations

Several conditions can result in an erosive arthropathy, but most are identified by the results of laboratory tests in addition to radiographic findings. Advanced imaging studies are not indicated unless laboratory data provide no clue to the diagnosis. Laboratory evaluation may include aspiration of the hip joint under fluoroscopy to rule out infection or to diagnose a crystal arthropathy.

Pitfalls

Infectious septic hip arthritis is a true emergency and always should be considered part of the differential diagnosis. The main pitfall is to miss a septic arthritis. A patient who has severe pain with any motion, a fever, and significantly limited motion with a partially flexed and externally rotated position (because of capsular distention) requires hip aspiration to rule out infection immediately after radiographs are obtained.

IMAGE DESCRIPTIONS

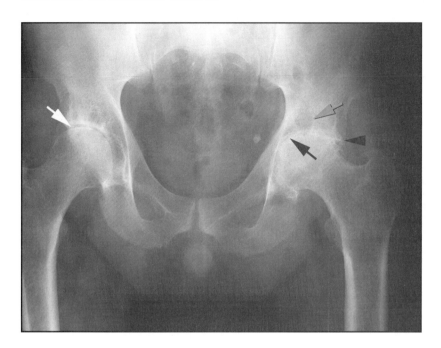

Figure 7-34

Rheumatoid arthritis (hips)—AP view

AP view of an adult patient shows advanced erosive arthritis in the left hip with degenerative changes. Moderate erosive changes are evident in the right hip (white arrow). Note the presence of marginal osteophytes (arrowhead), along with medial and superior migration of the left femoral head (black arrow). The joint space on the left side is also completely obliterated, and there are cystic changes visible on the acetabulum (gray arrow). The right hip shows some cystic changes, but some joint space remains and marginal osteophytes are not readily evident.

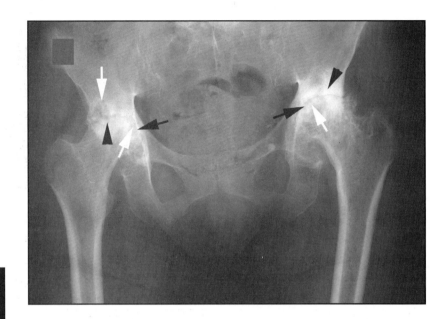

Figure 7-35

Rheumatoid arthritis (hips)—AP view

AP view of the pelvis of an adult patient shows a typical inflammatory arthritic pattern in the hip joints. Note the medial and superior migration of the femoral heads (black arrows), with periarticular cystic and erosive changes involving both sides of the joint (white arrows). Sclerosis is readily evident as well (arrowheads), especially in areas where cystic changes are not seen.

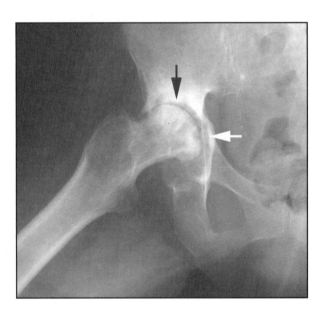

Figure 7-36

Erosive arthritis (hips)— Frog-lateral view

Frog-lateral view of the hip in an adult patient shows an erosive arthritic pattern with sclerosis (black arrow) and clear medial migration (white arrow) with remodeling of the medial wall of the acetabulum. Cystic changes are apparent on both sides of the joint, and loss of joint space is noted as well.

DIFFERENTIAL DIAGNOSIS

Midlumbar disk disease (clinical history of pain, weakness, and numbness in a dermal distribution; herniated disk impinging on a nerve root seen on MRI)

Primary osteoarthritis with an erosive pattern (normal laboratory tests, typical radiographic evidence of osteoarthritis)

Septic joint (fluid in the joint on MRI, positive Gram stain and culture on joint aspirate)

OSTEOARTHRITIS

SYNONYMS

Degenerative arthrosis
Degenerative joint disease
Osteoarthrosis
Primary osteoarthritis
Secondary osteoarthritis

DEFINITION

The progressive loss of cartilage at the hip joint as a consequence of wear and tear or aging is typically referred to as osteoarthritis or degenerative joint disease. Degenerative joint disease is the most common form of arthritis and is the most common reason for hip replacement surgery. Osteoarthritis generally is considered a condition of the elderly, but idiopathic primary osteoarthritis occasionally can develop in younger patients. Trauma can result in a condition called posttraumatic arthritis, which can occur at any age. Osteoarthritis is characterized by progressive segmental loss of cartilage, with joint space narrowing usually superiorly, formation of marginal osteophytes, intraosseous cysts, and subchondral sclerosis.

HISTORY AND PHYSICAL FINDINGS

Symptoms may initially occur only with high-impact activities such as jogging. Typically, patients report stiffness and aching, especially in the groin region and with internal and external rotation of the limb. Occasionally aching is noted in the trochanteric buttock or anterior thigh region, but symptoms rarely radiate to the medial aspect of the knee. Patients who point to the back of the hip as they describe their pain generally have some type of sciatic nerve irritation rather than pain within the hip joint itself.

In younger patients, especially those younger than 50 years, a history of trauma is common. Stiffness and pain are frequently noted in the morning yet the pain may be worse in the evening, especially if patients spend considerable time on their feet. Loss of motion is common, especially in limited rotation, which causes pain at the limits of rotation. This loss of motion is reflected in everyday activities such as difficulty putting on shoes or trousers.

On physical examination hip flexion contracture is usually evident. The gait may be antalgic or Trendelenburg-like (abductor insufficiency) and in advanced cases may suggest a limb-length discrepancy. An existing limb-length discrepancy can also exacerbate osteoarthritis, especially if the involved joint is on the

SECTION 7 ■ HIP AND THIGH

long side. Early symptoms may be relieved with aspirin or nonsteroidal anti-inflammatory drugs (NSAIDs) such as ibuprofen and by limiting high-demand activities. Extra-articular manifestations other than those described above may include exacerbation of related back or ipsilateral knee conditions.

IMAGING STUDIES

Required for diagnosis
An AP radiograph of the pelvis is standard in establishing the diagnosis.

Required for comprehensive evaluation
A low AP view of the hip (to include the proximal 8 to 10 inches of the femur) and a lateral view (either frog-lateral or cross-table lateral) are added for comprehensive evaluation, especially in secondary osteoarthritis of the hip. For a patient with loss of joint motion, the cross-table lateral view is less uncomfortable for the patient and easier to obtain than the frog-lateral view.

Special considerations
Shielding of the gonads in children and young adults is suggested. When a patient has both osteoarthritis of the hip and low back pain, the primary cause of the patient's symptoms may be difficult to determine. An anesthetic injection into the hip, which often is done by a specialist, may help resolve this dilemma.

Pitfalls
Herniated lumbar disk with sciatic irritation may cause symptoms similar to that of osteoarthritis of the hip. An abscess of the psoas muscle may also present as hip pain.

IMAGE DESCRIPTION

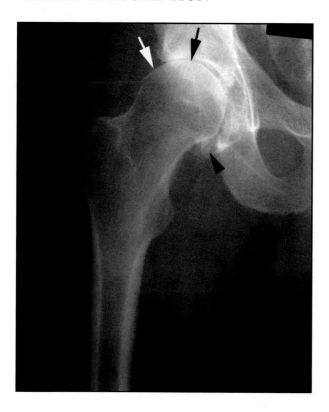

Figure 7-37

Osteoarthritis of the hip (posttraumatic)—AP view

AP view of the hip in an adult patient shows fairly classic signs of posttraumatic osteoarthritis, particularly loss of superolateral joint space (black arrow). Note the lateral subluxation of the femoral head (white arrow) and large medial acetabular osteophyte (arrowhead). This patient has obvious sclerosis of the acetabulum, especially in the area of lost joint space.

DIFFERENTIAL DIAGNOSIS

Developmental arthropathy (abnormal configuration of the acetabulum or femoral head)

Inflammatory arthropathy (erosive changes seen on radiographs, abnormal laboratory tests)

Midlumbar disk disease (nerve root impingement seen on MRI)

Osteonecrosis and Transient Osteoporosis

ICD-9 Codes

733.09
Osteoporosis, other

733.42
Aseptic necrosis of the
femoral head and neck

Synonyms

Aseptic necrosis
Avascular necrosis (AVN)

Definition

Osteonecrosis and transient osteoporosis are different disease processes of the hip that have similar early presentations but significantly different outcomes. Osteonecrosis (literally, bone death) is a painful condition involving the weight-bearing portion of the femoral head. Bone death results from the loss of local blood supply and can occur with many conditions, including trauma, prolonged corticosteroid use, alcohol abuse, chemotherapy, a history of diving and nitrogen toxicity (the bends), or sickle cell disease. The natural history of osteonecrosis is painful collapse of the femoral head followed by development of significant osteoarthritis. Significant disability usually results if osteonecrosis is left untreated. Transient osteoporosis is an uncommon idiopathic condition of the hip characterized by painful osteoporosis in the femoral neck and intertrochanteric region. Unlike osteonecrosis, transient osteoporosis usually completely resolves within 6 to 12 months.

History and Physical Findings

Both conditions are characterized by insidious onset, with pain in both the hip and groin that is exacerbated with weight bearing and activity and is relieved with rest. With osteonecrosis, pain increases as the femoral head collapses. Conversely, with transient osteoporosis, pain gradually improves with time.

Results of the physical examination are also similar in the early stages. Patients have an antalgic gait and pain at the limits of hip motion. With osteonecrosis, however, progressive loss of motion is associated with increased pain as the disease advances.

Imaging Studies

Required for diagnosis

AP and bilateral frog-lateral views of the pelvis should be obtained so that the affected joint can be compared with the opposite joint. In the early stages of both conditions, radiographs may appear normal. The radiographic appearance, however, becomes diagnostic with progression of the disease.

Osteonecrosis is characterized radiographically by sclerosis of the superior femoral head. As the disease progresses, a dark lucent line (the crescent sign), will appear around the area of sclerosis; this line is best seen on the frog-lateral view. With late-stage disease, radiographs will show collapse of the femoral head. End-stage disease is characterized by signs of osteoarthritis, such as loss of joint space, osteophyte formation, and formation of cysts on the femoral head and acetabulum.

Radiographs of a patient with transient osteoporosis will show osteopenia in the femoral neck and head, particularly at the inferior calcar, on the affected side. No sclerosis or femoral head collapse will be observed.

Required for comprehensive evaluation

MRI is indicated if radiographs are normal, show early-stage disease, or if a diagnosis of either condition is suspected. MRI is a sensitive and specific modality for both conditions and will aid in ruling out tumor, infection, and stress fracture.

Osteonecrosis will appear on T1-weighted images as low signal intensity in the superior femoral head. Transient osteoporosis will appear on T1-weighted images as diffuse low signal intensity throughout the femoral neck, extending into the femoral head and intertrochanteric region. The corresponding T2-weighted image shows diffuse high signal intensity in the same location.

Special considerations

None

Pitfalls

CT and bone scans may detect osteonecrosis and transient osteoporosis, but neither is as specific as MRI and therefore not recommended.

SECTION 7 ■ HIP AND THIGH

IMAGE DESCRIPTIONS

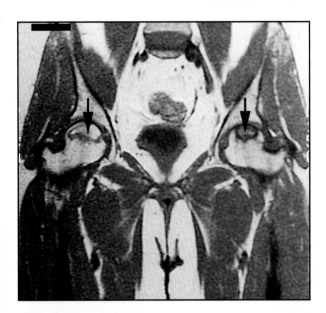

Figure 7-38

Osteonecrosis (early)—Coronal MRI

Coronal T1-weighted MRI scan of both hips shows bilateral serpentine areas of low signal intensity consistent with osteonecrosis in the superior aspect of both femoral heads (black arrows). Note that the lesions are geographic and that there is no evidence of femoral head collapse.

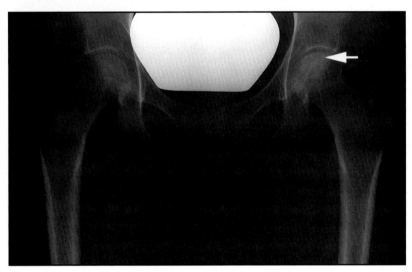

Figure 7-39

Osteonecrosis (early)—AP view

AP view of the pelvis reveals sclerosis in the left superior femoral head (arrow). Note the right femoral head appears normal.

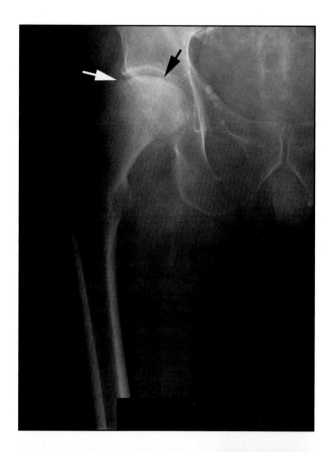

Figure 7-40

Osteonecrosis—AP view

AP view of the right hip shows early collapse of the right femoral head (black arrow). Note also sclerosis and notching of the lateral aspect of the femoral head (white arrow). The joint space does not appear to be affected.

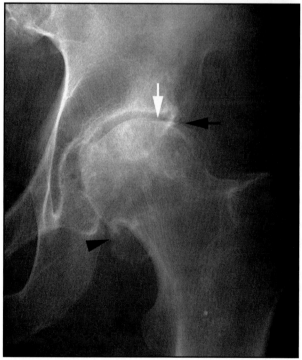

Figure 7-41

Osteonecrosis (late)—AP view

AP view of the left hip shows narrowed superolateral joint space (black arrow), collapse of the femoral head (white arrow), and formation of osteophytes on the inferior femoral head (arrowhead); the latter is the result of secondary osteoarthritis.

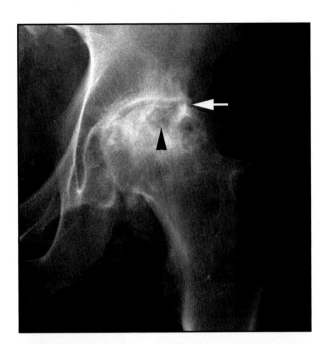

Figure 7-42

Osteonecrosis (end stage)—AP view

AP view of the left hip shows formation of osteophytes on the inferior femoral head (black arrow) and acetabulum and no joint space (white arrow). Note also that cysts have formed on the femoral head (arrowhead).

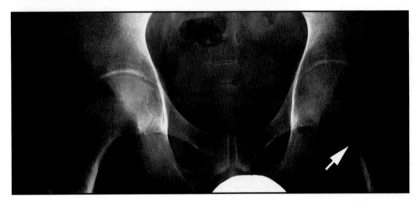

Figure 7-43

Transient osteoporosis—AP view

AP view of the pelvis shows significant osteopenia of the left femoral head and neck (arrow). This is quite apparent when compared with the opposite hip.

DIFFERENTIAL DIAGNOSIS

Infection (painful, limited motion; fever; elevated white blood cell count)

Osteoarthritis (gradual loss of motion, evident on radiograph)

Stress fracture (history of increased vigorous activity, groin pain, evident on MRI or radiograph)

Tumor (pain in groin, thigh, buttock; evident on radiograph and/or MRI)

KNEE AND LOWER LEG

Section Editor
Andrew Haims, MD

Section Co-Editor
Peter Jokl, MD

Imaging the Knee and Lower Leg—An Overview

Anatomy

The knee is made up of three bones (the femur, the tibia, and the patella) that form two joints, the tibiofemoral and patellofemoral articulations. The tibiofemoral articulation, which is the main joint of the knee, relies primarily on four main ligaments for stability: the anterior cruciate ligament (ACL) and posterior cruciate ligament (PCL), located in the center of the joint; and the medial collateral ligament (MCL) and the lateral collateral ligament (LCL), located outside the tibiofemoral articulation. These ligaments provide for anteroposterior, mediolateral, and rotational stability. The joint surfaces are separated by two C-shaped menisci that absorb shock from axial loads.

The normal knee has a range of motion of 0° to 140°. Some rotatory motion of the joint within its full range of flexion and extension is also apparent. The knee displays minimal valgus and varus motion, normally only 3° to 4°. The second joint of the knee is the patellofemoral articulation. Viewed end on, the patella is triangular, with medial and lateral facets separated by a central ridge. The patella tracks on a groove in the femur (the trochlea) during flexion and extension of the knee. The patella increases the lever arm of the quadriceps mechanism, thereby increasing its power.

Being weight-bearing, the knee joint is susceptible to various pathologic conditions, including dysfunction of the patellofemoral joint caused by the large loads that this articulation transmits across the knee during ambulation and squatting activities. Multiple bursae line the ligamentous structures about the periphery of the knee joint. The most commonly affected bursa is the prepatellar bursa, which is a subcutaneous structure between the skin and patella at the anterior aspect of the knee.

Ossification Centers

Ossification centers about the knee appear, on average, at the following ages: (1) distal epiphysis of the femur, present at birth; (2) proximal epiphysis of the tibia, present at birth; (3) proximal epiphysis of the fibula, at 3 to 4 years; (4) tibial tuberosity, at 7 to 15 years. For the patella, several primary centers appear at 3 to 6 years, and secondary centers appear at 12 years. These most often occur in the superolateral aspect of the patella.

STANDARD IMAGING VIEWS

Radiographs

AP and lateral views are standard. In older individuals in whom arthritis may be suspected, these views should be weight bearing. A weight-bearing AP view with the knee flexed 30°, also called a tunnel view, is helpful in detecting joint space narrowing of the knee. Merchant and sunrise axial views of the knee are ordered to evaluate the patellofemoral articulation. Oblique views are also sometimes obtained to identify subtle fractures of the articular surface.

Computed tomography

CT is most useful in studying the characteristics of intra-articular fractures to plan for surgical correction. CT arthrography can be performed in place of MRI in patients with pacemakers and other contraindications to MRI.

Magnetic resonance imaging

MRI, which easily visualizes ligament and meniscus tears, is the imaging study of choice to evaluate soft-tissue injuries about the knee. In addition, effusions, bone bruises, and osteochondral defects are evident on MRI.

Arthrography

Knee arthrograms, formerly used to study meniscus tears, have been replaced by MRI.

EMERGENCIES

Knee dislocations represent true emergencies and require urgent referral to a specialist. These injuries are associated with a significant rate of vascular and nerve injuries.

Fractures of the tibial plateau can cause a compartment syndrome of the leg. Pain out of proportion to the injury and increased pain with passive dorsiflexion of the foot should raise suspicion of a possible compartment syndrome. In these instances, specialty referral is mandatory.

A third emergency is a septic joint. Joint swelling, pain, redness, warmth, and fever are warning signs. Although radiographs obtained early on may be normal, joint aspiration will confirm the diagnosis. Prompt referral to a specialist is indicated.

NORMAL VARIANTS

Several findings on imaging studies can be mistaken for signs of trauma or another type of problem in the knee when they are in fact simply normal anatomic variants. First, medial and lateral condylar irregularities in children and adolescents can be mistaken for osteochondritis dissecans. Second, variations in ossification of the epiphyses of the distal femur can be confused with fractures and osteochondral defects. Third, the fabella, a normal variant seen in roughly 10% of the population, is a small sesamoid bone found in the posterior lateral aspect of the knee in the tendon of origin of the lateral head of the gastrocnemius. A fabella may be confused with a free-floating or intra-articular fragment within the knee joint. Fourth, when the ossification centers of the patella, located superolaterally along the patella, fail to unite completely, these nonunion sites appear as lucent lines within the patella on radiographs. These normal variants appear as a patella with two fragments (a bipartite patella) or, less commonly, three patellar fragments (a tripartite patella). These can be confused with fractures. Clinical examination should help eliminate this confusion. Finally, lateral views of the knee occasionally will show a circular opacity over the anterior aspect of the knee joint. This represents an en face projection of the transverse meniscal ligament, which can be mistaken for a loose body or lytic area in the anterior aspect of the knee adjacent to the tibial spine.

IMAGING TIPS

1. In individuals having sustained acute trauma to the knee joint in whom the standard views are negative and clinical suspicion for a fracture is high, oblique views should be obtained. If these are normal, CT or MRI should be ordered.

2. In patients having anterior knee pain with suspected maltracking of the patellofemoral joint, Merchant views at 20°, 40°, and 60° of knee flexion are recommended. Tilting or subluxation of the patella in its trochlear groove can be seen on these views.

3. When a patient presents with locking of the knee and a loose body in the knee joint is suspected, repeat radiographs following flexion and extension of the knee will often show a change in location of the fragment.

4. In patients with a suspected intra-articular fracture or significant swelling within the knee joint, the lateral view of the soft-tissue structures should be carefully examined to assess accumulation of fluids in the prepatellar bursa, which will confirm the diagnosis of an effusion within the knee joint. Differential density layering is indicative of an intra-articular fracture because medullary fat will rise to the top of an effusion.

ADULT OSGOOD-SCHLATTER DISEASE

SYNONYM
Tibial apophysitis

ICD-9 Code

732.4
Juvenile osteochondrosis of lower extremity, excluding foot

DEFINITION
The residual of juvenile Osgood-Schlatter disease is manifested by the formation of a bony ossicle occurring within the patellar tendon near its insertion into the tibia. These ossicles can be acutely tender as they form a pseudoarticulation or indention in the tibial cortex at their site of insertion with the anterior aspect of the tibial tubercle.

HISTORY AND PHYSICAL FINDINGS
In adult Osgood-Schlatter disease, tenderness can occur at the residual tibial ossicle secondary to overuse or local trauma. Diagnosis is confirmed by compression of the tibial ossicle against the tibia, eliciting the pain as described by the patient.

IMAGING STUDIES

Required for diagnosis
AP (standing or supine), lateral (routine or cross-table), and axial (Merchant or sunrise) views are required for diagnosis. The distal femur, the entire patella, and the proximal tibia must be included on all views. Of these views, the most useful is the lateral because it will show swelling of the distal patellar tendon and any bony irregularity or fragmentation of the tibial tuberosity (insertion site of the patellar tendon) or ossification in the distal patellar tendon.

Required for comprehensive evaluation
MRI is generally not required to diagnose adult Osgood-Schlatter disease, unless radiography and clinical examination have failed to do so. If radiographs show no abnormalities, MRI may be helpful in further evaluation.

Special considerations
None

Pitfalls
None

IMAGE DESCRIPTION

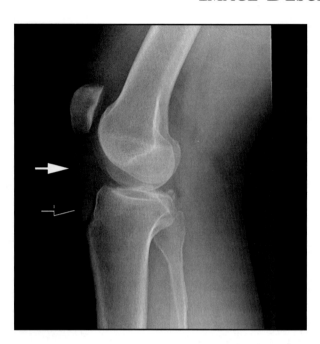

Figure 8-1

Adult Osgood-Schlatter disease— Lateral view

Lateral view shows bony fragmentation at the tibial insertion of the patellar tendon (black arrow). Mild swelling of the distal patellar tendon is apparent as well (white arrow).

DIFFERENTIAL DIAGNOSIS

Patellar tendinosis/jumper's knee (swelling of the proximal or distal patellar tendon without irregularity of the tibial tubercle)

Patellofemoral malalignment (subluxation and abnormal patellar tilt)

PATELLOFEMORAL INSTABILITY AND MALALIGNMENT

SYNONYM
Patellar subluxation

ICD-9 Code

718.36
Recurrent dislocation of joint
(lower leg)

DEFINITION
Patellofemoral instability and malalignment occur when the patella subluxates laterally out of the trochlear groove.

HISTORY AND PHYSICAL FINDINGS
Patellofemoral instability and malalignment are common causes of anterior knee pain in children and adolescents. This condition may be a result of an imbalance in the thigh musculature, which regulates normal tracking of the patella within the trochlear groove. Occasionally patellar instabilities are congenital, secondary to hypoplastic patellae or a shallow trochlear groove.

On physical examination, the patellofemoral joint should be observed for tracking. The alignment of the patellar tendon (also called the patellar ligament) and its insertion onto the tibial tubercle should be measured to assess the Q angle (normal = 10° to 15°). The Q angle is measured to assess the angle of insertion of the patellar tendon onto the tibia. If it is greater than 15°, lateral alignment of the patella within the trochlear groove with abnormal tracking of the patella tends to force the patella into a lateral position with extension of the knee. In extreme cases, realignment of the patellar tendon is often needed to correct patellar motion in the trochlear groove and to alleviate pain. Assessment for the presence of an effusion and crepitation on flexion and extension of the knee is necessary as well. Hypermobility of the joint and elevation of the patella (called patella alta) are also associated with patellofemoral instability.

IMAGING STUDIES

Required for diagnosis
AP (standing or supine), lateral (routine or cross-table), and Merchant axial views are required for diagnosis. The distal femur, the entire patella, and the proximal tibia must be included on all views. Of these images, the most useful is the axial view of the patella because both patellar subluxation and increased lateral tilt can be seen. These findings can be seen either alone or in combination with patellofemoral malalignment.

Required for comprehensive evaluation

MRI is generally not required to evaluate patellofemoral instability, unless radiography and clinical examination have failed to identify the source of the pain. In these cases, either MRI or CT can be helpful in establishing the diagnosis, but they must be done with the knee in different degrees of flexion to evaluate changes in the position of the patella in these positions. Note that these advanced studies are usually requested by orthopaedic surgeons.

Special considerations

MRI is generally needed for a suspected patellar dislocation to evaluate the extent of soft-tissue and bony injuries and to evaluate for cartilage injury or defects that may require surgical intervention.

Pitfalls

Occasionally the axial view of the patella will appear normal at high degrees of flexion (60° to 90°). For this reason, axial views are sometimes obtained with the knee at several different angles to evaluate the alignment at various degrees of flexion. If the axial view appears normal, views at lower degrees of flexion are commonly helpful to further evaluate suspected patellar subluxation.

IMAGE DESCRIPTIONS

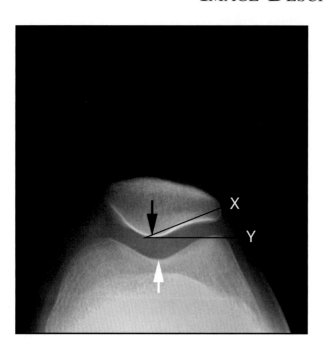

Figure 8-2

Patellofemoral malalignment (normal comparison view)— Axial view

Axial view demonstrates the normal position of the patella. The median ridge (lowest point) of the patella (black arrow) is just medial to the lowest point of the trochlear groove (white arrow). In this case, there is no patellar subluxation. Also on this image, the angle made by the lines drawn through the lateral facet of the patella (X) and across the femoral condyles (Y) opens laterally. If the lines form an angle that opens medially or if the lines are parallel, this is consistent with abnormal patellar tilt.

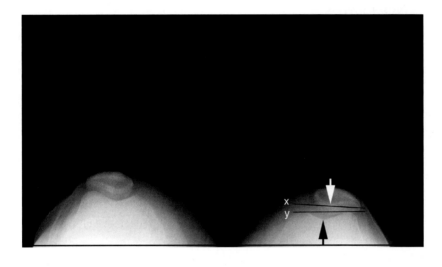

Figure 8-3

Patellofemoral malalignment— Axial view

Axial view shows left-sided patellofemoral malalignment. The median ridge of the patella (white arrow) is lateral to the lowest point of the trochlea (black arrow), consistent with subluxation. Also, the angle made by a line drawn along the lateral facet of the patella (X) and across the femoral condyles (Y) opens medially, consistent with abnormal patellar tilt. Compare the abnormal left side with the normal right side.

DIFFERENTIAL DIAGNOSIS

Adult Osgood-Schlatter disease (swelling of the distal patellar tendon and irregularity of the tibial tubercle)

Chondromalacia of the patella (cartilage defects on MRI)

Stress fracture of the patella (bone marrow edema and incomplete fracture line seen in patella)

SECTION 8 ■ KNEE AND LOWER LEG

Bone Bruise

Synonym
Contusion

Definition
The diagnosis of a bone bruise is considered relatively new and is defined by changes in the osseous structures seen on MRI or three-phase bone scans. As its name implies, there is swelling of the bone.

History and Physical Findings
Clinically, a bone bruise is associated with acute, localized pain within the bony structures and commonly occurs with ligament injuries. The areas associated with bone bruise usually are secondary to direct trauma or compression of the knee joint following an injury. Localized pain over the area of the bone bruise is common and can persist for weeks or months.

Imaging Studies

Required for diagnosis
Radiographs of the affected areas will not show any bony abnormality, although joint effusion may be seen on the lateral view. Therefore, MRI is the study of choice for confirming the diagnosis. The entire area of pain should be imaged because of the characteristic marrow edema (indicated by high signal intensity in the medullary space) that appears on T2-weighted images.

Required for comprehensive evaluation
None

Special considerations
None

Pitfalls
Although a three-phase bone scan will show increased activity, it will not provide the anatomic detail to adequately characterize the bone bruise and the commonly associated ligamentous abnormalities.

IMAGE DESCRIPTION

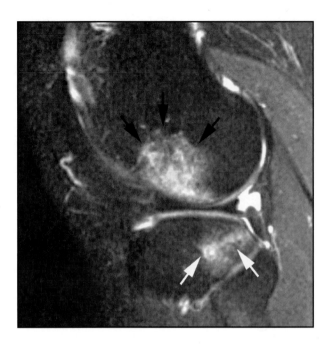

Figure 8-4

Bone bruise— Sagittal MRI

Sagittal T2-weighted, fat-suppressed image shows increased signal intensity (indicating marrow edema) in the anterior lateral femur (black arrows) and the posterior tibial plateau (white arrows). Note that there is no fracture line or evidence of cortical disruption on the image. Radiographs (not shown) showed no evidence of fracture.

DIFFERENTIAL DIAGNOSIS

Meniscal tear (abnormal signal intensity in the meniscus on MRI)

Muscle injury (edema within the muscle on MRI)

Stress fracture (marrow edema usually associated with a fracture line on MRI, but not in the acute setting)

SECTION 8 ■ KNEE AND LOWER LEG

Extensor Mechanism Injuries

Synonym

Jumper's knee

Definition

Extensor mechanism injuries are injuries to the extensor mechanism of the knee, which consists of the quadriceps tendon, patella, and patellar tendon (also called the patellar ligament).

History and Physical Findings

Injuries to the structures that comprise the extensor mechanism of the knee are commonly associated with overuse. Less common is acute disruption of the extensor tendons secondary to chronic degenerative changes and culminating in sudden failure. Young persons, athletically active persons, and manual laborers are more likely to experience these injuries from overuse. Elderly or debilitated persons will usually have pain in the extensor tendons about the knee secondary to degenerative changes within the tendon defined as tendinosis. This represents a breakdown of the tendon's collagen structure. The degeneration of this connective tissue is a precursor to acute disruption and breakdown of the extensor tendons.

In overuse injury, the pain develops gradually and can be localized by palpation. The history will indicate a rapid increase in loading of the involved extremity through athletic or occupational demands.

With acute failure, the medical history may include prior localized pain, suggesting existing ligament degeneration. More frequently, however, the knee joint simply collapses following physiologic loading such as climbing stairs or playing recreational sports. Acute failure of the extensor tendons also can be associated with steroid use.

Following the incident, the patient will be incapable of normal ambulation and unable to actively extend the knee. Disruption of the quadriceps or patellar tendon should be suspected in these cases.

IMAGING STUDIES

Required for diagnosis

MRI is the study of choice to evaluate most extensor mechanism injuries. The images must include the distal quadriceps tendon, the entire patella, and the patellar tendon (including its insertion onto the tibia).

Jumper's knee/patellar tendinosis MRI shows abnormal signal intensity and/or thickening of the patellar tendon.

Patellar tendon tear MRI shows disruption of the patellar tendon with fluid signal within the tendon defect. This may also be associated with elevation of the patella (patella alta).

Quadriceps tendinosis MRI shows abnormal signal intensity and/or thickening of the distal quadriceps tendon.

Quadriceps tendon tear MRI shows disruption of the quadriceps tendon with fluid signal within the tendon defect.

Patellar dislocation Because the dislocation is usually transient, MRI usually shows the sequelae of this condition, typically bone marrow edema in the lateral femoral condyle and in the medial patella from bone impaction. The medial soft-tissue restraints of the patella (medial retinaculum) usually are edematous from disruption.

Chondromalacia MRI shows abnormal signal intensity or defects of the patellar cartilage.

Required for comprehensive evaluation

AP, lateral, and axial views are usually obtained initially. Of these, the lateral view is usually the most helpful because it best visualizes the soft tissues of the extensor mechanism.

Jumper's knee/patellar tendinosis Radiographs are commonly normal, but they may show thickening in the region of the patellar tendon.

Patellar tendon tear Plain radiographs commonly show thickening or soft-tissue swelling in the region of the patellar tendon. These findings may be associated with elevation of the patella (patella alta).

Quadriceps tendinosis Radiographs are commonly normal, but they may show thickening in the region of the quadriceps tendon.

Quadriceps tendon tear Radiographs commonly show thickening or soft-tissue swelling in the region of the patellar tendon.

Patellar dislocation Axial views may show (1) avulsion fractures at the medial soft-tissue attachments of the patella, (2) osteochondral fractures on the lateral femoral condyle, and/or (3) fracture of the medial patella. Acutely, a joint effusion may be seen on the lateral view.

Chondromalacia Radiographs are commonly normal, but they may show evidence of patellofemoral malalignment (see Patellofemoral Instability and Malalignment).

Pitfalls

Some of these conditions, such as patellar tendon and quadriceps tendon tears, may be clinically apparent, and occasionally imaging is not necessary for definitive treatment. Patients with total loss of extensor mechanism function and a palpable gap in the region of the patellar or quadriceps tendon require specialty evaluation.

IMAGE DESCRIPTIONS

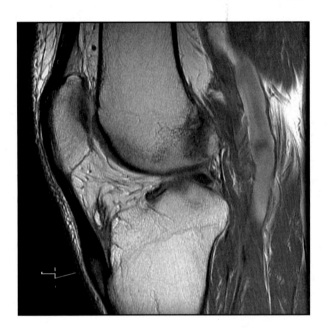

Figure 8-5

Jumper's knee/patellar tendinosis—Sagittal MRI

Sagittal proton-density–weighted MRI scan shows thickening of the distal patellar tendon (arrow) with increased signal intensity within the tendon.

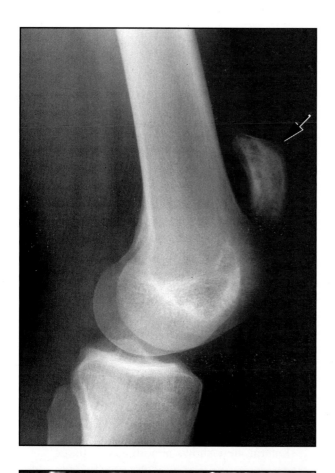

Figure 8-6

Patellar tendon tear—Lateral view

Lateral view of the knee shows elevation of the patella (patella alta) (arrow) consistent with a patellar tendon tear.

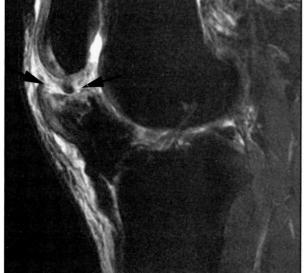

Figure 8-7

Patellar tendon tear—Sagittal MRI

Sagittal T2-weighted, fat-suppressed MRI scan shows disruption of the proximal patellar tendon just inferior to the patella (arrows). Note the abnormal signal intensity in the region of the tendon disruption, indicative of fluid.

SECTION 8 ■ KNEE AND LOWER LEG

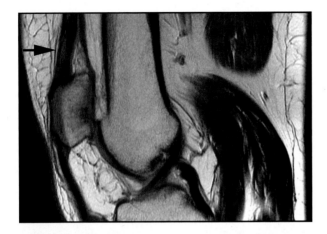

Figure 8-8

Quadriceps tendinosis—Sagittal MRI

Sagittal proton-density–weighted MRI scan shows increased signal intensity and thickening in the distal quadriceps tendon (black arrow), consistent with tendinosis.

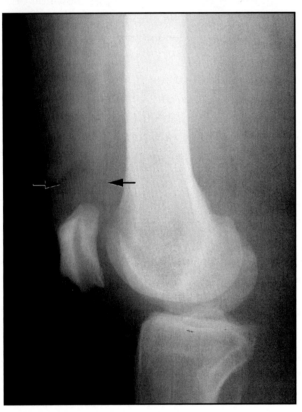

Figure 8-9

Quadriceps tendon tear— Lateral view

Lateral view shows abnormal soft-tissue density in the region of the distal quadriceps tendon (arrows). Note that the tendon is ill defined, and loss of the normal fat planes in this region is apparent. These findings suggest a quadriceps tendon tear.

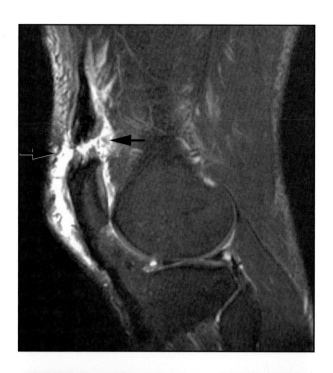

Figure 8-10

Quadriceps tendon tear—Sagittal MRI

Sagittal T2-weighted, fat-suppressed MRI scan shows disruption of the distal quadriceps tendon just superior to the patella (arrows). Note the area of abnormal signal intensity indicative of fluid in the region of the tendon gap.

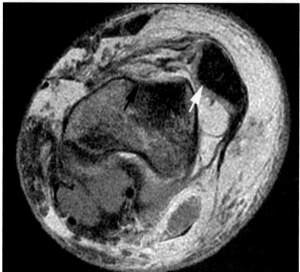

Figure 8-11

Patellar dislocation—Axial MRI

Axial gradient echo MRI scan shows a dislocated patella. The median ridge of the patella (white arrow) is out of the trochlear groove (black arrow) and is touching the lateral femoral condyle.

SECTION 8 ■ KNEE AND LOWER LEG

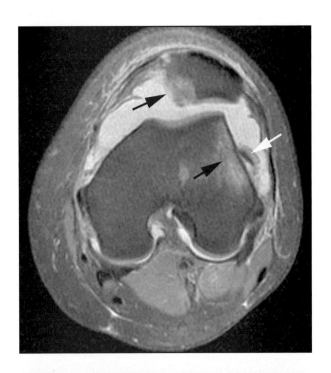

Figure 8-12

Patellar dislocation (postreduction)— Axial MRI

Axial T2-weighted, fat-suppressed MRI scan shows increased signal intensity indicating marrow edema in the lateral femoral condyle and the medial patella (black arrows), consistent with impaction injury. Note the joint effusion with an osteocartilaginous fragment in the lateral joint space (white arrow).

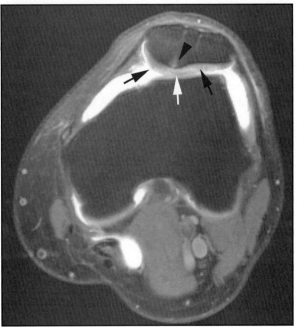

Figure 8-13

Chondromalacia of the patella— Axial MRI

Axial proton-density–weighted, fat-suppressed MRI scan shows increased signal intensity in the median ridge (central aspect of the patellar cartilage) of the patella (white arrow), consistent with chondromalacia (black arrows). Note also the marrow edema immediately adjacent to the patellar defect (arrowhead).

DIFFERENTIAL DIAGNOSIS

Adult Osgood-Schlatter disease (swelling of the distal patellar tendon and irregularity of the tibial tubercle)

Patellofemoral malalignment (subluxation and abnormal patellar tilt)

Stress fracture (marrow edema usually associated with a fracture line on MRI, but not in the acute setting)

FRACTURE OF THE PATELLA

SYNONYMS
None

DEFINITION
Fractures of the patella result from direct trauma to the anterior aspect of the knee. Such trauma occurs commonly in motor vehicle accidents, when the knee hits the dashboard. Because the patella is a major load transmitter across the knee joint, it is also susceptible to stress fractures. Stress fractures must be differentiated from congenital variants, such as bipartite and tripartite patellae. Diagnosis of these conditions may not be possible by clinical examination or from plain radiography. Specialized imaging studies may be necessary in these cases.

HISTORY AND PHYSICAL FINDINGS
These fractures are characterized by pain on palpation and with resisted extension of the knee. Usually, localized pain and swelling are diagnostic of an acute patellar fracture.

IMAGING STUDIES

Required for diagnosis
AP (standing or supine), lateral (routine or cross-table), and axial (Merchant or sunrise) views are generally required for diagnosis of the conditions listed below. The patella must be included in its entirety in each view.

Fracture of the patella Radiographs are the imaging modality of choice. A fracture line extending through the patella is required for diagnosis. Because the patella overlies the distal femur, visualization of the fracture line can sometimes be difficult on the AP view. In these cases, the lateral view can often be helpful in confirming the diagnosis.

Stress fracture of the patella MRI is the modality of choice because the fracture line is not commonly seen on plain radiographs. Marrow edema (indicated by increased signal intensity on T2-weighted images) is seen in a bandlike distribution in the patella.

Bipartite patella An AP view will show an oblique linear lucency in the superior and lateral aspects of the patella. This characteristic location and orientation help to distinguish this congenital anomaly from a fracture.

ICD-9 Codes

733.95
Stress fracture of other bone

755.64
Congenital deformity of knee (joint)

822.0
Fracture of patella (closed)

SECTION 8 ■ KNEE AND LOWER LEG

Tripartite patella As with the bipartite patella, an AP view is the modality of choice. In this condition, instead of a single fragment superiorly and laterally, there are two bony fragments. This characteristic location and orientation help to distinguish this condition from a fracture. Also, if these fragments are assembled, they do not form a normal patella.

Required for comprehensive evaluation

Radiographs are usually all that is required for the above conditions, with the exception of the stress fracture of the patella. In rare cases, physical examination and radiographs are not sufficient to confirm the diagnosis. If there is a question, special imaging studies may be necessary to distinguish a congenital bipartite or tripartite patella from an acute fracture. Bone scan or MRI should be definitive in differentiating between these conditions.

Fracture of the patella Radiographs are sufficient to diagnose this condition.

Stress fracture of the patella Initial imaging usually consists of plain radiographs. Unfortunately, these are commonly negative or inconclusive for these fractures. MRI is the imaging modality of choice, but three-phase bone scans can be used alternatively to confirm the diagnosis.

Bipartite patella and tripartite patella No additional imaging is usually required. However, patients with these conditions can have abnormal motion between the bony fragments, which can cause pain. Increased signal intensity (indicating bone marrow edema) on MRI can document the latter.

Special considerations

None

Pitfalls

Bipartite and tripartite patellae occasionally can be confused with fractures if images are not scrutinized for the characteristic location and appearance of these congenital anomalies.

IMAGE DESCRIPTIONS

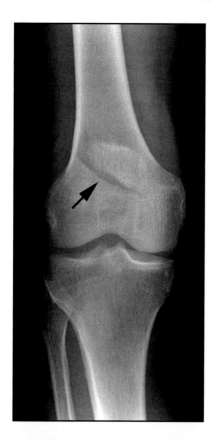

Figure 8-14

Fracture of the patella—AP view

AP view shows an oblique lucency extending through the superior aspect of the patella (black arrow), consistent with a fracture.

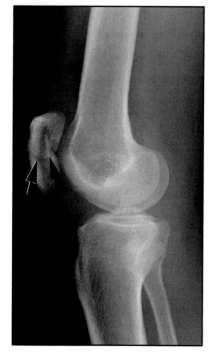

Figure 8-15

Fracture of the patella—Lateral view

Lateral view shows a vague lucency through the patella (black arrows). Note the cortical step-off at the articular surface. Both findings confirm the presence of the fracture.

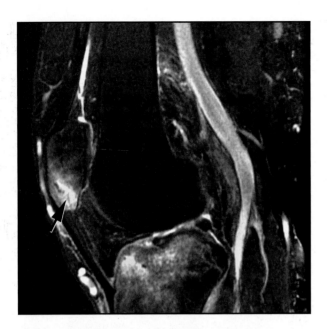

Figure 8-16

*Stress fracture of the patella—
Sagittal MRI*

Sagittal T2-weighted, fat-suppressed MRI scan
shows increased signal intensity (indicating
marrow edema) in the inferior aspect of the
patella (black arrow), consistent with a stress
fracture.

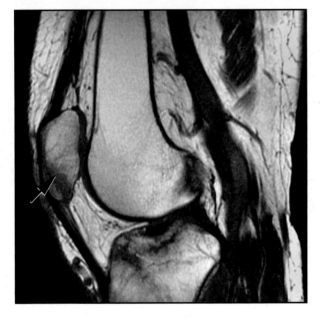

Figure 8-17

*Stress fracture of the patella—
Sagittal MRI*

Sagittal T1-weighted MRI scan shows low
signal intensity (indicating marrow edema) in
the inferior aspect of the patella (black arrow),
consistent with a stress fracture.

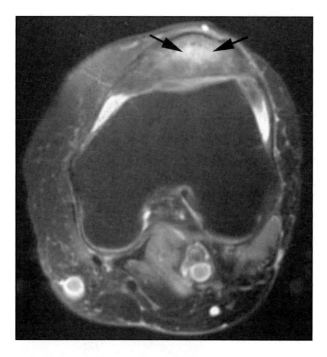

Figure 8-18

Stress fracture of the patella—Axial MRI

Axial T2-weighted, fat-suppressed MRI scan shows increased signal intensity (indicating marrow edema) in the inferior aspect of the patella (black arrows), consistent with a stress fracture.

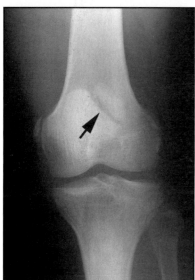

Figure 8-19

Bipartite patella—AP view

AP view shows an oblique lucency in the superior lateral aspect of the patella (black arrow), consistent with a bipartite patella. The characteristic appearance and location help differentiate this condition from a fracture.

SECTION 8 ■ KNEE AND LOWER LEG

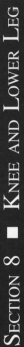

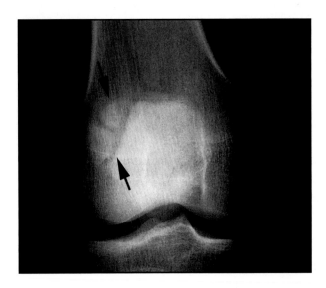

Figure 8-20

Tripartite patella—AP view

AP view shows two bony fragments in the superior and lateral aspects of the patella (black arrows), consistent with a tripartite patella. Note the sclerotic margins and smooth edges between the bony fragments, illustrating the chronic nature of this condition.

DIFFERENTIAL DIAGNOSIS

Chondromalacia (cartilage defects seen on MRI)

Patellofemoral malalignment (subluxation and abnormal patellar tilt)

FRACTURE OF THE TIBIAL PLATEAU

SYNONYMS

Bumper fracture

Fender fracture

Fracture of the proximal tibia

ICD-9 Code

823.0
Fracture of tibia and fibula
(upper end, closed)

DEFINITION

Fractures of the proximal tibia occur most commonly in the lateral and medial tibial plateaus. The most commonly accepted classification of these fractures is by Hohl (Table 1). These are high-impact injuries, often resulting from a motor vehicle accident or a fall from a height, so associated injuries to the chest and abdomen are common, as are neurovascular injuries about the knee. Fractures of the proximal tibia are serious injuries that can result in significant morbidity if not treated properly. Tears of the menisci and of the cruciate and collateral ligaments are commonly associated with these fractures.

Table 1 Hohl Classification of Fractures of the Proximal Tibia	
Type	**Percentage of fractures**
Nondisplaced fracture	25%
Central depression fracture	25%
Fracture of the fibula with a split compression fracture of the lateral tibial plateau	30%
Depression of the lateral tibial plateau	10%
Fractures of both tibial plateaus	10%

HISTORY AND PHYSICAL FINDINGS

Typically, the history includes a fall or a motor vehicle accident. Fractures of the proximal tibia may be open, or compound. Decreased distal pulses and/or decreased sensation may be present. Care must be taken to evaluate other associated chest and abdominal injuries. Associated fractures of the femur are also common. The knee is usually swollen because of a hemarthrosis, and any motion is painful. Deformity is usually obvious, and the patient cannot bear weight on the affected limb.

IMAGING STUDIES

Required for diagnosis

AP and lateral views, along with two oblique views in the AP plane, are required to confirm the diagnosis. The two additional oblique views help to evaluate the articular surface and identify fractures that may otherwise be missed. Fractures of the tibial plateau can manifest as lucencies extending into the tibial articular surface or areas of step-off or depression of the articular surface.

Required for comprehensive evaluation

Fractures of the tibial plateau may not be obvious on radiographs. CT is often obtained for preoperative planning to (1) evaluate the degree of articular depression and (2) identify the number and position of the bony fragments. Two-dimensional reformatted CT images are helpful to better evaluate the articular surface. MRI has the advantage of revealing associated ligamentous and meniscal injuries, which are commonly associated with fractures of the tibial plateau.

Special considerations

None

Pitfalls

These fractures can be difficult to visualize on radiographs. Depressed tibial plateau fractures can be missed easily if CT or MRI is not ordered, with the resultant sequelae of osteoarthritis and pain.

IMAGE DESCRIPTIONS

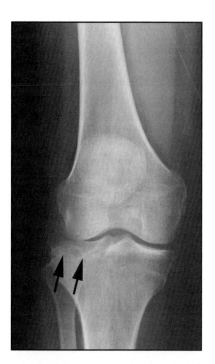

Figure 8-21

Depressed fracture of the tibial plateau—AP view

AP view of the knee shows an irregularity of the lateral tibial plateau (arrows) consistent with a fracture.

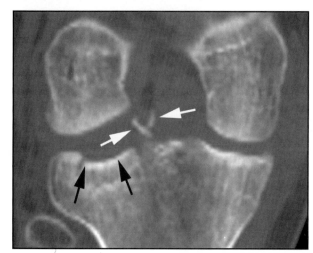

Figure 8-22

Depressed fracture of the tibial plateau—Coronal CT

Coronal reformatted CT scan of the knee shows depression of the posterior lateral articular surface (black arrows) consistent with a fracture. Note the two intra-articular fracture fragments about the tibia (white arrows).

SECTION 8 ■ KNEE AND LOWER LEG

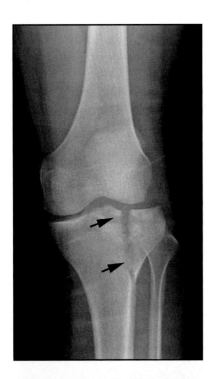

Figure 8-23

Split fracture of the tibial plateau—AP view

AP view shows a vertically oriented lucency extending through the lateral tibial plateau (arrows) consistent with a split-type fracture.

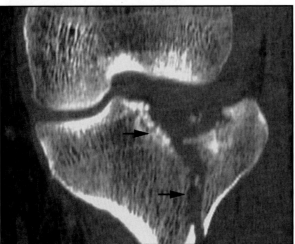

Figure 8-24

Split fracture of the lateral tibial plateau—Coronal CT

Coronal reformatted CT scan shows a split-type fracture of the lateral plateau extending to the articular surface (arrows).

DIFFERENTIAL DIAGNOSIS

Anterior cruciate and medial meniscal tear (abnormal signal intensity in the meniscus on MRI)

Fracture of the femoral condyle (fracture seen on radiographs)

Meniscal tear (seen on MRI)

FRACTURE OF THE TIBIAL SHAFT

ICD-9 Code

823.0
Fracture of tibia and fibula
(upper end, closed)

SYNONYMS
None

DEFINITION
Fracture of the tibia usually requires a significant force to disrupt the osseous integrity of this bone. Of importance in fractures of the proximal tibia, which include the tibial plateau, are those that enter the articular surface of the knee. Disruption of the articular surface is important to identify because these injuries often require aggressive treatment. Fractures of the tibial shaft can occur in various degrees of severity. Deformities of the legs are typically clearly seen, indicating a loss of the tibial diaphyseal integrity. More subtle fractures, as occur in low-energy injuries, will cause fractures of various configurations without disrupting the anatomic alignment of the tibial shaft. These should be recognized and treated appropriately.

HISTORY AND PHYSICAL FINDINGS
Fracture of the tibial shaft is typically associated with major trauma. Findings on physical examination depend on the severity of the injury. Gross malalignment suggests a major disruption of the bone, whereas localized pain without deformity may indicate a stress fracture.

IMAGING STUDIES

Required for diagnosis
AP and lateral views, including the entire tibia extending from the knee joint to the ankle joint, are needed to confirm the diagnosis.

Required for comprehensive evaluation
No additional imaging studies are required for acute traumatic fractures of the tibial shaft. Stress fractures can be evaluated with MRI or three-phase bone scans.

Pitfalls
The main pitfalls associated with imaging this type of fracture are failure to include the entire tibia and failure to order the proper views. Both can lead to missed fractures.

SECTION 8 ■ KNEE AND LOWER LEG

IMAGE DESCRIPTIONS

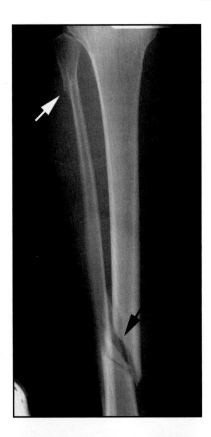

Figure 8-25

Fracture of the tibial shaft—AP view

AP view of the tibia and fibula shows an oblique fracture through the distal third of the tibial diaphysis (black arrow), with slight lateral translation of the distal fragment. Note also the fracture of the proximal fibula (white arrow).

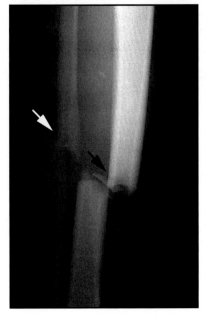

Figure 8-26

Fracture of the tibial shaft—AP view

AP view of the tibia and fibula shows a transverse fracture through the mid-diaphysis of the tibia (black arrow). Note also the transverse fracture through the midshaft of the fibula (white arrow) with lateral displacement of the distal fragments.

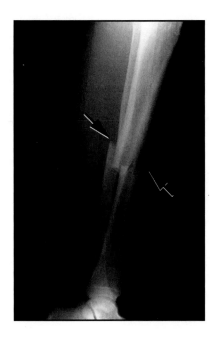

Figure 8-27

Fracture of the tibial shaft—Lateral view

Lateral view of the tibia and fibula shows transverse fractures of the midshafts of the tibia and fibula (black arrows). Note the anterior displacement of the distal tibial fragment.

DIFFERENTIAL DIAGNOSIS

Fracture of the tibial plateau (fracture of the proximal tibia extends to the articular surface)

LOOSE BODY

ICD-9 Code

717.6
Loose body in knee

SYNONYMS
Chondral loose body
Joint mouse
Osteochondral loose body

DEFINITION
A loose body (sometimes called an intra-articular body) is a free-floating fragment within the knee joint. These can result from previous trauma, or they can occur as a spontaneous growth of osteocartilaginous fragments within the joint cavity. When radiographs show multiple loose bodies within the knee joint, synovial osteochondromatosis (SO) should be considered. The etiology of these loose bodies is more often related to trauma and cartilage damage and less often secondary to metaplastic formation of cartilaginous fragments by the synovium.

HISTORY AND PHYSICAL FINDINGS
History and physical examination typically reveal recurrent locking, giving way, and effusions of the knee. Fragments can sometimes be felt on palpation of the knee joint.

IMAGING STUDIES

Required for diagnosis
AP (standing or supine) and lateral (routine or cross-table) views are needed to confirm the diagnosis. The entire articular space, including the synovial recesses of the joint, must be included on the image. On radiographs, loose bodies appear as ossified or calcified fragments that project over the joint space on two orthogonal views. A donor site (bony defect) in the underlying bone is also a helpful sign.

Required for comprehensive evaluation
Unfortunately, loose bodies sometimes consist of cartilage, in which case they will not be visible on radiographs, and additional imaging modalities will be necessary. In patients who have symptoms of intermittent locking, loose bodies are in the differential diagnosis. MRI is excellent in these instances and in identifying articular defects or donor sites.

Special considerations

CT arthrography or MR arthrography can be helpful in identifying loose bodies. These are minimally invasive studies that are more specific for identifying intra-articular loose bodies and are most commonly ordered by specialists.

Pitfalls

A fabella is a small sesamoid bone (bone within a tendon) that can look like a loose body on radiographs. This normal variant is always seen on the AP and lateral views in a characteristic location posterolaterally. Knowledge of its appearance and location can be helpful in distinguishing it from intra-articular pathology.

IMAGE DESCRIPTIONS

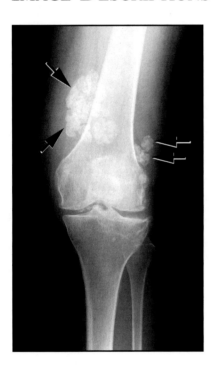

Figure 8-28

Synovial osteochondromatosis with multiple loose bodies—AP view

AP view shows multiple calcified cartilaginous fragments in the medial and lateral aspects of the suprapatellar recess of the knee (black arrows). These findings are characteristic of SO with multiple intra-articular loose bodies.

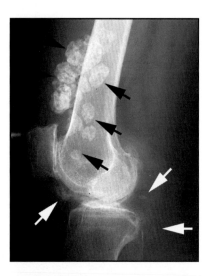

Figure 8-29

Synovial osteochondromatosis with multiple loose bodies—Lateral view

Lateral view shows multiple calcified cartilaginous fragments in the suprapatellar recess of the knee joint (black arrows) and in the anterior and posterior knee joint (white arrows). These findings are characteristic of SO with multiple loose bodies.

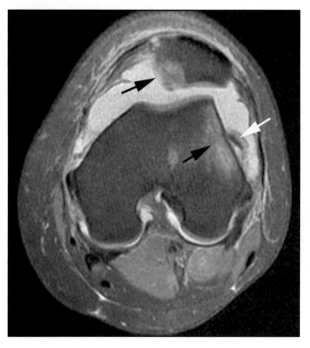

Figure 8-30

Posttraumatic loose body from patellar dislocation—Axial MRI

Axial T2-weighted, fat-suppressed MRI scan shows increased signal intensity indicating marrow edema in the lateral femoral condyle and the medial patella (black arrows), consistent with impaction injury. Note the joint effusion and the osteocartilaginous fragment in the lateral joint space (white arrow).

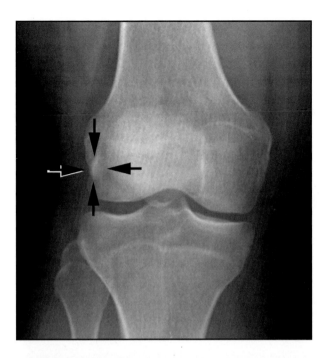

Figure 8-31

Fabella—AP view

AP view of the knee shows a well-defined area of bony density projecting over the lateral femoral condyle (black arrows), consistent with a fabella.

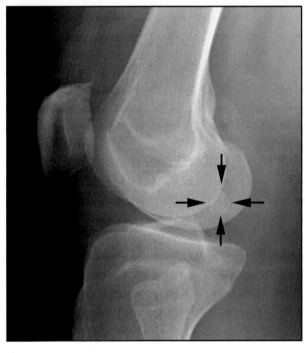

Figure 8-32

Fabella—Lateral view

Oblique lateral view of the knee shows a well-defined bony fragment projecting posterior to the lateral femoral condyle (black arrows), consistent with a fabella. Note that the characteristic posterior and lateral position of this bony density helps to confirm that it is a normal variant.

DIFFERENTIAL DIAGNOSIS

Fabella (well-defined bony fragment projecting posterior to the lateral femoral condyle)

Pigmented villonodular synovitis (PVNS) (MRI needed to differentiate; PVNS does not calcify)

OSTEOCHONDRITIS DISSECANS

ICD-9 Code

732.7
Osteochondritis dissecans

SYNONYM

Osteochondral fracture

DEFINITION

Osteochondritis dissecans (OCD) is characterized by localized osteonecrosis (bone death) of subchondral bone. It is thought to be caused by chronic repetitive trauma. OCD can occur in people of all ages, but it most commonly affects adolescent boys. OCD in patients who have reached skeletal maturity rarely heals spontaneously. In the knee the lesions commonly involve the lateral aspect of the medial femoral condyle. OCD varies in severity, from in situ OCD with the cartilage intact to a completely displaced osteochondral loose body.

HISTORY AND PHYSICAL FINDINGS

Patients typically report diffuse knee pain with OCD, which can be a precursor to a loose body. However, there are no specific findings on physical examination.

IMAGING STUDIES

Required for diagnosis

AP, lateral, tunnel (or notch), and axial (Merchant or sunrise) views are obtained if OCD is suspected. All articular surfaces of the knee joint must be included in each view.

Osteochondritis dissecans The key finding is a crescent-shaped lucency extending to the subchondral bone. These lesions characteristically appear on the lateral aspect of the medial femoral condyle but also can be seen on any aspect of the subchondral bone in the knee, including the patella. Occasionally, OCD lesions are extremely subtle on radiographs.

Osteochondral injury These injuries are best visualized on MRI rather than on radiographs. MRI shows increased signal intensity in the articular cartilage with an underlying bone bruise. Occasionally, a crack can be seen in the articular cartilage.

Required for comprehensive evaluation

MRI is generally helpful for a definitive diagnosis.

Osteochondritis dissecans MRI can be used not only to definitively document and size the lesion but also to evaluate the overlying articular cartilage, which also can be damaged. MRI and MR arthrography are also valuable for identifying signs that the lesion is becoming unstable, as OCD lesions can occasionally dislodge and become loose bodies.

Osteochondral injury MRI is used to document these injuries, because they are infrequently seen on radiographs, and to identify associated injuries. Osteochondral injuries are frequently associated with ligamentous injuries.

Special considerations
None

Pitfalls
A normal femoral ossification center occasionally has the same appearance as an OCD lesion. However, the ossification center is characteristically located in the lateral femur, whereas OCD lesions are typically medial.

IMAGE DESCRIPTIONS

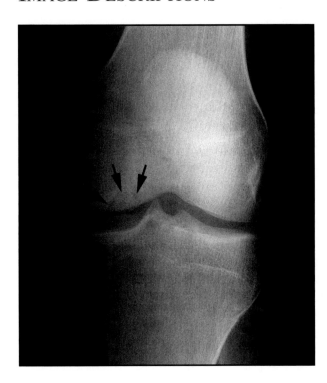

Figure 8-33

Osteochondritis dissecans—AP view

AP view shows a crescent-shaped lucency in the lateral aspect of the medial femoral condyle (black arrows), which is characteristic of the location and appearance of an OCD lesion.

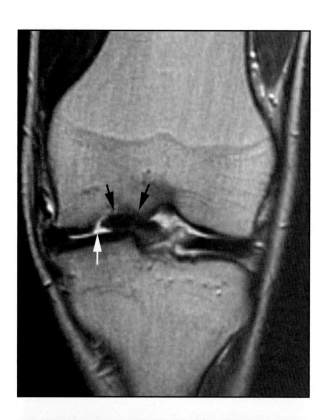

Figure 8-34

Osteochondritis dissecans— Coronal MRI

Coronal T2-weighted MRI scan shows an area of low signal intensity in the lateral aspect of the medial femoral condyle (black arrows), characteristic of an OCD lesion. Note the fluid signal extending through the articular cartilage (white arrow), which is consistent with a cartilage break.

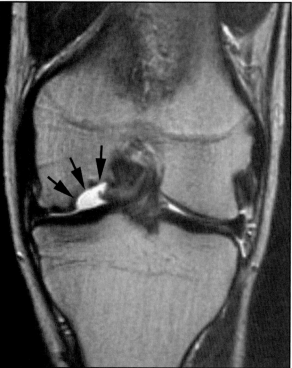

Figure 8-35

Osteochondritis dissecans with multiple loose bodies—Coronal MRI

Coronal T2-weighted MRI scan of the same patient several months later shows that the OCD fragment has been dislodged from the underlying femur (black arrows).

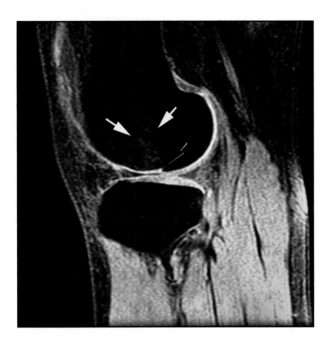

Figure 8-36

Osteochondral injury—Sagittal MRI

Sagittal gradient echo MRI scan shows disruption of the articular cartilage (black arrow) and subtle marrow edema (white arrows), characteristic of an osteochondral injury. The patient has an associated anterior cruciate ligament injury (not shown).

DIFFERENTIAL DIAGNOSIS

Meniscal tear (abnormal high signal intensity in the meniscus on MRI)

Stress fracture (fracture line or marrow edema seen on MRI)

SEGOND FRACTURE

ICD-9 Code

823.0
Fracture of tibia and fibula
(upper end, closed)

SYNONYMS
Avulsion fracture of the proximal lateral tibia
Lateral capsular sign

DEFINITION
A Segond fracture is an avulsion of the posterior lateral capsule attachment from the tibia. The injury is caused by external rotation of the femur on the fixed tibia with the knee flexed and in varus. The anterior cruciate ligament (ACL) is invariably torn. The patient will experience anterior subluxation of the lateral tibial plateau.

HISTORY AND PHYSICAL FINDINGS
A Segond fracture is typically the result of a forceful rotatory injury to the knee joint. This fracture is almost always associated with a joint effusion, given its frequent association with ACL tears. The patient reports lateral joint line pain, which is often caused by disruption of the posterior capsule and the ACL. Physical examination reveals a prominent, acute knee effusion and laxity of the posterior lateral capsule. Results of a Lachman test frequently are positive. A positive pivot shift is almost always present.

IMAGING STUDIES

Required for diagnosis
An AP view, including the lateral aspect of the tibia just below the joint surface, best confirms the diagnosis. The characteristic appearance of this fracture is a small, irregular bony fragment adjacent to the lateral tibia that has avulsed from the lateral capsular insertion.

Required for comprehensive evaluation
MRI is also helpful for these fractures because there is usually an associated ACL tear and should always be obtained in this situation to confirm the diagnosis and frequently to identify any meniscal pathology. For these conditions, surgery may be considered; therefore, consultation with a specialist is advised.

Special considerations
None

Pitfalls
None

IMAGE DESCRIPTIONS

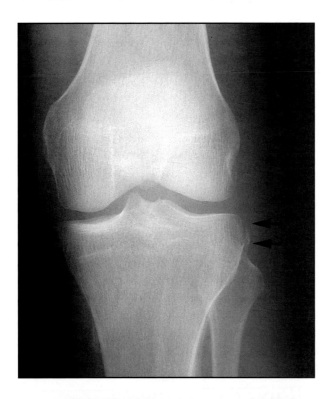

Figure 8-37

Segond fracture—AP view

AP view of the knee shows a small avulsion (flake) fracture of the lateral tibia just below the articular surface of the tibia (black arrows).

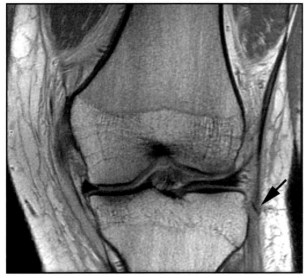

Figure 8-38

Segond fracture—Coronal MRI

Coronal proton-density–weighted MRI scan shows an avulsion of the lateral capsular attachment (black arrow), consistent with a Segond fracture.

DIFFERENTIAL DIAGNOSIS

This differential diagnosis stems from the associated injuries.

STRESS FRACTURES

ICD-9 Code

823.0
Fracture of tibia and fibula
(upper end, closed)

SYNONYMS
Shin-splints
Periostitis

DEFINITION
Overuse injuries of bone occur following high-impact activities such as running or jumping. Stress fractures can occur in normal bone that is subjected to an unusual load. These are referred to as fatigue fractures. Insufficiency fractures are a second type of stress fracture in which a bone weakened by disease such as osteoporosis or rheumatoid arthritis is subjected to a normal load that ordinarily would not cause a fracture. In the lower extremity, both the tibia and fibula can be involved. Competitive runners such as marathon runners are prone to develop stress fractures in the proximal posteromedial aspect of the tibia as well as in the distal fibula. Stress fractures also occur in the tibial plateaus.

HISTORY AND PHYSICAL FINDINGS
Stress fractures often occur at the start of a sports season as individuals begin strenuous activity to which they are not accustomed. Examples are cross-country running and basketball, which involve repetitive running and jumping. Overuse injuries of the tibia comprise a continuum of symptoms, ranging from diffuse pain caused by periosteal reaction to tendinosis and occasionally culminating in failure of the bone with associated localized swelling and tenderness on palpation of the tibial margins. Patients report a history of rapidly progressive activity such as running associated with increased localized leg pain that typically is relieved by rest. Examination reveals localized tenderness over the involved area of the tibia and/or fibula.

IMAGING STUDIES

Required for diagnosis
AP and lateral views should be ordered, but frequently they will be normal. Bone changes may not be present on radiographs for weeks to months after the onset of symptoms. Early changes seen on radiographs include a periosteal reaction and/or sclerosis in the region of reported pain. Occasionally, a fracture line may be apparent.

Required for comprehensive evaluation

Because radiographs are frequently normal, especially early, three-phase bone scan or MRI is commonly required for a definitive diagnosis. A bone scan will show increased radiotracer uptake in the region of reported pain in all three phases (perfusion, blood-pool, and delayed). MRI will show marrow edema, periosteal edema, and occasionally a fracture line in the region of reported pain. For years, the gold standard was the bone scan. However, MRI is becoming the imaging modality of choice. MRI and bone scans are equally sensitive, but MRI is more specific in diagnosing stress fractures.

Special considerations

CT is not routinely used to diagnose stress fractures, but it occasionally can be helpful in difficult cases, as fracture lines through the cortex are best seen with this modality.

Pitfalls

Either MRI or three-phase bone scan is adequate to diagnose this condition. Both are not required for the diagnosis. Infection and osteoid osteoma can have a similar appearance on radiographs and cross-sectional imaging.

IMAGE DESCRIPTIONS

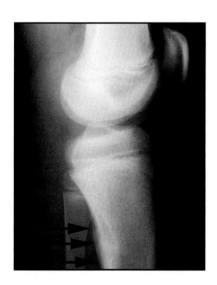

Figure 8-39

Stress fracture of the tibia—Lateral view

Lateral view shows sclerosis and periosteal reaction in the posterior tibia (black arrows), consistent with a stress fracture.

SECTION 8 ■ KNEE AND LOWER LEG

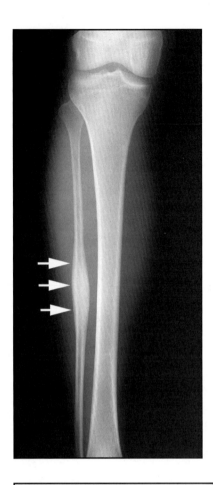

Figure 8-40

Stress fracture of the fibula—AP view

AP view of the tibia and fibula shows increased bony density (sclerosis) in the midfibula (arrows), characteristic of a stress fracture.

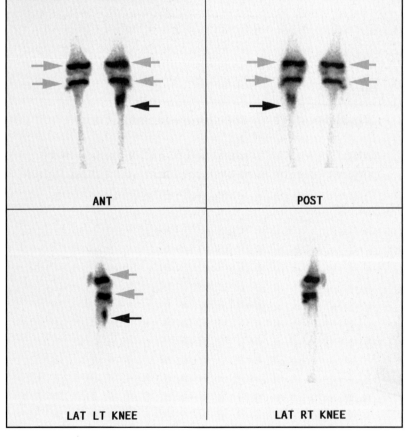

Figure 8-41

Stress fracture of the tibia—Bone scan

Three images from this three-phase bone scan show increased activity in the left proximal tibia (black arrows), consistent with a stress fracture. Note the increased activity normally seen in the open growth plates (gray arrows). Note the normal growth plates without evidence of fracture on the lateral view of the right knee.

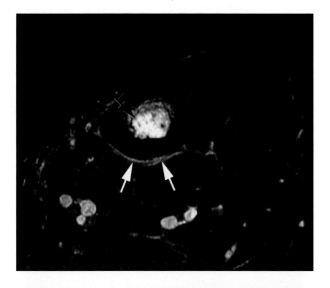

Figure 8-42

Stress fracture of the tibia— Axial MRI

Axial T2-weighted, fat-suppressed MRI scan shows increased signal intensity indicating marrow edema (black arrows), as well as edema in the posterior periosteum (white arrows), characteristic of a stress fracture.

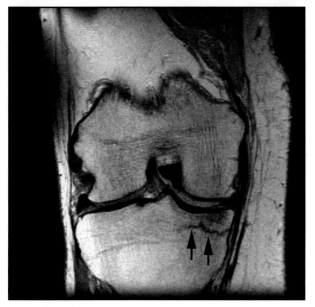

Figure 8-43

Stress fracture of the tibial plateau— Coronal MRI

Coronal proton-density–weighted MRI scan shows a linear area of low signal intensity consistent with an incomplete fracture line (black arrows), characteristic of a stress fracture.

DIFFERENTIAL DIAGNOSIS

Ligament tear (disruption of a ligament seen on MRI)

Meniscal tear (abnormal signal in the meniscus on MRI)

Shin-splints (delayed phase of bone scan shows longitudinal area of increased uptake along cortex)

SECTION 8 ■ KNEE AND LOWER LEG

SUPRACONDYLAR FRACTURE OF THE FEMUR

ICD-9 Code

821.23
Supracondylar fracture of femur

SYNONYMS
None

DEFINITION
Fracture of the distal femur above the femoral condyles is often a sequela of high-velocity injuries, typically from motor vehicle accidents. Occasionally, these fractures are seen in the elderly with failure of osteoporotic bone in the supracondylar region following a fall.

HISTORY AND PHYSICAL FINDINGS
Traumatic disruption of the distal femur often involves extension of the fracture into the knee joint. The history is characterized by severe local trauma. Physical examination reveals swelling in the distal thigh, acute tenderness, and pain that precludes flexion and extension of the knee and weight bearing.

IMAGING STUDIES

Required for diagnosis
AP and cross-table lateral views of the distal aspect of the femur, including the knee joint, are needed to make the diagnosis. Radiographs usually show cortical disruption of the distal femur, commonly extending into the knee joint. When the fracture extends into the knee joint, bone marrow fat and blood can typically be found in the joint (lipohemarthrosis). This is best seen as a fat-fluid level (a characteristic layering of these substances, where the fat, being of lower density than the blood, rises to the top) on the cross-table lateral view of the knee.

Required for comprehensive evaluation
Radiographs are usually the only imaging study necessary to confirm the diagnosis.

Special considerations
CT is occasionally obtained for preoperative planning, usually when the fracture is intra-articular.

Pitfalls
None

IMAGE DESCRIPTIONS

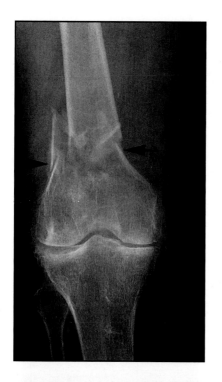

Figure 8-44

Supracondylar fracture of the femur—AP view

AP view shows disruption of the femoral cortex above the femoral condyles (black arrows) with associated comminution (bony fragmentation), consistent with a supracondylar fracture.

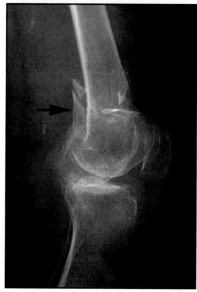

Figure 8-45

Supracondylar fracture of the femur—Lateral view

Lateral view shows disruption of the femoral cortex above the femoral condyles (black arrows), diagnostic of a supracondylar fracture.

DIFFERENTIAL DIAGNOSIS

Patellar fracture (cortical disruption of the patella)

Tibial plateau fracture (cortical disruption of the tibial plateau)

SECTION 8 ■ KNEE AND LOWER LEG

BURSITIS

SYNONYM
Housemaid's knee

DEFINITION
Bursitis of the knee is inflammation of any of the multiple bursae of the knee, as shown in the figure below.

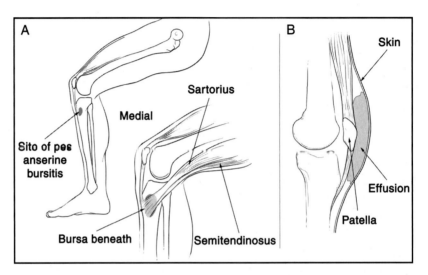

Areas affected by bursitis. **A,** Medial view showing the region of tenderness with pes anserine bursitis. **B,** Involved region with prepatellar bursitis.

HISTORY AND PHYSICAL FINDINGS
Bursitis can be caused by trauma, overuse, arthritis, or localized infection. Physical examination will reveal swelling and tenderness over the affected bursa.

IMAGING STUDIES

Required for diagnosis
MRI or ultrasound of all the bursae that surround the knee joint is helpful to establish the diagnosis.
Prepatellar bursitis MRI will show fluid signal anterior to the patella and patellar tendon.
Popliteal cyst MRI will show an oval area of fluid signal in a characteristic location between the medial gastrocnemius muscle and the tendon of the semimembranosus muscle in the medial aspect of the knee.
Pes anserine bursitis MRI will show fluid signal surrounding the distal pes anserine tendons (semitendinosus, gracilis, and sartorius) just below the joint.

Required for comprehensive evaluation
Radiographs usually are not helpful in making the diagnosis.

Special considerations
None

Pitfalls
None

IMAGE DESCRIPTIONS

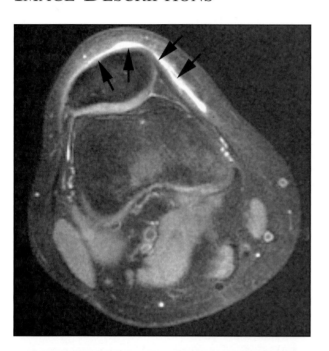

Figure 8-46

Prepatellar bursitis—Axial MRI

Axial T2-weighted, fat-suppressed MRI scan shows fluid signal anterior to the patella that extends medially (black arrows). The location of the fluid is characteristic for prepatellar bursitis.

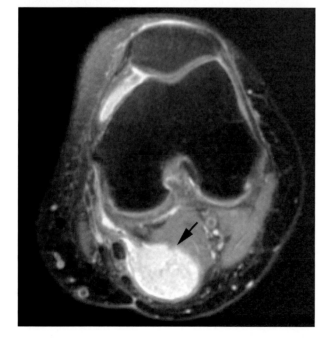

Figure 8-47

Popliteal cyst—Axial MRI

Axial T2-weighted, fat-suppressed MRI scan shows an oval area of fluid signal between the semimembranosus tendon and the medial head of the gastrocnemius muscle (black arrow), characteristic of a popliteal cyst.

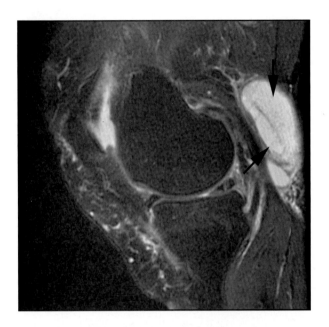

Figure 8-48

Popliteal cyst—Sagittal MRI

Sagittal T2-weighted, fat-suppressed MRI scan shows an oval area of fluid signal behind the knee (black arrows) in the characteristic location of a popliteal cyst.

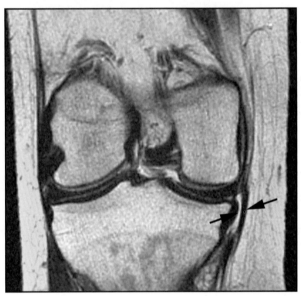

Figure 8-49

Pes anserine bursitis—Coronal MRI

Coronal T2-weighted MRI scan shows fluid signal just below the joint surface (black arrows) in the region of the pes anserine tendons.

DIFFERENTIAL DIAGNOSIS

Joint effusion (soft-tissue density in the suprapatellar recess on lateral radiograph)

Soft-tissue tumor (tumors are more often solid with different MRI characteristics)

SECTION 8 ■ KNEE AND LOWER LEG

CHONDROCALCINOSIS

SYNONYMS
Calcium pyrophosphate deposition disease (CPPD)
Crystalline arthritis
Pseudogout

ICD-9 Code
712.3
Chondrocalcinosis,
unspecified

DEFINITION
Chondrocalcinosis is calcification of cartilage, either articular or meniscal, caused by accumulation of calcium pyrophosphate (CP) within the cartilaginous and, to a lesser degree, the soft-tissue structures of the knee joint.

HISTORY AND PHYSICAL FINDINGS
Accumulation of CP commonly occurs with degenerative changes. CP also accumulates, although less commonly, in association with metabolic conditions affecting calcium metabolism. A history of recurrent acutely painful effusions is common. Physical examination can reveal variable degrees of swelling within the knee joint. Often the knee is acutely painful, and a differential diagnosis of crystalline synovitis or acute infection needs to be considered. When these diagnoses are considered, analysis of joint aspirate is necessary to differentiate between the two conditions.

IMAGING STUDIES

Required for diagnosis
AP (standing or supine), lateral (routine or cross-table), tunnel, and axial (Merchant or sunrise) views should be obtained initially to image the articular surfaces of the joint. Increased density between the tibia and femur in the region of the menisci or adjacent to the subchondral bone in the region of the articular cartilage is considered a positive finding.

Required for comprehensive evaluation
Radiographs are the only imaging study necessary to make the diagnosis.

Special considerations
None

Pitfalls
MRI is not only unnecessary to make the diagnosis but also can be misleading because calcification in the menisci can be misinterpreted as a meniscal tear.

IMAGE DESCRIPTIONS

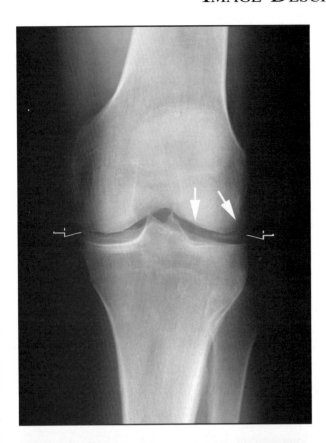

Figure 8-50

Chondrocalcinosis—AP view

AP view shows increased density (calcification) between the femur and the tibia in the region of the medial and lateral menisci (black arrows) as well as the hyaline cartilage (white arrows), which is characteristic of chondrocalcinosis.

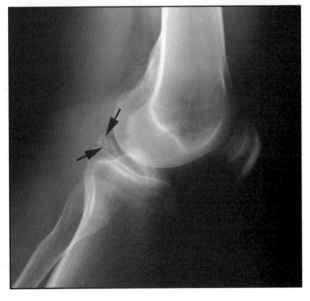

Figure 8-51

Chondrocalcinosis—Lateral view

Lateral view shows increased density between the tibia and femur posteriorly (black arrows), consistent with chondrocalcinosis of the menisci.

DIFFERENTIAL DIAGNOSIS

Gout (uric acid crystals present)

Septic joint (effusion with loss of the normal white cortical lines surrounding the joint; primarily a clinical diagnosis)

JOINT EFFUSION

SYNONYM
Water on the knee

ICD-9 Code

719.06
Effusion of joint (lower leg)

DEFINITION
Accumulation of fluid within the knee joint can be caused by trauma, infection, arthritis, and collagen diseases.

HISTORY AND PHYSICAL FINDINGS
Knee effusion is readily apparent on physical examination of the knee because of the characteristic swelling, which masks the normal anatomic landmarks. Effusions can be painless in some conditions such as psoriasis or synovial osteochondromatosis; they also can be quite painful in others such as septic arthritis and chondrocalcinosis. Palpation of the joint and ballottement of the patella will confirm the presence of fluid within the joint cavity.

IMAGING STUDIES

Required for diagnosis
Both AP and lateral views of the articular space, particularly the synovial recesses of the joint, are generally obtained to make the diagnosis. Of these, the lateral view is the most valuable because fluid can easily be seen collecting in the suprapatellar recess. An area of soft-tissue density measuring 1 cm or more between the fat planes behind the quadriceps tendon and anterior to the femur (suprapatellar recess of the joint) is a positive sign.

Required for comprehensive evaluation
No additional imaging studies are required to make the diagnosis. Physical examination and radiographs are sufficient to diagnose joint effusion. However, MRI is helpful to identify the cause of the effusion.

Special considerations
Although MRI can confirm the presence of an effusion, it is generally not required for this purpose.

Pitfalls
None

IMAGE DESCRIPTIONS

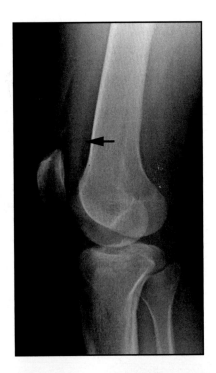

Figure 8-52

Joint effusion—Lateral view

Lateral view shows an area of soft-tissue density in the region of the suprapatellar recess (black arrows), which is diagnostic of a joint effusion.

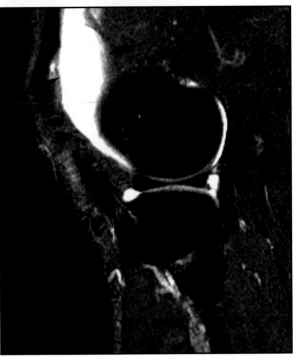

Figure 8-53

Joint effusion—Sagittal MRI

Sagittal T2-weighted, fat-suppressed MRI scan shows high signal intensity in the suprapatellar recess (black arrows), diagnostic of a joint effusion.

DIFFERENTIAL DIAGNOSIS

None

OSTEOARTHRITIS

SYNONYMS

Degenerative arthritis
Degenerative arthrosis
Degenerative joint disease (DJD)
Osteoarthrosis

ICD-9 Code

715.16
Osteoarthrosis, localized,
primary (lower leg)

DEFINITION

Osteoarthritis (OA) is characterized by degenerative joint changes. Degenerative joint disease (DJD) is a better term to describe the changes that occur in the cartilage, synovium, and fibrous soft-tissue structures in and about the knee. The "-itis" in osteoarthritis is a misnomer because histologic studies of the tissues about the knee in OA do not reveal inflammatory changes.

OA has many causes. The Mitchell-Cruess classification is useful and is based on two general mechanisms: (1) abnormal concentration of force on a normal joint and (2) normal concentration of force on an abnormal joint. Examples of the first mechanism are obesity, especially in women; malunited fractures of the femoral or tibial shafts; epiphyseal injuries; and limb-length discrepancies. Examples of the second mechanism are meniscal tears or absent menisci (postoperative), loose bodies, osteochondritis dissecans, osteonecrosis, gout, calcium pyrophosphate deposition disease (CPPD), and osteoporosis. Regardless of the mechanism, abnormalities develop in the cartilage and subchondral bone with eventual thinning and ultimately total loss of cartilage, resulting in bone-on-bone contact. The knee joint is the most common site for OA.

HISTORY AND PHYSICAL FINDINGS

Patients may report a history of trauma, previous knee surgery such as meniscectomy, or fracture about the knee. They may also have noted a gradual deformity of the knee, usually genu varum (bowlegs) or, less commonly, genu valgum (knock-knees). Pain that is aggravated by getting up from a chair and by weight bearing is the main and initial presenting symptom. Often the pain is relieved only partially by rest. Weather changes (changes in barometric pressure) exacerbate the symptoms. Stiffness is also common, and the patient may report intermittent swelling.

On physical examination, a varus or valgus deformity of the knee may be seen. Localized tenderness at the joint line may be present. Flexion and extension of the knee often reveals patellofemoral crepitation. The range of motion of the knee may be limited, and an antalgic (limping) gait may be observed. A joint effusion may be present, but not to the degree seen with rheumatoid arthritis.

IMAGING STUDIES

Required for diagnosis

Weight-bearing AP and lateral views of the knee are usually sufficient to make the diagnosis. A weight-bearing AP view with the knee flexed 30° (a standing tunnel view) can show bone-on-bone contact, which may not be seen on a weight-bearing view with the knee fully extended. Patellofemoral arthritis can be studied with an axial (Merchant) view. Loss of articular cartilage (joint space narrowing), osteophyte formation, subchondral sclerosis, and subchondral cyst formation are diagnostic findings typical of OA.

Required for comprehensive evaluation

MRI generally is not required in the evaluation of OA; however, it is occasionally helpful in identifying early articular cartilage changes not seen on radiographs.

Special considerations

None

Pitfalls

Weight-bearing views are necessary when assessing for joint space narrowing because non–weight-bearing views can mask this finding. A weight-bearing tunnel view can also show bone-on-bone contact when routine weight-bearing views are normal.

IMAGE DESCRIPTIONS

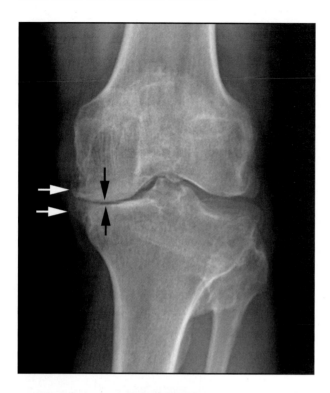

Figure 8-54

Osteoarthritis (knee)—AP view

AP view shows joint space narrowing in the medial compartment (black arrows) and osteophyte formation (white arrows), characteristic of OA.

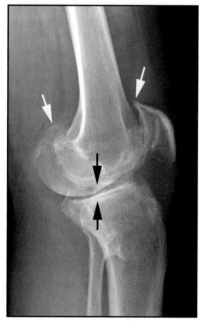

Figure 8-55

Osteoarthritis (knee)—Lateral view

Lateral view shows joint space narrowing (black arrows) and osteophyte formation (white arrows) in the posterior femur and off the superior aspect of the patella.

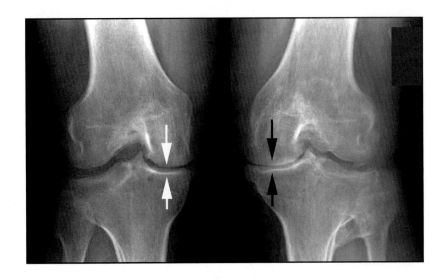

Figure 8-56

Osteoarthritis (knee)— Tunnel view

Tunnel view of both knees shows joint space narrowing in the medial compartment of the left knee (black arrows). Note the more subtle joint space narrowing in the medial compartment of the right knee (white arrows) with less obvious degenerative change.

DIFFERENTIAL DIAGNOSIS

CPPD (chondrocalcinosis present within the joint)

Gout (bony erosions, normal joint space, elevated serum uric acid level)

Meniscal tear (abnormal signal in the meniscus on MRI)

Rheumatoid arthritis (medial and lateral femorotibial compartments both narrowed; synovial cysts)

Stress fracture (marrow edema and possibly a fracture line on MRI)

Pigmented Villonodular Synovitis

Synonym
PVNS

ICD-9 Code
696
Psoriasis and similar disorders

Definition
Pigmented villonodular synovitis (PVNS) is a pathologic condition involving the synovial lining of the knee joint. A bloody effusion and localized hemosiderin deposition within the synovium are noted.

History and Physical Findings
Patients report gradual spontaneous onset of recurring effusions in the knee joint. These effusions often precede reports of pain or discomfort and are not related to a history of trauma, infection, or other iatrogenic cause. Physical examination reveals the presence of a prominent effusion and a diffusely boggy synovium on palpation. Aspirate obtained from the knee is found to be blood-tinged on analysis.

Imaging Studies

Required for diagnosis
AP and lateral radiographs are obtained initially, although they may be nonspecific. However, they can show a joint effusion, bony erosion, and subchondral cysts. PVNS does not calcify.

Required for comprehensive evaluation
MRI of the articular surfaces and the extent of the synovial recesses is required for diagnosis. Lesions of low signal intensity in the joint space on both T1- and T2-weighted images, especially with gradient echo–weighted sequences, are diagnostic. These findings are the result of artifacts associated with the presence of hemosiderin from blood products.

Special considerations
None

Pitfalls
None

IMAGE DESCRIPTIONS

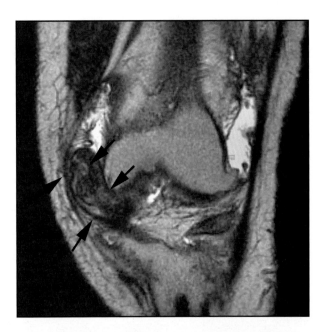

Figure 8-57

Pigmented villonodular synovitis— Coronal MRI

Coronal T2-weighted MRI scan shows a large area of low signal intensity in the anterior medial aspect of the joint (black arrows), consistent with a large focus of PVNS.

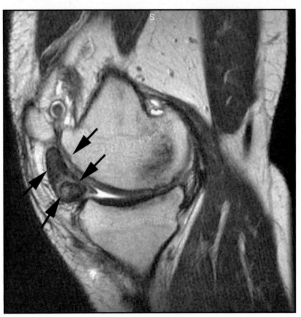

Figure 8-58

Pigmented villonodular synovitis— Sagittal MRI

Sagittal T2-weighted MRI scan shows a large area of low signal intensity anteriorly and medially (black arrows), consistent with PVNS.

DIFFERENTIAL DIAGNOSIS

Synovial osteochondromatosis (multiple calcified lesions within the joint on radiographs)

Psoriatic Arthritis

Synonyms

None

Definition

Psoriatic arthritis occurs in 2% to 7% of patients with psoriasis. The condition occurs occasionally in children, but patients age 55 to 60 years are most commonly affected, with men and women affected equally. Areas typically affected are the interphalangeal joints of the hands and feet, the sacroiliac joints, and the spine; the knee is less commonly involved. Onset usually follows the appearance of the skin lesions, but in 10% to 20% of patients, the arthritis precedes or is simultaneous to the appearance of the lesions. Five subgroups of psoriatic arthritis have been described.

Radiographs show normal bone density, in contrast to the osteopenia and osteoporosis seen in rheumatoid arthritis. Marked joint space narrowing is typical, as with rheumatoid arthritis. Bone proliferation occurs at tendon and ligament insertions. Joint involvement is bilateral but asymmetric. Resorption of the tufts of the distal phalanges is typical.

History and Physical Findings

Patients with psoriatic arthritis usually have a long history of skin involvement before the articular component manifests itself. The arthritis is more prevalent in patients with severe skin involvement. A high correlation exists between the presence of fingernail changes in psoriasis and the presence of psoriatic arthritis. Individual or multiple joints may be involved, especially the small joints of the hands and feet. Soft-tissue swelling may be marked, especially in the fingers. Systemic symptoms associated with a flare of the arthritis include eye changes such as conjunctivitis and iritis, as well as fatigue and low-grade fever. Laboratory studies are negative for rheumatoid factor. HLA-B27 antigen tests are often positive, especially if sacroiliac involvement is present. Elevated erythrocyte sedimentation rate and a mild anemia may be present.

ICD-9 Codes

696.0
Psoriatic arthropathy

696.1
Other psoriasis

SECTION 8 ■ KNEE AND LOWER LEG

IMAGING STUDIES

Required for diagnosis

Weight-bearing AP and lateral views of the articular surfaces and the extent of the synovial recesses are needed to make the diagnosis. Uniform loss of articular cartilage, along with normal bone density and bone proliferation at the tendon and ligament insertions, is characteristic of this condition.

Required for comprehensive evaluation

Radiographs, along with the typical skin lesions seen on physical examination, are adequate for diagnosis. MRI and three-phase bone scan are not helpful.

Special considerations

None

Pitfalls

The radiographic findings of this condition can resemble rheumatoid arthritis, Reiter's syndrome, or ankylosing spondylitis.

IMAGE DESCRIPTIONS

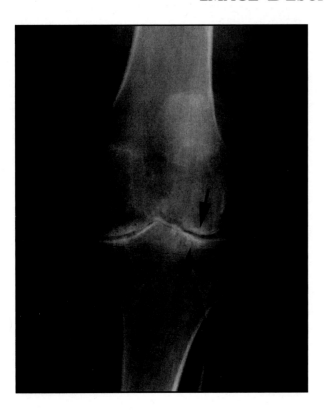

Figure 8-59

Psoriatic arthritis—AP view

AP view shows marked symmetric loss of articular cartilage in the tibiofemoral compartment (arrows), consistent with psoriatic arthritis. The bone density appears normal.

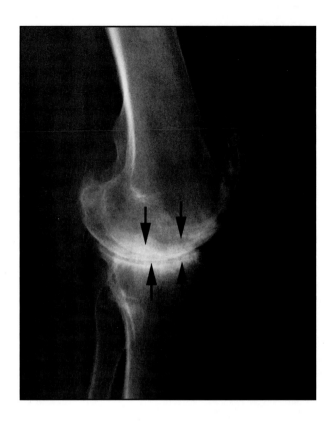

Figure 8-60

Psoriatic arthritis—Lateral view

Lateral view shows marked joint space narrowing with subchondral sclerosis (arrows), consistent with psoriatic arthritis.

DIFFERENTIAL DIAGNOSIS

Ankylosing spondylitis (axial skeletal involvement)

Reiter's syndrome (asymmetric involvement of joints of the lower extremity)

Rheumatoid arthritis (symmetric joint space narrowing with associated osteoporosis)

SECTION 8 ■ KNEE AND LOWER LEG

RHEUMATOID ARTHRITIS

ICD-9 Code

714.0
Rheumatoid arthritis

SYNONYM
RA

DEFINITION
Rheumatoid arthritis (RA) is an immune-mediated inflammatory condition of the synovium that affects women three to four times as often as men. Increasing evidence supports the hypothesis that RA is triggered by an infectious agent, possibly one of the viruses. The knee is surrounded by an extensive synovial lining, so it is not surprising that this joint is commonly affected in patients with RA. Early in the course of the disease, pain and swelling in the knee are common. The diseased synovium attacks cartilage, bone, and the ligamentous structures about the knee. Symmetric narrowing of all three compartments (medial and lateral femorotibial and patellofemoral) is typical. The bony and cartilaginous lesions tend to appear at the margins first and progress inward. The proximal tibiofibular joint can also be affected. Osteoporosis is common, as are subchondral cysts. As the cruciate and collateral ligaments are destroyed, marked instability and deformity can result. In advanced cases, complete loss of articular cartilage occurs.

HISTORY AND PHYSICAL FINDINGS
Pain and swelling in multiple joints, both large and small, is typical of RA. The course of the disease is characterized by exacerbations and remissions. Less than 10% of patients go into permanent remission; most progress to chronic polyarticular RA. The presence of certain antibodies called rheumatoid factors in the blood and joint fluid help to make the diagnosis, but up to 25% of patients with RA test negative for these factors.

IMAGING STUDIES

Required for diagnosis
Weight-bearing AP and lateral views of the articular surfaces and the extent of the synovial recesses can be helpful to establish the diagnosis. Tunnel views can be helpful to evaluate for early joint space narrowing. The characteristic findings of RA include symmetric loss of articular cartilage without the osteophyte formation or sclerosis typically seen with osteoarthritis. Erosive changes are possible but less likely in large joints such as the knee.

Required for comprehensive evaluation
MRI and other advanced imaging techniques usually are not necessary for the evaluation of RA. The diagnosis is typically made with radiographs and clinical and laboratory evaluations.

Special considerations
None

Pitfalls
Secondary osteoarthritic changes can develop with long-standing RA, presenting a mixed picture radiographically.

IMAGE DESCRIPTION

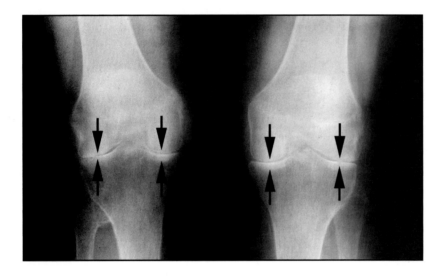

Figure 8-61

Rheumatoid arthritis (knee)—Tunnel view

Bilateral tunnel view demonstrates symmetric joint space loss in the medial and lateral compartments of both knees (black arrows) without sclerosis or osteophyte formation.

DIFFERENTIAL DIAGNOSIS

Osteoarthritis (asymmetric loss of joint space, osteophyte formation, and subchondral sclerosis on radiographs)

Psoriatic or reactive arthritis (symmetric loss of joint space with maintenance of bone mineral density; bony proliferation at the tendon and ligament insertions on radiographs)

SEPTIC ARTHRITIS

ICD-9 Code

711.0
Pyogenic arthritis

SYNONYM
Infectious arthritis

DEFINITION
Septic arthritis of the knee joint represents an acute process in which multiple causative organisms (eg, bacterial, viral, or fungal) are possible. The infecting organism can be delivered to the knee either from an iatrogenic process such as a laceration or a cutaneous lesion. Other etiologies include prior aspiration or injection into the knee joint. Blood-borne pathogens can also be a source of infection.

HISTORY AND PHYSICAL FINDINGS
The diagnosis of septic arthritis generally is not made based on imaging but on clinical evaluation and laboratory analysis of joint aspirate. The systemic findings of infection, including fever, localized pain, and malaise, are key components of the diagnosis. On physical examination, acute tenderness about the knee joint, limited range of motion, and an effusion are common. This condition is always considered a surgical emergency, so diagnosis should not be delayed awaiting imaging studies if they cannot be obtained in a timely manner.

IMAGING STUDIES

Required for diagnosis
Weight-bearing AP and lateral views of the articular surfaces and the extent of the synovial recesses are adequate to make the diagnosis, but confirmation with cross-sectional imaging studies is not advisable in this condition as it may delay diagnosis and immediate treatment. The presence of a joint effusion on the radiographs, in the clinical setting of fever and joint pain, is diagnostic. Joint space narrowing and osteopenia may follow. Occasionally cortical erosions and loss of the normal white subchondral bone can be seen, although these are considered late findings.

Required for comprehensive evaluation
MRI can show a joint effusion, enhanced synovium, reactive marrow edema, and possible osteomyelitis. Patients with recurrent fevers following surgery for a septic arthritis may have an underlying osteomyelitis. MRI is crucial to make this diagnosis.

Special considerations
None

Pitfalls
Septic arthritis is considered a surgical emergency; therefore, the diagnosis should not be delayed awaiting confirmation with imaging studies if they cannot be obtained in a timely manner.

IMAGE DESCRIPTIONS

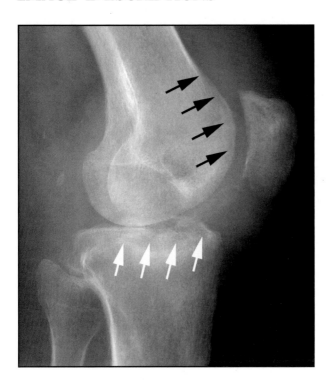

Figure 8-62

Septic arthritis (knee)—Lateral view

Lateral view shows a joint effusion (black arrows) and loss of the subchondral white line (white arrows) seen on normal radiographs. These findings suggest a diagnosis of septic arthritis in the correct clinical setting.

SECTION 8 ■ KNEE AND LOWER LEG

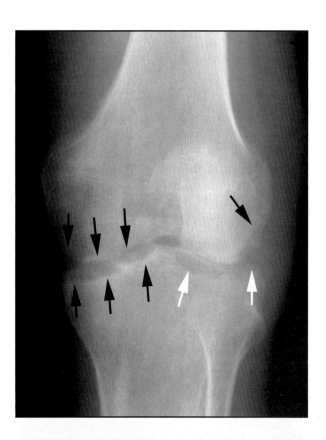

Figure 8-63

Septic arthritis (knee)—AP view

AP view shows loss of the normal subchondral white line (black arrows) and subtle cortical erosions in the proximal tibial articular surface (white arrows). These findings are diagnostic in a patient with fever and joint pain.

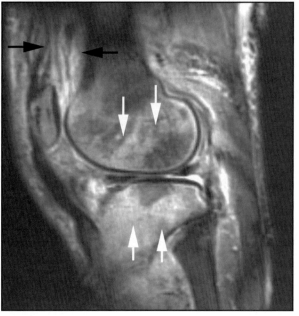

Figure 8-64

Septic arthritis (knee)—Sagittal MRI

Sagittal T1-weighted, fat-suppressed MRI scan with gadolinium contrast medium shows enhancement of the synovium in the region of the suprapatellar recess (black arrows) and enhancement in both the tibia and the femur (white arrows), consistent with not only a septic arthritis but also an associated osteomyelitis.

DIFFERENTIAL DIAGNOSIS

CPPD (chondrocalcinosis, cartilage calcification, and an associated joint effusion)

Spontaneous Osteonecrosis

Synonyms
Avascular necrosis (AVN)
SONC

Definition
Osteonecrosis literally means "bone death." Loss of the blood supply to a localized area of the bone, usually involving the distal femur, is associated with progressively severe knee pain. Often the etiology of the acute loss of blood supply is unknown. Some believe that spontaneous osteonecrosis is actually related to stress fracture rather than osteonecrosis. Spontaneous osteonecrosis of the knee typically involves the weight-bearing surface of the medial femoral condyle. Less commonly it affects the lateral femoral condyle and proximal tibia. In contrast to other forms of osteonecrosis, this condition is not typically associated with predisposing factors such as corticosteroid use, alcohol use, or some forms of systemic disease, which also supports the stress fracture hypothesis.

History and Physical Findings
Spontaneous osteonecrosis most commonly occurs in middle-aged and elderly patients, more commonly women, who report a sudden onset of knee pain. The principal symptoms include progressively severe bone pain, usually localized to the distal femur on the medial or lateral femoral condyles.

Imaging Studies

Required for diagnosis
AP and lateral views of the distal femur and proximal tibia can sometimes make the diagnosis. Sclerosis and an area of lucency and a contour deformity associated with collapse of the subchondral bone are diagnostic but commonly not present.

Required for comprehensive evaluation
MRI usually is required because radiographs are commonly normal, and if findings are nonspecific, MRI will show a relatively extensive area of marrow edema, most commonly in the medial femoral condyle, which can be associated with a subchondral area of low signal intensity. A three-phase bone scan can also show an area of increased uptake in the region of necrosis.

Special considerations
MRI or bone scan can confirm the diagnosis in the presence of normal or nonspecific findings on radiographs.

Pitfalls
None

IMAGE DESCRIPTIONS

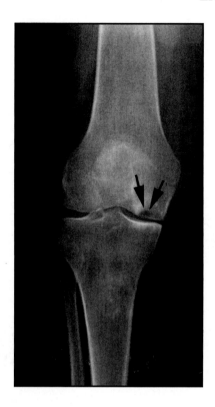

Figure 8-65

Osteonecrosis—AP view

AP view shows subchondral sclerosis in the medial femoral condyle with subchondral lucency (black arrows), suggestive of spontaneous osteonecrosis.

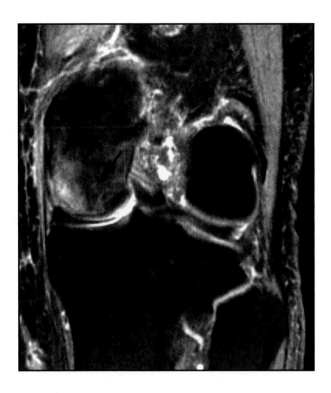

Figure 8-66

Osteonecrosis—Coronal MRI

Coronal T2-weighted, fat-suppressed MRI scan shows extensive edema in the medial femoral condyle (black arrows) characteristic of spontaneous osteonecrosis.

DIFFERENTIAL DIAGNOSIS

Meniscal tear (high signal intensity in the meniscus on MRI)

Osteoarthritis (joint space narrowing, subchondral sclerosis, and osteophyte formation on radiographs)

Osteochondritis dissecans (younger patients, different location on medial femoral condyle)

SECTION 8 ■ KNEE AND LOWER LEG

LIGAMENT INJURIES

ICD-9 Codes

717.81
Old disruption of lateral collateral ligament

717.82
Old disruption of medial collateral ligament

717.83
Old disruption of anterior cruciate ligament

717.84
Old disruption of posterior cruciate ligament

717.85
Old disruption of other ligaments of knee

SYNONYMS

Torn anterior cruciate ligament
Torn lateral collateral ligament
Torn medial collateral ligament
Torn posterior cruciate ligament

DEFINITION

The major ligamentous structures of the knee provide the attachments of the femur to the tibia. The most important structures are the medial (MCL) and lateral (LCL) collateral ligaments, which provide side-to-side (medial-lateral) stability to the knee joint, and the anterior (ACL) and posterior (PCL) cruciate ligaments, which are the primary stabilizers in all other planes. Tears of the ACL and MCL are the most common ligamentous injuries of the knee. These two tears frequently occur together, along with a tear of the medial meniscus; this combination is sometimes referred to as O'Donoghue's unhappy triad. Tears of the PCL are much less common. A tear of the ACL along with a tear of the lateral and posterolateral capsule will give rise to a disabling anterolateral instability of the knee in which the knee gives way. Injuries to both the ACL and PCL in combination with injuries to either the MCL or LCL or both suggest a transient knee dislocation; in such cases, neurovascular injury may be present.

HISTORY AND PHYSICAL FINDINGS

Patients often report an acute twisting injury associated with subluxation of the femur on the fixed tibia. They usually describe hearing a "snap" or "pop." Onset of pain is immediate, and the knee swells within a few hours after the injury. Weight bearing is often impossible. Physical examination will reveal an effusion; joint motion may be limited. Drawer tests, including the Lachman test, will be positive. Varus and valgus stress views of the knee may show widening of the joint space medially or laterally, depending on the structures that are torn. Tests for anterolateral instability such as the MacIntosh test or Losee test may be positive, although a large effusion may give a false-negative result.

IMAGING STUDIES

Required for diagnosis

Although AP and lateral views are usually not helpful in the diagnosis of ligament tears, they should be obtained to rule out any bony injury. An AP view can show a small avulsion fracture from the lateral tibia (Segond fracture), which is invariably accompanied by a torn ACL. An avulsion of bone at the site of the insertion of the ACL into the intercondylar eminence also is indicative of an ACL rupture. AP stress views in varus and valgus may show widening of the medial or lateral joint space, depending on the ligaments that are torn. MRI of all the ligamentous structures around the knee is necessary to identify the particular structures that have been disrupted.

ACL tear MRI will show disruption of the fibers and associated edema in the region of the ACL. These injuries are commonly associated with bone bruising and a joint effusion acutely.

PCL tear MRI will show disruption of the fibers and edema in the region of the PCL. Bone bruising is less common in these tears unless there is an associated posterior lateral corner injury.

LCL tear MRI will show edema around the ligament, usually associated with disruption of the fibers of the ligament. A tear of the LCL can be either isolated or associated with posterior lateral corner injuries.

MCL tear MRI will show edema around the ligament, usually associated with disruption of the fibers of the ligament. These tears generally occur proximally around the femoral attachment of the MCL.

Posterior lateral corner injuries MRI will show ligamentous disruption of many of the posterior lateral ligaments that attach onto the fibula. These injuries commonly occur in conjunction with tears of the LCL, ACL, and PCL.

Required for comprehensive evaluation

MRI is required for comprehensive evaluation of all ligamentous injuries about the knee.

Special considerations

Knee dislocations may be associated with injuries to the popliteal artery. Assessment of vascular injury is frequently necessary.

Pitfalls

None

SECTION 8 ■ KNEE AND LOWER LEG

IMAGE DESCRIPTIONS

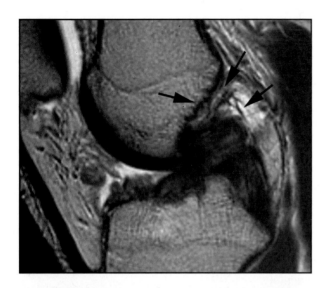

Figure 8-67

Anterior cruciate ligament tear—Sagittal MRI

Sagittal T2-weighted MRI scan shows disruption of the proximal fibers of the ACL (black arrows), typical of an ACL tear.

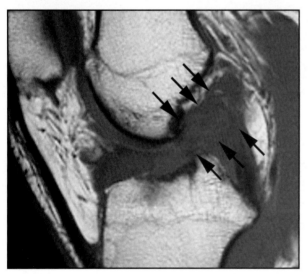

Figure 8-68

Anterior cruciate ligament tear—Sagittal MRI

Sagittal T1-weighted MRI scan shows edema and poor definition of the normal fibers of the ACL (black arrows), characteristic of an ACL tear.

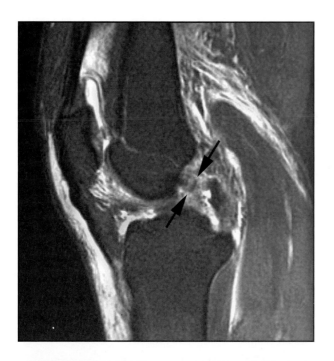

Figure 8-69

Posterior cruciate ligament tear—Sagittal MRI

Sagittal T2-weighted, fat-suppressed MRI scan shows disruption and edema at the femoral attachment of the PCL (black arrows), diagnostic of a PCL tear.

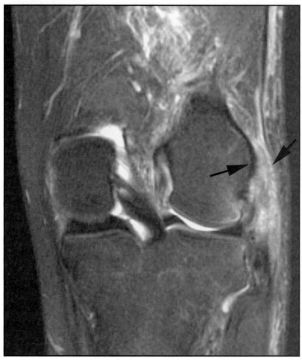

Figure 8-70

Lateral collateral ligament tear—Coronal MRI

Coronal T2-weighted, fat-suppressed MRI scan shows edema around the femoral attachment of the LCL (black arrows), with disruption of the fibers of the ligament.

SECTION 8 ■ KNEE AND LOWER LEG

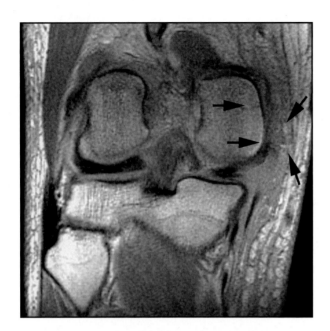

Figure 8-71

Medial collateral ligament tear— Coronal MRI

Coronal proton-density–weighted MRI scan shows complete disruption of the fibers of the MCL (black arrows), consistent with a severe tear.

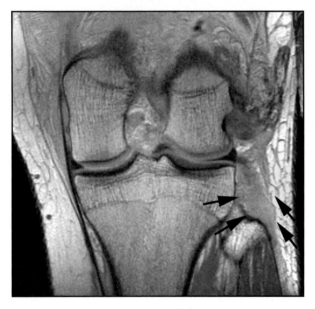

Figure 8-72

Posterolateral corner tear— Coronal MRI

Coronal proton-density–weighted MRI scan shows an avulsion of the fibular insertion of multiple tendons and ligaments (black arrows), including the LCL and biceps femoris tendon, characteristic of a posterior lateral corner tear.

DIFFERENTIAL DIAGNOSIS

Meniscal tear (abnormal signal intensity in the meniscus on MRI)

Meniscal Tear

Synonym
Torn cartilage

Definition
Meniscal pathology is one of the most common causes of knee pain and mechanical dysfunction in patients of all ages. The menisci are semicircular structures within the periphery of the knee joint, located between the femoral and tibial joint surfaces. They are fibrocartilaginous in nature and therefore are not visible on radiographs. The medial and lateral menisci act as shock absorbers and weight distributors in the knee joint. Damage to or absence of these structures will induce progressive degeneration of the articular surfaces in the knee joint, culminating in osteoarthritis.

Tears of the medial meniscus are most common. Meniscal tears may be of several types, with a vertical tear being the most common. A vertical tear that is sufficiently large may displace into the joint, causing the knee to "lock" and limiting movement. This is called a "bucket handle" tear. Horizontal tears are common in older adults and are often associated with osteoarthritis. A developmental anomaly that can occur in the lateral meniscus is called a discoid meniscus. With this condition, the meniscus is thicker and wider than normal and extends into the center of the knee. Because of its shape, it is prone to tears. On radiographs the lateral joint space appears wider than normal.

History and Physical Findings
The mechanism of injury in young patients usually is trauma involving twisting of the knee. In the elderly, symptoms often develop as a result of degenerative changes, which can cause a tear or breakdown. The history often includes reports of clicking, locking, buckling, and giving way. Recurrent effusions and pain are often associated with these episodes. The physical examination reveals swelling, joint line tenderness, and loss of motion. Clicking with flexion and extension and in internal and external rotation (McMurray's sign) also is noted. A vigorous anterior drawer test can displace a bucket handle tear of the meniscus (Finochietto's sign).

ICD-9 Codes

717.5
Derangement of meniscus, not elsewhere classified

836.0
Tear of medial cartilage or meniscus of knee, current

836.1
Tear of lateral cartilage or meniscus of knee, current

SECTION 8 ■ KNEE AND LOWER LEG

Imaging Studies

Required for diagnosis

Weight-bearing AP and lateral radiographs should be ordered initially, even when a meniscus injury is suspected, to rule out osteoarthritis or fracture.

Required for comprehensive evaluation

The meniscus is not a bony structure; therefore, imaging studies that best visualize soft-tissue structures, such as MRI, are indicated. Sagittal and coronal MRI of the knee, including the joint line, are needed to make the diagnosis. MRI has replaced the arthrogram as the imaging modality of choice.

Meniscal tear MRI will show increased signal intensity at the articular surface on T1-weighted images. In addition, with a displaced meniscal tear such as a bucket handle tear, the area of signal that represents the meniscus will be displaced from its normal location.

Discoid meniscus This condition is a normal variation in which the meniscus lacks its typical C-shaped configuration. It is more common in the lateral meniscus. MRI may or may not show abnormal signal intensity.

Special considerations

MR arthrography is helpful for evaluation of the postoperative meniscus, as meniscal signal abnormality (or a meniscal tear in a native knee) normally can be seen in a postoperative meniscus.

Pitfalls

Patients who have had prior meniscal surgery can have signal abnormalities suggestive of a meniscal tear. A discoid meniscus may not be appreciated. Also, a bucket handle tear that has displaced into the notch can be missed.

IMAGE DESCRIPTIONS

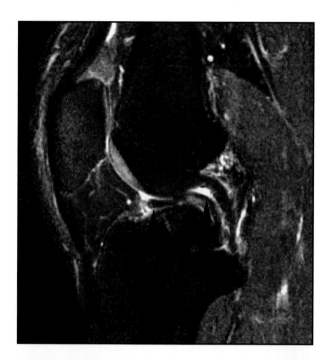

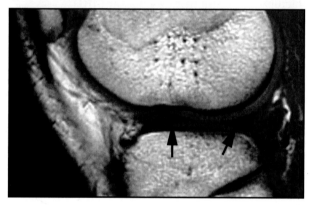

Figure 8-73

Meniscal (bucket handle) tear— Sagittal MRI

Sagittal T2-weighted, fat-suppressed MRI scan shows an area of meniscal signal intensity in the region of the intercondylar notch (black arrows), consistent with a displaced bucket handle tear. Typically, there is no meniscus in the intercondylar notch in the region of the posterior cruciate ligament.

Figure 8-74

Meniscal (lateral) tear— Sagittal MRI

Sagittal T1-weighted MRI scan shows abnormal signal intensity at the articular surface in both the anterior and posterior horns (black arrows) of the lateral meniscus.

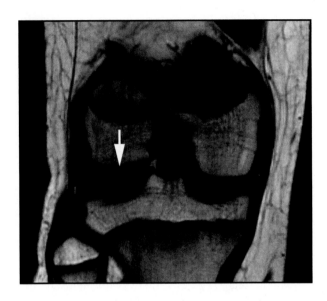

Figure 8-75

Discoid meniscus—MRI

T1-weighted MRI scan shows a discoid lateral meniscus. Note that the lateral meniscus measures more than 12 mm in width (arrow) and is much larger than the medial meniscus.

DIFFERENTIAL DIAGNOSIS

Ligament tear (increased signal intensity and ligament fiber disruption on MRI)

Stress fracture (fracture line or marrow edema on MRI)

Muscle Strain

Synonyms
Charley horse
Myotendinous strain
Plantaris tendon tear
Pulled muscle
Tennis leg

ICD-9 Code
728.83
Rupture of muscle, nontraumatic

Definition
Muscle strain is quite common in individuals who participate in sports and recreational activities. Typically, these injuries are tears that occur at the musculotendinous junction and represent a failure of the muscle-tendon unit under tensile loading. The muscles in the lower extremity that are most commonly affected are the hamstrings (Charley horse), the rectus femoris, the medial head of the gastrocnemius (tennis leg), and the plantaris. The hamstring muscles (biceps femoris, semitendinosus, and semimembranosus) are the most commonly injured muscles in track athletes. Of these muscles, the biceps femoris is the most frequently injured. Tears of the medial head of the gastrocnemius muscle commonly occur in middle-aged tennis players or runners; this injury is referred to as tennis leg. Although most of these injuries are incomplete tears, healing can be unexpectedly long, from 3 months to 1 year or longer.

History and Physical Findings
Athletes involved in running and jumping report acute pain in the back of the leg or calf associated with swelling and difficulty in moving the leg. On physical examination, localized tenderness over the affected muscle is noted. If a complete tear is present, a palpable defect is found.

Imaging Studies

Required for diagnosis
Radiographs will not show the pathology. MRI of the posterior aspect of the thigh in the region of pain is needed to make the diagnosis. Edema within the injured musculature confirms the diagnosis. Ultrasound has also proven useful in diagnosing tennis leg and plantaris tendon tear.

Required for comprehensive evaluation
None

SECTION 8 ■ KNEE AND LOWER LEG

Special considerations

Intramuscular tumors can sometimes present as increased signal intensity within muscle on MRI. The addition of gadolinium contrast medium can be helpful to distinguish these conditions in equivocal cases.

Pitfalls

Failure to order MRI may result in a missed diagnosis.

IMAGE DESCRIPTIONS

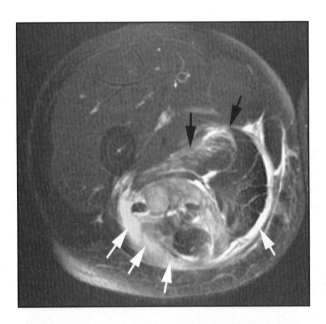

Figure 8-76

Muscle (hamstring) strain—Axial MRI

Axial T2-weighted, fat-suppressed MRI scan shows fluid in the fascial planes (white arrows) and high signal intensity (black arrows) in the hamstring musculature, consistent with a muscle strain.

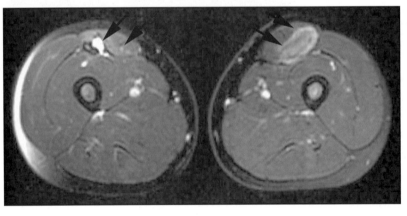

Figure 8-77

Muscle (rectus femoris) strain—Axial MRI

Axial T2-weighted, fat-suppressed MRI scan shows high signal intensity in the rectus femoris muscles bilaterally (arrows), consistent with a muscle strain.

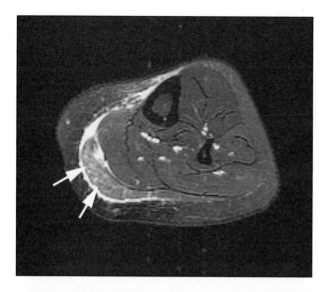

Figure 8-78

Muscle strain (medial gastrocnemius edema)—Axial MRI

Axial T2-weighted, fat-suppressed MRI scan shows high signal intensity in the medial gastrocnemius musculature (arrows), consistent with a muscle strain.

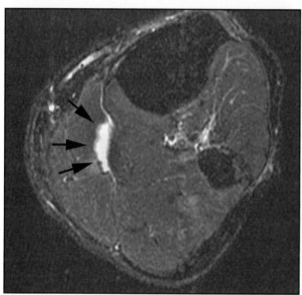

Figure 8-79

Plantaris tendon tear—Axial MRI

Axial T2-weighted, fat-suppressed MRI scan shows edema in the region of the plantaris muscle, between the soleus and the medial head of the gastrocnemius muscles (arrows), consistent with a muscle tear.

DIFFERENTIAL DIAGNOSIS

Achilles tendinitis (tenderness over the Achilles tendon)

Achilles tendon rupture (lack of plantar flexion of the foot)

Deep venous thrombosis (DVT) (positive venogram or ultrasound)

Delayed-onset muscle soreness (DOMS) (symptoms develop 1 to 2 days after exercise and subside in 7 to 10 days)

Muscle contusion (history of direct trauma)

Ruptured popliteal cyst (apparent on MRI)

Stress fracture (positive bone scan or MRI)

SECTION 8 ■ KNEE AND LOWER LEG

FOOT AND ANKLE

Section Editor
Carol Frey, MD

Contributors
Aaron A. Bare, MD
Gregory C. Berlet, MD
Michael E. Brage, MD
Vincent A. Fowble, MD
Jessica Gallina, MD
Steven L. Haddad, MD
Thomas H. Lee, MD
Richard M. Marks, MD
Andrew K. Sands, MD

IMAGING THE FOOT AND ANKLE— AN OVERVIEW

ANATOMY

The foot consists of the hindfoot, midfoot, and forefoot and is composed of 26 bones. The hindfoot is composed of the talus and the calcaneus; the midfoot consists of the navicular, three cuneiforms, and the cuboid bone; and the forefoot consists of five metatarsals and the phalanges.

The extrinsic muscles to the foot originate in the leg, and their tendons cross the ankle. The extrinsic muscles include the anterior tibial, the extensor hallucis longus, the extensor digitorum longus, and the peroneus tertius. On the flexor surface, the extrinsic muscles include the gastrocnemius, the soleus, the plantaris, the flexor hallucis longus, the flexor digitorum longus, the posterior tibial, the peroneus longus, and the peroneus brevis muscles.

The intrinsic muscles that originate from the dorsal surface of the foot consist of the extensor hallucis brevis, which has its origin on the dorsum of the os calcis and inserts on the base of the great toe proximal phalanx, and the extensor digitorum brevis, which originates with the extensor hallucis brevis and inserts into the extensor expansion of toes two through four.

Intrinsic muscles that originate on the plantar surface of the foot are arranged in layers. The superficial layer originates from the calcaneus and extends to the toes. The superficial layer consists of the abductor hallucis muscle, which inserts on the proximal phalanx; the flexor digitorum brevis muscle, which inserts on the middle phalanx of the lesser toes; and the abductor digiti quinti muscle, which inserts on the lateral surface of the proximal phalanx of the fifth toe.

The second layer includes the extrinsic tendons—the flexor hallucis longus and the flexor digitorum longus. The intrinsic muscles in this layer are the quadratus plantae and the lumbrical muscles. The medial head of the quadratus plantae originates from the calcaneus and plantar fascia, and the lateral head originates from the lateral surface of the calcaneus. Both heads insert on the flexor digitorum longus tendons. The lumbricals originate on the long flexor to the lesser toes and insert into the tibial surface of the extensor expansion.

The third layer consists of the short muscles to all the toes. The flexor hallucis brevis has its origin from the cuboid and lateral cuneiform bones and inserts through two tendons onto the base of the proximal phalanx of the great toe. The medial head inserts with the abductor hallucis and the lateral head with the adductor hallucis. Each of the heads of the flexor hallucis brevis has a sesamoid bone within the tendon. The flexor hallucis longus tendon runs between the two sesamoids. The adductor hallucis has an oblique head, which originates from the second, third, and fourth metatarsals and the sheath of the peroneus longus and then inserts on the lateral aspect of the base of the proximal phalanx. The transverse head originates from the plantar ligaments of the metatarsophalangeal (MTP) joints and has the same insertion site as the oblique head. The origin of the flexor digiti quinti is off the base of the fifth MTP joint and attaches to the base of the proximal phalanx.

The deep layer contains three plantar and four dorsal interosseous muscles. The plantar interosseous muscles come from and course on the medial side off of toes three through five and insert into the bases of proximal phalanges and extensor expansions of respective toes. The dorsal interosseous muscles originate from the third and fourth toes. They insert on both sides of the second proximal phalanx and the lateral side of the third and fourth proximal phalanges and extensor expansions.

OSSIFICATION CENTERS

Ossification centers about the foot and ankle appear, on average, in the following sequence: (1) distal fibula and lateral cuneiform at 1 year; (2) base of the distal phalanx at 1 to 3 years; (3) medial cuneiform at 2 years; (4) distal tibia, base of the first metatarsal and proximal phalanx, and middle cuneiform at 2 to 3 years; (5) capital epiphysis (toes two to four) and navicular at 2 to 4 years; (6) capital epiphysis (toe five) at 3 to 4 years; (7) posterior os calcis at 5 to 8 years; (8) os trigonum at 8 to 12 years; (9) lateral sesamoid at 9 to 11 years; and (10) base of the fifth metatarsal at 9 to 14 years.

STANDARD IMAGING VIEWS

Foot problems can result from trauma, congenital abnormalities, overuse, and the effects of ill-fitting shoes. The standard radiographic views of the foot for all these problems are AP, lateral, and 45° oblique views. The ankle has been reported to be the most commonly injured joint of the body. The most common injury occurs with supination, adduction, and internal rotation, the so-called twisted ankle. Depending on the direction and amount of force, this "twisting" may result in a minor sprain or a severe fracture. Standard radiographic views of the ankle are the AP, lateral, and mortise views.

Radiographs

Non–weight-bearing views In addition to the standard views for the foot and ankle, an additional forefoot view (tangential sesamoid view) is sometimes needed to evaluate the position of of the sesamoids and the integrity of the transverse arch. In the hindfoot, a Harris view may be used to evaluate the os calcis.

The subtalar joint may be better visualized with Broden's views because these views better visualize the posterior articular facets and joint.

Weight-bearing views Weight-bearing (sometimes called standing) views are helpful in the evaluation of many foot and ankle conditions. A weight-bearing AP view of the foot is necessary to measure the 1-2 intermetatarsal (IM) angle, which is important in the evaluation of hallux valgus. The 4-5 IM angle is useful in the evaluation of a bunionette. With a potential splayfoot or flexible flatfoot, the IM angle is more accurately measured with a weight-bearing AP view.

A weight-bearing lateral view is helpful when evaluating the medial longitudinal arch, especially in flatfoot. A cavus foot also is more accurately evaluated with a weight-bearing lateral view. A weight-bearing lateral view of the ankle in which the ankle is in maximum dorsiflexion can show whether there is an impinging bony lesion of the ankle.

Stress views Stress views can help determine the extent of ligament damage; thus, comparison views of the opposite, uninjured side should be obtained. For the AP talar tilt view, the foot should be held in neutral to slight plantar flexion. With this view, a difference of 6° is considered positive. The anterior drawer test should be performed in about 10° of plantar flexion. With this test, an anterior translation of the talus of more than 4 mm is usually considered abnormal.

Computed tomography

In general, CT is useful in the evaluation of calcaneus or talus fractures, nonunions, fracture patterns, tarsal coalition, and osteochondral lesions of the talus.

Magnetic resonance imaging

The anatomy of the foot and ankle is complex and lends itself well to imaging in multiple planes. MRI is of value in the workup of chronic foot and ankle pain. It is also useful for showing the extent of osseous and soft-tissue infection.

Bone scans

Generally, bone scans will be abnormal in the presence of infection, tumor, or fracture. These studies also are very useful for the evaluation of stress fractures of the foot and ankle.

EMERGENCIES
None

NORMAL VARIANTS
Accessory bones are developmental anomalies, and many may be present in the foot. Some occur commonly in the normal, pain-freepain-free foot. They are unilateral in more than one half of

affected individuals; in others, they may be multipartite. The most common accessory bones are the os trigonum, os tibiale, os intermetatarseum (1-2), os navicularis, and os peronei. Other accessory bones are the os susentaculi, os calcaneus secundarius, os talonaviculare dorsale, os intercuneiforme, os cuboids secundarium, os cuneometatarsale I plantare, os vesalianum, os subtibiale, and os subfibulare.

IMAGING TIPS

1. The hindfoot is denser than the forefoot and either can be overexposed or underexposed on an AP view. The use of a tapered thickness wedge, which is thicker under the forefoot, will provide a more uniform image and reduce this effect.
2. Look at the global alignment and image of the foot and ankle, not just the suspected pathology. Obtain a comparison view of the uninjured foot, if needed. Comparison views are very helpful in children and when evaluating subluxations and dislocations.
3. The width of the joint space should be constant around the entire ankle mortise.
4. On the mortise view, a space of 5 mm or greater between the medial malleolus and the talus indicates a deltoid ligament tear. This space can change a stable fibula fracture into an unstable one.
5. A fibula fracture above the level of the tibial plafond should be considered a complex injury, which may involve disruption of the syndesmosis and a bone, or ligament injury on the medial side of the ankle joint.
6. A failure to recognize and subsequently treat a widened mortise can result in osteoarthritis of the ankle.
7. A syndesmosis injury is thought to have occurred if there is more than 5 mm of space between the tibia and the fibula on the mortise view. This is measured 1 cm up from the plafond. If in doubt, a definitive evaluation is available with CT using axial cuts across the syndesmosis with comparison views of the opposite side.
8. When evaluating a calcaneus fracture, remember that concurrent fractures of the lumbar spine occur in 10% of patients and other lower extremity fractures in 25%. A careful physical and radiographic examination is required in these patients.
9. Initial radiographs of a metatarsal stress fracture are usually negative. Periosteal reaction may not appear until 3 to 4 weeks after the injury. A technetium Tc 99m bone scan will be positive before the radiographs. Stress fractures are commonly missed because of delays in radiographic findings.
10. To accurately evaluate hallux valgus, bunionette, flatfoot, cavus foot, and alignment disorders, weight-bearing views are required.

SECTION 9 ■ FOOT AND ANKLE

HEEL SPUR

SYNONYMS

Heel pain syndrome
Proximal plantar fasciitis (PPF)

DEFINITION

Heel pain is common and at times very disabling, but its etiology is not well understood. Pain is typically found in two areas, the inferior medial heel and the posterior superior heel. Pain in both locations often coexists, and symptoms overlap.

The presence of plantar heel spurs, however, does not correlate directly with heel pain. In fact, a heel spur will appear on radiographs in only 50% of patients with proximal plantar fasciitis and in 15% of patients who have no history of heel pain. A heel spur is a projection of bone arising from the plantar distal aspect of the calcaneal tuberosity. A plantar heel spur usually occurs at the origin of the flexor digitorum brevis from the calcaneal tuberosity, not at the origin of the plantar fascia.

Plantar heel spurs are believed to be secondary to degenerative changes and inflammation surrounding the calcaneal origin of the plantar fascia. Microruptures and collagen degeneration may occur in the Sharpey's fibers, which anchor the fascia to the calcaneus. Fibrosis, ossification, and periosteal inflammation commonly cause the pain in plantar fasciitis.

Proximal plantar fasciitis has a gradual onset and lacks a specific traumatic etiology. One extremity is usually affected, although bilateral involvement can occur in up to 30% of patients. The condition is thought to predominate in women, although this has not been confirmed in statistically sound studies. Proximal plantar fasciitis has been associated with obesity, prolonged standing, distance running, and systemic inflammatory disease.

HISTORY AND PHYSICAL FINDINGS

Patients typically report localized heel pain that is often worse in the morning and after long periods of rest. They also can usually isolate the area on the heel of the most intense pain. Patients with long-standing pain will have an antalgic gait, with preferential weight bearing to the lateral border of the foot to prevent placing weight on the medial heel.

Physical examination reveals localized tenderness over the medial plantar aspect of the calcaneal tuberosity. Pain over the heel must be differentiated from medial pain over the abductor tendon;

ICD-9 Codes

726.73
Enthesopathy of ankle and tarsus, calcaneal spur

728.71
Disorders of muscle, ligament, and fascia; plantar fascial fibromatosis

SECTION 9 ■ FOOT AND ANKLE

the latter may signify local nerve irritation as a component of distal tarsal tunnel syndrome.

IMAGING STUDIES

Required for diagnosis
Proximal plantar fasciitis is a clinical diagnosis; therefore, imaging studies are not needed to establish the diagnosis.

Required for comprehensive evaluation
A lateral view of the heel is obtained to rule out other causes of heel pain. The bony architecture is usually normal, but it is not uncommon to see an indistinct medial border at the calcaneus signifying a small heel spur.

Special considerations
MRI may be useful only as a follow-up to radiographs that appear abnormal or if the diagnosis remains unclear. Serious lesions that warrant further investigation include lytic lesions of the calcaneus, rapidly growing nodular lesions of the plantar fascia, and suspected stress fractures of the calcaneus.

The most common lytic lesion of the calcaneus is a unicameral bone cyst. MRI is useful to evaluate the matrix, periosteal reaction, and lytic borders that define whether the lesion is passive or aggressive.

Nodular lesions of the plantar fascia, such as plantar fibromatosis, may occasionally mimic proximal plantar fasciitis. With rapidly growing lesions, MRI may be indicated to rule out a neoplasm.

Radiographs of calcaneal stress fractures will appear normal until the periosteum has mounted a healing response. Bone scan is the most sensitive way to detect a stress fracture. Repeat radiographs 2 weeks after the onset of pain may reveal resorption of the fracture line, endosteal thickening, or localized periostitis. On MRI, a stress fracture may appear as an intramedullary or cortical region of decreased signal intensity on T1-weighted images. On T2-weighted images, a stress fracture will appear as increased signal intensity; increased signal intensity may also appear in adjacent soft tissue.

Pitfalls
Bone scans are rarely useful in the evaluation of plantar heel pain, although they often show increased uptake at the medial calcaneal tuberosity. MRI will often show thickening of the plantar fascia origin and marrow edema at the medial calcaneal tuberosity. MRI, however, is not necessary for treatment or diagnosis.

IMAGE DESCRIPTIONS

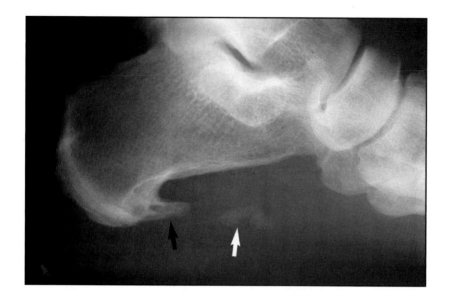

Figure 9-1

Proximal plantar fasciitis—Lateral view

Lateral view of a patient with heel pain shows a large heel spur emanating from the distal plantar calcaneal tuberosity (black arrow). Several small soft-tissue calcifications are distal to the heel spur (white arrow). These calcifications may represent dystrophic calcification within a degenerative plantar fascia ligament or an acute fracture of a preexisting heel spur. The bony anatomy of the calcaneus is otherwise unremarkable.

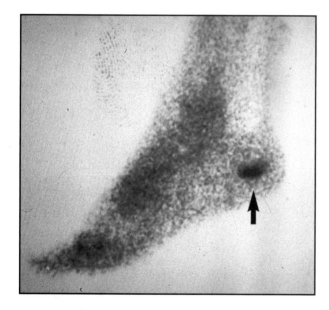

Figure 9-2

Proximal plantar fasciitis— Bone scan

A bone scan of a patient with proximal plantar fasciitis shows tracer uptake at the plantar aspect of the calcaneus (arrow), which suggests focal inflammation at the plantar fascia origin on the calcaneus. Note that there are no changes within the body of the calcaneus, ruling out a stress fracture of the tuberosity.

SECTION 9 ■ FOOT AND ANKLE

Differential Diagnosis

Calcaneal stress fracture (rare, pain with side-to-side compression of the calcaneus)

Compression of the first branch of the lateral plantar nerve (tenderness on percussion or a positive Tinel's sign over the first branch of the lateral plantar nerve in the distal tarsal tunnel)

Heel pad atrophy (thin fat pad with poor rebound on compression, pain more centrally located)

Neoplastic changes of the calcaneus (rare, pain at night and/or at rest)

Plantar fibromatosis (nodules, may not be painful)

Ruptured plantar fasciitis (ecchymosis, swelling, and possible palpable gap)

PUMP BUMP

SYNONYMS

Haglund's syndrome or deformity
Pretendon bursitis

DEFINITION

Also known as pretendon bursitis, pump bumps are a soft-tissue
response that develops over the proximal posterolateral aspect of
the calcaneus. This condition affects both soft tissue and bone and
is most common in women who wear pump-style high-heeled
shoes.

The stiff heel counter of some shoes is often responsible for the
development of bursitis. The heel counter is often curved inward on
its superior aspect to enhance fit; often this design will irritate the
posterolateral calcaneus (Haglund's process). The bone itself may
undergo reactive change but more commonly the pre-Achilles bursa
becomes inflamed. Soft-tissue inflammation is the primary finding
of a pump bump. Irritation of the inflamed bursa can make shoe
wear intolerable.

HISTORY AND PHYSICAL FINDINGS

Physical examination will reveal a thickening and inflammation of
the soft tissue on the posterior aspect of the calcaneus. A bony
prominence often can be palpated in the area of pain. The Achilles
tendon is noted to be intact.

IMAGING STUDIES

Required for diagnosis

Pump bump is a clinical diagnosis. Radiographs are not needed.

Required for comprehensive evaluation

A lateral view of the foot can evaluate the size of the posterior
superior aspect of the calcaneus, but often no abnormalities are
noted. Soft-tissue swelling posterior to the calcaneus may be seen
in advanced cases.

Special considerations

MRI can identify areas of edema and can help evaluate the status
of the retrocalcaneal bursa, pre-Achilles bursa, and the Achilles
tendon.

ICD-9 Codes

726.91
Unspecified enthesopathy of
ankle and tarsus, exostosis
of unspecified site

727.82
Other disorders of synovium,
tendon, and bursa; calcium
deposits in tendon and bursa

SECTION 9 ■ FOOT AND ANKLE

Pitfalls

The bursae may be filled with radiopaque dye and radiographs taken to obtain a bursogram. However, bursograms are rarely indicated. An inflamed bursa accepts more fluid and therefore will have an irregular appearance on a bursogram.

Image Description

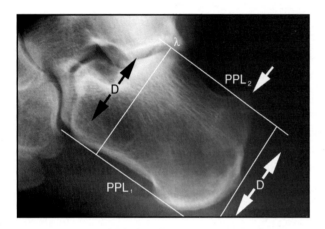

Figure 9-3

Haglund's deformity—Lateral view

Lateral view shows a prominent calcaneal projection consistent with a Haglund's deformity. This condition is defined radiographically as the bony projection above the parallel pitch lines (PPL). These lines can be drawn on a weight-bearing lateral view. The lower PPL (PPL_1) is the baseline and is drawn along the plantar aspect of the calcaneus from the anterior to the posterior plantar tubercles. A perpendicular line (D) is drawn from the posterior lip of the talar articular facet to the baseline. The upper PPL (PPL_2) is drawn parallel to the baseline at a distance of D. A posterior process of the calcaneus that touches or is below PPL_2 is normal. A posterior process (white arrow) that projects above PPL_2 is excessively prominent.

Differential Diagnosis

Insertional Achilles tendinitis/tendinosis (pain on palpation directly over the site)

Retrocalcaneal bursitis (pain on palpation anterior to the Achilles tendon in the area of the retrocalcaneal bursa)

RETROCALCANEAL BURSITIS

SYNONYM

Haglund's syndrome or deformity

DEFINITION

Retrocalcaneal bursitis is an inflammation of the bursa, a structure that lies between the posterior calcaneus and the Achilles tendon. It often occurs in conjunction with insertional Achilles tendinitis and is a component of Haglund's syndrome. Retrocalcaneal bursitis occurs secondary to overuse, repetitive trauma, impingement from the calcaneus, or increased dorsiflexion. The retrocalcaneal bursa is lined with synovial cells; therefore, mechanical irritation can cause painful swelling. Arthritides such as psoriasis, Reiter's disease, rheumatoid arthritis, gout, and ankylosing spondylitis can also cause retrocalcaneal bursitis.

HISTORY AND PHYSICAL EXAMINATION

Patients typically report pain at rest that increases with activity. The key physical finding is pain on palpation over the retrocalcaneal bursa that lies anterior to the Achilles tendon. Swelling can be felt with pressure on both the medial and lateral sides of the bursa. Ankle dorsiflexion typically exacerbates the pain in the posterior heel as the bursa is compressed between the calcaneus and the Achilles tendon.

IMAGING STUDIES

Required for diagnosis

The diagnosis is clinical; therefore, radiographs are not needed to make the diagnosis.

Required for comprehensive evaluation

A lateral view can be used to evaluate the size of the posterior superior aspect of the calcaneus (Haglund's process). Calcifications are often identified at the insertion of the Achilles tendon, and occasionally calcification within the Achilles tendon itself is seen. The os trigonum, also seen well on the lateral view, is located at the posterior aspect of the talus.

Special considerations

MRI can identify areas of edema and help identify whether the pathologic process is confined to the retrocalcaneal bursa or whether it involves the Achilles tendon. The flexor hallucis longus tendon and the os trigonum are best visualized with MRI.

ICD-9 Codes

726.71
Achilles bursitis or tendinitis

726.79
Enthesopathy of ankle and tarsus, other

726.91
Unspecified enthesopathy; Exostosis of unspecified site

Pitfalls

Bursograms have been advocated as an invasive means of diagnosing retrocalcaneal bursitis. An inflamed bursa accepts more fluid and therefore has an irregular appearance on the bursogram. Impingement at the posterior aspect of the calcaneus also can be seen. This modality is rarely used, however, because the diagnosis can be made by physical examination and with other noninvasive tests.

IMAGE DESCRIPTIONS

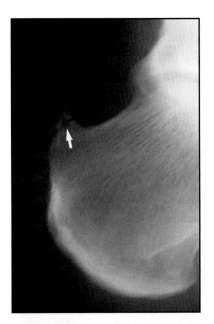

Figure 9-4

Inflamed calcaneal process—Lateral view

Close-up lateral view of the calcaneus shows an enlarged Haglund's process. Note the cystic changes (white arrow) and fragmentation (black arrow) in the calcaneus secondary to chronic inflammation. Soft-tissue inflammation also is noted posterior to the Achilles insertion.

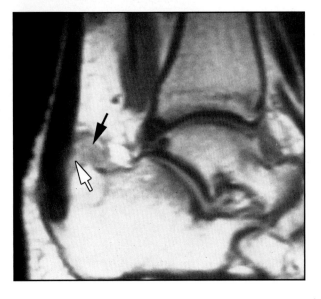

Figure 9-5

Retrocalcaneal bursitis— Sagittal MRI

Sagittal MRI scan shows an enlarged retrocalcaneal bursa (black arrow) with superficial inflammation of the anterior aspect of the Achilles tendon (white arrow). The Achilles tendon shows focal inflammation at the point of contact with the Haglund's process.

SECTION 9 ■ FOOT AND ANKLE

DIFFERENTIAL DIAGNOSIS

Ankle synovitis (swelling with an effusion; pain with dorsiflexion and plantar flexion; normal radiographs)

Flexor hallucis longus tendinitis (pain on palpation over the site; pain worse with plantar flexion and dorsiflexion of the great toe)

Insertional Achilles tendinitis (pain on palpation directly over the site of insertion)

Painful os trigonum (pain on palpation over the site; pain worse with plantar flexion; os trigonum apparent on radiographs)

SECTION 9 ■ FOOT AND ANKLE

ACCESSORY NAVICULAR

ICD-9 Code

755.67
Anomalies of foot, not
elsewhere classified

SYNONYMS

Accessory scaphoid
Os naviculare
Os tibiale externum
Prehallux

DEFINITION

The accessory navicular, a nonfused ossicle and a normal variant of
the navicular bone, is present in 3% to 14% of the normal
population and may be associated with posterior tibial tendon
dysfunction. It is more common in females than in males. Three
types of accessory navicular have been defined. Type I is a small
sesamoid bone within the posterior tibial tendon, without
attachment to the body of the navicular. With type II, the most
common type, the accessory navicular is attached to the medial
aspect of the navicular by a cartilaginous connection, or
synchondrosis. This type frequently becomes symptomatic and must
be differentiated from an acute fracture of the navicular tuberosity.
Type III is the same as type II except that instead of being attached
by cartilage, the accessory navicular is fused to the navicular,
creating a cornuate, or horn-shaped, navicular.

HISTORY AND PHYSICAL FINDINGS

Patients typically exhibit point tenderness at the insertion of the
posterior tibial tendon that is exacerbated by resisted inversion with
plantar flexion. The overlying skin may be inflamed as a result of
rubbing of the enlarged accessory bone on shoe wear. Some
patients report a history of antecedent trauma; however, this is most
frequently associated with an eversion injury, or an injury in which
the foot is turned outward. Patients with a symptomatic accessory
navicular may have associated pes planus and inflammation or
dysfunction of the posterior tibial tendon. With a type II accessory
navicular, symptoms are a result of tension or compression forces at
the synchondrosis. With a type III accessory navicular, symptoms
are usually caused by direct pressure from shoe wear.

IMAGING STUDIES

Required for diagnosis

AP, lateral, and internal oblique views should be obtained to establish the diagnosis. Weight-bearing radiographs are recommended because they are more helpful in evaluating associated capsuloligamentous instability and in accurately assessing concomitant pes planus. A 30° external oblique radiograph of the foot best assesses the medial tuberosity and accessory navicular. The accessory navicular will have smooth margins with a well-defined cortex.

Required for comprehensive evaluation

None

Special considerations

A technetium Tc 99m bone scan should be ordered when a fracture is suspected and will show increased uptake with either an accessory navicular or a tuberosity avulsion fracture. MRI can help differentiate an accessory navicular from a tuberosity avulsion fracture by revealing the presence or absence of bone edema.

Pitfalls

The standard foot series (AP, lateral, internal oblique) may obscure the accessory navicular because of bony overlap. The irregular margins of the ossification center of the navicular bone can resemble an acute fracture. This ossification center typically appears at 3 to 4 years of age.

IMAGE DESCRIPTIONS

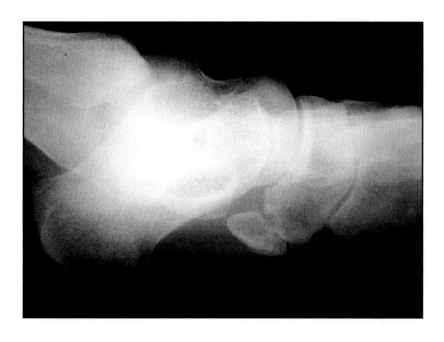

Figure 9-6

Accessory navicular—External oblique view

External oblique view reveals a type II accessory navicular (arrow), as indicated by the rounded, regular margins. This may be differentiated from the irregular appearance of the navicular seen in Figure 9-7.

SECTION 9 ■ FOOT AND ANKLE

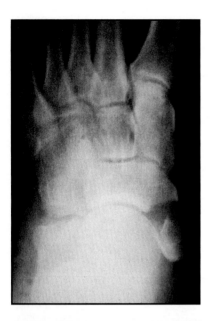

Figure 9-7

Navicular fracture—AP view

AP view of the foot shows an avulsion fracture of the navicular tuberosity with irregular margins (arrow). MRI will reveal edema at the fracture margins.

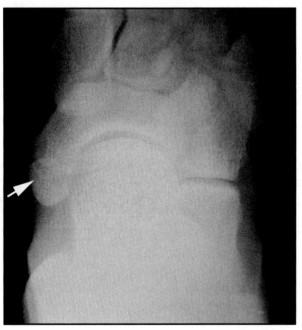

Figure 9-8

Accessory navicular—Reverse oblique view

Reverse oblique view of the forefoot shows an accessory navicular bone (arrow).

DIFFERENTIAL DIAGNOSIS

Navicular tuberosity avulsion fracture (sharp, irregular margins; MRI will reveal edema at the fracture margins)

ANKLE FRACTURES

SYNONYMS

Ankle fracture-dislocation
Bimalleolar fracture
Dupuytren fracture
Lateral malleolus fracture
Maisonneuve fracture
Medial malleolus fracture
Pilon fracture
Trimalleolar fracture

ICD-9 Codes

824.0
Fracture of ankle, medial malleolus, closed

824.4
Fracture of ankle, bimalleolar, closed

824.7
Fracture of ankle, trimalleolar, open

DEFINITION

The ankle is one of the most frequently injured joints. The many types of ankle fractures include lateral malleolus fractures, isolated medial malleolus fractures, bimalleolar fractures, trimalleolar fractures, fracture-dislocations, and intra-articular pilon fractures. The radiographic findings produced by these injuries are directly related to the mechanism that produced the injury.

Several fracture classification systems are in use. The AO (Weber) classification system, based on the level of the fibular fracture, is illustrated below. Another system, the Lange-Hansen classification, is based on the mechanism of injury, as defined by a combination of foot position (supination or pronation) and the

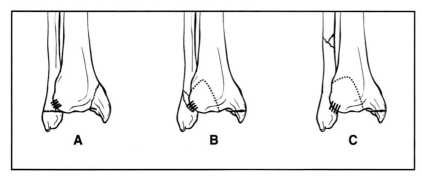

AO (Weber) classification of ankle fractures. Type A is a transverse avulsion fracture of the fibula at or below the level of the ankle joint. The fracture line in the medial malleolus lies between the horizontal and the vertical. In a type B injury, an oblique fracture of the fibula passes up and back from the level of the ankle joint. It is accompanied by a transverse avulsion fracture of the medial malleolus or a rupture of the deltoid ligament. A posterolateral fracture fragment of the tibia (Volkmann's triangle) is frequently sheared off. A type C injury is characterized by a fibular fracture above the level of the syndesmosis and an avulsion fracture of the medial malleolus or a tear of the deltoid ligament. There may be a fracture at the posterior edge of the tibia. With type C injuries, the syndesmotic ligaments connecting the tibia and fibula are ruptured. (Adapted with permission from Müller ME, Allgöwer M, Schneider R, Willenegger H (eds): *Manual of Internal Fixation*, ed 2. Berlin, Germany, Springer-Verlag, 1979, p 244.)

direction of the force on the talus (abduction, adduction, or eversion). These categories are then further subdivided based on the sequential involvement of the supporting soft-tissue structures.

HISTORY AND PHYSICAL FINDINGS

A thorough patient history is important when caring for patients with ankle injuries. The most important information to obtain is when and where the injury occurred, how it happened, any preexisting foot or ankle pathology, and the patient's overall medical condition.

The ankle should be inspected for open wounds, swelling, blisters, and bony deformity. Tenderness should be localized by palpation. The vascular examination should include palpation of the posterior tibial and dorsalis pedis pulses. If swelling or deformity interferes with palpation of the pulses, a Doppler device may be useful. The function of the nerves that cross the ankle is assessed by testing sensation in the specific areas that they innervate.

The function of the tendons that cross the ankle should be tested. This includes checking the Achilles tendon, the peroneus longus and brevis, the anterior compartment muscles that dorsiflex the ankle and toes, and the deep posterior compartment muscles that flex the hallux and lesser toes.

It is important to recognize that ankle pain may be the initial symptom of a developing compartment syndrome. Early signs of a compartment syndrome include calf tenderness, induration, and pain with passive motion of the involved muscle groups.

IMAGING STUDIES

Required for diagnosis

Localized malleolar tenderness or the inability to bear weight is the best indication for obtaining radiographs of the ankle. AP, lateral, and mortise views are obtained to evaluate ankle fractures. The mortise view, taken in internal rotation, is a true AP radiograph of the ankle joint. The mortise and lateral views are adequate to confirm the diagnosis in 92% to 96% of patients.

Required for comprehensive evaluation

Although the mortise and lateral views are sufficient in most cases, the addition of the AP view is recommended. This view helps in understanding the fracture orientation and in planning surgical intervention when indicated.

With some isolated lateral malleolus fractures, stress views of the ankle are obtained to assess the integrity of the deltoid ligament. The tibia is stabilized with one hand, and the ankle is everted with the other hand. The resulting eversion stress radiographs are scrutinized for shifting of the talus. If the deltoid ligament is intact, the talus will remain reduced in the mortise despite the eversion stressing. If the deltoid ligament is disrupted, the talus will shift laterally, resulting in an abnormal widening of the space between the talus and the medial malleolus. In this scenario, the ankle is considered unstable and the patient should be referred for surgery consult.

Special considerations

CT can be helpful in the case of unusual fracture patterns because it supplies more detail. In addition, CT is essential in evaluating intra-articular displacement and in planning the reconstruction of pilon fractures.

MRI is useful if the physical examination raises suspicion of a tendon rupture or articular surface disruption.

Pitfalls

None

IMAGE DESCRIPTIONS

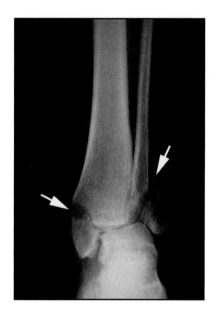

Figure 9-9

Displaced bimalleolar fracture—AP view

AP view of the ankle shows a displaced bimalleolar fracture (arrows). Note that the talus has shifted laterally (toward the fibula).

SECTION 9 ■ FOOT AND ANKLE

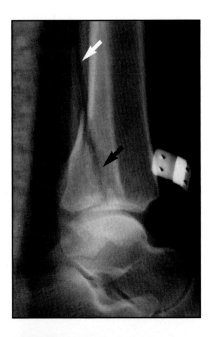

SECTION 9 ■ FOOT AND ANKLE

Figure 9-10

Fractures of the posterior and lateral malleolus—Lateral view

Lateral view of the ankle shows fractures of the posterior malleolus (black arrow) and lateral malleolus (white arrow). The posterior malleolus fracture is an intra-articular fracture and, in this case, is displaced.

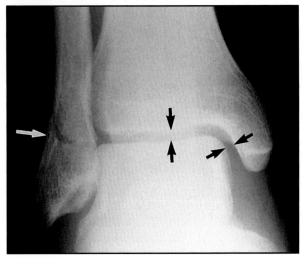

Figure 9-11

Fracture of the lateral malleolus— Mortise view

This eversion stress radiograph reveals a lateral malleolus fracture (white arrow) without widening of the mortise (black arrows).

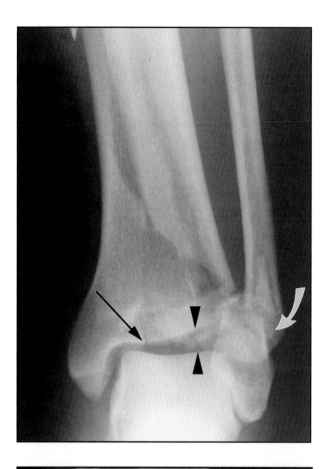

Figure 9-12

*Intra-articular pilon fracture—
AP view*

AP view reveals an intra-articular pilon
fracture (black arrow) and fibula fracture
(white arrow). The ankle mortise is unstable
with lateral widening (arrowheads).

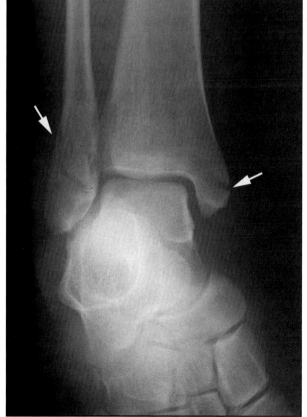

Figure 9-13

Bimalleolar fracture—AP view

AP view of the ankle shows a bimalleolar
ankle fracture (arrows) with minimal
displacement.

SECTION 9 ■ FOOT AND ANKLE

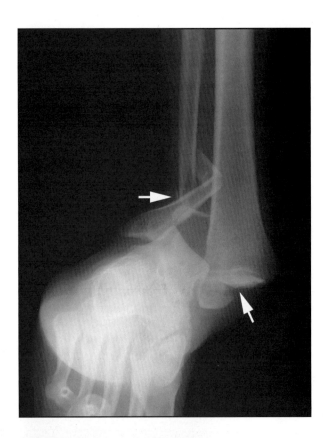

Figure 9-14

Bimalleolar fracture-dislocation—AP view

AP view shows a bimalleolar fracture-dislocation of the ankle (arrows).

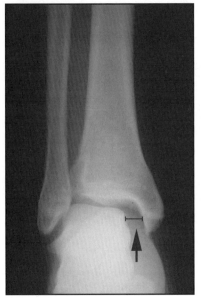

Figure 9-15

Maisonneuve fracture—AP view

AP view of the ankle view reveals a widening of the medial ankle mortise (arrow, line) with a normal appearing medial malleolus; for this to occur, the deltoid ligament and distal tibiofibular syndesmosis must be disrupted. This combination associated with a fracture of the proximal fibula is known as a Maisonneuve fracture.

DIFFERENTIAL DIAGNOSIS

Fractures of the base of the fifth metatarsal, lateral process of the talus, or anterior process of the calcaneus (pain over fracture site, bony involvement apparent on radiographs)

Ligament injuries, including the lateral collateral ligament complex and medial collateral ligament (pain on palpation over the involved ligaments, soft-tissue findings on MRI, normal radiographs)

Osteochondral fracture (apparent on radiographs and MRI)

Syndesmosis injuries (> 5 mm spread between the tibia and fibula measured 1 cm above the joint line on AP or mortise view; pain over syndesmosis with compression of the tibia and fibula at the midcalf level)

Tendon injuries, including peroneal tendon dislocation or rupture (normal radiographs, positive findings on MRI, pain on palpation over the involved tendon)

SECTION 9 ■ FOOT AND ANKLE

FIFTH METATARSAL APOPHYSIS

ICD-9 Codes
None

SYNONYMS
None

DEFINITION
A fifth metatarsal apophysis is a normal variant that appears in boys between the ages of 11 and 14 years and in girls between the ages of 9 and 11 years. It is sometimes confused with a nondisplaced tuberosity fracture. Closure of the apophysis occurs 2 to 3 years after its appearance, although infrequently, it will fail to unite.

HISTORY AND PHYSICAL FINDINGS
The apophysis is a normal variant, so physical examination will be benign. If tenderness is present over the fifth metatarsal base, apophysitis or concomitant avulsion fracture should be suspected.

IMAGING STUDIES

Required for diagnosis
AP, lateral, and oblique views are the standard imaging studies for this condition. The apophysis will appear smooth and longitudinally oriented, running parallel to the metatarsal shaft.

Required for comprehensive evaluation
None

Special considerations
None

Pitfalls
A fifth metatarsal apophysis may be confused with a nondisplaced tuberosity fracture.

IMAGE DESCRIPTION

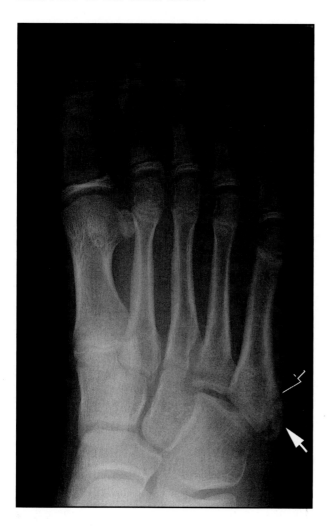

Figure 9-16

*Fifth metatarsal apophysis—
AP view*

AP view of the foot of a skeletally immature
patient shows a fifth metatarsal apophysis.
Note the longitudinally oriented line (black
arrow) and slight fragmentation (white arrow)
at the base of the fifth metatarsal, indicative of
an apophysis.

DIFFERENTIAL DIAGNOSIS

Os peroneum or os vesalianum (smooth, regular edges located
just proximal to the tip of the tuberosity)

Tuberosity fracture (irregular fracture line in skeletally mature
individual; runs more obliquely or transversely than an
apophysis)

FRACTURE OF THE CALCANEUS

ICD-9 Code

825.0
Fracture of calcaneus, closed

SYNONYMS
None

DEFINITION
Fractures of the calcaneus account for approximately 60% of all tarsal fractures. They are usually caused by a sudden, high-velocity impact to the heel. The most common mechanisms of injury are motor vehicle accidents and falls from a height of 6 feet or more. Most of these fractures (80% to 90%) occur in physical laborers between the ages of 20 and 40 years. Those that extend into the subtalar joint can cause severe functional disability.

HISTORY AND PHYSICAL FINDINGS
Physical examination should include inspection of the foot for open wounds and swelling. Any foot deformity should be noted, including a widened or varus heel, which signifies a displaced fracture. The ankle and subtalar range of motion should be assessed. The opposite, uninjured foot also should be examined because of the possibility of bilateral fractures. Injuries associated with a fall from a height, such as vertebral compression fractures, should be ruled out.

Follow-up examination after a calcaneus fracture should include assessment for compartment syndrome as it develops in up to 25% of patients with calcaneus fractures. Compartment syndrome is characterized by severe swelling and inordinate pain on passive stretch of the toes.

IMAGING STUDIES

Required for diagnosis
AP, oblique, lateral, and axial Harris views of the foot are needed to establish the diagnosis. The oblique view is used to evaluate the calcaneocuboid joint. Measurement of Böhler's angle, which normally is 20° to 40°, on the lateral view will show step-off and depression in the posterior facet. The axial Harris view will demonstrate lateral wall displacement, fibular abutment, and the direction of displacement of the tuberosity along the primary fracture line.

Required for comprehensive evaluation

CT is very helpful in assessing calcaneus fractures. The bone should be imaged in two planes: a semicoronal plane perpendicular to the posterior facet, and transversely, parallel to the plantar surface of the foot. CT should be ordered to assess damage to the subtalar and calcaneal cuboid joints, as well as tendon entrapment in the fracture fragments.

Special considerations

None

Pitfalls

None

IMAGE DESCRIPTIONS

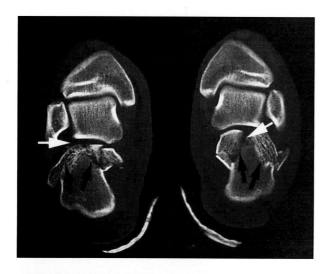

Figure 9-17

Fracture of the calcaneus—Coronal CT

Coronal CT scan of the calcaneus shows bilateral displaced, comminuted, intra-articular fractures (black arrows) and depression of the posterior facet (white arrows).

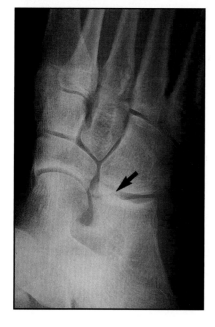

Figure 9-18

Fracture of the calcaneus—Oblique view

Oblique view of the heel shows a fracture of the anterior process of the calcaneus (black arrow).

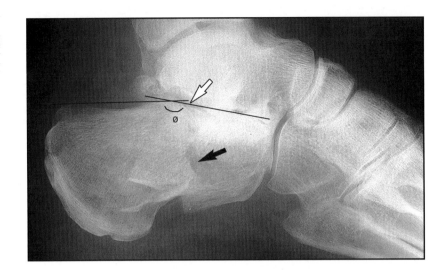

Figure 9-19

Fracture of the calcaneus— Lateral view

Lateral view of the foot shows an intra-articular fracture of the calcaneus (black arrow) and depression of the posterior facet (white arrow). There is flattening of Böhler's angle (lines), which is formed by the intersection between a straight line drawn along the upper surface of the tuber calcanei and a straight line connecting the highest points of the anterior upper and posterior joint surfaces of the calcaneus.

DIFFERENTIAL DIAGNOSIS

None

FRACTURE OF THE FIFTH METATARSAL BASE

SYNONYMS
Tennis fracture
Tuberosity avulsion fracture

ICD-9 Code
825.25
Fracture of other tarsal and metatarsal bones, closed; metatarsal bone(s)

DEFINITION
A fifth metatarsal base fracture involves a fracture of the tuberosity. This is distinct from a Jones fracture, which occurs at the metaphyseal-diaphyseal junction, and from a diaphyseal stress fracture, which occurs more distally. Tuberosity fractures are typically extra-articular, but they may extend into the cuboid-metatarsal joint.

HISTORY AND PHYSICAL FINDINGS
Fractures of the fifth metatarsal base occur secondary to a sudden inversion of the foot that causes the lateral band of the plantar aponeuroses or peroneus brevis to contract, avulsing a portion of the tuberosity. The fracture fragment should not be confused with the os peroneum, which lies within the peroneus longus tendon, or the os vesalianum, which lies within the peroneus brevis tendon, at the tip of the tuberosity. Palpation over the fifth metatarsal base will elicit pain, as will resisted eversion of the foot.

IMAGING STUDIES

Required for diagnosis
AP, lateral, and oblique views of the foot should be obtained to establish the diagnosis. This fracture, which occurs at the tuberosity, must be distinguished from a Jones fracture, which occurs at the metaphyseal-diaphyseal junction, or diaphyseal stress fracture, which occurs more distally.

Required for comprehensive evaluation
None

Special considerations
None

SECTION 9 ■ FOOT AND ANKLE

Pitfalls

In the skeletally immature individual, the apophysis may be confused with a nondisplaced tuberosity fracture. A displaced avulsion fragment must also be distinguished from the os peroneum or os vesalianum. These sesamoid bones, which are situated in the peroneus longus tendon and peroneus brevis tendon, respectively, are recognized by their smooth, regular edges.

IMAGE DESCRIPTION

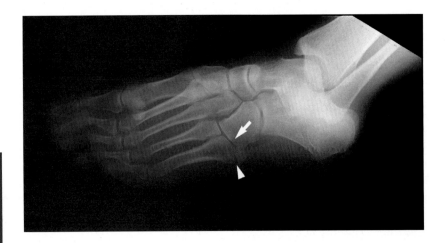

Figure 9-20

Fracture of the fifth metatarsal base— Oblique view

Oblique view reveals a minimally displaced tuberosity fracture (white arrowhead) with intra-articular extension into the cuboid (white arrow). Note the transverse orientation of the fracture.

DIFFERENTIAL DIAGNOSIS

Apophysis (smooth line running parallel to shaft of bone in skeletally immature individual)

Os peroneum or os vesalianum (smooth, regular edges)

FRACTURE OF THE METATARSAL NECK

SYNONYMS
None

ICD-9 Code

825.25
Fracture of other tarsal and metatarsal bones, closed; metatarsal bone(s)

DEFINITION
Fractures of the metatarsal neck occur just proximal to the metatarsal head. The degree of displacement is often related to the force of injury and associated soft-tissue disruption. Damage to the intrinsic musculature and capsuloligamentous attachments may result in plantar and proximal displacement because of the attachments of the relatively stronger flexor tendons at the base of the proximal phalanx.

Plantar displacement will result in metatarsalgia under the affected metatarsal. Significant medial-lateral displacement may create an interdigital neuroma.

HISTORY AND PHYSICAL FINDINGS
Fractures of the metatarsal neck can be caused by either direct or indirect forces. Direct forces, such as from an object dropped on the dorsum of the foot or a crush injury, can result in multiple, "across-the-board" neck fractures. Indirect, twisting forces may create sufficient mediolateral torque to produce a fracture. Ecchymosis is invariably present, and swelling may be dramatic in direct crush injuries. Forefoot compartment syndrome can occur with these injuries. Direct palpation and/or axial compression of the affected metatarsal will elicit pain.

IMAGING STUDIES

Required for diagnosis
A standard series consisting of AP, lateral, and internal oblique views should be obtained. The x-ray beam should be centered on the forefoot to avoid overexposure of the affected area. The AP and oblique views are most helpful for fracture diagnosis; however, the lateral view can help reveal any significant dorsal-plantar displacement or angulation.

Required for comprehensive evaluation
In the acute setting, additional imaging modalities are not helpful. If a stress fracture is suspected, a technetium Tc 99m bone scan is 100% sensitive. If questions still exist, MRI can identify the presence of bony edema or cortical disruption.

SECTION 9 ■ FOOT AND ANKLE

Special considerations
None

Pitfalls
None

Image Descriptions

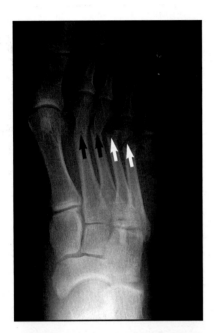

Figure 9-21

Fractures of the metatarsal neck—AP view

AP view shows minimally displaced fractures of the necks of the second and third metatarsals with valgus angulation (black arrows). Note the complete lateral displacement and shortening of the necks of the fourth and fifth metatarsals (white arrows).

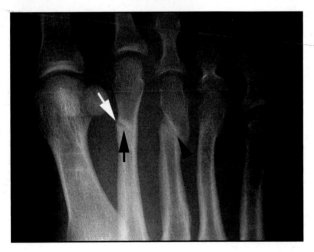

Figure 9-22

Fractures of the metatarsal neck (healed)—AP view

AP view shows an oblique, nondisplaced fracture of the neck of the second metatarsal with probable healing. Note the persistent fracture line with surrounding sclerosis (black arrow) and apparent medial cortical bridging (white arrow). Also note the healed oblique third metatarsal neck fracture with bayoneting of the distal fragment (arrowhead).

Differential Diagnosis

Lisfranc fracture-dislocation (lateral displacement of the second through fifth metatarsal bones, fracture of the base of the second metatarsal)

Section 9 ■ Foot and Ankle

FRACTURE OF THE NAVICULAR

SYNONYM
Fracture of the tarsal navicular

DEFINITION
Fractures of the navicular can be grouped into cortical avulsion fractures, tuberosity fractures, body fractures, and stress fractures. Cortical avulsion fractures are caused by a twisting force (as occurs with eversion, or turning outward of the foot) and occur more frequently in women. The dorsal talonavicular capsule and anterior fibers of the deltoid ligament may avulse a dorsal portion of bone. The size of the portion varies. This fracture must be differentiated from an os supranaviculare or os supratalare.

Tuberosity fractures occur as a result of an acute eversion or abduction force on the foot that results in increased tension on the anterior fibers of the deltoid ligament and particularly on the insertion of the posterior tibial tendon. This fracture is sometimes seen in conjunction with a compression fracture of the cuboid, indicative of a severe abduction force.

Fractures of the body of the tarsal navicular are frequently associated with additional midfoot injuries, indicative of high-energy trauma. Comminution may result in talonavicular joint subluxation.

Stress fractures result from repetitive high-impact loading and are seen most often in young male athletes. The fracture line occurs in the middle third of the bone and is typically vertically oriented. This corresponds to the region of the navicular that is relatively avascular.

HISTORY AND PHYSICAL FINDINGS
Patients with cortical avulsion fractures report a history of a twisting injury and present with point tenderness over the dorsal talonavicular capsule. Various degrees of swelling and ecchymosis may be present.

Tuberosity fractures, which occur as a result of an eversion force, are typically associated with point tenderness over the insertion of the posterior tibial tendon at the navicular tuberosity. With higher energy injuries, there may be associated tenderness along the lateral aspects of the cuboid, indicative of cuboid compression fracture. Resisted inversion or passive eversion of the foot may elicit pain.

Fractures of the navicular body are commonly caused by high-energy injuries and are often associated with midfoot injuries.

ICD-9 Code

825.22
Fracture of other tarsal and metatarsal bones, closed; navicular (scaphoid), foot

SECTION 9 ■ FOOT AND ANKLE

Diffuse swelling and ecchymosis are typical. The dorsal midfoot may be diffusely tender. Physical examination should include assessment for associated midfoot injuries and should rule out the possibility of compartment syndrome.

Stress fractures of the navicular, which are found most commonly in runners and basketball players, are more insidious in nature. Patients report dull, nonspecific pain over the midfoot. Pain may be accentuated by having the patient stand on the toes.

IMAGING STUDIES

Required for diagnosis
Imaging of navicular fractures should include AP, lateral, and oblique views of the foot. The lateral view best reveals cortical avulsion fractures. The 30° external oblique view best assesses tuberosity fractures. The 45° internal oblique view best visualizes the lateral portion of the navicular. The os will appear with a smooth margin and well-defined cortex. The fracture will have irregular margins with little or no sclerosis at the margin.

Required for comprehensive evaluation
In patients with a suspected stress fracture and unremarkable radiographs, a coned-down AP radiograph centered on the navicular may provide a better view. CT or MRI is recommended to evaluate a possible navicular stress fracture. MRI can reveal the earliest stress changes, but CT is a better choice for follow-up of fracture healing.

Special considerations
None

Pitfalls
The irregular margins of the ossification center of the navicular bone can resemble an acute fracture. Onset of ossification of the navicular bone is age 3 to 4 years.

IMAGE DESCRIPTIONS

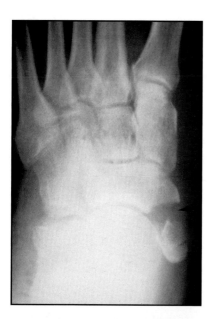

Figure 9-23

Navicular fracture—AP view

AP view shows an avulsion fracture with comminution of the tarsal navicular (black arrow). Proximal migration of the fragments reveals retraction of the insertion of the posterior tibial tendon. The fracture margins are irregular and reveal no sclerosis.

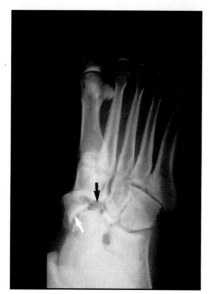

Figure 9-24

Navicular fracture—AP view

AP view shows a comminuted, displaced navicular fracture (black arrow). Note the medial subluxation of the medial two thirds of the navicular (white arrow). Assessment for associated midfoot injury is indicated when this fracture pattern is seen.

SECTION 9 ■ FOOT AND ANKLE

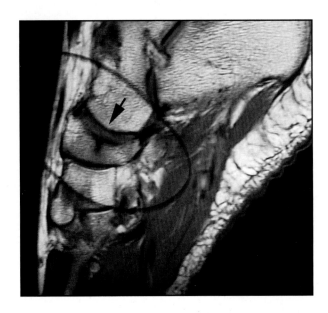

Figure 9-25

Stress fracture of the navicular—Sagittal MRI

Sagittal T1-weighted MRI scan of the foot shows a stress fracture at the midsection of the navicular bone (arrow).

DIFFERENTIAL DIAGNOSIS

Accessory navicular (smooth, sclerotic border on radiographs; no marrow edema on MRI)

Os supranaviculare (nonfused ossicle superior to navicular bone, smooth margins and well-defined cortex on radiographs)

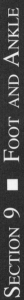

FRACTURE OF THE PHALANGES

SYNONYM
Tuft fracture

ICD-9 Code

826.0
Fracture of one or more
phalanges of foot, closed

DEFINITION
Fractures of the phalanges typically occur either as a result of direct trauma from dropped objects or from "jamming" the toe, typically with the foot unprotected. Fractures are described relative to pattern (transverse, oblique, spiral), degree of displacement, angulation, and/or shortening. The phalanx involved should be identified (proximal, middle, distal), as should the location of the fracture and the presence of any rotation or intra-articular involvement.

HISTORY AND PHYSICAL FINDINGS
Patients typically present with significant swelling and ecchymosis. Subungual hematoma may be present with distal phalanx fractures. Patients may report paresthesia and/or numbness secondary to swelling and/or direct nerve injury. Angular deformity of the toe is rarely seen.

IMAGING STUDIES

Required for diagnosis
AP, lateral, and oblique views of the involved digit should be taken. For the oblique and lateral views, the affected digit should be isolated by taping the uninvolved toes out of the field.

Required for comprehensive evaluation
None

Special considerations
None

Pitfalls
None

SECTION 9 ■ FOOT AND ANKLE

IMAGE DESCRIPTION

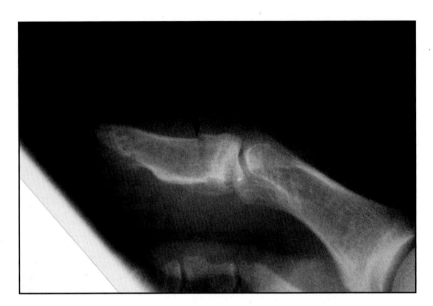

Figure 9-26

Fracture of the phalanx—Lateral view

Lateral view of the hallux reveals a transverse fracture of the proximal third of the distal phalanx (arrow).

DIFFERENTIAL DIAGNOSIS

Gout (no fracture seen on radiograph)

Osteoarthritis (joint changes seen on radiograph)

FRACTURE OF THE SESAMOID

SYNONYMS
None

DEFINITION
The first metatarsophalangeal (MTP) joint has two sesamoids, a tibial and fibular sesamoid. Each possesses a dorsal facet that articulates with the metatarsal head. The plantar surface is enveloped by fibers of the flexor hallucis brevis and plantar plate. The flexor hallucis longus lies between the two sesamoids. The tibial sesamoid bears more weight and therefore is more vulnerable to mechanical trauma. The fibular sesamoid sits in a more protected position in the lateral soft tissues and therefore is fractured less frequently. The sesamoids may fracture secondary to direct trauma, avulsion forces (particularly in hyperdorsiflexion injuries), or repetitive stress. An acute fracture must be differentiated from a bipartite sesamoid, which is a normal variant.

HISTORY AND PHYSICAL FINDINGS
Most fractures of the sesamoid are associated with acute trauma. However, repetitive stress to the flexor tendon complex, such as occurs during distance running or ballet dancing, can also create avulsion or stress fractures. Patients report pain that is localized under the fractured sesamoid and may be elicited with dorsiflexion of the MTP joint. Swelling is variable, and ecchymosis is rare.

IMAGING STUDIES

Required for diagnosis
AP, lateral, and axial views should be obtained to establish the diagnosis. The fibular sesamoid is best visualized on an internal oblique view.

Required for comprehensive evaluation
A technetium Tc 99m bone scan can help differentiate an acute fracture or stress fracture from a bipartite sesamoid and is considered to be 100% sensitive. MRI can also be helpful in differentiating a fracture from a bipartite sesamoid or osteonecrosis. A bone scan will demonstrate increased uptake in the fractured sesamoid, and MRI will show marrow edema. MRI can also provide information about the condition of the plantar plate, the intersesamoid ligament, and the flexor tendons.

ICD-9 Code
825.20
Fracture of other tarsal and metatarsal bones, closed; unspecified bone(s) of foot (except toes)

SECTION 9 ■ FOOT AND ANKLE

Special considerations

Accessory sesamoids (usually tibial) may occur under any of the lesser metatarsal heads.

Pitfalls

A bipartite sesamoid can be mistaken for a fracture of the sesamoid. The fracture line is usually transverse and can be difficult to distinguish from a bipartite sesamoid. However, the fracture line will be more irregular than the smooth, sclerotic margin of a bipartite sesamoid.

IMAGE DESCRIPTIONS

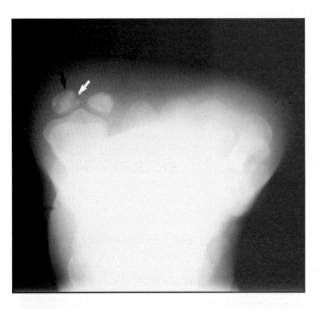

Figure 9-27

Sesamoid fracture—Axial view

Axial view of a tibial sesamoid fracture shows a nondisplaced oblique fracture (black arrow) and an avulsion fracture along the lateral aspect of the sesamoid (white arrow).

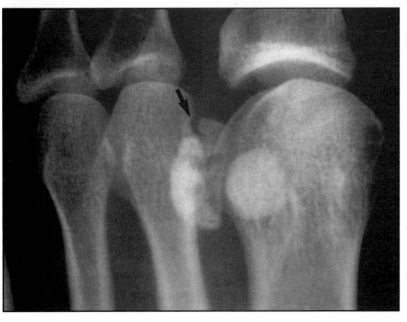

Figure 9-28

Sesamoid fracture— Internal oblique view

Internal oblique view shows a comminuted fracture of the fibular sesamoid (arrow).

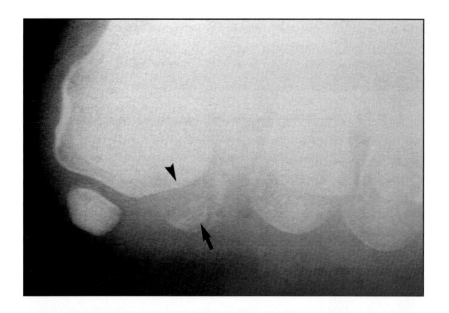

Figure 9-29

Sesamoid fracture—Axial view

Axial view of the same comminuted fracture of the fibular sesamoid (black arrow) shown in Figure 9-28. Note that despite comminution, the fibular sesamoid still lies within the crista of the first metatarsal head (arrowhead).

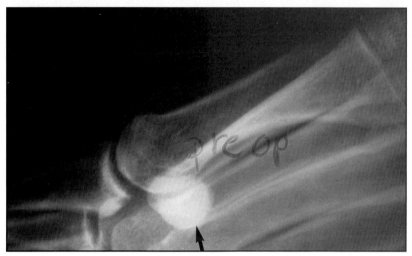

Figure 9-30

Osteonecrosis of the hallux sesamoid—Lateral view

Lateral view of the hallux demonstrates a sclerotic appearance of the sesamoid (arrow), indicative of osteonecrosis.

SECTION 9 ■ FOOT AND ANKLE

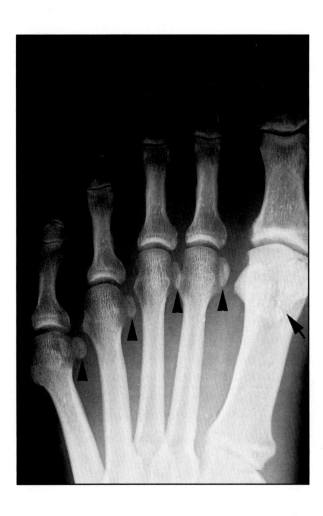

Figure 9-31

*Bipartite sesamoid (tibial)—
AP view*

AP view of the forefoot shows a bipartite tibial sesamoid (arrow) and accessory sesamoids under the second through fifth metatarsal heads (arrowheads). The accessory sesamoids can become symptomatic if overloaded.

DIFFERENTIAL DIAGNOSIS

Bipartite sesamoid (smooth, sclerotic edges; negative bone scan)

Osteonecrosis (sclerotic appearance of entire sesamoid or irregularity with fragmentation)

Plantar plate disruption (proximal migration of sesamoid)

Fracture of the Talus

ICD-9 Code

825.21
Fracture of other tarsal and metatarsal bones, closed; talus

Synonyms

Aviator's astragalus
Aviator's fracture

Definition

The talus is a bone of the hindfoot that has unique anatomic features that make it vulnerable to injury and difficult to treat. Because it articulates with the tibia, calcaneus, and navicular, approximately 60% of the surface of the talus is covered with articular cartilage. Normal motion in each of these joints contributes to normal gait.

The talus is vulnerable to osteonecrosis because it relies chiefly on direct blood supply from three arterial sources: branches of the posterior tibial artery, the tibialis anterior artery, and the peroneal artery. Indirect perfusion is limited because the talus lacks muscular or tendinous insertions.

History and Physical Findings

The mechanism of injury of talus fractures varies widely. The type of talus fracture most commonly seen in trauma centers is a fracture of the neck or anterior body. The injury is usually caused by impaction of the foot during a high-energy collision in which the ankle is forced into severe dorsiflexion and excessive axial loads are applied to the foot. The Hawkins classification is used to grade the severity of the injury and to help determine the best treatment. Type I fractures are nondisplaced vertical fractures of the talar neck; type II fractures are displaced fractures with a subluxated or dislocated subtalar joint; and type III fractures are displaced fractures in which the body of the talus is dislocated from both the ankle and subtalar joints.

Fractures of the head of the talus are less common but may occur as a result of axial loads or high-energy trauma such as from motor vehicle accidents. These fractures are usually associated with more complex injuries, and partial dislocation or subluxation of the talus is common.

A fracture of the lateral process of the talus usually results from low- to moderate-energy trauma. It is a common injury among snowboarders and is typically caused by axial loading with elements of dorsiflexion and eversion.

SECTION 9 ■ FOOT AND ANKLE

The patient should be examined for open wounds, foot or ankle deformity, and swelling. Palpation should be performed sequentially to localize specific areas of tenderness. A neurovascular examination of the foot should be performed.

IMAGING STUDIES

Required for diagnosis
AP, lateral, and modified AP views of the foot are necessary to identify the fracture pattern. An AP or mortise view of the ankle is necessary to assess the congruency of the tibiotalar joint. Fractures of the lateral process or posterior process often require hindfoot oblique views.

Required for comprehensive evaluation
CT is often used instead of special radiographic views because CT is able to detect nondisplaced fractures and osteochondral injuries. Images in the coronal plane are best for visualizing fractures of the talar body or the posterior or lateral process. Images in the transverse or sagittal planes best visualize vertical fractures of the talar neck and talar dome.

Bone scans are useful to evaluate occult talus fractures. This test is sensitive but not specific for such fractures.

Special considerations
At 6 to 12 weeks after a talar neck fracture, a subchondral radiolucency may form (Hawkins sign), indicating disuse osteoporosis. This finding on radiographic images confirms that there is intact blood flow. In general, this finding rules out osteonecrosis, which can occur after talar neck fractures.

Pitfalls
Radiographic changes consistent with osteonecrosis following a talar neck fracture may take 3 months or longer to develop. Increased density in the body of the talus may be seen. Diffuse disuse osteoporosis will be seen in the surrounding vascularized bone. MRI will usually identify osteonecrosis earlier.

IMAGE DESCRIPTIONS

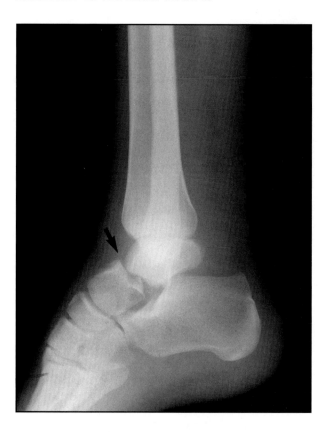

Figure 9-32

Fracture of the talus—Lateral view

Lateral view of the ankle demonstrates a displaced talar neck fracture (arrow).

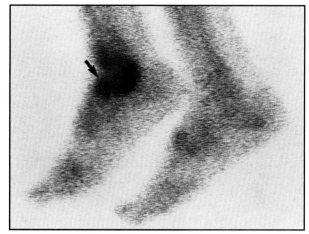

Figure 9-33

Fracture of the talus—Bone scan

Bone scan shows increased uptake in an area of the talus, suggesting a fracture (arrow).

SECTION 9 ■ FOOT AND ANKLE

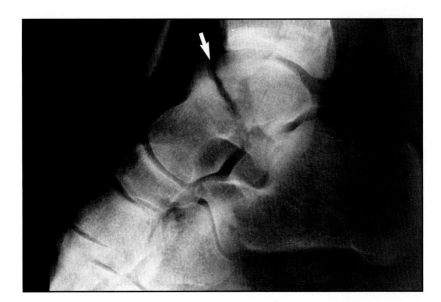

Figure 9-34

*Fracture of the talus—
Lateral view*

Lateral view of the foot shows a displaced fracture of the anterior talar body (arrow).

DIFFERENTIAL DIAGNOSIS

Fracture-dislocation of the subtalar joint (dislocation seen on radiographs)

Ligament injuries (normal radiographs and bone scan, soft-tissue findings on MRI, pain on palpation over the involved ligaments)

Osteochondral fracture of the talus (apparent on radiographs and MRI)

Tendon injuries (normal radiographs and bone scan, soft-tissue findings on MRI, pain on palpation over the involved tendon)

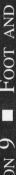

FREIBERG'S INFRACTION

ICD-9 Code

732.5
Juvenile osteochondrosis of
foot

SYNONYMS

Freiberg's disease
Osteochondrosis of the metatarsal head
Osteonecrosis of the metatarsal head

DEFINITION

Freiberg's infraction is an osteochondrosis of the second or, less
commonly, the third or fourth metatarsal head. It is typically found
in adolescent girls and is presumed to be osteonecrosis of the
subchondral bone of the metatarsal head. Repetitive stress that
causes microfractures and subsequent compromise of blood supply
may play a role in the etiology.

HISTORY AND PHYSICAL FINDINGS

The patient usually reports pain at the involved metatarsophalangeal
(MTP) joint that is aggravated with activity. Physical examination
reveals signs of inflammation with increased warmth, swelling,
palpable tenderness over the joint or metatarsal head, and limited
range of motion in the affected MTP joint. Deformity may be
evident in late stages of the disease.

IMAGING STUDIES

Required for diagnosis

Weight-bearing AP, lateral, and oblique views of the forefoot are
needed for evaluation. Characteristic radiographic changes include
increased density of the metatarsal head, flattening, collapse, cystic
changes, and changes of the MTP joint. Fragmentation may develop
later in the course of the disease.

Required for comprehensive evaluation

Because radiographs may appear normal in the early stages of
Freiberg's infraction, MRI may be helpful to show osteonecrotic
changes. Although not specific, bone scan may be useful in
localizing the pathologic process in the metatarsal head, aiding in
the diagnosis.

Special considerations

None

Pitfalls

Radiographs may appear normal in the early stages of the disease.

IMAGE DESCRIPTIONS

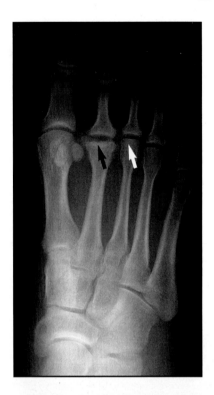

Figure 9-35

Freiberg's infraction—AP view

AP view of the mid- and forefoot shows severe flattening and collapse of the second metatarsal head with subchondral sclerosis (black arrow). The third metatarsal head (white arrow) shows mild flattening and increased density in the subchondral bone.

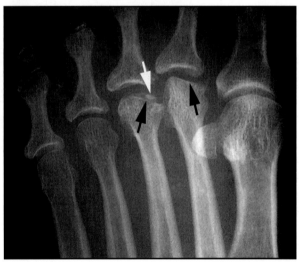

Figure 9-36

Freiberg's infraction—AP view

AP view of the forefoot of a patient with Freiberg's infraction shows collapse and flattening (black arrows) of the second and third metatarsal heads, and fragmentation at the third metatarsal head is also apparent (white arrow). Minimal subchondral sclerosis is present.

DIFFERENTIAL DIAGNOSIS

Inflammatory arthritis (negative radiographs in early stage, soft-tissue swelling, osteopenia, subchondral erosions, and malalignment in later stages)

Metatarsal head osteomyelitis (negative radiographs in early stage; increased uptake on bone scan in later stages before radiographic changes apparent)

MTP joint synovitis syndrome (negative radiographs usually, occasional subluxation at the MTP joint as condition progresses)

MTP septic arthritis (negative radiographs in early stage, destructive changes and osteolysis consistent with infection)

Neuroma (negative radiographs, plantar pain on compression and palpation of the involved webspace)

JONES FRACTURE

ICD-9 Code

825.25
Fracture of other tarsal and metatarsal bones, closed; metatarsal bone(s)

SYNONYM
Proximal fracture of the fifth metatarsal

DEFINITION
The Jones fracture is a transverse fracture at the proximal metaphyseal-diaphyseal junction of the fifth metatarsal, typically 15 mm (3/4 inch) from the base. Jones fractures are distinct from diaphyseal stress fractures, which occur more distally, and from tuberosity avulsion fractures.

HISTORY AND PHYSICAL FINDINGS
The mechanism of injury involves an adduction force applied to the forefoot with the ankle plantar flexed. Palpation over the fifth metatarsal base will elicit pain, as will resisted eversion of the foot. Swelling and ecchymosis are typically present. In the past, Jones fractures have been mistakenly referred to as "dancer's fractures." A true dancer's fracture, which is a spiral fracture of the mid to distal shaft, occurs when a dancer is on demipoint and inverts the foot. Tenderness and swelling are more distal than with a Jones fracture.

IMAGING STUDIES

Required for diagnosis
AP, lateral, and oblique views should be obtained. A Jones fracture can be identified by its location at the metaphyseal-diaphyseal junction, 15 mm distal to the tip of the tuberosity. Fractures in more distal locations are diaphyseal stress or acute fractures.

Required for comprehensive evaluation
None

Special considerations
None

Pitfalls
None

IMAGE DESCRIPTIONS

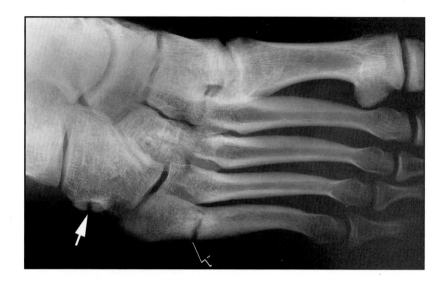

Figure 9-37

Jones fracture with bipartite os peroneum—AP view

AP view of the foot shows a transverse, incomplete fracture line with intact medial border at the metaphyseal-diaphyseal junction (black arrow), a location characteristic of a Jones fracture. A bipartite os peroneum (white arrow) is also present.

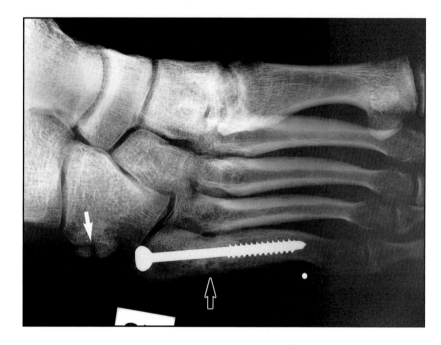

Figure 9-38

Jones fracture— AP view

AP view of the foot of the same patient in Figure 9-37 shows a Jones fracture that required open reduction and internal fixation. The fracture appears to have healed (black arrow). The bipartite os peroneum (white arrow) is seen again.

DIFFERENTIAL DIAGNOSIS

Diaphyseal stress fracture (more distal than a Jones fracture; ie, 15 to 30 mm from tip of tuberosity)

Tuberosity avulsion fracture (more proximal than a Jones fracture; metaphyseal location)

LISFRANC INJURY

SYNONYM

Tarsometatarsal fracture-dislocation

DEFINITION

The Lisfranc injury (fracture-dislocation) is a lateral dislocation of the second through fifth metatarsal bones. A fracture of the base of the second metatarsal and the cuboid may also be present. Lisfranc joint, or tarsometatarsal, injuries represent approximately 0.2% of all fractures. The tarsometatarsal articulations are referred to as the Lisfranc joint complex. The Lisfranc ligament is a stout, more plantarly based ligament that connects the base of the second metatarsal to the medial cuneiform. The Lisfranc joint complex is stabilized by the dorsally based trapezoidal shape of the metatarsal bases, particularly the recessed second metatarsal base. The first, second, and third metatarsals articulate with the corresponding cuneiforms, and the fourth and fifth metatarsal bases articulate with the cuboid. The investing capsuloligamentous structures also provide stability to this joint complex. The dorsalis pedis artery and deep peroneal nerve course between the first and second metatarsal bases and are prone to associated injury. Most (81%) of these injuries are associated with other injuries, and males are affected two to four times more often than are females. Lisfranc injuries are either missed or misdiagnosed 20% of the time.

HISTORY AND PHYSICAL FINDINGS

Injury to the Lisfranc joint complex can occur through either direct or, more frequently, indirect forces. Injury patterns are quite variable and, with an indirect injury, may be subtle. Direct injuries are often associated with fractures, soft-tissue injury, and compartment syndrome. With direct crush injuries, swelling and ecchymosis may be quite extensive; therefore, evaluation for possible neurovascular compromise is indicated. Indirect injuries result from a combination of twisting and axial loading on a plantar flexed foot. These injuries will present with more variable swelling. Plantar ecchymosis may be present. Sagittal stressing of the individual tarsometatarsal joints helps delineate the location and extent of the injury. Abduction stressing of the midfoot may also elicit symptoms, but this may be difficult in the acute setting.

IMAGING STUDIES

Required for diagnosis

AP, lateral, and internal oblique views should be obtained at the time of injury. Although weight-bearing radiographs are preferable because they allow evaluation of tarsometatarsal diastasis, these may not be possible to obtain in the acute setting. In addition, 30° and 45° internal oblique views, which better delineate the lateral tarsometatarsal joints, are recommended. The x-ray beam may be angled 10° cephalad to better visualize the tarsometatarsal joints. Normal radiographs will reveal an uninterrupted line between the medial aspect of the second metatarsal base and the middle cuneiform, as well as an uninterrupted line between the medial aspect of the fourth metatarsal base and the medial aspect of the cuboid. Additionally, the third metatarsal-lateral cuneiform articulation should be colinear. Any dorsal displacement of the metatarsal bases, as seen on the lateral view, is indicative of Lisfranc injury. More than 2 mm of space between the first and second metatarsal bases and their corresponding cuneiforms is indicative of a Lisfranc ligament tear.

Comparison views of the contralateral foot may be helpful. The "fleck sign" represents an avulsion injury of the medial aspect of the base of the second metatarsal, indicative of Lisfranc ligament tear and instability.

Required for comprehensive evaluation

If a Lisfranc injury is suspected but non–weight-bearing radiographs are negative, the foot may be immobilized for 5 to 7 days to allow for swelling to subside, at which time weight-bearing views should be obtained. Alternatively, stress views may be obtained with the patient under anesthesia.

If the patient reports persistent pain after a midfoot injury and radiographic findings are negative, further studies are indicated. MRI is the best choice because it can delineate any ligamentous or soft-tissue disruption.

Special considerations

When radiographs are normal but there is a possible injury to the Lisfranc joint complex, stress views of the midfoot with the patient under local anesthesia are indicated. If these views are negative, MRI of the midfoot should be ordered.

Pitfalls

Lisfranc injuries are frequently missed. Even minimal displacement in this area may require surgical correction. Therefore, there should be a high index of suspicion when evaluating these injuries.

SECTION 9 ■ FOOT AND ANKLE

IMAGE DESCRIPTIONS

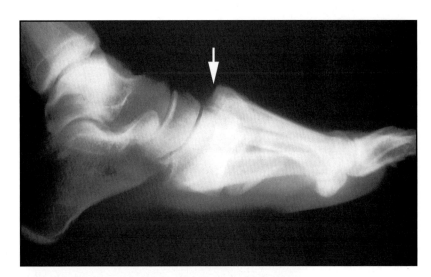

Figure 9-39

Lisfranc joint complex injury—Lateral view

Non–weight-bearing lateral view of the foot reveals dorsal displacement of the base of the first and second metatarsals (arrow), indicative of significant Lisfranc joint complex injury.

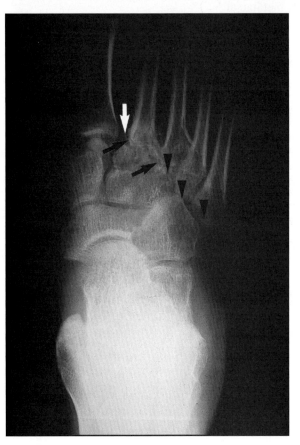

Figure 9-40

Lisfranc fracture-dislocation— AP view

AP view of the foot reveals a displaced fracture of the base of the second and third metatarsals (black arrows). Note the diastasis between the first and second tarsometatarsal joints (white arrow), as well as the lateral displacement of the metatarsal bases (arrowheads).

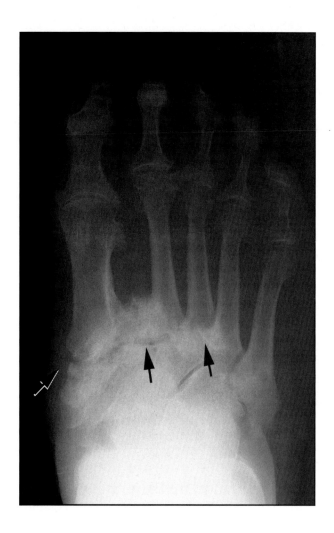

Figure 9-41

Charcot arthropathy—AP view

AP view of the foot reveals a Charcot arthropathic process of the midfoot (black arrows). This condition should be distinguished from either an acute Lisfranc complex injury or the posttraumatic sequelae of such an injury.

DIFFERENTIAL DIAGNOSIS

Charcot arthropathy of the midfoot (greater bony destruction, peripheral neuropathy, absence of antecedent trauma)

Metatarsal fracture (local tenderness over the metatarsal, positive radiographs)

Midfoot arthritis (chronic pain and tenderness in the midfoot, no history of recent injury)

Navicular fracture (local tenderness over the navicular, positive radiographs)

SECTION 9 ■ FOOT AND ANKLE

Osteochondral Lesions of the Talus

ICD-9 Code

733.44
Aseptic necrosis of bone,
talus

Synonyms

Osteochondral fracture
Osteochondritis dissecans (OCD)

Definition

Osteochondral lesions of the talus are intra-articular injuries to the dome of the talus involving the articular cartilage and the underlying subchondral bone. Most cases are caused by trauma, but osteonecrosis is sometimes responsible, and some cases are idiopathic. Medial lesions, which are more common than lateral lesions, tend to be posterior, nondisplaced, and cup-shaped. Lateral lesions tend to be anterior and are generally more shallow, wafer-shaped, displaced, and associated with trauma. Mechanisms of injury for medial lesions involve impaction of the talus into the tibial plafond/medial malleolus during an inversion/external rotation force while the foot is plantar flexed. With lateral lesions, the talus is impacted into the fibula during an inversion/dorsiflexion force to the ankle.

History and Physical Findings

Symptoms include pain, swelling that may be intermittent, possible catching, decreased range of motion, and stiffness. A history of repetitive sprains or trauma is common. Medial or lateral joint tenderness may localize the lesion.

Imaging Studies

Required for diagnosis

Initial radiographs should include AP, lateral, and mortise views of the involved ankle. Findings can be subtle; positioning the ankle in varying degrees of plantar flexion and dorsiflexion may bring the posteromedial and anterolateral lesions, respectively, into better view. Berndt and Hardy classified these lesions into four radiographic stages (Table 1).

Table 1	
Classification of Osteochondritis Dissecans Based on Radiographic Results	
Stage	**Description**
I	Small area of subchondral compression
II	Partially detached fragment
III	Completely detached fragment remaining within the crater, nondisplaced
IV	Completely detached fragment displaced out of the crater

Required for comprehensive evaluation

If a lesion is visible on the radiographs, CT is recommended for staging the lesion. Ferkel and Sgaglione developed a CT staging classification for osteochondral lesions of the talus (Table 2).

Table 2	
Classification of Osteochondritis Dissecans Based on Computed Tomography Results	
Stage	**Description**
I	Cystic lesion within dome of talus, intact roof on all views
IIA	Cystic lesion with communication to talar dome surface
IIB	Open articular surface lesion with overlying nondisplaced fragment
III	Nondisplaced lesion with lucency
IV	Displaced fragment

If the lesion is not visible on radiographs, MRI is recommended because of its increased sensitivity for overall pathology and ability to assess the soft-tissue structures around the ankle. In addition, MRI can accurately determine lesion stability and extent of talar dome involvement. Anderson and associates have proposed a classification system based on MRI results (Table 3).

Table 3	
Classification of Osteochondritis Dissecans Based on Magnetic Resonance Imaging Results	
Stage	**Description**
I	Subchondral trabecular compression; plain radiographs normal, positive bone scan; marrow edema on MRI
IIA	Formation of subchondral cyst
II	Incomplete separation of fragment
III	Unattached, nondisplaced fragment with synovial fluid around fragment
IV	Displaced fragment

Special considerations
None

Pitfalls
None

IMAGE DESCRIPTIONS

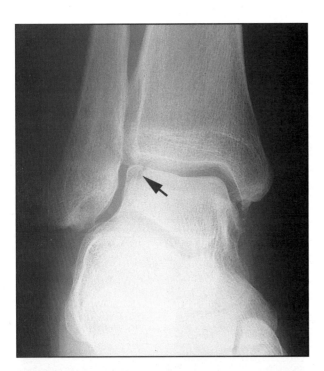

Figure 9-42

Osteochondral lesion of the talus— Mortise view

Mortise view of the ankle reveals a subchondral lucency in the lateral talar dome (arrow).

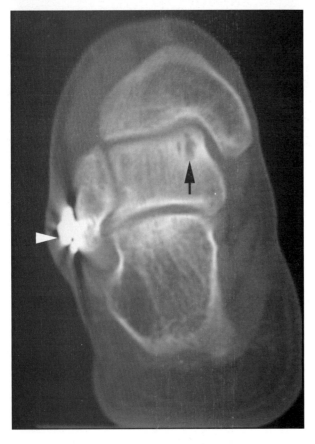

Figure 9-43

Osteochondral lesion of the talus— Coronal CT

Coronal CT scan of the ankle and subtalar joint reveals a lytic lesion beneath the dome of the medial talus (arrow) with surrounding sclerosis. Metallic artifact is noted on the lateral fibula (arrowhead).

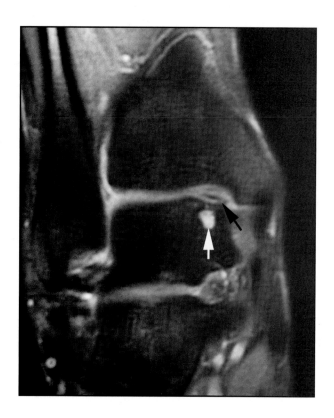

Figure 9-44

Osteochondral lesion of the talus—Coronal MRI

Coronal gradient echo MRI scan shows high signal intensity at the interface of the osteochondral defect with the talus (black arrow). The cyst underneath the defect (white arrow) makes this lesion more unstable.

DIFFERENTIAL DIAGNOSIS

Bone bruise (edema seen on MRI; resolves within 6 months)

Chondral avulsion (cartilage separation from underlying subchondral bone with no bone involvement seen on MRI)

Chronic ankle sprain (ligament pathology seen on MRI)

SECTION 9 ■ FOOT AND ANKLE

STRESS FRACTURES OF THE FOOT

ICD-9 Codes

733.94
Stress fracture of the metatarsals

733.95
Stress fracture of other bone

SYNONYMS

Fatigue fracture
Insufficiency fracture
March fracture

DEFINITION

A stress fracture is caused by repetitive stress that creates strain within the bone, exceeding its local strength and causing microfractures. Theoretically, stress fractures can occur in any bone, but they are seen most often in weight-bearing bones. The femur and tibia and the bones of the ankle and foot can be subject to high stress during repetitive activity. Within the foot and ankle, the calcaneus, navicular, and metatarsals are involved most often. The incidence of stress fractures is virtually identical in males and females. Most patients are young and have a history consistent with activity- or exercise-related pain. The diagnosis of stress fractures can be challenging because initial radiographs are often negative. This can necessitate further imaging.

HISTORY AND PHYSICAL FINDINGS

Most patients have a history of weight-bearing physical activity. On examination, discrete tenderness over the area of pain is common. Pain is associated with activity and relieved by rest. Risk factors include a rapid increase in exercise time or intensity, decreased lower extremity strength, low bone density, change in shoe wear, and a history of menstrual disturbances. One exception is stress fractures in the second metatarsal. Studies have shown that normal walking causes high stress in the second metatarsal. Therefore, a stress fracture may develop in the second metatarsal without a history of intense physical activity.

A bone developing a stress fracture undergoes a cycle of fracture progression and repair. Bone that is subjected to repetitive strain attempts to strengthen itself by remodeling, which involves bone resorption followed by bone formation. If high strain continues during the resorption phase, the microdamage in the bone may progress to a stress fracture. Stress fractures can progress to bicortical fractures if the stress continues.

IMAGING STUDIES

Required for diagnosis

AP, lateral, and oblique views of the involved bone should comprise the initial evaluation. Radiographic appearance is variable, depending on the stage of the process. Radiographs are often taken during the office visit when a stress fracture is initially suspected. These radiographs are often normal if the onset of symptoms is recent. In addition, when radiographic changes are present, they are often subtle and difficult to identify. Radiographic changes may reveal trabecular sclerosis, periostitis, cortical thickening, or cortical defects. If confusion exists as to whether a radiograph is abnormal, a contralateral comparison view should be ordered to help with the diagnosis.

Required for comprehensive evaluation

If further imaging is necessary, a technetium Tc 99m bone scan, MRI, or CT may be beneficial. When ordering radiographs, the physician should specify that a stress fracture is suspected and indicate its presumed location.

A bone scan will show increased uptake at the area of the stress fracture; this remains the secondary imaging study of choice according to most authors. Bone scanning also allows assessment of other osseous structures that may be under stress. The disadvantage of bone scans is that they expose the patient to increased radiation. However, it should be noted that the amount of radiation delivered during a single bone scan has not been shown to be hazardous. Bone scans have low specificity; ie, other conditions that involve increased blood flow, such as tumors, will also show increased uptake.

MRI is becoming more popular in the diagnosis of stress fractures. The primary finding of a stress fracture on MRI is marrow edema, which manifests as low signal intensity on T1-weighted images and high signal intensity on T2-weighted images. Occasionally, a fracture line is seen, confirming the diagnosis. At other times, as with bone scanning, MRI has low specificity because many conditions can cause marrow edema. However, in conjunction with a good clinical examination in which the findings are consistent with a stress fractures, MRI can be extremely helpful. A limited-sequence MRI study consisting of only T1- and T2-weighted images can be done quickly and at a relatively low cost. Whether MRI should supplant the traditionally preferred bone scan is subject to debate. Either study can be beneficial, but the bone scan costs substantially less. Consider discussing with the radiologist which study he or she prefers.

CT is rarely used for stress fractures. The most common use is for midfoot tarsal stress fracture (ie, navicular fracture) evaluation because these fractures are often sagittally oriented and are best demonstrated on coronal CT scans. CT can also be useful to evaluate healing of a stress fracture following treatment.

Special considerations

If symptoms are mild, repeat radiographs can be obtained 1 to 2 weeks later, at which time they will often reveal early callus, indicative of fracture healing.

Pitfalls

Stress fractures are often missed on initial radiographs. A clinical picture that includes persistent pain and swelling, especially on weight bearing, and a high level of suspicion for stress fracture are key in establishing the diagnosis. Sclerosis of a weight-bearing bone in a young, physically active patient is assumed to be a stress fracture until proven otherwise. Occasionally, a stress fracture may appear aggressive, with sclerosis and periostitis prevailing. The fracture may even be mistaken for a tumor and a biopsy performed. MRI is the best study to evaluate for a tumor.

IMAGE DESCRIPTIONS

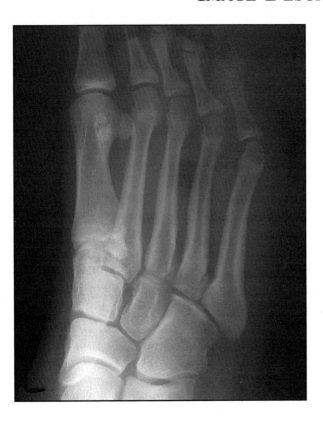

Figure 9-45

Stress fracture of the metatarsal (early)—Medial oblique view

AP view of the foot in a patient who reported a 2-day history of pain in the second metatarsal does not show an obvious fracture.

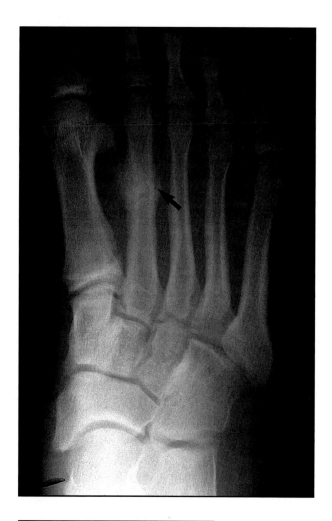

Figure 9-46

Stress fracture of the metatarsal (late)—AP view

AP view of the same patient in Figure 9-45 3 weeks later shows callus formation at the site of the stress fracture (black arrow).

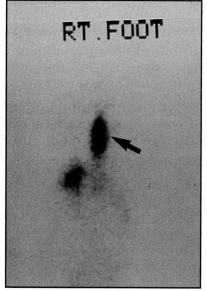

Figure 9-47

Stress fracture of the metatarsal (early)—Bone scan

Bone scan of the same patient taken 1 week after the initial onset of pain but before Figure 9-45 was obtained shows increased uptake at the fracture site (black arrow).

SECTION 9 ■ FOOT AND ANKLE

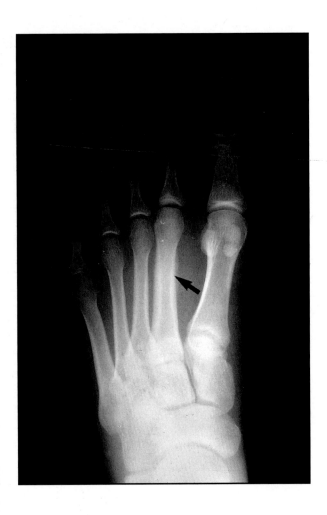

Figure 9-48

*Stress fracture of the
metatarsal—AP view*

AP view of a stress fracture of the second
metatarsal shows sclerosis and periosteal
reaction at the fracture site (black arrow).

DIFFERENTIAL DIAGNOSIS

Foot sprain (normal radiographs, even at 2 to 3 weeks; negative
bone scan)

Osteomyelitis (fever)

Neoplasm (pain persists despite rest)

GOUT

SYNONYM

Podagra (MTP joint of the great toe)

DEFINITION

Gout is a metabolic disorder of purine metabolism resulting in hyperuricemia and deposition of monosodium urate crystals into a variety of locations throughout the body. Joint cartilage is especially affected. Gout is characterized by the intra-articular presence of these crystals, which are needle-shaped and negatively birefringent (doubly refractive) under a polarizing microscope.

Gout more commonly affects men than women, and presenting symptoms typically include an acute arthritis or periarticular inflammatory reaction of the great toe metatarsophalangeal (MTP) joint. This joint is involved in 75% of initial episodes of gout and is ultimately affected in 90% of patients who have gout. Recurrent episodes of arthritis in the lower extremity are common in men between 40 and 60 years of age. Extra-articular manifestations develop as crystalline deposits, called tophi, which commonly occur in the ear helix, eyelid, olecranon, Achilles tendon, and kidneys.

HISTORY AND PHYSICAL FINDINGS

Hallmark signs and symptoms include acute, severe pain, swelling, erythema, and warmth about the involved joint that typically last for several days before subsiding. Physical examination and analysis of the crystals obtained from joint aspirate will confirm the diagnosis. Patients with gout often seek medical attention during or after the first episode because of the severe pain. Diagnosis, followed by medical management with allopurinol, often will prevent subsequent episodes and eventual development of gouty arthropathy. Serum uric acid levels and radiographs are often normal during the early stages of the disease.

Differentiating gout from a septic or infected joint may create confusion in the workup and diagnosis. If a septic joint is suspected, a CBC, erythrocyte sedimentation rate, and C-reactive protein should be obtained in conjunction with uric acid levels. If the joint aspirate appears cloudy (a sign of septic arthritis), Gram stain and culture, WBC with neutrophil count, acid-fast bacteria, and crystal analysis are necessary.

ICD–9 Codes

274.0
Gouty arthropathy

274.10
Gouty nephropathy, unspecified

274.81
Gouty tophi of ear

274.82
Gouty tophi of other sites

274.9
Gout, unspecified

SECTION 9 ■ FOOT AND ANKLE

IMAGING STUDIES

Required for diagnosis
Gout is a clinical diagnosis; therefore, imaging studies are not required for an initial episode, particularly when the MTP joint of the great toe is affected. Episodes in other joints, such as the knee, chronic involvement, or an atypical presentation warrant AP and lateral views of the affected areas. Additional imaging studies are seldom necessary.

Required for comprehensive evaluation
Radiographs are often normal, especially early in the disease. Only after 4 to 6 years of chronic gout will radiographic signs of the disease develop. At this time, the arthropathy caused by gout is very characteristic. Classic radiographic findings include well-defined erosions, often with sclerotic margins or overhanging edges. For long-standing disease or advanced stages, these erosions can be very deforming.

Special considerations
CT is usually not necessary unless advanced arthropathy is present. When warranted, however, CT further visualizes the articular surfaces and evaluates the extent of the bony erosions.

Pitfalls
A painful, swollen joint due to gout can mimic a septic joint, which can lead to unnecessary testing. Joint aspiration remains the gold standard in diagnosing gout. Additional imaging studies such as MRI and bone scanning are usually not necessary.

IMAGE DESCRIPTIONS

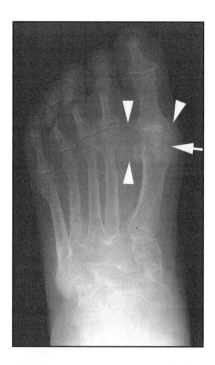

Figure 9-49

Gout (MTP joint of the great toe)—AP view

AP view of the foot shows erosions with sharp margins and an overhanging edge in the distal medial first metatarsal head (arrow). Note that the central joint space is not narrowed or compromised. There is a soft-tissue mass around the first metatarsal consistent with a tophus (arrowheads). A lateral view will further delineate the size and location of the erosion.

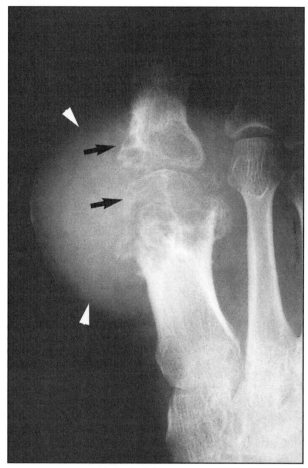

Figure 9-50

Gout (MTP joint of the great toe)—AP view

AP view of the great toe shows marked soft-tissue swelling throughout the MTP joint and destructive, large, well-marginated erosions on both sides of the joint (arrows). These findings are consistent with advanced gout. There is a large soft-tissue tophus (arrowheads). The focal areas of soft-tissue swelling are called tophi, some of which are calcified.

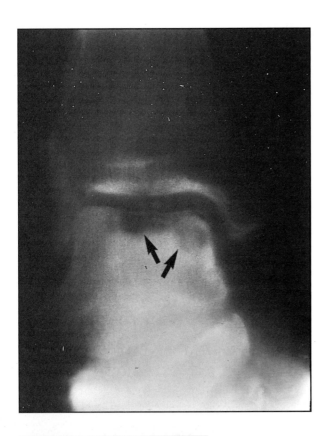

Figure 9-51

Gout (talus)—AP view

AP view of the ankle of a patient with chronic tophaceous gout shows several lytic lesions in the talar dome (arrows) with surrounding sclerosis. This could be caused by either an intraosseous uric acid deposit or a bony infarct. Biopsy at the time of surgery confirmed an intraosseous uric acid deposit.

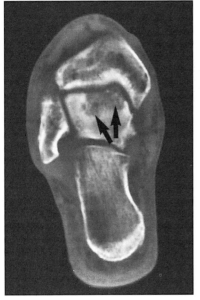

Figure 9-52

Gout (talus)—Coronal CT

Coronal CT scan of the same patient shown in Figure 9-51 shows sharply marginated erosions of the talus (arrows). The joint space is preserved despite the presence of these well-marginated erosions, a finding often seen in gout.

DIFFERENTIAL DIAGNOSIS

Osteoarthritis (decreased joint space, subchondral sclerosis)

Psoriasis (diffusely swollen toe with periostitis, may have toenail and skin changes)

Rheumatoid arthritis (periarticular erosions)

Septic arthritis (normal radiographs, possible metaphyseal abscesses)

OSTEOARTHRITIS

SYNONYMS

Degenerative joint disease
Hallux rigidus
OA
Primary/secondary arthritis
Traumatic arthritis

DEFINITION

Osteoarthritis (OA) is a noninflammatory degenerative joint disease that is characterized by articular cartilage degradation, subchondral sclerosis, osteophyte formation, and changes in the surrounding soft tissues. By the year 2020, OA is expected to affect nearly 60 million people in the United States. Women are approximately twice as likely to have OA as men. The pattern of joint involvement differs by sex, with women having a greater number of joints involved and more frequent complaints of morning stiffness, joint swelling, and night pain than men. More than 80% of patients older than 75 years of age report symptoms of OA.

OA most commonly affects weight-bearing joints such as the foot and ankle. After the age of 55 years, prevalence increases dramatically, especially with OA of the knee. Evidence has shown that the risk of knee and hip OA is lower than expected in postmenopausal women on estrogen replacement therapy. Posttraumatic arthritis is common in the foot and ankle after injuries and fractures. Altered mechanics in a single joint of the foot can cause increased stress and subsequent OA in adjacent joints in that foot.

HISTORY AND PHYSICAL FINDINGS

Despite the prevalence of OA, a complete understanding of its etiology, pathogenesis, and progression is elusive. It typically involves the articular joint surfaces, and its effects are evident throughout the entire synovial joint. Loss of motion and pain with motion and weight bearing are the principal symptoms. Joint space narrowing typically limits range of motion. Risk factors include age, sex, genetic predisposition, mechanical stress or trauma, and obesity. Disease progression varies, with no distinct correlation between findings on imaging studies and progression or clinical severity. Some patients have long-standing disease with mild symptoms, but others have severe symptoms with minimal evidence of clinical and radiographic disease.

ICD–9 Codes

715.1
Osteoarthrosis, localized, primary

715.2
Osteoarthrosis, localized, secondary

715.3
Osteoarthrosis, localized, not specified whether primary or secondary

715.37
Osteoarthrosis, localized, not specified whether primary or secondary; involving ankle and foot

715.8
Osteoarthrosis involving, or with mention of more than one site, but not specified as generalized

SECTION 9 ■ FOOT AND ANKLE

IMAGING STUDIES

Required for diagnosis

OA is diagnosed with weight-bearing AP and lateral views of the affected joint. These views will show complete involvement in two different planes. Hallmark radiographic features are joint space narrowing, sclerosis, and formation of osteophytes. All three features should be present on radiographs to make the diagnosis; if they are not, another diagnosis should be considered. Subchondral cysts are seen in later stages of the disease. In addition, the pathologic manifestations seen on radiographs should be confined to the involved joint spaces. No periarticular involvement surrounding the joint space should be noted.

Required for comprehensive evaluation

Comprehensive evaluation with a variety of imaging studies is rarely warranted. With evidence of diffuse sclerosis and joint space collapse, MRI may be warranted to evaluate for osteonecrosis. The history should delineate a prior traumatic event that may have led to the development of OA.

Special considerations

Additional imaging studies are rarely indicated. Following nonsurgical treatment of intra-articular fractures, CT will evaluate the congruity of the articular surface.

Pitfalls

In the foot and ankle, weight-bearing radiographs are required to simulate loading the respective joints in an attempt to identify joint collapse. Without weight-bearing radiographs, the amount of joint surface involvement is often underestimated.

IMAGE DESCRIPTIONS

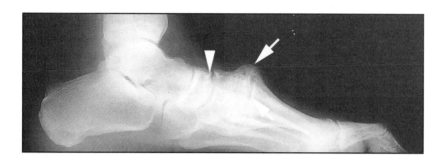

Figure 9-53

Osteoarthritis (foot)— Lateral view

Weight-bearing lateral view of the foot shows a dorsal osteophyte with joint space narrowing of the first tarsometatarsal joint (white arrow). This view illustrates a dorsal osteophyte, which is often not appreciated on an AP view. Early osteophytes are also seen dorsally at the naviculocuneiform joint (arrowhead).

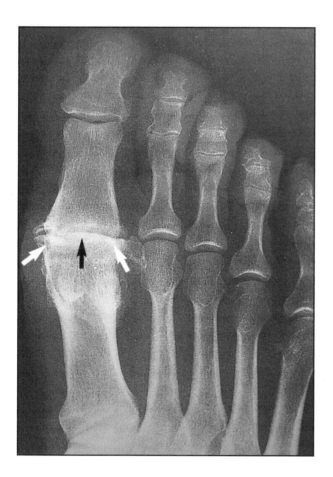

Figure 9-54

Hallux rigidus (MTP joint of the great toe)—AP view

Weight-bearing AP view of the forefoot shows hallux rigidus (or OA) of the MTP joint of the great toe. Note the joint space narrowing (black arrow), subchondral sclerosis, and medial and lateral osteophytes (white arrows).

SECTION 9 ■ FOOT AND ANKLE

DIFFERENTIAL DIAGNOSIS

Diffuse idiopathic skeletal hyperostosis (DISH) (osteophytes; no sclerosis or joint space narrowing; often ankylosis or joint autofusions)

Rheumatoid arthritis (periarticular erosions)

Psoriatic Arthritis

Synonyms
Inflammatory arthritis
Psoriasis
Seronegative spondyloarthropathy

ICD-9 Code
696.0
Psoriatic arthropathy

Definition
Psoriasis is an inflammatory arthritis or seronegative spondyloarthropathy that primarily involves the skin, with occasional psoriatic arthropathy. By definition, a seronegative spondyloarthropathy is characterized by a positive HLA-B27 locus and a negative rheumatoid factor.

Psoriasis generally affects younger patients, but sex is not a factor. Joint involvement is usually asymmetric, with distal joints such as the distal interphalangeal (DIP) joints of the hands and feet most commonly affected. Other manifestations involve the skin and include epidermal hyperplasia, pustules, and plaque formation. In severe cases, systemic symptoms such as fever and arthralgias can occur. More than 50% of patients have nail deformities such as pitting, primarily in the fingernails. Between 5% and 10% of patients have joint manifestations.

History and Physical Findings
Joint involvement produces pain and usually develops after the onset of cutaneous lesions. As the inflammatory condition progresses, symptoms worsen. Pain and limited activity are the most common symptoms. Physical examination will reveal a cutaneous rash, nail pitting, and swelling of the digits (sausage digits). Laboratory tests to evaluate for the HLA-B27 antigen and rheumatoid factor (negative in psoriasis) are necessary to confirm the diagnosis. Radiographs are the best way to confirm psoriatic arthropathy.

Imaging Studies

Required for diagnosis
A weight-bearing AP view of the forefoot will reveal the characteristic "pencil-in-cup" deformity of the distal joint, usually the DIP joint. This deformity appears as a rounded distal middle phalanx lodging into a distal phalanx with loss of joint space. The unique fit involves the full articular surface. Multiple joint involvement in the same foot can result in severe erosive

destructive changes, called arthritis mutilans. Corresponding nail pathology is often present.

Weight-bearing AP and lateral views of the involved joint will evaluate the joint space and the congruity of the bones, as well as the symmetry of involvement.

Required for comprehensive evaluation

Additional imaging studies are rarely indicated. However, MRI is occasionally needed when evaluating for refractory tendon inflammation (tenosynovitis), which can lead to destructive changes in the soft-tissue structures.

Special considerations

None

Pitfalls

With a painful, swollen digit, radiographs should be obtained prior to ordering a bone scan or MRI because the characteristic findings of psoriatic arthritis may negate the need for further tests.

IMAGE DESCRIPTIONS

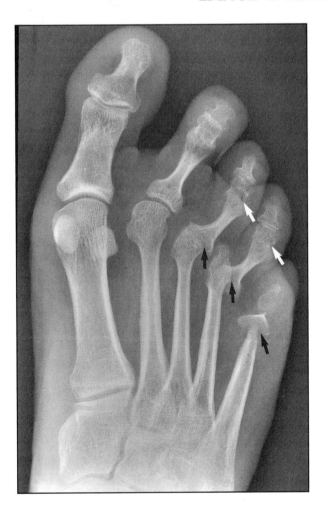

Figure 9-55

Psoriatic arthritis (metatarsals)— AP view

In this patient, psoriatic arthritis has progressed to a chronic destructive arthritis (black arrows), producing arthritis mutilans. Erosions at the proximal interphalangeal joints of the third and fourth metacarpals (white arrows) indicate significant involvement of the toes.

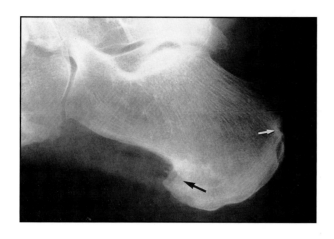

Figure 9-56

Psoriatic arthritis (calcaneus)— Lateral view

Lateral view of the foot shows plantar erosion (black arrow) and erosion of the posterior calcaneus (white arrow) in the region of the retrocalcaneal bursa. With psoriasis, chronic inflammation of the tendons, fascia, and retrocalcaneal bursa produce characteristic erosions seen here.

DIFFERENTIAL DIAGNOSIS

Osteoarthritis (joint space narrowing, osteophytes, subchondral sclerosis)

Reiter's syndrome (also called reactive arthritis; similar clinically, involves weight-bearing joints, urethritis, conjunctivitis)

Rheumatoid arthritis (periarticular erosions, positive rheumatoid factor)

Severe hallux valgus (bunion) (angular deformity at the first metatarsophalangeal joint, increased intermetatarsal angle between the first and second metatarsals)

RHEUMATOID ARTHRITIS

SYNONYMS

Inflammatory arthritis
RA

DEFINITION

Rheumatoid arthritis (RA) is the most common form of inflammatory arthritis, affecting approximately 1% of men and 3% of women. The prevalence increases with advancing age. The hallmark features include symmetric polyarthritis with joint swelling, tenderness, and morning stiffness that lasts for more than 1 hour. RA can affect any joint, but it is usually found in the metacarpophalangeal (MCP), proximal interphalangeal (PIP), and metatarsophalangeal (MTP) joints, with the wrist and knee joints also potentially involved. Foot and ankle involvement also is very common.

Despite intensive research efforts, the cause of RA is unknown. It has been viewed as an autoimmune disease from an unknown antigen. A viral etiology also has been hypothesized. In general, it is a connective tissue disorder that can affect any synovial-lined joint in the body. Inflammatory mediators initiate a destructive cascade that leads to joint space destruction.

HISTORY AND PHYSICAL FINDINGS

The natural history of the disease is believed to follow the exposure of genetically susceptible individuals to an unknown environmental agent with an autoimmune response. Symptoms correlate with the duration of the disease. Nearly one third of patients have a moderate or severe hallux valgus (bunion) deformity. The lesser toes are affected in nearly 50% of patients with long-standing disease. These processes often occur in tandem. As the great toe deforms, the lesser MTP joints dislocate dorsally. Symptoms tend to be progressive, with intermittent and variable remissions. The most common reported symptom in the forefoot is metatarsalgia, or pain underlying the metatarsal heads with ambulation or pressure.

Workup includes analysis of rheumatoid factor in the blood. Radiographs are helpful to evaluate musculoskeletal manifestations of the disease. Hallmark findings on radiographs include soft-tissue swelling, osteoporosis, joint space narrowing, and marginal (periarticular) erosions.

IMAGING STUDIES

Required for diagnosis

Radiographic evidence of RA varies widely and thus can be difficult to diagnose with any degree of certainty. Osteoporosis, joint space narrowing, marginal erosions, and soft-tissue swelling are often present but are nonspecific findings. The most specific radiographic evidence is the marginal or periarticular erosions. Unfortunately, erosions are not seen on every radiograph in every patient with RA who has musculoskeletal complaints. Thus, laboratory studies and clinical evaluation confirm the diagnosis.

RA in the foot and ankle is characterized by a significant bunion deformity at the great toe with a variable amount of degenerative arthritis. The synovitis involving the MTP joints of the lesser toes leads to plate destruction with dorsal joint dislocation. The lesser toes often develop rigid hammering, which makes shoe wear difficult. These characteristics are often easily identified on weight-bearing AP and lateral views of the forefoot. Early erosive changes and synovitis can also be assessed with MRI.

Required for comprehensive evaluation

Additional imaging studies often are not needed. Severe soft-tissue involvement may warrant MRI to evaluate the destruction but usually only in patients with chronic disease.

Special considerations

None

Pitfalls

Patients whose clinical picture and radiographs suggest RA should be diagnosed based on radiographs. Weight-bearing radiographs are necessary to accurately evaluate malalignment.

SECTION 9 ■ FOOT AND ANKLE

IMAGE DESCRIPTIONS

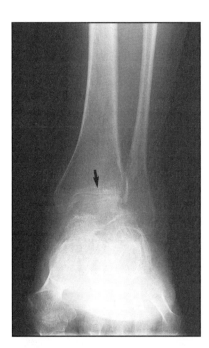

Figure 9-57

Rheumatoid arthritis (foot and ankle)—AP view

This AP view of the ankle demonstrates uniform narrowing of the tibiotalar joint (black arrow), typical of long-standing RA.

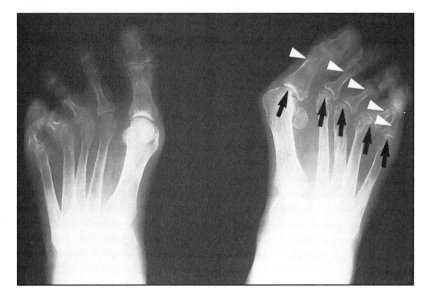

Figure 9-58

Rheumatoid arthritis (forefoot)—AP view

AP view of both feet in a patient with RA shows severe fibular deviation of the toes (white arrowheads) in both feet but notably worse in the right foot. Note also the narrowing of all MTP joints in the right foot (black arrows).

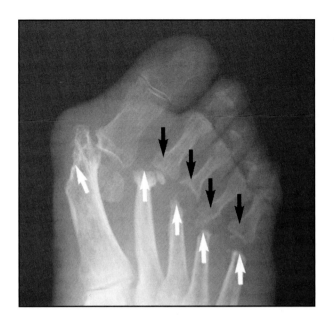

Figure 9-59

Rheumatoid arthritis (forefoot)—AP view

AP view of the forefoot in a patient with RA shows significant fibular drift of the toes (black arrows). Resection of the metatarsal heads (white arrows) was performed to correct the malalignment and to relieve pain.

DIFFERENTIAL DIAGNOSIS

Posttraumatic arthritis (history of trauma; joint space narrowing, osteophyte formation, subchondral sclerosis on radiographs)

Seronegative spondyloarthropathies (enthesopathies on radiographs, especially at the insertion of the plantar fascia and Achilles tendon)

SECTION 9 ■ FOOT AND ANKLE

ACHILLES TENDINITIS

ICD-9 Codes

726.71
Achilles bursitis or tendinitis

727.82
Calcium deposits in tendon and bursa

SYNONYMS

Achilles tendinosis
Calcific insertional Achilles tendinitis
Insertional Achilles tendinitis

DEFINITION

Achilles tendinitis is characterized by pain in the area where the Achilles tendon inserts on the calcaneus and can occur with or without calcification. Changes within the tendon are thought to result from chronic strain and inflammation. Fibrovascular degeneration and reparative fibrous stroma form within and around the tendon, causing a thickening in the posterior heel. Heterotopic calcification can result from chronic inflammation.

HISTORY AND PHYSICAL FINDINGS

Patients report a gradual onset of pain in the area where the Achilles tendon inserts on the calcaneus. Pain and inflammation increase with activity. Physical examination reveals a palpable thickening of the tendon. Often there is bony enlargement and periostitis at the posterior tuberosity, where the Achilles tendon inserts on the calcaneus. Examination must differentiate Achilles tendinitis from retrocalcaneal bursitis, pre-Achilles bursitis, chronic degeneration/tear of the tendon, and acute Achilles tendon tear. After the clinical diagnosis is made, appropriate tests and treatment can be ordered.

IMAGING STUDIES

Required for diagnosis
The diagnosis is clinical; therefore, imaging studies are not required to make the diagnosis.

Required for comprehensive evaluation
A lateral view is needed to evaluate the size of the posterior superior aspect of the calcaneus (Haglund's process) and/or the presence of insertional spurs or calcification. Other radiographic changes may include bony enlargement or cystic changes in the calcaneus secondary to chronic inflammation.

MRI will demonstrate the zone of injury of the Achilles tendon and any associated bursitis. Often partial tearing of the anterior surface of the Achilles tendon, where it makes contact with the calcaneus, may be seen. With MRI, the normal Achilles tendon appears with low signal intensity. On axial images, it appears as a plump, semilunar structure with a convex posterior contour and rounded margins on the medial and lateral sides. It is flattened or concave on the anterior margin. With tendinitis, the tendon increases in width and may demonstrate abnormal signal intensity.

Special considerations

Ultrasound can detect cystic changes and partial tears of the Achilles tendon.

Pitfalls

The quality of an ultrasound depends on the accuracy and skill of the technician. For MRI, positioning of the foot is important.

IMAGE DESCRIPTION

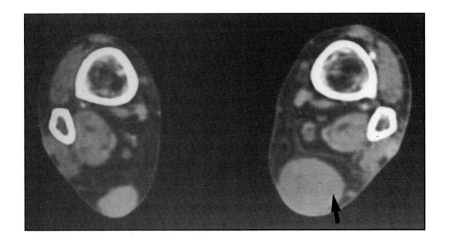

Figure 9-60

Achilles tendinitis—Axial CT

Axial CT scan of the distal tibia of both legs shows marked thickening of the Achilles tendon of the right leg (black arrow), compared with the left. No tear is noted in this view, although sequential images are necessary to rule out a tear and the zone of tendinosis.

DIFFERENTIAL DIAGNOSIS

Achilles tendon tear (palpable gap, weak or absent plantar flexion, probable history of "pop" or acute onset)

Medial gastrocnemius tear (proximal partial tear of the muscle and fascia of medial head of the gastrocnemius muscle) (pain located more proximally)

Retrocalcaneal bursitis (pain on palpation anterior to the Achilles tendon)

ANKLE INSTABILITY

ICD-9 Codes

718.87
Other joint derangement not elsewhere classified; ankle and foot

845.00
Sprains and strains of ankle; unspecified site

SYNONYMS

Acute ankle instability
Chronic ankle instability
Loose ankles
Sprained ankle
Strained ankle

DEFINITION

The term ankle instability includes a spectrum of conditions involving the dysfunction of the medial and lateral collateral ligaments of the ankle. Dysfunction of the medial collateral ligament (also called the deltoid ligament) is unusual and is generally associated with fractures. Deltoid ligaments are injured or ruptured during high ankle sprains. In these injuries, as the foot pronates and is subjected to an external rotation force (pronation-external rotation [PE] type injury), the deltoid ligament ruptures, followed by rupture of the anterior tibiofibular ligament and fracture of the midshaft of the fibula.

In contrast, lateral collateral ligament dysfunction is extremely common. Known to all of us as a "sprained" ankle, this injury is ubiquitous. The daily incidence of ankle sprains is estimated to be one out of every 10,000 people. This injury involves various degrees of tearing of the anterior talofibular ligament and the calcaneofibular ligament.

Several systems of grading ankle sprains are based on the magnitude of injury to these two ligaments. The grade of ankle sprain correlates with the recovery rate and with overall functional outcome. Late ankle instability can occur in the face of incompetent ligaments (mechanical instability) or in the face of normal ligamentous restraint (functional instability). Advanced diagnostic testing is frequently required to assess chronic injury and to develop an effective treatment plan.

HISTORY AND PHYSICAL FINDINGS

Ankle instability is invariably caused by trauma. Patients usually report an incident involving a twisting and rotational mechanism. The force and mechanism of the injury dictate whether a ligament ruptures or a fracture occurs. The mechanism of injury also helps differentiate a lateral ligament sprain from a high ankle sprain, in which the syndesmosis is injured. Internal rotation often results in an injury to the lateral collateral ligaments, whereas external rotation may result in an injury to the medial collateral ligaments and/or syndesmotic disruption.

Physical examination usually reveals pain and tenderness over the injured structures. It is important to differentiate pain over the anterior talofibular, calcaneofibular, deltoid, and syndesmotic ligaments. Tenderness over the deltoid ligament and pain with abduction of the dorsiflexed ankle while squeezing the distal tibiofibular joint indicates a high ankle sprain. This is in contrast to tenderness over the lateral collateral ligaments found in the more common lateral ankle sprain.

Clinical and radiographic stress tests are difficult to perform in the acute setting but can be useful in establishing a more accurate diagnosis. A positive anterior drawer test is often associated with an injury to the anterior talofibular ligament, while a varus tilt greater than the contralateral side may indicate an injury to the calcaneofibular ligament. Stress tests, both clinical and radiographic, do not affect the treatment plan in the acute setting but are useful in assessing chronic mechanical instability.

IMAGING STUDIES

Required for diagnosis

The diagnosis can be made by history and physical findings, but imaging studies are required as part of a comprehensive evaluation to rule out the presence of fracture.

Required for comprehensive evaluation

A weight-bearing AP radiograph of the ankle and a mortise view are necessary to reveal possible diastasis of the syndesmosis. Examination of the clear space between the tibia and fibula and the overlap of the tibia and fibula is necessary to properly evaluate a possible injury to the syndesmosis.

The clear space is measured between the medial border of the fibula and the lateral border of the posterior tibia as shown in the figure below. This measurement is made 1 cm above the plafond and should not exceed 5 mm on AP and mortise views of the ankle. The overlap of the fibula and the anterior tibial tubercle should be approximately 42% of the width of the fibula on AP views of the ankle.

If there is still doubt about a syndesmosis injury, an external rotation stress view can be ordered; with this view, local anesthesia may be necessary.

MRI is the best choice to evaluate occult injuries such as an osteochondral defect or fracture and injury to the posterior tibial tendon or flexor hallucis longus tendon. Although it is not useful in evaluating ankle instability, MRI is helpful in assessing chronic pain after an ankle sprain.

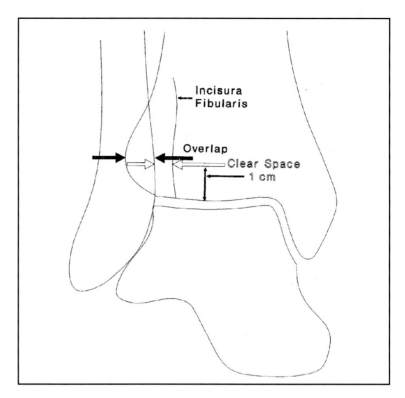

Normal syndesmotic relationships. The tibiofibular clear space between the hollow arrows, 1 cm above the tibial plafond, should be less than 6 mm. The tibiofibular overlap on this simulated anteroposterior view (solid arrows) should be greater than 6 mm or 42% of the fibular width and greater than 1 mm on the mortise view. (Reproduced from Lutter LD, Mizel MS, Pfeffer GB (eds): *Orthopaedic Knowledge Update: Foot and Ankle.* Rosemont, IL, American Academy of Orthopaedic Surgeons, 1994, pp 241-253.)

Stress radiographs are useful for evaluating chronic ankle instability but are not recommended in the acute setting. A positive anterior drawer test (> 5 mm anterior translation) and talar tilt test (> 5° variance from the contralateral side) are indicative of mechanical instability of the ankle. It should be kept in mind, however, that because the medial structures remain intact and the lateral structures are torn or attenuated, the instability pattern is actually an anterolateral rotatory instability. Each stress view of the ankle visualizes one component of the rotatory instability pattern seen in ankles with chronic ankle instability.

CT and MRI scans are helpful in assessing a diastasis of the syndesmosis. A bone scan is helpful in evaluating occult fractures of the ankle after an ankle sprain and in the workup of chronic ankle pain. If the bone scan is positive, follow-up CT can better visualize bone architecture. If the bone scan is negative, follow-up MRI better evaluates potential soft-tissue injury.

Special considerations
None

Pitfalls
Injuries to the syndesmosis are often missed; therefore, careful evaluation, as described above, is critical.

IMAGE DESCRIPTIONS

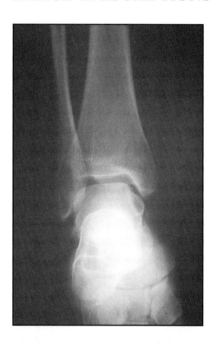

Figure 9-61

Ankle instability—AP view, unstressed

Ankle instability is difficult to assess on non–weight-bearing radiographs. In this unstressed view, radiographic findings are normal, though further studies (Figure 9-62) revealed evidence of ligament injury.

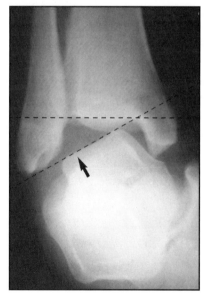

Figure 9-62

Ankle instability—AP view, stressed

In this AP view, manual varus stress is applied to the same ankle shown in Figure 9-61, revealing significant varus tilting (black arrow). This amount of instability is attributed to incompetence of both the anterior talofibular ligament and the calcaneofibular ligament.

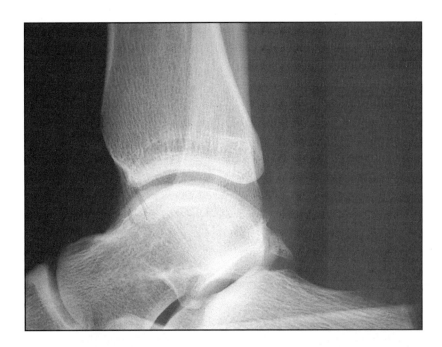

Figure 9-63

Ankle instability— Lateral view, unstressed

In this unstressed lateral view, the ankle appears normal, though further studies (Figure 9-64) revealed evidence of instability.

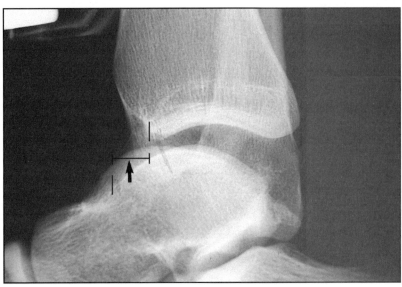

Figure 9-64

Ankle instability— Lateral view, stressed

In this lateral view, a forward drawer force has been applied. Translation of more than 5 mm or asymmetry to the contralateral side is indicative of anterior talofibular ligament instability (black arrow, lines). Note that this stress test cannot be performed weight bearing. Subtle instability may require a slightly plantar flexed position of the tibiotalar joint to offset the dome of the talus.

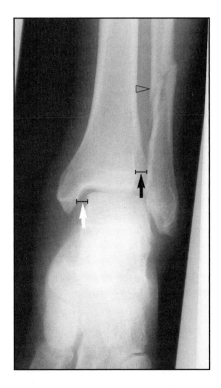

Figure 9-65

Pronation-eversion fracture of the ankle—AP view

Non–weight-bearing AP view shows a typical pronation-eversion type of ankle fracture. Note the increased space between the medial malleolus and talus, called the medial clear space (white arrow), that is indicative of a rupture of the deltoid ligament. Also, the space between the distal tibia and fibula (the tibiofibular clear space) is widened (black arrow). For this to occur, the anterior tibiofibular ligament and the syndesmosis must be ruptured. An oblique fracture of the fibula (arrowhead) can be seen above the level of the syndesmosis.

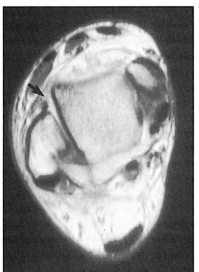

Figure 9-66

Ankle instability—Axial MRI

Axial T1-weighted MRI scan reveals a clear disruption of the anterior talofibular ligament (black arrow).

DIFFERENTIAL DIAGNOSIS

Avulsion fracture of the base of the fifth metatarsal (fracture apparent on radiographs, focal pain at site)

Bimalleolar fracture (fracture apparent on radiographs, focal pain over the malleoli)

Fracture of the anterior process of the calcaneus (fracture apparent on oblique view, focal pain over the fracture site)

Fracture of the fibula (fracture apparent on radiographs, focal pain over fracture site)

PERONEAL TENDON DYSFUNCTION

SYNONYMS

Dislocated peroneal tendon
Peroneal tendon tear
Subluxated peroneal tendon tear

DEFINITION

Pain posterior to the distal fibula is commonly associated with dysfunction of the peroneal tendon complex. Generally, the peroneus longus and brevis tendons traverse through a fibro-osseous tunnel at the distal aspect of the fibula. The tendons are held in place by the superior peroneal retinaculum (SPR), which is the primary stabilizer of the tendon complex. Tears of the peroneal tendons and/or SPR generally occur proximal to the tip of the fibula as they traverse through the fibular groove. Subluxation and dislocation can occur as a result of trauma to the SPR. Inframalleolar tears and tendinopathy occur less frequently. Impingement along the peroneal tubercle on the lateral wall of the calcaneus can cause peroneal injury at this level. Finally, tendinitis can occur at the insertion of the peroneus brevis tendon at the base of the fifth metatarsal.

Pain over the lateral border of the foot can be caused by inflammation of the peroneus longus or as a result of a "bowstring" effect, as the peroneus longus traverses the plantar aspect of the foot and crosses the lateral bands of the plantar fascia.

Os peroneum syndrome occurs secondary to injury to the os peroneum, an accessory ossicle in the peroneus longus tendon. The os peroneum is usually present plantar and lateral to the cuboid and can become painful from direct or indirect trauma.

Peroneal tendinitis occurs primarily as a result of overuse. In athletes, weak abduction of motion in the foot, as well as weak eversion strength, frequently causes inflammation of the peroneal tendons. Traumatic injuries rarely rupture the peroneal tendons; more commonly trauma (specifically forced dorsiflexion and inversion) causes a rupture of the SPR, which can subsequently evolve to peroneal subluxation or dislocation. Sometimes with an SPR rupture, a fragment of bone may avulse off of the anterior insertion, revealing a characteristic "fleck sign" on radiographs.

Rheumatologic conditions can cause primary inflammation within the tendon sheath, resulting in injury to either the tendon or the SPR. These conditions can also create a space-occupying mass that can cause pain. Rarely, primary soft-tissue tumors such as pigmented villonodular synovitis or giant cell tumors can create a similar effect.

HISTORY AND PHYSICAL FINDINGS

Peroneal tendon dysfunction is associated with a history of ankle sprains or ankle instability in many patients. The location of the pain, however, differs. With peroneal tendon dysfunction, the pain is posterior to the distal fibula. If the peroneal tendon injury is at the peroneal tubercle level, the pain will be over the peroneal tubercle, inferior to the lateral malleolus and below the typical location of a sprained ankle.

With insertional peroneal tendinitis, pain and inflammation are present at the base of the fifth metatarsal. The lateral contour of the foot will be asymmetric, characterized by a lateral bulge and callus formation.

Injuries to the SPR are associated with violent, forceful dorsiflexion and inversion. These injuries are often associated with Alpine skiing. Patients typically report a specific traumatic episode and are frequently able to dislocate or subluxate the tendon at will.

Generalized ligamentous laxity needs to be excluded by examining the opposite, unaffected ankle.

IMAGING STUDIES

Required for diagnosis

Peroneal tendon dysfunction is a clinical diagnosis and can be made by history and physical examination; therefore, imaging studies are not required to make the diagnosis.

Required for comprehensive evaluation

Although the diagnosis is considered clinical, a comprehensive evaluation requires AP, lateral, and oblique views of the ankle, along with MRI to exclude other potential causes of lateral ankle pain. Exostosis, osteochondroma, and space-occupying lesions frequently mimic tendinopathy.

MRI is the most comprehensive imaging modality because it not only identifies the presence of mucoid degeneration and the loss of tendinous integrity but also helps with anatomic mapping of the pathology. Axial images with fluid-sensitive sequences are the most valuable. In acute tenosynovitis, the tendon sheath is distended with synovial fluid. On T2-weighted images, the low signal intensity tendon is enveloped by high signal intensity fluid. Ultrasound may also be used to evaluate the peroneal tendons.

Special considerations

Because the primary pathology is soft tissue, CT and bone scans are rarely helpful. Tenograms with contrast can provide elegant views of retinacular tears but may be considered impractical in the age of MRI.

Pitfalls

Chronic tendinitis, as in all cases of tendinitis, can result in diffuse or focal thickening of the tendon with or without an associated change in signal intensity. A comparison to the opposite, unaffected side can help make the diagnosis.

With ultrasound, there is a steep learning curve, and the test can be time consuming.

IMAGE DESCRIPTIONS

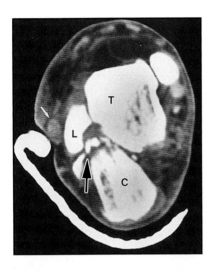

Figure 9-67

Fracture of the calcaneus with dislocated peroneal tendons—Coronal CT

Coronal CT scan of the ankle shows a soft-tissue window of a calcaneal fracture (L = lateral malleolus, T = talus, C = calcaneus). Note the clear fracture with subluxation of the subtalar joint (black arrow). The fractured calcaneus is compressed against the tip of the distal fibula, and comminution is seen within the fibular groove. Note also that the peroneal tendons are dislocated laterally (white arrow).

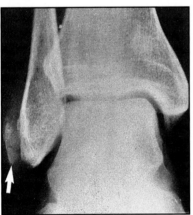

Figure 9-68

Rupture of the superior peroneal retinaculum (fleck sign)—AP view

AP view of the ankle shows the "fleck sign" associated with rupture of the SPR (arrow). As the SPR avulses off of the anterior insertion to the fibula, a fleck of bone may come off. In addition to causing peroneal tendon instability and dislocation, a palpable mass may be noted on physical examination laterally and anteriorly to the fibula.

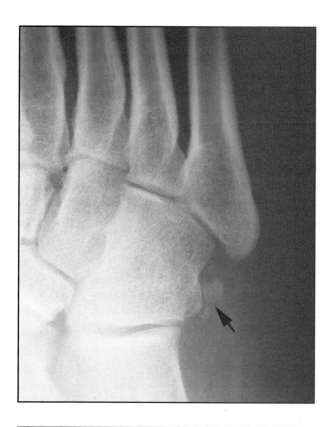

Figure 9-69

Fracture of the os peroneum—Oblique view

Oblique view of the foot shows an acute fracture of the os peroneum (arrow). This fracture should be distinguished from a diastasis of a multipartite os peroneum.

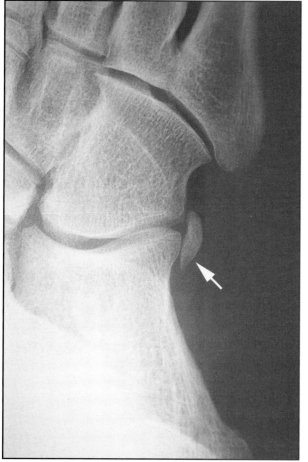

Figure 9-70

Os peroneum (normal)—Oblique view

Oblique view of the foot shows an intact os peroneum (arrow). The os peroneum exists within the peroneus longus tendon.

DIFFERENTIAL DIAGNOSIS

Anterior lateral impingement syndrome (pain worse with dorsiflexion in the anterior lateral gutter of the ankle)

Chronic ankle instability (chronic giving way, pain in the lateral collateral ligaments with each episode of giving way)

Subtalar arthrosis (focal pain over the subtalar joint)

Subtalar ligament injury (pain over the sinus tarsi area of the subtalar joint)

POSTERIOR TIBIAL TENDON DYSFUNCTION

SYNONYMS

Acquired adult flatfoot
Acquired flatfoot deformity
Posterior tibial tendinitis
Posterior tibial tendon insufficiency
Posterior tibial tendon tear

DEFINITION

The function of the posterior tibial tendon is to invert, adduct, and plantar flex the foot while supporting the longitudinal arch during middle and terminal stances of gait. By allowing the midfoot joints to lock up, the gastrocnemius-soleus complex can act through a longer lever arm, creating an efficient push-off phase of gait.

Asymmetric acquired adult flatfoot is generally caused by progressive dysfunction of the posterior tibial tendon. Although frank rupture of this tendon is unusual, progressive mucoid degeneration and expansion can occur, followed by gradual longitudinal tearing. A vascular etiology for this condition is possible because most tears occur directly in the inframalleolar region where the blood flow is most tenuous. As the tendon begins to fail, its antagonist muscle (the peroneal brevis) begins to pull unopposed, creating a typical flatfoot deformity.

The incidence of this condition is high in middle-aged women. Posterior tibial tendon dysfunction also has been associated with rheumatoid arthritis, smoking, vascular insufficiency, hypertension, diabetes mellitus, and obesity.

HISTORY AND PHYSICAL FINDINGS

Posteromedial ankle pain often signals posterior tibial tendon dysfunction. However, only about 50% of patients report a precipitating injury. Over time, lateral pain becomes progressively worse, as does associated stiffness and arthrosis of adjacent joints. Presenting signs and symptoms include hindfoot valgus, forefoot abduction, and loss of arch height. Patients cannot initiate the movement to stand on their tiptoes but can maintain the position once attained because the function of their Achilles tendon is not altered. Late presentation includes lateral ankle and hindfoot pain.

Physical examination reveals inflammation and point tenderness from the inframalleolar region to the insertion on the medial tuberosity of the navicular bone. As the foot continues to abduct and evert, the lateral wall of the calcaneus can impinge on the tip of the distal fibula and cause pain. Fractures of the fibula can occur

ICD–9 Codes

726.72
Tibialis tendinitis

726.79
Enthesopathy of ankle and tarsus; other

736.73
Cavus deformity of foot

845.00
Sprains and strains of ankle, unspecified site

SECTION 9 ■ FOOT AND ANKLE

in severe cases. Paradoxically, medial pain may disappear with complete rupture of the tendon.

Imaging Studies

Required for diagnosis

Posterior tibial tendon dysfunction is a clinical diagnosis made by history and physical examination; therefore, imaging studies are not required to make the diagnosis.

Required for comprehensive evaluation

Weight-bearing AP and lateral views of both feet, weight-bearing AP views of both ankles, and MRI are important to grade the severity of the deformity and to assist in surgical planning. Radiographs are also helpful in excluding other causes of asymmetric flatfoot deformities such as tarsal coalitions, Charcot fracture, subtalar arthrosis, rheumatoid arthritis, and malunion. The weight-bearing lateral views help evaluate the amount of longitudinal collapse. The weight-bearing AP views of the foot are helpful in assessing talonavicular subluxation and the amount of uncovering of the talar head by the navicular bone. Weight-bearing AP views of both ankles are mandatory prior to any surgical reconstruction. Talar tilt on a weight-bearing AP view of the ankle will reveal concomitant deltoid insufficiency. For patients with concurrent deltoid insufficiency, reconstruction of the posterior tibial tendon or a triple arthrodesis will frequently exacerbate ankle deformity and make the clinical outcome worse.

Although the diagnosis is clinical, a comprehensive evaluation will require radiographs and MRI to exclude other etiologies of medial ankle pain. Exostosis, osteochondroma, and space-occupying lesions will frequently mimic tendinopathy. MRI is the most comprehensive test as it will reveal not only the presence of mucoid degeneration and the loss of tendinous integrity but also will assist in anatomic mapping of the pathology.

Because the primary pathology is soft tissue, CT and bone scans are rarely helpful. Tenograms with contrast can provide elegant views of retinacular tears but may be considered impractical in the age of MRI.

MRI is helpful in excluding primary tendinous pathology such as soft-tissue tumors (pigmented villonodular synovitis, giant cell tumor, or rheumatoid arthritis), as well as to grade the amount of destruction of these typically attritional tears.

Special considerations

Ultrasound provides certain advantages by giving a dynamic assessment of posterior tibial tendon function. Classic early findings include a normal hyperechoic tendon surrounded by a hypoechoic halo or the "target sign."

Pitfalls

Bone scans are not helpful, although they do reveal secondary changes to the ankle region. Increased activity in the blood-pool phase can be seen along the tendon, and focal uptake at the medial malleolus on the delayed view can be seen.

With ultrasound, there is a steep learning curve, and the test can be time consuming.

IMAGE DESCRIPTION

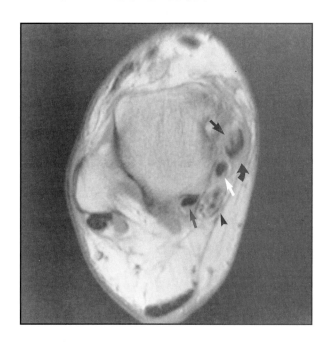

Figure 9-71

Posterior tibial tendon dysfunction— Axial MRI

Axial T1-weighted MRI scan of the ankle shows the tibial posterior tendon (black arrow), flexor digitorum longus (white arrow), the posterior tibial neurovascular bundle including the artery (arrowhead), and the flexor hallucis longus (gray arrow); the mnemonic for these is Tom, Dick, And, Harry. Note the longitudinal tearing and splitting of the posterior tibial tendon. Surrounding tenosynovitis is also seen (curved black arrow).

DIFFERENTIAL DIAGNOSIS

Congenital pes planus (bilateral and present throughout life)

Lisfranc fracture-dislocation (history of trauma and pain in midfoot)

Medial malleolus stress fracture (focal pain at the site)

Tarsal coalition (fixed deformity, onset at early age)

SECTION 9 ■ FOOT AND ANKLE

BUNION

ICD-9 Codes

727.1
Bunion

735.0
Hallux valgus (acquired)

754.52
Metatarsus primus varus

SYNONYMS

Hallux valgus
Metatarsus primus varus

DEFINITION

A bunion, also known as hallux valgus, involves the metatarsophalangeal (MTP) joint of the great toe and is characterized as a lateral deviation of the phalanx with an increased angle between the first and second metatarsals. It is also associated with pronation of the first ray and a prominent medial eminence. The degree of deformity is variable but important because the degree of deformity often influences treatment and is important in the surgical plan.

Bunions affect women much more frequently than men. They are believed to be caused by or aggravated by modern shoes, especially those with narrow toe boxes. Other causes include trauma, diabetes mellitus, rheumatoid arthritis, and a variety of connective tissue disorders. Bunions have a weak genetic linkage.

HISTORY AND PHYSICAL FINDINGS

Patients often report either a cosmetic deformity or pain at the medial eminence of the first metatarsal head associated with mechanical irritation from shoe wear. In some cases, medial eminence bursitis or skin ulceration may be present. Occasionally, the deformity may be associated with a crossover lesser toe. Examination should include assessment of the deformity by inspection, range of motion of the first MTP joint, tenderness over the medial eminence, and reducibility of the deformity. Pain with dorsal and plantar flexion suggests possible associated arthrosis of the joint, which will influence treatment.

The natural history of a bunion is variable. Shoes with narrow toe boxes can exacerbate the deformity and lead to progression of symptoms. However, altering shoe wear does not guarantee that the disease will stop progressing. Nonsurgical measures should be exhausted prior to consideration of surgical management.

IMAGING STUDIES

Required for diagnosis

Weight-bearing AP and lateral radiographs will reveal bony malalignment, a prominent medial eminence, and arthrosis within the joint. The AP view will show the severity of the deformity, while the lateral view illustrates the congruity of the joint and the presence of arthritis or osteophyte formation dorsally.

Radiographs will allow for quantitative assessment of the bunion. Four important parameters should be documented in the initial radiographs of a patient with a bunion. (1) The hallux valgus (HV) angle represents the relationship of the long axis of the proximal phalanx to the long axis of the first metatarsal. Up to 15° of lateral deviation is considered normal. (2) The intermetatarsal (IM) angle is the relationship between the first and second metatarsals. Lines are drawn through each metatarsal shaft and the angle is measured. In general, this angle is less than 10°. (3) The congruency of the joint should then be assessed. A congruent joint is one in which there is no lateral deviation or subluxation of the proximal phalanx upon the metatarsal head. (4) The presence of arthrosis should be evaluated. Signs of arthrosis include joint space narrowing, sclerosis, and possible subchondral cyst formation.

Required for comprehensive evaluation

Additional imaging studies are infrequently warranted.

Special considerations

The presence of a mass in an area other than the medial eminence, along with signs of neurovascular compromise, is unusual and warrants further evaluation.

Pitfalls

The severity of hallux valgus is measured by forefoot angles on weight-bearing AP views of the foot. Non–weight-bearing radiographs are useless for this evaluation.

IMAGE DESCRIPTIONS

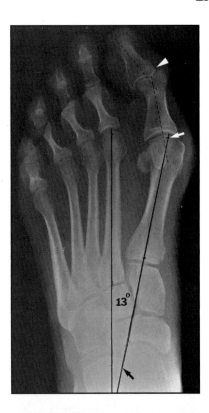

Figure 9-72

Bunion (grading severity)—AP view

The severity of the hallux valgus deformity is graded by measuring forefoot angles, as shown on this AP view. The IM angle (black arrow) is measured by lines bisecting the longitudinal axes of the first and second metatarsals. The IM angle in a normal foot is < 10°. The HV angle is measured by lines bisecting the proximal phalanx and first metatarsal (white arrow). The normal HV angle is < 15°. The hallux valgus interphalangeus (HVI) angle is measured by lines bisecting the proximal phalanx and the distal phalanx (arrowhead). The normal HVI angle is < 5°.

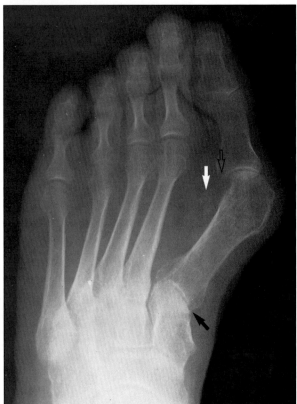

Figure 9-73

Bunion—AP view

Weight-bearing AP view of the forefoot shows an increased IM angle, increased HV angle, and angulation at the first metatarsocuneiform joint (black arrow). The lateral sesamoid is subluxated in a lateral direction (white arrow). Note the clear subluxation at the first MTP joint (open arrow).

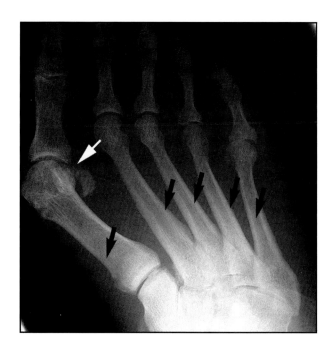

Figure 9-74

Bunion—AP view

AP view of the forefoot shows hallux valgus
(white arrow) in association with generalized
metatarsus adductus (black arrows).

DIFFERENTIAL DIAGNOSIS

Hallux rigidus (peripheral articular spurs, narrowing of the first
MTP joint, predominantly dorsal and lateral spurs)

Hallux varus (medial deviation of the great toe)

Inflammatory arthritis (soft-tissue swelling, osteopenia,
subchondral erosion, articular malalignment on radiographs)

BUNIONETTE

ICD-9 Code

727.1
Bunion

SYNONYM

Tailor's bunion

DEFINITION

Bunionette, or tailor's bunion, is the abnormal lateral prominence of the fifth metatarsal head, usually accompanied by medial deviation of the fifth toe. The condition is similar to a bunion in that it is associated with shoe wear. Thus, women are more frequently affected than men. Symptoms generally arise from pressure on the lateral prominence, creating a lateral, or plantar lateral, callus. Several anatomic variants of the fifth metatarsal have been identified as an underlying cause, including an enlarged metatarsal head, a curved fifth metatarsal, and a straight but laterally deviated fifth metatarsal. A bunionette is limited to the fifth toe metatarsophalangeal (MTP) joint.

HISTORY AND PHYSICAL FINDINGS

Symptoms usually are isolated to the lateral prominence and are exacerbated with shoe wear. Constant pressure often leads to a painful callus laterally at the metatarsal head. Again, ascertaining from the patient whether the complaint is a cosmetic issue, or secondary to pain, is important in the history. Similar to bunions, the clinical course is also variable.

IMAGING STUDIES

Required for diagnosis

Weight-bearing AP and lateral views of the foot are necessary to evaluate the mechanical alignment of the fifth MTP joint. Evaluation of the metatarsal for the following three anatomic variants is important for planning treatment: (1) an enlarged metatarsal head; (2) a bowed metatarsal; or (3) a widened intermetatarsal (IM) angle. The normal 4-5 IM angle is between 6° to 8°. Again, assessing for joint congruity and arthrosis is important in the initial evaluation.

Required for comprehensive evaluation

Additional imaging studies usually are not necessary.

Special considerations

None

Pitfalls
None

IMAGE DESCRIPTION

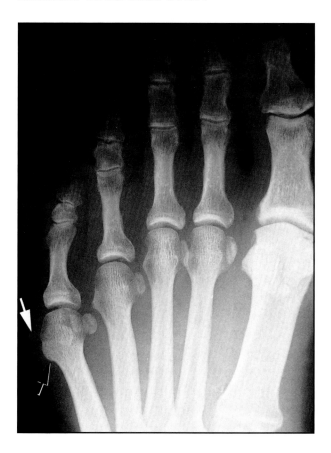

Figure 9-75

Bunionette—AP view

Weight-bearing AP view of the forefoot shows an enlarged fifth metatarsal head (black arrow). The soft-tissue outline also shows the bunionette (white arrow).

DIFFERENTIAL DIAGNOSIS

Cavovarus foot (excessive weight bearing and pain over the fifth metatarsal head; radiograph consistent with cavus foot)

Inflammatory arthritis (soft-tissue swelling, periarticular erosions on radiographs)

CLAW TOE

ICD-9 Code

735.5
Claw toe (acquired)

SYNONYM
Lesser toe deformity

DEFINITION
Claw toe is a deformity of the lesser toes in which there is flexion of the proximal interphalangeal (PIP) joint and hyperextension of the metatarsophalangeal (MTP) joint. The MTP joint may also subluxate dorsally. The distal interphalangeal (DIP) joint is typically flexed, but it may be extended or in a neutral position. Classically, claw toe has been linked to a neurologic disorder that creates an imbalance between the extrinsic and intrinsic muscles. The deformity may be dynamic with passive correctability, or it may be fixed with joint contractures. Claw toe is exacerbated if the patient also has a tight calf (equinus contracture).

HISTORY AND PHYSICAL FINDINGS
Patients typically report painful callosities and/or pain under the metatarsal heads. With a claw toe, dorsal subluxation of the proximal phalanx can cause the fatty cushion under the metatarsal heads to displace distally. With the loss of this protective cushioning, a painful plantar keratosis can occur. Callosities on the dorsum of the PIP joint or at the tip of the toe may be present as well.

Physical examination should include an evaluation of the neurovascular status of the lower extremity in severe deformities. Both weight-bearing and non–weight-bearing alignment of the toe should be assessed. The deformity's correctability should also be assessed. An effort should be made to pinpoint the diagnosis. If necessary, a thorough neurologic examination should be conducted because claw toes usually are present in all the lesser toes and can be secondary to neurologic disorders such as Charcot-Marie-Tooth disease.

IMAGING STUDIES

Required for diagnosis
The diagnosis is clinical; therefore, imaging studies are not necessary to establish the diagnosis. They are helpful, however, in planning surgery to rule out bone pathology.

Required for comprehensive evaluation
Weight-bearing AP and lateral views are needed to make the
diagnosis. On the AP view, a severe claw toe deformity may
have a "gun barrel sign," which is the proximal phalanx seen
end-on. The AP view also is helpful in evaluating the MTP joint
for congruency, subluxation, dislocation, and arthritic changes.
The lateral view helps to assess the magnitude of the deformity
at the PIP and DIP joints.

Special considerations
None

Pitfalls
None

IMAGE DESCRIPTIONS

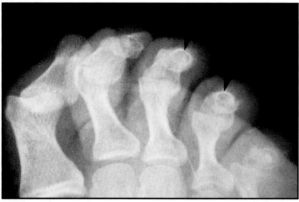

Figure 9-76

Claw toes—Oblique view

Oblique view of claw toe deformity shows
involvement of all the toes. Although usually
seen at the proximal phalanx on the AP view,
the gun barrel sign (arrows) is seen on the
third and fourth toes and is the distal phalanx
seen end-on.

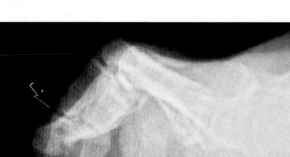

Figure 9-77

Claw toes—Lateral view

Weight-bearing lateral view of the forefoot
shows claw toe deformity involving all the
toes. Note the mild flexion at the DIP joint
(arrow).

SECTION 9 ■ FOOT AND ANKLE

DIFFERENTIAL DIAGNOSIS

Hammer toe (flexion deformity of the PIP joint with no significant deformity of the DIP or interphalangeal joints)

Neuropathic toe deformity (muscle weakness or imbalance)

Posttraumatic toe deformity (including deformity from foot compartment syndrome) (history of trauma)

CROSSOVER TOE

SYNONYM
Lesser toe deformity

ICD-9 Code

838.05
Dislocation of foot, closed,
metatarsophalangeal (joint)

DEFINITION
Crossover toe deformity of the lesser toes (typically the second) occurs when joint instability leads to progressive dorsal subluxation and medial deviation. The etiology is primarily traumatic, with disruption of the plantar plate, capsule, and metatarsophalangeal (MTP) collateral ligaments. Systemic and inflammatory arthritides, other connective tissue disorders, and chronic synovitis may lead to capsular insufficiency with eventual deterioration of the collateral ligaments and joint capsule and subsequent MTP joint instability. Hallux valgus may be associated with the deformity and becomes worse when the second toe is no longer in the same plane. This deformity is exacerbated if the patient has a tight calf (equinus contracture).

HISTORY AND PHYSICAL FINDINGS
Patients often report a history of a traumatic injury, along with pain and deformity at the affected MTP joint. Pain in the intermetatarsal space with ambulation is not uncommon. Physical examination reveals inflammation over the MTP joint. Weight-bearing toe alignment should be observed, along with correctability of the deformity. Instability should be assessed by dorsoplantar manipulation of the MTP joint (MTP Lachman's test). This will often elicit characteristic pain.

IMAGING STUDIES

Required for diagnosis
Weight-bearing AP and lateral views are needed to assess the severity of the deformity. The AP view is helpful to evaluate the MTP joint for congruency, subluxation, dislocation, arthritic changes, and to determine the length of the second metatarsal. The lateral view will show the dislocated or hyperextended MTP joint.

Required for comprehensive evaluation
MRI may be useful and reliable in the diagnosis of plantar plate abnormalities. A bone scan may help to differentiate nonspecific forefoot pain.

Special considerations
None

Pitfalls
None

IMAGE DESCRIPTIONS

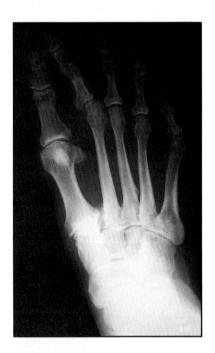

Figure 9-78

Crossover toe deformity—AP view

Weight-bearing AP view of the forefoot shows subluxation of the second MTP joint (arrow). The base of the proximal phalanx is overlapping the medial head of the second metatarsal.

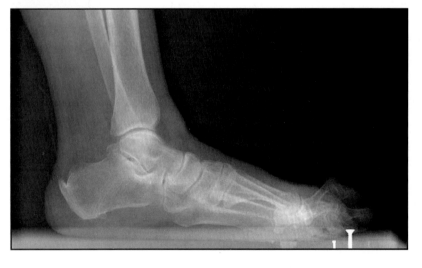

Figure 9-79

Crossover toe deformity— Lateral view

Weight-bearing lateral view shows dorsal subluxation of the second MTP joint (arrow). The second toe is crossing over the great toe.

DIFFERENTIAL DIAGNOSIS

Inflammatory arthritides (soft-tissue swelling and possible periarticular erosions on radiographs)

Posttraumatic MTP injury (history of trauma, swelling, and ecchymosis)

Mallet/Hammer Toe

Synonym

Lesser toe deformity

ICD-9 Code

735.4
Other hammer toe (acquired)

Definition

Mallet and hammer toes are deformities of the lesser toes, but hammer toe is much more common (ratio of 9:1). A mallet toe is an isolated flexion deformity of the distal interphalangeal (DIP) joint and may be a result of trauma. It usually occurs in a longer toe and is typically a fixed deformity. Hammer toe involves flexion deformity of the proximal interphalangeal (PIP) joint, with the DIP joint in neutral or extension. The metatarsophalangeal (MTP) joint may be in extension but not hyperextension; this difference distinguishes hammer toe from claw toe.

Shoe wear plays an important role in the etiology of these deformities. Neuromuscular diseases may cause muscle imbalances resulting in hammer toe deformities. The systemic and inflammatory arthritides may also play a role. Hammer toe deformity is exacerbated by a tight calf (equinus contracture).

History and Physical Findings

Patients typically report pain over callosities as a result of the deformity. Mallet toe causes a callosity to form at the tip of the toe, which develops as a result of increased pressure from striking the ground (end-bearing callus). With a hammer toe deformity, a painful callosity develops on the dorsum of the PIP joint from impingement within the toe box of a shoe. MTP joint symptoms are common as well.

Physical examination should include evaluation of the neurovascular status of the foot, especially in severe deformities. Weight-bearing and non–weight-bearing toe alignment should be observed. The deformity's correctability should also be assessed.

Imaging Studies

Required for diagnosis

AP and lateral views of the feet are needed to make the diagnosis. The AP view may show a severe hammer deformity with a "gun barrel sign," which is the proximal phalanx seen end-on. The AP view also is helpful to evaluate the MTP joint for congruency, subluxation, dislocation, and arthritic changes. The lateral view helps to assess the magnitude of the contracture at the DIP and PIP joints.

Required for comprehensive evaluation
None

Special considerations
None

Pitfalls
None

IMAGE DESCRIPTION

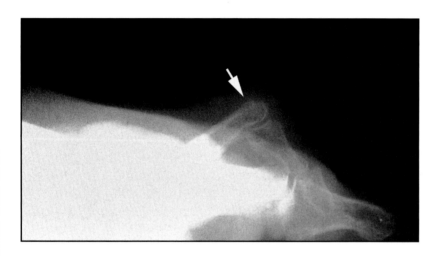

Figure 9-80

*Hammer toe—
Lateral view*

Lateral view shows a flexion deformity involving the PIP joint (arrow), with the DIP joint in a neutral position. The MTP joints are not clearly visible; however, based on the position of the toe, the MTP joint may be extended but not hyperextended.

DIFFERENTIAL DIAGNOSIS

Claw toe (flexion of the PIP joint and hyperextension of the MTP joint; DIP joint typically flexed but may be extended or in neutral)

Neuropathic toe deformity (muscle weakness or imbalance)

Posttraumatic toe deformity (including deformity from foot compartment syndrome) (history of trauma)

MORTON'S NEUROMA

SYNONYMS
Interdigital neuritis
Plantar interdigital neuroma

ICD-9 Code
355.6
Lesion of plantar nerve

DEFINITION
Morton's neuroma is a nerve entrapment of the common digital nerve to the affected toes as it passes beneath the transverse metatarsal ligament. It is not a neoplastic process. The nerve becomes compressed beneath the ligament when the toes are dorsiflexed. Histologic studies confirm that changes in the nerve occur distal to the ligament, while proximally the nerve is normal. Perineural thickening and fibrosis are commonly seen. The condition typically involves the web space between the third and fourth toes and, to a lesser degree, the space between the second and third toes. This is thought to be due to the smaller relative space in the metatarsal head/transverse ligament region in which the nerve passes. The incidence in women is up to 10 times greater than in men, implicating extrinsic sources, such as shoe wear (dorsiflexion of the metatarsophalangeal joint). Shoes with constricting toe boxes are also thought to play a role.

HISTORY AND PHYSICAL FINDINGS
Patients report plantar pain at the level or just distal to the metatarsal heads. The pain is characterized as "burning" or "electrical" and radiates into the affected toes. The symptoms are typically worse with activity and shoe wear. Physical examination reveals tenderness in the plantar web space, with occasional reproduction of the radiating pain into the toe. A firm, mobile mass may be present as well.

IMAGING STUDIES

Required for diagnosis
Even though the diagnosis of Morton's neuroma is principally clinical, soft-tissue imaging techniques may be helpful in confirming the diagnosis. MRI with gadolinium using fat suppression enhancements helps detect these lesions and rules out other possible etiologies.

SECTION 9 ■ FOOT AND ANKLE

Required for comprehensive evaluation
Ultrasound with high resolution has been used successfully to diagnose these lesions. There is a reportedly high predictive value regarding the presence, size, and location without false-positive results.

Special considerations
None

Pitfalls
With any ultrasound study, the quality of the images and their interpretation is technician dependent.

IMAGE DESCRIPTION

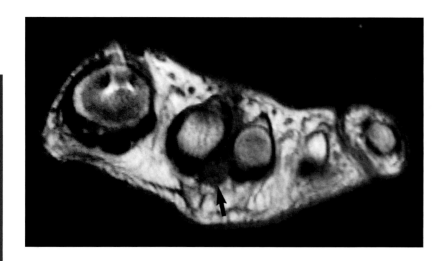

Figure 9-81

Morton's neuroma— Axial MRI

Axial T1-weighted MRI scan of the forefoot shows a soft-tissue mass between the second and third metatarsals (arrow), consistent with Morton's neuroma.

DIFFERENTIAL DIAGNOSIS

Ganglion cyst (MRI should differentiate with high signal intensity)

Lesser toe overload syndrome (a thick periosteum of the affected metatarsal on radiographs and callus under the metatarsal head)

Metatarsophalangeal synovitis (tenderness and swelling directly over the joint, pain will be plantar and dorsal on palpation over the joint)

Stress fracture (MRI should differentiate with signal void within the bone)

CHARCOT JOINT

SYNONYMS
Charcot foot
Charcot neuropathy
Diabetic foot
Diabetic neuroarthropathy
Neuroarthropathy
Neuropathic arthrosis

ICD-9 Code
713.5
Arthropathy associated with
neurological disorders

DEFINITION
Charcot arthropathy is a progressive disease characterized by painful or painless progressive bone and joint destruction in limbs that have lost sensory innervation. It is most frequently seen in patients with diabetic polyneuropathy. Diabetic neuroarthropathy involves the ankle and midfoot almost exclusively.

HISTORY AND PHYSICAL FINDINGS
Most patients with Charcot arthropathy are at least 40 years of age and have a history of diabetes mellitus of at least 10 years' duration. Initial symptoms include discomfort and persistent swelling. Previous trauma is probably underreported because of the lack of associated pain in the insensate foot.

In the acute setting, the foot is often swollen, warm, and erythematous. It may be tender on palpation. Patients who present with chronic Charcot arthropathy will have an established foot deformity. Charcot arthropathy is most common in the midfoot, where it causes collapse of the arch. This results in a rocker-bottom deformity of the foot, predisposing the patient to ulceration of the plantar surface of the foot.

IMAGING STUDIES

Required for diagnosis
Weight-bearing AP, lateral, and oblique views are useful initially to provide anatomic information. In the acute phase, radiographs can show bone destruction, demineralization, and periosteal reaction. Radiographs are not sufficient for definitive diagnosis, however, because these findings may also be present in osteomyelitis. In the chronic phase of Charcot arthropathy, radiographs may reveal the "pencil-in-cup" deformity at the metatarsophalangeal joints, fragmentation of the metatarsal heads, Lisfranc fracture or dislocation, bony fragmentation and eburnation at the

tarsometatarsal joints, talocalcaneal dislocation, talar collapse, or atypical calcaneal fractures.

Required for comprehensive evaluation

Radionuclide imaging can be helpful in diagnosing Charcot arthropathy. A three-phase bone scan will be positive in all three phases. Because this test is very sensitive but not specific, a combination of three-phase bone scan and indium-labeled white blood cell scan can be used to differentiate infection from Charcot arthropathy. A labeled white cell scan will show increased activity at the site of infection, whereas there will not be increased signal intensity where new bone is forming without infection.

Special considerations

MRI is the most sensitive imaging tool that may be ordered by the specialist. However, it is difficult to differentiate Charcot arthropathy from osteomyelitis using MRI alone. Routine sequences include T1-weighted spin echo, T2-weighted fast spin echo, and either a short-tau inversion recovery or T2-weighted fat-suppressed sequence. Chronic Charcot arthropathy is characterized by low signal intensity of the joint and the marrow on T1-weighted imaging. With acute Charcot arthropathy, the signal intensity on T2-weighted images might be high because of edema and high bone turnover. However, these findings would be the same for osteomyelitis, osteonecrosis, and recent surgery. Gadolinium enhancement does not enable differentiation between osteomyelitis and Charcot arthropathy, but it can be used to identify abscess collections.

Pitfalls

There is often a delay in diagnosing Charcot arthropathy, which may result in irreversible damage because the progression from the acute to chronic phase can occur in 6 months or less.

IMAGE DESCRIPTIONS

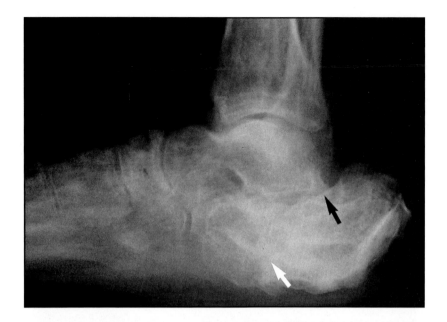

Figure 9-82

Charcot foot— Lateral view

Lateral view of a foot with chronic neuropathic fracture of the calcaneus shows hindfoot collapse (black arrow) and bony fragmentation (white arrow).

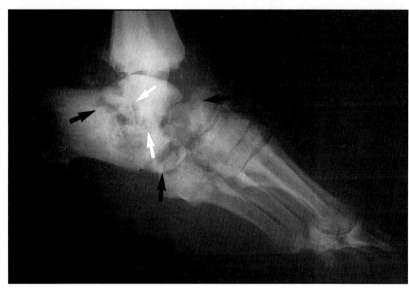

Figure 9-83

Charcot foot— Lateral view

Non–weight-bearing lateral view shows bony fragmentation (black arrows) and eburnation of the subtalar and transverse tarsal joints (white arrows), consistent with chronic Charcot hindfoot and midfoot.

SECTION 9 ■ FOOT AND ANKLE

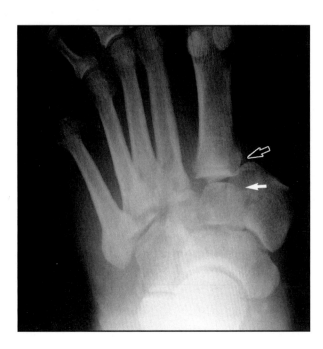

Figure 9-84

Charcot foot—AP view

Non–weight-bearing AP view of a Charcot midfoot shows an acute neuropathic Lisfranc fracture-dislocation (black arrow). Bony fragmentation (white arrow) and eburnation at the tarsometatarsal joints are minimal in this early stage of disease.

DIFFERENTIAL DIAGNOSIS

Cellulitis (soft-tissue infection, swelling, possible skin breakdown)

Deep vein thrombosis (positive venous ultrasound)

Gout (painful lesion, increased serum uric acid)

Inflammatory arthritis (soft-tissue swelling, periarticular erosions, enthesopathy)

Osteomyelitis (primarily occurs beneath an open skin ulcer)

SPINE

Section Editor
Daniel Gelb, MD

Section Co-Editor
Louis G. Jenis, MD

Contributors
Timothy A. Garvey, MD
Steven C. Ludwig, MD
Robert W. Molinari, MD
Raymond A. Pensy, MD
Charles N. Seal, MD
Kern Singh, MD
Alexander R. Vaccaro, MD
Kirkham B. Wood, MD

IMAGING THE SPINE—AN OVERVIEW

ANATOMY

The spine is a flexible, particulate column responsible for supporting the head and upper extremities in space during upright stance. The three-dimensional anatomy is fairly complex, containing a multitude of articulations, any of which can present with pathology. A careful, systematic analysis of radiographs is necessary to identify whatever pathology might be present. However, in addition to its biomechanical function, the spine also acts as a conduit for the neural elements. The soft-tissue structures within the spinal canal are not easily visualized on radiographs. Advanced imaging studies such as MRI play a frequent role in the complete evaluation of spinal pathology.

The functional unit of spinal anatomy is the motion segment: two adjacent vertebrae and their interposed articulations (intervertebral disk and paired facet joints). Each vertebra is composed of a body and a neural arch formed by paired pedicles and lamina. The articular processes, which comprise the facet joints, project superiorly and inferiorly from the base of the pedicle to form an array of interlocking joints to control motion and rotation in the sagittal plane. These are typical synovial joints. The neural arch also serves as the origin for several bony processes—the transverse processes and spinous process—that serve as muscle attachment sites. Each pair of adjacent vertebral bodies is also connected by an intervertebral disk, a flexible synchondrosis that permits flexibility and absorbs load.

The spinal canal acts as a conduit for the neural elements. The spinal cord enters the canal through the foramen magnum and terminates at about the level of the L1-L2 disk in the adult. At each vertebral level, paired nerve roots exit the spine beneath the pedicles to supply motor power and sensation to the trunk and limbs.

Viewed as a composite, the spine is straight in the frontal plane but presents a series of reciprocal curves in the sagittal plane. The cervical spine is normally lordotic (convex anterior), whereas the thoracic spine generally demonstrates kyphosis. The lumbar spine should have sufficient lordosis such that in the standing position, a plumb line dropped from C7 or T1 will pass through the thoracolumbar junction, posterior to L3, and through or behind the lumbosacral disk. The vertebrae are arranged in a gentle harmonious curve without acute angular or translational discontinuities.

The most cranial and caudal ends of the spine contain significant anatomic variations. The atlas (C1) is a ring with two lateral masses to support the occipital condyles but no body. Likewise, the axis

(C2) contains a superior projection (dens) into the ring of C1. Half of cervical motion occurs between the occiput and C2. At the caudal end of the spinal column, the sacrum results from the fusion of five vertebral segments, is generally kyphotic, and participates in the formation of the pelvic ring at the sacroiliac joints. In this manner, load is transferred from the spine to the lower extremities. Two or three vestigial coccygeal segments can be subject to traumatic injury and become a source of pain.

Ossification Centers

The ossification centers for the vertebrae are as follows. The atlas has three centers of ossification; the axis has seven, including five primary and two secondary centers; and a typical vertebra has eight centers, three primary and five secondary.

The ossification centers for the atlas include one for the anterior body, which appears at age 6 months to 2 years, and one in each neural arch, which are present at birth.

The centers for the axis are as follows: the five primary centers include two in the neural arch, which are present at birth; one in the vertebral body, also present at birth; and two in the odontoid, which are usually fused at birth. The two secondary centers are at the apex of the odontoid, which appears in the second year, and the lower aspect of the vertebral body, which appears at puberty.

In the typical vertebra, the three primary ossification centers, one in the body and two at the root of the transverse process, are present at birth. The five secondary centers, which include one at the tip of each transverse process, one at the tip of the spinous process, and two ringlike bony apophyses at the top and bottom of the vertebra, appear at puberty.

Standard Imaging Views

Low back pain is the most frequent cause of disability among adults younger than age 45 years. Up to 80% of adults will experience an episode of low back pain at some point in their lives. Note that changes present on radiographs, and even on advanced imaging studies such as MRI, are commonly seen even in asymptomatic individuals. Therefore, any findings on imaging studies must be correlated with an accurate history and physical examination to ensure that the changes seen are related to the patient's symptoms.

Radiographs

In most cases, AP and lateral views of the area of interest are sufficient for initial evaluation. Whenever possible, radiographs should be obtained with the patient in an upright position to assess the effect of gravity on spinal alignment. For each motion segment, each individual anatomic feature should be evaluated (ie, vertebral body, pedicle, lamina, transverse process, spinous process). Assessment also should include an evaluation of the overall frontal and sagittal plane alignment. Acute rotational or sagittal malalignment may be the only evidence of significant traumatic instability that has spontaneously reduced with the patient supine on a backboard.

Several specialized views are useful in demonstrating specific pathologies, primarily in the setting of trauma. Although most traumatic cervical spine injuries can be diagnosed with a lateral view, the open mouth odontoid view is useful for demonstrating abnormalities of the craniocervical junction, including occipital condyle fractures, C1 ring fractures, and odontoid fractures. Evaluation of a traumatic cervical spine injury requires evaluation of the entire cervical spine, including the C7-T1 motion segment. This area can be difficult to image because of overlying shadows from the shoulders. A swimmer's view obtained with one arm abducted to 180° degrees can allow for visualization of the lower cervical spine. Thin-slice CT with sagittal reformations provides an excellent means for assessing lower cervical spine alignment and anatomy. Flexion-extension views demonstrate dynamic instability but should be performed only in alert, cooperative, neurologically intact patients in whom static radiographs are normal. The efficacy of oblique views is limited but can be used to demonstrate fractures of the pars interarticularis in cases of suspected spondylolisthesis.

Computed tomography
Patients unable to undergo MRI can be evaluated with either CT or CT myelography.

Magnetic resonance imaging
MRI is the imaging modality of choice to demonstrate occult spinal pathology and to assess the neural elements. Patients with significant neurologic deficits require MRI evaluation, as do patients with suspected spinal infection or tumor. MRI is unnecessary, however, for routine evaluation of acute-onset low back pain or radiculopathy without significant neurologic deficits. Rather, MRI should be reserved for patients whose symptoms do not spontaneously resolve after 4 to 6 weeks of nonsurgical treatment.

EMERGENCIES
Patients being evaluated for traumatic spinal injury should be maintained supine in a spine-neutral position for initial radiographic evaluation.

Normal Variants

Minor congenital bony abnormalities are common, especially at the lumbosacral junction (eg, spina bifida occulta). Most of these abnormalities are asymptomatic. However, any congenital bony abnormality may potentially signify an occult abnormality of the neural axis such as syringomyelia or a tethered spinal cord. In the appropriate clinical situation, advanced imaging studies such as MRI may be necessary to fully evaluate this possibility, but this rarely needs to be done on an emergency basis.

The following is a partial list of anomalies that occur within the cervical, thoracic, and lumbar spine: (1) the posterior arch of C1 may articulate with the base of the skull; (2) C1 may be assimilated into the base of the skull; (3) the neural arch of C1 may be incompletely developed and mistaken for a fracture; (4) in children, it is normal for the interval between C1 and the dens to change with flexion and extension; (5) the accessory ossicles of the anterior arch of C1 may be mistaken for a fracture; (6) an open mouth view of patients with spina bifida occulta of C1 may show widening of C1 on C2, which is suggestive of a Jefferson fracture in the general population but normal in these patients; (7) os odontoideum, an overgrowth of the os terminale, may simulate a fracture of the odontoid; (8) C5 may have abnormal shapes that can mimic a fracture, such as wedging or irregularity of the anterosuperior end plate; (9) on an oblique view, a bifid spinous process may simulate a fracture; (10) spina bifida occulta of the thoracic and lumbar spine may be mistaken for a fracture; (11) failure of segmentation of a thoracic vertebra may look like ankylosing spondylitis; (12) on CT, normal vascular channels may be mistaken for a comminuted vertebral fracture; (13) notochordal remnants can produce radiolucencies on radiographs and CT scans; (14) normal variations in the transverse processes can range from complete absence to a developmental bridge; (15) bowel gas overlying the pedicle and superimposition of the iliac crest can simulate spondylolysis; (16) a limbus vertebra, which is created by the uniting of secondary lumbar ossification centers off the anterosuperior and anteroinferior aspects of the lumbar vertebral body, may mimic a fracture; and (17) the unilateral or bilateral fusion of L5 to S1 (sacralization) may be a cause of pain.

Imaging Tips

1. Radiographs are not a particularly cost-effective way to evaluate acute low back pain or neck pain of short duration. The high prevalence of asymptomatic degenerative change makes this imaging modality relatively insensitive and nonspecific. However, several specific risk factors mandate early imaging: history of significant trauma or prior malignancy; constitutional

symptoms such as fever or recent infection; neurologic deficits; patient age older than 50 years; history of substance abuse or chronic steroid use; or pain unrelieved by rest.

2. Whenever possible, radiographs should be obtained in the upright position to show the effect of gravity on vertebral alignment. Significant abnormalities related to instability or deformity (eg, kyphosis, deformity) may reduce spontaneously in the supine position. Flexion-extension views can be used to demonstrate dynamic instability but should be obtained only in alert, cooperative, neurologically intact patients with static radiographs that are normal.

3. MRI is required in any patient who presents with significant neurologic deficits.

4. C7 must be visualized when evaluating suspected injury to the cervical spine. If C7 is not adequately seen on a lateral view, a swimmer's view should be obtained.

5. Carefully evaluate open mouth views of the odontoid. If the lateral masses are displaced, a Jefferson fracture is likely present. CT will confirm this diagnosis.

6. Fractures of the occipital condyles are easily missed. Injuries to cranial nerves IX and XII, indicated by loss of taste and loss of tongue movement, respectively, suggest a condyle fracture, which may be seen only on CT images.

7. Soft-tissue extension injuries to the cervical spine are often difficult to detect on radiographs. Radiographs should be carefully examined for prevertebral soft-tissue swelling, a vacuum sign, horizontal or angular displacement of one vertebra on an adjacent vertebra, and widened disk space, signs that suggest a soft-tissue injury. MRI will document the degree of injury.

8. An AP view of the cervical spine will show a double spinous process (or ghost sign) in patients with fractures of the spinous processes of C6 or C7 (clay-shoveler's fracture).

9. Paraspinous swelling on an AP chest radiograph may be secondary to a thoracic spine fracture.

10. If widening of the distance between the pedicles is seen on an AP view of the thoracolumbar spine, which may indicate a burst fracture, CT should be obtained.

11. Fractures of the transverse process of L5 may be associated with sacral fractures.

12. Transverse process fractures are frequently associated with intra-abdominal injury.

SECTION 10 ■ SPINE

ADULT SPONDYLOLISTHESIS

SYNONYMS
None

DEFINITION
Spondylolisthesis is the forward displacement of a cranial vertebra on the adjacent caudal vertebra. The most common types of spondylolisthesis seen in adult patients are (1) isthmic (defect in the pars interarticularis allowing anterolisthesis of the vertebral body while the posterior elements remain in place) and (2) degenerative (related to incompetence of the facet joints and intervertebral disk in older individuals in which anterolisthesis occurs with an intact posterior arch). Progressive forward subluxation may lead to mechanical low back pain, nerve root irritation and lower extremity radiculopathy, spinal stenosis with symptoms of neurogenic claudication, and, rarely, cauda equina syndrome.

HISTORY AND PHYSICAL FINDINGS
Spondylolisthesis may be asymptomatic and be identified as an incidental finding. Pain, when it occurs, is usually localized to the lumbosacral area with referred pain to the thighs and buttocks. The symptoms are usually initiated or aggravated by strenuous activity involving repetitive flexion and extension of the spine. The pain may last for varying amounts of time and be relieved by rest and avoidance of the particular activities. Leg pain resulting from nerve root impingement in either type of spondylolisthesis may be intermittent and positional. Radiculopathy will follow a specific nerve root distribution. Spinal stenosis, which is more commonly seen in degenerative spondylolisthesis, may lead to bilateral leg discomfort associated with walking or standing and relieved by sitting.

Physical examination is usually unremarkable in adult patients with spondylolisthesis as high-grade slips rarely present at this stage of life. Typically, patients will show varying degrees of diminished range of lumbar motion, tension signs, motor weakness, or loss of sensation.

ICD-9 Codes

738.4
Acquired spondylolisthesis

756.11
Spondylolysis, lumbosacral region

756.12
Spondylolisthesis

SECTION 10 ■ SPINE

IMAGING STUDIES

Required for diagnosis

AP and weight-bearing lateral radiographs should be ordered to establish the diagnosis. Weight-bearing lateral views of the lumbar spine are usually sufficient to demonstrate the malalignment. Forward subluxation is best measured along the posterior border of the vertebral bodies. Supine studies may miss the diagnosis, as the subluxation may spontaneously reduce when the patient is in a recumbent position. Flexion-extension lateral radiographs may also reveal instability.

Required for comprehensive evaluation

MRI of the lumbar spine is useful primarily in patients with radiculopathy associated with spondylolisthesis. It, however, is not indicated in patients with low back pain alone unless nonmechanical symptoms are present or if the pain does not respond to nonsurgical measures. T2-weighted sagittal images of the spine can illustrate the status of the disk involved in the spondylolisthesis. Compression of the nerve root in the foramen, under an isthmic defect, by fibrocartilage can be a cause of radiculopathy. T1-weighted parasagittal images can identify nerve root compression in the foramen. Axial images can define the extent of lateral recess and central canal stenosis present in patients with degenerative spondylolisthesis.

CT myelography of the lumbar spine is indicated in patients who are unable to undergo MRI or if significant instability is a potential cause of spinal stenosis not appreciated on MRI. CT myelography may be able to demonstrate nerve root compression.

Special considerations

None

Pitfalls

Failure to obtain weight-bearing views may underestimate the degree of translation present because the slip may reduce when the patient is in a recumbent position. In addition, lateral views should center on the area of the slip, not on the entire lumbar spine.

IMAGE DESCRIPTIONS

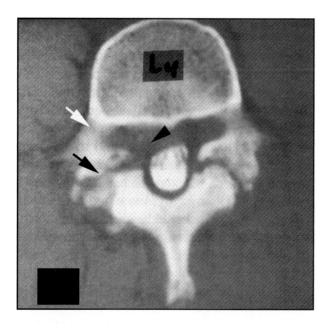

Figure 10-1

Spondylolisthesis—CT myelogram

CT myelogram of a patient with spondylolisthesis shows a pars interarticularis defect (black arrow) at the level of the pedicle (white arrow), as opposed to the disk space, that is irregular and transverse rather than smooth and oblique like the facet joint. Nerve root compression under the pars defect is shown as a filling void on myelography (arrowhead).

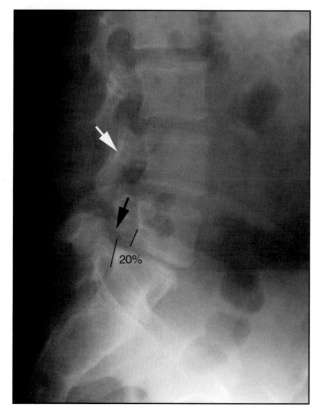

Figure 10-2

Spondylolisthesis—Lateral view

Lateral view of the lumbar spine shows a 20% slip of L5 on S1 (lines). The defect in the pars interarticularis (black arrow) is readily seen on this view. Compare this with the normal pars seen in the vertebra above (white arrow).

SECTION 10 ■ SPINE

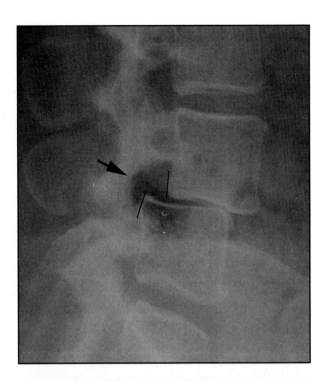

Figure 10-3

Spondylolisthesis—Lateral view

Lateral view of a patient with degenerative L4-L5 spondylolisthesis shows anterolisthesis (lines). Note also the intact posterior arch and pars area (arrow).

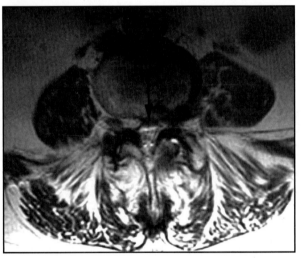

Figure 10-4

Spondylolisthesis—Axial MRI

Axial T2-weighted MRI scan of L4-L5 shows central canal stenosis at the level of the intervertebral disk space (arrow). Note the loss of cerebrospinal fluid and the compressed thecal sac.

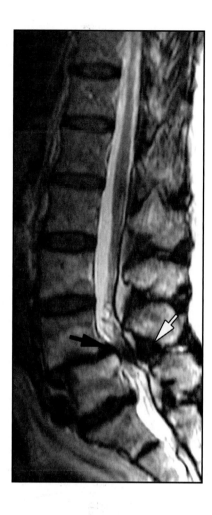

Figure 10-5

Spondylolisthesis—Sagittal MRI

Sagittal T2-weighted MRI scan of a patient with lumbar spinal stenosis shows focal stenosis as a result of spondylolisthesis (black arrow) and ligamentum flavum hypertrophy (white arrow).

DIFFERENTIAL DIAGNOSIS

Acute fracture-dislocation (fractures of posterior elements other than pars interarticularis)

Congenital vertebral anomaly (congenital abnormalities in upper part of sacrum and arch of lumbar vertebrae)

Discogenic compression (extruded or bulging disk pressing on nerve root, seen on MRI)

BURST FRACTURE

ICD-9 Codes

805.2
Fracture of vertebral column without mention of spinal cord injury, thoracic, closed

805.4
Fracture of vertebral column without mention of spinal cord injury, lumbar, closed

806.4
Fracture of vertebral column with spinal cord injury, lumbar, closed

806.25
Fracture of vertebral column with spinal cord injury, thoracic, closed, T7-T12 with unspecified spinal cord injury

806.26
Fracture of vertebral column with spinal cord injury, thoracic, closed, T7-T12 with complete lesion of cord

806.27
Fracture of vertebral column with spinal cord injury, thoracic, closed, T7-T12 with anterior cord syndrome

806.28
Fracture of vertebral column with spinal cord injury, thoracic, closed, T7-T12 with central cord syndrome

806.29
Fracture of vertebral column with spinal cord injury, thoracic, closed, T7-T12 with other specified spinal cord injury

SYNONYMS

None

DEFINITION

Burst fractures of the thoracolumbar spine commonly result from a direct axial load combined with a forward bending moment. Characteristically, the fracture affects the entire vertebral body, including both the anterior and posterior cortices, with varying degrees of retropulsion of bone into the spinal canal. Burst fractures typically result from high-energy trauma, with L1 the most commonly fractured. Nearly 50% of all vertebral body fractures occur from T11 to L2, which represents a high-stress transition zone from the rigid thoracic to the flexible lumbar spine. Along with the fractured anterior vertebral body, some burst fractures will have posterior laminar fractures as well. Young men are twice as likely to sustain these fractures as women. A noncontiguous fracture elsewhere in the spinal column is present in approximately 15% of patients. Burst fractures with intact posterior ligamentous structures (interspinous and supraspinous ligaments) and facet capsules are considered stable, whereas those with disruption or dislocation of these elements are considered relatively unstable and may require surgical stabilization. Roughly half of patients with burst fractures will also have some type of neurologic deficit.

HISTORY AND PHYSICAL FINDINGS

Motor vehicle accidents and falls from a height are two common presenting histories. Direct trauma from a heavy falling object is another common mechanism of injury. Because of the high association of neurologic injuries, a careful neurologic examination is mandatory, including a rectal examination to rule out conus medullaris or spinal cord injury.

IMAGING STUDIES

Required for diagnosis

AP and lateral radiographs of the injured segment and at least one segment above and below are needed to establish the diagnosis. Because most of these injuries are associated with an acute traumatic injury, patients should be imaged in a supine position.

Required for comprehensive evaluation

CT of the injured vertebra and at least one segment above and one below is required to confirm the diagnosis of a burst-type fracture. Axial images best show the retropulsion of bone into the spinal canal. Sagittal reformatted images can aid in further visualization of the fracture with its characteristic loss of vertebral body height anteriorly. Sagittal images also can be used to assess any interspinous widening or facet subluxation/ dislocation. MRI is not typically necessary to evaluate burst-type injuries, although it may be helpful to assess any potential damage to the interspinous ligaments (edema), the spinal cord (edema, hemorrhage), or to the intervertebral disks (herniation).

Pitfalls

Burst-type fractures can easily be misdiagnosed as compression fractures on radiographs. CT will eliminate this error. The entire spine must be imaged to prevent missing any noncontiguous injuries.

IMAGE DESCRIPTION

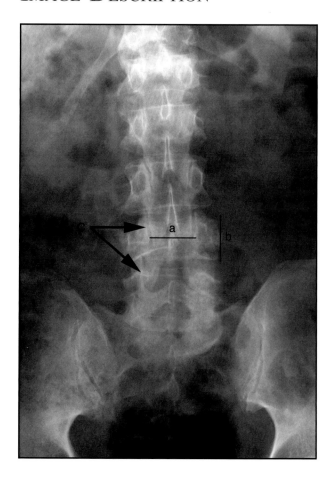

Figure 10-6

Burst fracture—AP view

AP view of a burst fracture of a lumbar vertebra shows the characteristic widening of the interpedicular distance (a) associated with the loss of vertebral height (b). The facet joints appear to be normally aligned (c).

SECTION 10 ■ SPINE

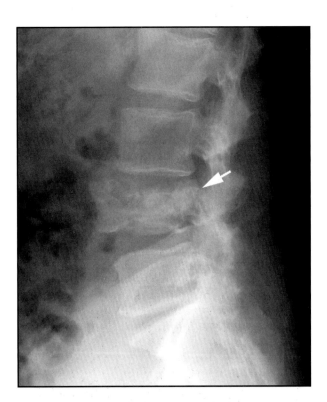

Figure 10-7

Burst fracture—Lateral view

Lateral view shows a burst fracture at L4. The essential characteristic is retropulsion of bone into the spinal canal (arrow) associated with shortening of the posterior vertebral body wall.

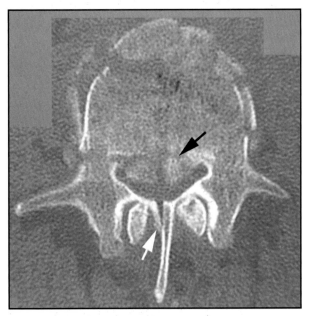

Figure 10-8

Burst fracture—Axial CT

Axial CT scan of a lumbar burst fracture shows the degree of spinal canal compromise by the retropulsed fracture fragments (black arrow). A fracture of the lamina extending into the base of the spinous process (white arrow) is a common finding and can result in nerve root entrapment and neurologic deficit.

DIFFERENTIAL DIAGNOSIS

Compression fracture (posterior vertebral body height remains intact; axial CT fails to demonstrate retropulsion of bone into the canal)

Flexion-distraction (Chance; seat belt) type injuries (posterior element disruption apparent on CT; trauma to the posterior ligamentous structures seen on MRI)

CHANCE FRACTURE

SYNONYMS
Lap belt injury
Seat belt injury

DEFINITION
The classic injury described by Chance, and hence, its name, is a bone injury that passes through the neural arch and the vertebral body. These injuries are also referred to as seat belt or lap belt injuries. The mechanism of injury is a sudden shearing and distraction that typically occurs as a result of a sudden flexion force to a fulcrum anterior to the thoracolumbar spine. These fractures commonly occur at the thoracolumbar junction and upper two lumbar vertebrae in adults and at the midlumbar area in children.

The Chance fracture involves purely bony structures with healing potential, making nonsurgical treatment with a hyperextension cast a sufficient treatment in most circumstances. Seat belt injuries include ligamentous disruption of the spinal ligaments, the intervertebral disk, and anulus fibrosus. Usually when the fracture extends through the primarily soft-tissue ligamentous structures or combinations of bony and ligamentous sites, the injury is considered unstable and rarely heals without surgical stabilization and fusion. Since the advent of shoulder-lap belt combinations and air bags, however, the incidence of seat belt injuries has been reduced considerably.

HISTORY AND PHYSICAL FINDINGS
A typical history is of a motor vehicle accident in which the patient is riding on the passenger side wearing a lap belt. Back and abdominal pain is commonly reported, but neurologic involvement is rare. Up to half of patients, however, will have associated intra-abdominal trauma, such as a ruptured spleen or torn viscus.

IMAGING STUDIES

Required for diagnosis
AP and lateral radiographs of the spine are needed to establish the diagnosis. The AP view will show a characteristic widening between the posterior elements. The lateral view will outline the kyphosis secondary to posterior element disruption. Increased space between the spinous processes or fracture through the spinous processes and neural arch also can be seen on the lateral view.

ICD-9 Codes

805.2
Fracture of vertebral column without mention of spinal cord injury, thoracic, closed

805.4
Fracture of vertebral column without mention of spinal cord injury, lumbar, closed

806.4
Fracture of vertebral column with spinal cord injury, lumbar, closed

806.25
Fracture of vertebral column with spinal cord injury, thoracic, closed, T7-T12 with unspecified spinal cord injury

806.26
Fracture of vertebral column with spinal cord injury, thoracic, closed, T7-T12 with complete lesion of cord

806.27
Fracture of vertebral column with spinal cord injury, thoracic, closed, T7-T12 with anterior cord syndrome

806.28
Fracture of vertebral column with spinal cord injury, thoracic, closed, T7-T12 with central cord syndrome

806.29
Fracture of vertebral column with spinal cord injury, thoracic, closed, T7-T12 with other specified spinal cord injury

SECTION 10 ■ SPINE

Required for comprehensive evaluation
CT will show the injury on sagittal reformations but may miss the injury on transaxial cuts because of the horizontal orientation of the fracture. MRI is obtained increasingly more often because it better shows posterior ligament and intervertebral disk injuries as well as bony injury.

Special considerations
None

Pitfalls
Transaxial CT may miss the fracture; therefore, sagittal reconstructions are necessary.

IMAGE DESCRIPTIONS

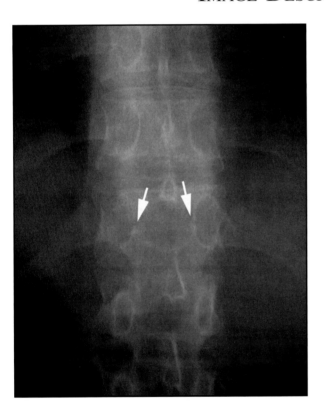

Figure 10-9

Chance fracture—AP view

AP view of the lower thoracic/upper lumbar spine shows bilateral pedicle fractures (arrows).

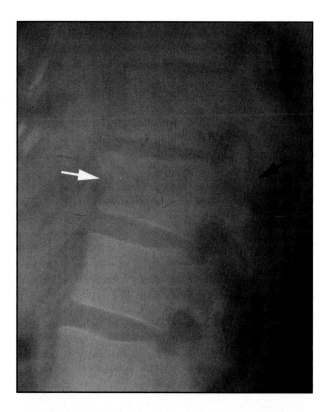

Figure 10-10

Chance fracture—Lateral view

Lateral view of the lower thoracic/upper lumbar spine shows a fracture line extending from the posterior aspect of the pedicle (black arrow) to the anterior cortex of the vertebral body (white arrow).

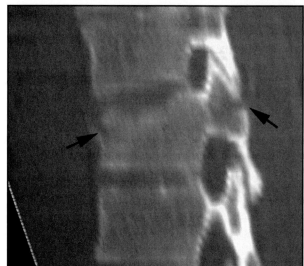

Figure 10-11

Chance fracture—Sagittal CT

Sagittal CT reconstruction shows a Chance fracture of T12, extending from the spinous process through the vertebral body (arrows).

DIFFERENTIAL DIAGNOSIS

Burst fracture (displacement of bony fragments apparent on CT)

Fracture-dislocation (displacement of one vertebra onto another apparent on radiographs)

SECTION 10 ■ SPINE

FRACTURE-DISLOCATION

ICD-9 Codes

805.2
Fracture of vertebral column without mention of spinal cord injury, thoracic, closed

805.4
Fracture of vertebral column without mention of spinal cord injury, lumbar, closed

806.4
Fracture of vertebral column with spinal cord injury, lumbar, closed

806.8
Fracture of vertebral column with spinal cord injury, unspecified, closed

SYNONYMS

None

DEFINITION

A fracture-dislocation of the spine represents failure of all soft-tissue and ligamentous structures of the spine, along with varying degrees of bony injury. The fractures are seen with the most violent degrees of trauma, often incorporating flexion, distraction, extension, and other significant forces. These fractures are unstable and commonly have concomitant neurologic injuries for which surgical stabilization is typically required. The main goals of surgical intervention are to limit pain, prevent spinal deformity, and prevent deterioration of neurologic status.

HISTORY AND PHYSICAL FINDINGS

Most patients with a spinal fracture-dislocation are involved in high levels of trauma and often have other musculoskeletal or soft-tissue injuries, including pulmonary or abdominal injuries. Patients may report extreme pain and/or exhibit varying degrees of neurologic injury, ranging from lower motor neuron pain or dysfunction to frank and complete paralysis.

Clinical manifestations of neurologic injury depend on the level and extent of injury to the spinal column. Spinal shock is present for 24 to 48 hours after injury; when resolved, the severity of spinal cord injury can be determined. Incomplete spinal cord injury is diagnosed by the presence of sacral sparing where perianal sensation or the bulbocavernosus reflex has recovered. Absence of sacral sparing signifies complete spinal cord injury and poor prognosis for further neurologic recovery.

Acute management includes routine care of the trauma ABCs, including hemodynamic stabilization from spinal shock and loss of sympathetic tone or other injuries. Spinal precautions are emphasized until radiographic evaluation is completed and the diagnosis is established to prevent additional iatrogenic spinal cord injury.

IMAGING STUDIES

Required for diagnosis

AP and lateral radiographs of the affected area will show a characteristic lack of continuity from the superior to inferior vertebra, along with varying degrees of bony injury. The lateral view is especially helpful in showing not only the degree of bony injury but also the lack of continuity of the anterior and posterior vertebral walls across the fracture site.

Required for comprehensive evaluation

CT is very helpful in illustrating the degree of structural damage. Sagittal reformations identify whether any anterior or posterior translation exists due to failure of the osseous or ligamentous structures.

MRI of the affected area also may be used to assess the integrity of the intervertebral disk (ie, herniated disk may retropulse into the canal with spontaneous reduction of a fracture-dislocation), the interspinous ligaments, the contents of the spinal canal, and the spinal cord itself.

Special considerations

None

Pitfalls

None

IMAGE DESCRIPTIONS

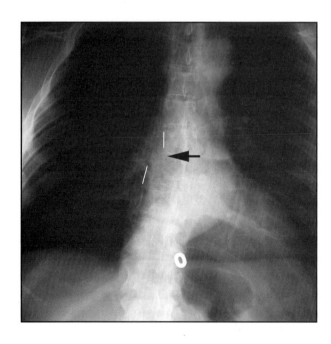

Figure 10-12

Vertebral fracture-dislocation— AP view

AP view of the thoracic spine shows a comminuted fracture of the body of T9 (arrow). Note the lateral step-off between T8 and T9 (lines). The patient had a complete paralysis below this level.

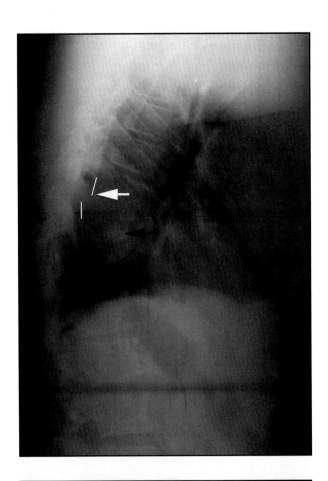

Figure 10-13

*Vertebral fracture-dislocation—
Lateral view*

Lateral view of the thoracic spine of the same
patient shown in Figure 10-12 shows the
comminuted fracture of T9 (black arrow) and
the anterior displacement of the body of T8 on
T9 (white arrow, lines).

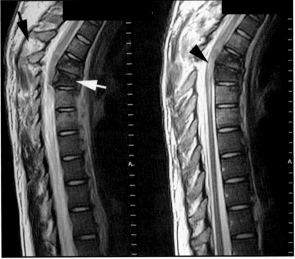

Figure 10-14

*Vertebral fracture-dislocation—
Sagittal MRI*

Sagittal T2-weighted MRI scan of the thoracic
spine shows posterior ligamentous damage
characterized by high signal intensity and
widening in the interspinous ligament (black
arrow), thoracic vertebral body collapse with
marrow signal change indicating acute injury
(white arrow), and spinal cord impingement at
the apex of the kyphosis with cord swelling
and signal change (arrowhead). The patient
presented with complete paraplegia at that
level.

DIFFERENTIAL DIAGNOSIS

Congenital deformities of the spine (differentiated with imaging
studies that show the chronicity of deformity; lack of edematous
marrow changes consistent with an acute injury seen on MRI)

Fracture of the Atlas

Synonym

Jefferson fracture

Definition

Fractures of the atlas (C1) are relatively uncommon, accounting for only 13% of all cervical spine fractures. Atlas fractures are divided into seven subgroups, the most common of which is the burst-type fracture in which the anterior and posterior rings are fractured and spread apart. This type of fracture is called a Jefferson fracture and results from an axial load to the superior ring of C1. Because these fractures tend to spread and thus decompress the spinal canal, neurologic injury is not common. However, neurapraxia of the greater occipital nerve can occur as it courses through the atlantoaxial membrane. Injuries to the vertebral artery are also possible. Fractures of the posterior arch of C1 are often associated with fractures of the odontoid. Comminuted fractures through the lateral mass may lead to nonunion or posttraumatic arthritis and poor clinical outcomes.

History and Physical Findings

Fractures of the atlas result from high-energy injuries such as a motor vehicle accident or a fall from a height in which the patient sustains a blow to the top of the head. Severe neck pain and an occipital headache are commonly reported. As noted earlier, neurologic injury is uncommon. If the vertebral artery has been injured, the patient may experience blurred vision, vertigo, and nystagmus.

Imaging Studies

Required for diagnosis

AP, lateral, and open mouth odontoid views of the cervical spine are ordered first. A C1 ring burst fracture (Jefferson fracture) is not easily visualized on a lateral view. However, the open mouth odontoid view will show lateral displacement of the lateral masses of C1. If the combined lateral displacement of the lateral masses exceeds 7 mm on radiographs, the transverse ligament, which courses between the C1 medial tubercles and maintains C1-C2 stability, is likely disrupted.

ICD-9 Codes

805.01
Fracture of vertebral column without mention of spinal cord injury, closed, first cervical vertebra

805.11
Fracture of vertebral column without mention of spinal cord injury, open, first cervical vertebra

806.01
Fracture of vertebral column with spinal cord injury, closed, C1-C4 level with complete lesion of cord

806.11
Fracture of vertebral column with spinal cord injury, open, C1-C4 level with complete lesion of cord

Section 10 ■ Spine

Required for comprehensive evaluation
Thin-cut CT reconstructions of the cervical spine will identify facet fractures and displacements. If a patient has a neurologic injury, MRI is indicated to visualize any cord damage or potential epidural hematoma.

Special considerations
None

Pitfalls
The entire cervical spine (including the cervicothoracic junction) should be carefully scrutinized for injury at additional levels, which occurs frequently.

IMAGE DESCRIPTION

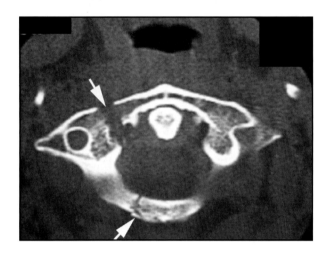

Figure 10-15

Fracture of the atlas—Axial CT

Axial CT scan at C1 shows the nature of fractures involving the atlas (arrows) and the minimal displacement of fracture fragments.

DIFFERENTIAL DIAGNOSIS

Atlantoaxial rotatory subluxation and dislocation (open mouth view may show asymmetry of lateral masses)

C2 fracture (apparent on CT)

FRACTURE OF THE ODONTOID

SYNONYM

Dens fracture

DEFINITION

Fracture of the odontoid is a common upper cervical spine injury, accounting for up to 14% of all cervical spine fractures. It may be seen in younger patients involved in significant trauma or elderly individuals following an innocuous fall. It is considered an unstable injury at the C1-C2 articulation and carries a 5% to 10% mortality due to spinal cord injury. Unfortunately, odontoid fractures are commonly missed on radiographs given their subtle presentation.

Several variables such as patient age, neurologic status, fracture type, degree of displacement, comminution, angulation, and delay in diagnosis are predictive of healing potential and useful in selecting an approach for initial intervention.

Odontoid fractures are classified as one of three types according to the anatomic level of injury on the dens. Type I injuries (5%) are small oblique fractures of the superior tip of the odontoid and are generally considered to be stable injuries; however, an association with occipitocervical dislocation has been described, and careful evaluation is required. Type II fractures, which occur at the base of the dens, are the most common (60%). Healing potential is unpredictable; rates of nonunion are reported to be as high as 60%. Type III fractures (30%) occur through the body of C2 and have a much better healing potential than type II fractures due to the large exposed cancellous surface area.

HISTORY AND PHYSICAL FINDINGS

The most common presentation is that of a patient who reports severe neck pain after striking his or her head in a fall or following other traumatic events. The presence of a frontal or occipital contusion in an elderly patient should always raise concern for an odontoid fracture. Incomplete neurologic injury is relatively rare.

IMAGING STUDIES

Required for diagnosis

Lateral and open mouth AP views of the cervical spine are necessary to establish the diagnosis. A fracture line may be difficult to detect, and displacement of the dens on the C2 body should be evaluated.

ICD-9 Codes

805.12
Fracture of vertebral column without mention of spinal cord injury, open, second cervical vertebra

806.12
Fracture of vertebral column with spinal cord injury, open, C1-C4 level with anterior cord syndrome

SECTION 10 ■ SPINE

Required for comprehensive evaluation

Thin-slice CT with sagittal and coronal reconstructions allows for detection of the fracture line and will also show with greater detail any translation or angulation of the dens on the body of C2. MRI is rarely needed for evaluation of odontoid fractures unless a concomitant spinal cord injury is suggested.

Special considerations

Evaluation of the entire spine is necessary to identify any noncontiguous injuries.

Pitfalls

Complex craniocervical anatomy may be difficult to interpret on lateral views of the cervical spine. Therefore, a lateral view of the skull centered closer to C2 may show the anatomy more clearly. Also, because these fractures are often in the transverse plane, CT may miss the fracture if the cuts are not sufficiently thin.

IMAGE DESCRIPTIONS

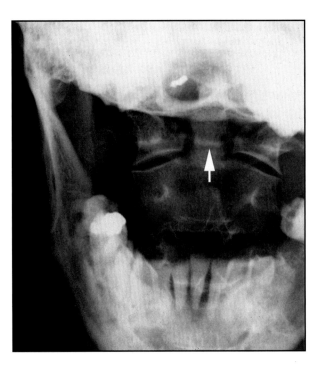

Figure 10-16

Fracture of the odontoid— Open mouth view

Open mouth view of the cervical spine in an adult patient shows a type II odontoid fracture at the base of the dens (arrow).

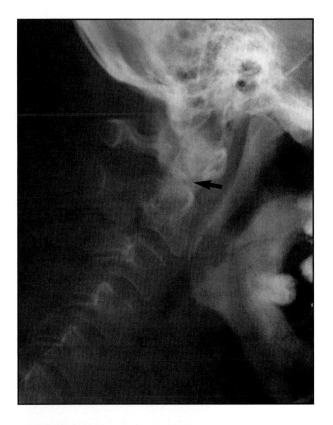

Figure 10-17

Fracture of the odontoid— Lateral flexion view

Lateral flexion view of the cervical spine in the patient shown in Figure 10-16 shows the fracture site (arrow).

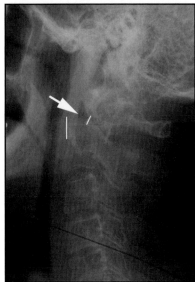

Figure 10-18

Fracture of the odontoid—Lateral view

Lateral view of the cervical spine shows posterior translation of the odontoid process, consistent with a fracture (arrow).

SECTION 10 ■ SPINE

DIFFERENTIAL DIAGNOSIS

Chronic nonunion of a dens fracture (appears with more evidence of chronicity on radiographs, including rounded edges of the odontoid, separation from the dens, and lack of anterior soft-tissue swelling)

Congenital malformation (lack of fracture lines apparent on CT with reformatted images)

Ossicle (os odontoideum) (congenital ossicle above C2 instead of dens that is continuous)

Rheumatoid arthritis (bones appear more osteopenic, associated subluxation of rheumatoid instability may be noted)

Hangman's Fracture

Synonyms

Fracture of the pedicles of C2

Spondylolisthesis of the pars interarticularis of C2

Definition

Hangman's fracture is a traumatic spondylolisthesis of the pars interarticularis of the axis (C2) and accounts for up to 20% of all cervical spine fractures. The name comes from the similarity of the bony injury that occurs after an execution by hanging.

The Levine and Edwards classification system divides hangman's fractures into three types. In type 1 injuries, the fracture line extends through the pedicle of C2 from the superior facet to the inferior facet. Type 2 injuries are similar to type 1 injuries but have a disruption of the intervertebral disk between C2 and C3. If angulation is present at the fracture site but there is no significant translation, the injury is classified as a type 2A injury. A type 3 injury includes the above injuries plus a facet dislocation between C2 and C3. Type 3 injuries likely result from a flexion injury, in contrast to types 1 and 2, which are extension injuries.

History and Physical Findings

The mechanism of injury usually is a motor vehicle accident or a fall in which the patient lands with the neck in hyperextension. Fortunately, neurologic injury is uncommon because separation of the fracture fragments decompresses the spinal canal. However, a small percentage of patients may die immediately. Vertebral artery injuries can accompany hangman's fractures but usually are asymptomatic, and facial wounds are common. These fractures are unstable and require evaluation and treatment by a spine specialist.

ICD-9 Code

805.02
Fracture of vertebral column without mention of spinal cord injury, closed, second cervical vertebra

SECTION 10 ■ SPINE

IMAGING STUDIES

Required for diagnosis

AP, open mouth odontoid, and lateral views of the cervical spine should be obtained initially. The lateral view shows more than 90% of these fractures. In patients with type 2 and 3 injuries, a prevertebral hematoma often can be seen. The hematoma results from a disruption of the intervertebral disk. The swelling reaches its peak roughly 72 hours after injury. The normal maximum width of the prevertebral soft tissues at the level of the upper four cervical vertebrae is 4 to 5 mm, but the width is somewhat variable. Any swelling of more than 7 mm should be considered abnormal. C2 often can be seen to be subluxated anteriorly on C3, and the posterior elements of C2 may be displaced posteriorly relative to the posterior elements of C3.

Required for comprehensive evaluation

CT should be ordered for patients with a suspected hangman's fracture to better define the character of the fracture. Nondisplaced fractures will be seen on CT. If neurologic injury is present, MRI will reveal the extent of the soft-tissue injury, including any injury to the vertebral artery, as well as prevertebral soft-tissue swelling.

Special considerations
None

Pitfalls

Children have increased motion in the upper cervical spine. Pseudosubluxation seen at C2–C3 with cervical flexion may be confused with a hangman's fracture. The spinolaminar line is helpful in differentiating these two conditions. This line outlines the posterior margin of the spinal canal and is drawn along the anterior margin of the bases of the spinous processes. In the presence of a hangman's fracture, the line at C2 is displaced more than 2 mm posteriorly.

IMAGE DESCRIPTION

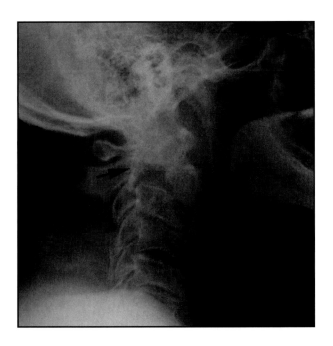

Figure 10-19

Hangman's fracture—Lateral view

Lateral view of the cervical spine shows a major subluxation of C2 on C3 related to a fracture of the posterior elements of C2 (arrow).

DIFFERENTIAL DIAGNOSIS

Atlanto-occipital dislocation (apparent on coronal and sagittal CT)

Extension teardrop fracture (triangular-shaped fragment at the anterior-inferior margin of the axis [C2] apparent on a lateral view)

Fracture of the atlas (C1) (apparent on CT or MRI)

Fracture of the odontoid (apparent on open mouth view and CT)

TRANSVERSE PROCESS FRACTURE

ICD-9 Code

805.8
Fracture of vertebral column without mention of spinal cord injury, unspecified, closed

SYNONYMS
None

DEFINITION
The transverse processes of the lumbar vertebrae arise from the junction of the pedicles and lamina and project laterally and slightly posteriorly. They serve as attachments for two of the strong back muscles, the quadratus lumborum and the aponeurosis of the transversus abdominis. The transverse process at L3 tends to be the longest. Fractures of the transverse processes are often avulsion-type fractures that result from severe contractions of the attached muscles. Blunt abdominal trauma and rotational injuries are common mechanisms of injury. Although these fractures are often thought of as minor injuries, up to half of patients will have associated intra-abdominal organ injuries. These fractures are considered stable injuries and, when in isolation, require no specific treatment. Nonunion is common given the constant pull of the attached muscles, but this seems to be of relatively little functional significance.

HISTORY AND PHYSICAL FINDINGS
A history of blunt abdominal trauma or a direct blow to the back as in a football injury is common. Falls while snowboarding have become an increasingly common cause of transverse process fractures. The patient will report localized pain and muscle spasm, which can be palpated on physical examination. Patients who report abdominal pain require thorough assessment for an abdominal organ injury.

IMAGING STUDIES

Required for diagnosis
AP and lateral radiographs of the lumbar spine should be ordered initially.

Required for comprehensive evaluation
CT is quite accurate in diagnosing transverse process fractures. It is also helpful in identifying subtle fractures, especially in the thoracic spine where radiographs are difficult to interpret due to overlapping shadows. MRI is seldom indicated unless signs of nerve root irritation are present.

Special considerations

None

Pitfalls

These fractures are easily missed on plain radiographs; CT needs to be obtained if suspicion of transverse process fracture is raised.

IMAGE DESCRIPTION

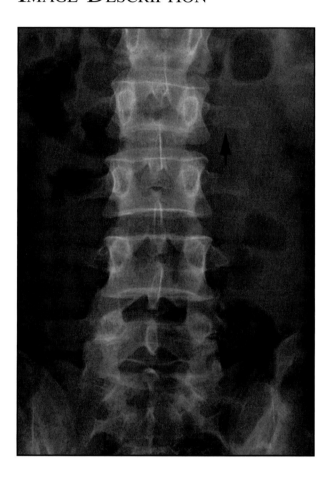

Figure 10-20

Fracture of the transverse process—AP view

AP view of the lumbar spine shows a nondisplaced fracture of the left transverse process of L2 (arrow).

DIFFERENTIAL DIAGNOSIS

Benign tumor (CT should differentiate)

Transitional vertebra (junction of thoracic and lumbar spine, may have transverse process on one side and small articulating rib on the other)

SECTION 10 ■ SPINE

VERTEBRAL COMPRESSION FRACTURE

ICD-9 Code

733.13
Pathologic fracture of
vertebrae

SYNONYM

Osteoporotic compression fracture

DEFINITION

Compression fracture of the vertebral body is defined as failure of the anterior aspect of the body under a compression or flexion force while the posterior part of the body, including the posterior vertebral wall (which forms the anterior aspect of the spinal canal), remains intact.

Compression fractures typically represent those involving the least degree of trauma. The two principal situations are when relatively normal bone fails due to sudden compression and flexion severe enough to fracture the anterior body but not severe enough to include the posterior wall. The other typical scenario is in the older, relatively osteoporotic population, wherein even less force is applied; yet due to the fragile nature of the bone, it fails into a fracture. Because no bone retropulses into the canal, the vast majority of patients remain neurologically intact.

HISTORY AND PHYSICAL FINDINGS

Patients may report localized pain at the site of the compression fracture without neurologic symptoms. The treatment of compression fractures is nonsurgical, including pain management, brace immobilization, or even observation. More recently, surgical options have been developed for osteoporotic compression fractures in the elderly with the main indication being intractable pain that does not respond to nonsurgical treatment. Surgical treatment options include percutaneous vertebral augmentation such as vertebroplasty or kyphoplasty.

IMAGING STUDIES

Required for diagnosis

AP and lateral radiographs of the spine in the area of pain are needed to establish the diagnosis. The conversion of the typically square-shaped vertebral body into a wedged compression fracture can be seen on the lateral radiograph. The AP radiograph may appear normal or with subtle loss of vertebral body height. Splaying apart of the spinous processes on the AP view should raise concern for a potential ligamentous injury or burst fracture.

Required for comprehensive evaluation

MRI may show the characteristic edematous changes under the fractured end plate on the T2-weighted images that are indicative of an acute injury. In addition, marrow replacement processes and retropulsion of the posterior vertebral wall may be seen. MRI is indicated with an acute compression fracture in a patient with a known history of carcinoma or intractable pain.

CT may confirm the lack of retropulsion of bone into the canal, thus excluding the diagnosis of a burst fracture. CT is indicated when MRI cannot be obtained for various reasons. Bone scan is possibly indicated to classify the age of a fracture as acute, subacute, or chronic; bone scans, however, are principally used to identify occult injuries or to plan surgical intervention.

Special considerations

None

Pitfalls

The main differential diagnosis of an osteoporotic compression fracture is a pathologic fracture caused by a marrow replacement process such as myeloma or metastatic disease. MRI is essential to differentiate these processes, but may not always be specific.

IMAGE DESCRIPTIONS

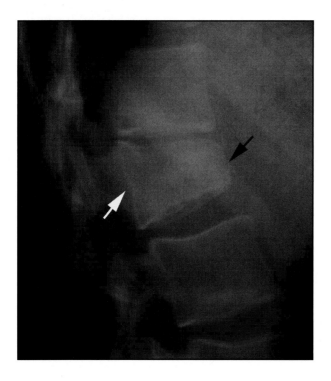

Figure 10-21

Vertebral compression fracture—Lateral view

Lateral view of the thoracolumbar junction shows a typical wedge-shaped vertebral compression fracture. Note the loss of anterior body height (black arrow), but the posterior aspect of the body and the posterior wall remain intact (white arrow).

SECTION 10 ■ SPINE

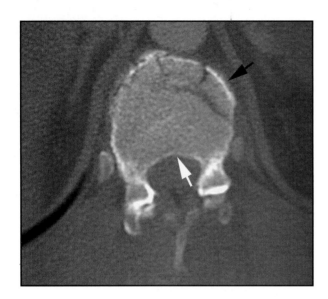

Figure 10-22

Vertebral compression fracture—CT

CT scan of a thoracic vertebral compression fracture shows damage to the anterior portion of the vertebral body (black arrow) without retropulsion of bone into the spinal canal (white arrow) or pedicle fracture.

DIFFERENTIAL DIAGNOSIS

Burst fracture (confirmed by CT or MRI)

Congenital deformity (other anomalies may be seen on radiographs)

Flexion-distraction (Chance; seat belt) type fractures (lateral radiograph and CT will show the difference)

ANKYLOSING SPONDYLITIS

SYNONYMS
Bamboo spine
Marie-Strumpell's disease
Pelvospondylitis ossificans
Rhizomelic spondylitis
Rugger jersey spine

ICD-9 Code
720.0
Ankylosing spondylitis

DEFINITION
Ankylosing spondylitis is a disease of chronic synovitis, which causes cartilage destruction, joint erosions, and ultimately ankylosis of a given joint. The *sine qua non* is bilateral sacroiliac joint inflammatory erosive change. The spine typically will become stiffened and undergo spontaneous fusion. Other joints can be involved, particularly the hips. The etiology is unknown, although there is an association with the HLA-B27 antigen. While HLA-B27 is present in the Caucasian population at a rate of about 8% to 10%, it is felt to be present in 90% of symptomatic patients with ankylosing spondylitis and in 50% of their relatives. Family members of patients with ankylosing spondylitis are 20 times more likely to have the condition. Men are four to ten times more likely to have ankylosing spondylitis than are women.

HISTORY AND PHYSICAL FINDINGS
The characteristic presentation is of young men (age 15 to 35 years) with insidious onset of low back pain radiating into the buttocks and posterior thigh. Typically, pain and stiffness are worse in the morning than later in the day. Spine involvement generally progresses from the pelvis (sacroiliac joints) cranially. As the disease progresses, significant kyphosis of either the thoracolumbar spine or cervical spine may develop. Patients assume a characteristic posture, with hips and knees flexed. In severe cases, even these postural accommodations are insufficient to maintain horizontal gaze. The rigid spine is extremely brittle, and these patients may sustain highly unstable spinal fractures with even minimal trauma. This is an emergency situation, as these patients are prone to neurologic compromise secondary to subluxation and/or to epidural hematoma. Limited chest expansion (less than 2 cm) is a possible finding on physical examination secondary to costovertebral joint involvement. Laboratory testing will screen for

inflammatory arthritides and may or may not include the HLA-B27 test. If HLA-B27 is positive, it does not mean the patient has the disease. Likewise, a small percentage of patients who have the disease do not have the HLA-B27 antigen.

IMAGING STUDIES

Required for diagnosis

AP radiographs of the pelvis will depict bilateral sacroiliitis.
AP and lateral views of the affected portion of the spine will show characteristic squaring of the vertebral bodies and linear syndesmophytes (ossification of the anulus fibrosus).

Required for comprehensive evaluation

Weight-bearing long-cassette AP and lateral views of the entire spine are useful to evaluate the extent of deformity. In cases of suspected fracture or unexplained neurologic deficit in a patient with ankylosing spondylitis, MRI will demonstrate disruption of the disk space anteriorly and may demonstrate epidural hematoma.
CT is useful in demonstrating bony detail of a fracture.

Special considerations

A history of trauma, or a fall with pain, should raise concern for fracture. If the patient has an ankylosed spine, what may look like minimal subluxation suggests a serious fracture-dislocation. These fractures are always three-column injuries and should be considered highly unstable. Widening of a single disk space in comparison to the rest of the spine is almost always an indication of an acute fracture.

Pitfalls

None

IMAGE DESCRIPTIONS

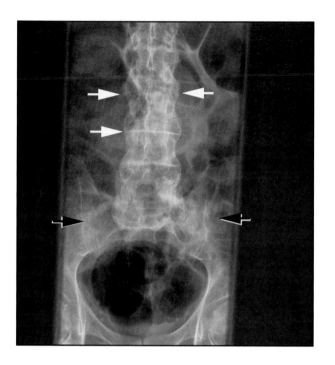

Figure 10-23

Ankylosing spondylitis—AP view

AP view of the lower thoracolumbar spine and pelvis shows complete obliteration of the bilateral sacroiliac joints with ankylosis (black arrows). Segmental bamboo bridging syndesmophytes are noted (white arrows).

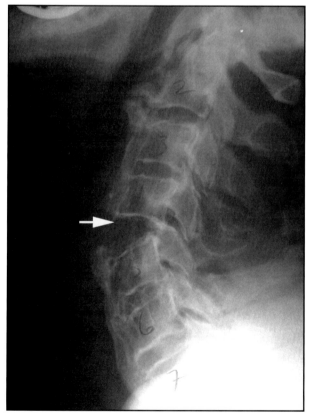

Figure 10-24

Ankylosing spondylitis—Lateral view

Lateral view of the cervical spine shows a fracture-dislocation at C4-C5 (arrow). The rigid nature of the ankylosed spine combined with characteristic osteopenia make it particularly susceptible to trauma. Because the spinal column is rigid, all fractures represent injury to all three columns of the spine. These fractures are extremely unstable.

SECTION 10 ■ SPINE

DIFFERENTIAL DIAGNOSIS

Posttraumatic and infectious diskitis (absence of multilevel involvement, lack of sacroiliac joint involvement)

Psoriatic arthritis (hip joint rarely involved, interphalangeal and metacarpophalangeal joints of hand involved)

Reiter's syndrome (involvement of knee and small joints of foot, hip joint rarely involved)

Rheumatoid arthritis (osteoporosis, symmetric involvement, lack of bony proliferation)

CERVICAL SPONDYLOSIS

SYNONYMS
Cervical discogenic syndrome
Degenerative cervical arthritis
Degenerative cervical disk disease

ICD-9 Code
721.0
Cervical spondylosis without myelopathy

DEFINITION
Cervical spondylosis is the generic term for degenerative arthritic changes seen in the cervical spine. Spondylotic changes are a biomechanical response to disk degeneration and manifest as disk desiccation, loss of disk height, osteophyte formation, subchondral sclerosis, and facet arthropathy. Cervical spondylosis is ubiquitous, occurs in the third to fourth decades, and becomes more prevalent with advancing age. These adaptations may lead to compression of the exiting nerve roots (radiculopathy) and/or spinal cord (myelopathy) and neurologic dysfunction.

HISTORY AND PHYSICAL FINDINGS
Symptoms from cervical spondylosis are, generally speaking, slowly progressive and insidious in nature. There may or may not be a history of trauma. The most common features are mechanical neck pain and restricted range of cervical motion.

Symptoms of cervical spondylotic radiculopathy are typically monoradicular, with pain described as sharp or lancinating following a specific nerve root distribution. Decreased deep tendon reflexes, muscle weakness, and variable sensory loss are suggestive of nerve root impingement. Neck extension and ipsilateral rotation may exacerbate symptoms (Spurling's test), whereas placing the ipsilateral hand on the head may relieve symptoms (shoulder abduction test).

Presenting symptoms may include upper and lower extremity weakness, gait ataxia, paresthesias, loss of manual dexterity, and, rarely, loss of bladder or bowel sphincter control. Neck pain is not typically a common problem on presentation in patients with myelopathy. On physical examination, patients may exhibit a wide based gait, hyperreflexia, motor weakness, sensory loss, and pathologic reflexes such as the Babinski sign or Hoffmann's reflex.

IMAGING STUDIES

Required for diagnosis

AP and lateral radiographs of the cervical spine are needed to establish the diagnosis.

Required for comprehensive evaluation

MRI of the cervical spine is indicated for patients with neurologic symptoms. CT myelogram is useful in patients in whom MRI cannot be obtained.

Special considerations

A patient who has had an acute onset of myelopathy requires emergent evaluation with MRI or CT myelogram.

Pitfalls

None

IMAGE DESCRIPTIONS

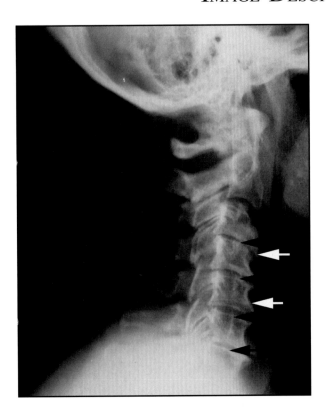

Figure 10-25

Cervical spondylosis—Lateral view

Lateral view of a patient with cervical spondylosis shows loss of disk space at each of the levels from C3-C7 (black arrows). Note the anterior and posterior osteophyte formation with hypertrophic anterior osteophyte formation (white arrows). This view gives classic information for loss of disk height and the arthritic mechanism.

SECTION 10 ■ SPINE

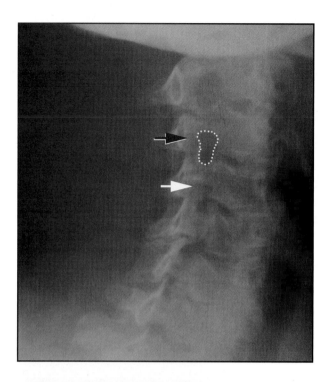

Figure 10-26

Cervical spondylosis—Oblique view

Oblique view of the cervical spine shows the neural foramen where the nerve root exits the spine (black arrow, dotted circle). Disk height loss and uncovertebral spurring lead to narrowing of the foramen and impingement on the exiting root (white arrow).

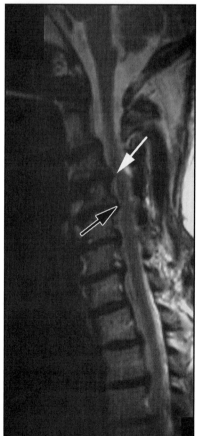

Figure 10-27

Cervical spondylosis—Parasagittal MRI

Parasagittal T2-weighted MRI scan of the cervical spine shows multiple-level cervical spondylosis. Posterior bulging of the anulus fibrosus and osteophyte formation from the vertebral body (black arrow) leads to loss of subarachnoid space (white arrow).

SECTION 10 ■ SPINE

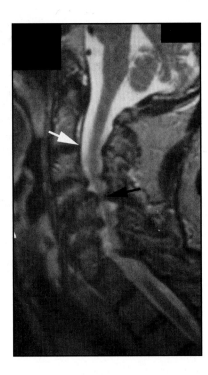

Figure 10-28

Cervical spondylosis with myelopathy— Sagittal MRI

Sagittal T2-weighted MRI scan of a patient with cervical spondylosis with myelopathy shows narrowing with spinal cord compression (black arrow). Proximally at C2 and C3, the wide open cerebrospinal fluid space is noted (white arrow).

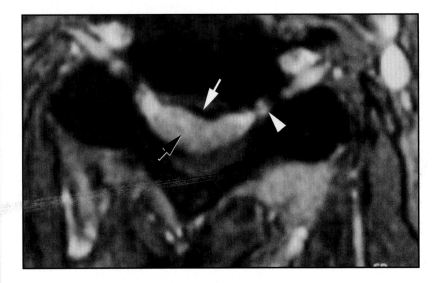

Figure 10-29

Cervical spondylosis with myelopathy— Axial MRI

Axial T2-weighted MRI scan shows ventral compression of the spinal cord (black arrow) by the posterior disk and vertebral end plate margin (white arrow). Note the lack of subarachnoid space and foraminal narrowing between the facet and uncovertebral joints (arrowhead).

DIFFERENTIAL DIAGNOSIS

Cervical spondylotic myelopathy (cervical stenosis that is narrowing with compression of the spinal cord noted on advanced imaging) (also includes spinal cord tumor, multiple sclerosis, amyotrophic lateral sclerosis, peripheral neuropathy, cerebrovascular accident, normal pressure hydrocephalus)

Cervical spondylotic radiculopathy (bony osteophyte narrowing on oblique radiographs or more particularly on transverse MRI or CT myelogram) (also includes shoulder arthropathy, peripheral nerve entrapment syndrome [carpal tunnel, cubital tunnel, radial tunnel])

Diskitis (differentiated by lack of significant osteophyte formation, intradiscal signal on MRI)

SECTION 10 ■ SPINE

LUMBAR DISK DEGENERATION

ICD-9 Code

722.52
Degeneration of lumbar or
lumbosacral intervertebral
disk

SYNONYMS

Black disk disease
Lumbar degenerative disk disease
Lumbar discogenic disease
Lumbar spondylosis

DEFINITION

Lumbar disk degeneration is an age-related, ubiquitous phenomenon that can be identified in essentially all individuals as time progresses. The intervertebral disk consists of the inner nucleus pulposus, outer anulus fibrosus, and the vertebral body end plate cartilage. The nucleus pulposus contains highly aggregated proteoglycans, which avidly bind water, in a loose stromal matrix. The anulus fibrosus consists of interwoven sheets of primarily type I collagen that contain the nucleus pulposus to form a "hydraulic shock absorber." With age, the proteoglycan content of the nucleus changes in both content and character with the end result that it becomes less hydrophilic. Stress transfer is shifted and the anulus begins to develop radial tears. Loss of disk height can result in annular bulging into the spinal canal and occasionally focal protrusion of disk material into the canal—a lumbar disk herniation. Concurrently, biomechanical forces are altered in the facet articulations leading to hypertrophy and further spinal canal narrowing. Clinical symptoms and radiographic findings do not universally correlate, leading to the difficulty in managing patients with these problems.

HISTORY AND PHYSICAL FINDINGS

The history may include an injury with acute onset of pain, or patients may report an insidious onset of pain. Some patients may be completely asymptomatic, and findings may be incidental to examination performed for other reasons. Approximately 80% of adults will experience an episode of low back pain during their lifetimes, and this is probably the most frequent presenting complaint resulting in radiographic examination. Pain generally is limited to the lumbosacral area, although referred or radicular leg pain may occur as well. Physical examination may reveal tenderness, muscle spasm, and limited lumbar motion in all planes of motion. In patients with nerve root impingement from a disk herniation, leg pain will follow a dermatomal distribution, and examination may reveal diminished reflexes, weakness or sensory abnormalities (depending on the degree of spinal canal compromise present), and tension signs.

IMAGING STUDIES

Required for diagnosis

AP and lateral radiographs of the lumbar spine will reveal disk space narrowing, end plate sclerosis, and spurring typical of degenerative processes. Osteophytes are oriented horizontally (traction osteophytes) as opposed to the linear syndesmophytes of ankylosing spondylitis or the flowing syndesmophytes of DISH syndrome.

Since there is a high degree of asymptomatic degenerative change present in the general population, the utility of screening radiographs for common low back pain is questionable. The radiographic findings rarely provide information that will have any effect on initial nonsurgical treatment. Most patients do not require routine imaging unless they have been symptomatic for 4 to 6 weeks or fulfill specific criteria to indicate early imaging. The main reason to obtain images early is to detect and prevent irreversible neurologic deterioration or progressive bone destruction from either tumor or infection. Still, radiographs should continue to be the initial diagnostic imaging modality of choice. Criteria for early imaging include:

- Age over 50 years
- History of malignancy
- Constitutional symptoms (fever, chills, weight loss)
- Significant trauma (motor vehicle accident, fall from a height)
- History of steroid or IV drug use
- Significant neurologic deficits
- Pain unrelieved by supine bed rest/night pain

Required for comprehensive evaluation

Sagittal T2-weighted MRI best quantifies the loss of disk height compared with uninvolved segments, along with varying degrees of disk dehydration or posterior bulging. T1-weighted para-sagittal images demonstrate the exiting nerve roots surrounded by high signal intensity where there may be impingement from lateral disk herniations or facet degeneration. Axial images are useful to evaluate the actual degree of canal compromise. MRI is also useful to rule out other potential sources of axial low back pain such as tumor or infection.

Special considerations

None

Pitfalls

It is critical to use imaging studies for confirmation of clinical diagnosis only.

SECTION 10 ■ SPINE

IMAGE DESCRIPTIONS

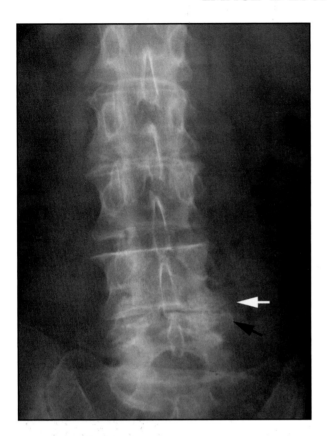

Figure 10-30

Lumbar disk degeneration—AP view

AP view of the lumbar spine shows disk space narrowing (white arrow) and horizontal marginal osteophyte formation (black arrow), both of which are the hallmarks of degenerative disease of the lumbar spine.

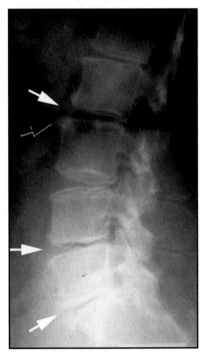

Figure 10-31

Lumbar disk degeneration—Lateral view

Lateral view of the patient in Figure 10-30 shows multiple-level disk involvement with narrowing (white arrows) and marginal osteophytes (black arrow) at all levels.

SECTION 10 ■ SPINE

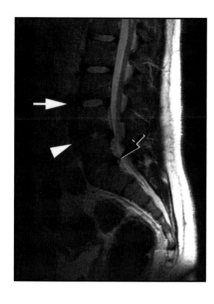

Figure 10-32

Lumbar disk degeneration—Sagittal MRI

Sagittal T2-weighted MRI scan of the lumbar spine is an excellent example of the stages of disk degeneration. Normal disks have high signal intensity within the nucleus pulposus and signal void in the anulus fibrosus (white arrow). Disk degeneration at L4-L5 shows loss of high signal intensity within the nucleus and posterior disk bulging (white arrowhead). At L5-S1 there is loss of disk height and an area of high signal intensity within the posterior anulus, indicative of an annular tear (black arrow).

DIFFERENTIAL DIAGNOSIS

Abdominal aneurysm (abdominal tenderness, pulsation, or palpable masses)

Extremity muscle strain (normal lumbar MRI)

Herniated disk (seen on lumbar MRI)

Low back pain

Lumbar disk degeneration (narrowed disk space, marginal osteophytes)

Muscle strain (history of trauma, self-limited course)

Osteoarthritis (hip/knee) (AP radiograph of the pelvis shows hip joint space narrowing)

Pathologic/metastatic disease (nonmechanical or night pain, constitutional symptoms)

Peripheral nerve entrapment) (Normal lumbar MRI, abnormal nerve conduction studies

Sciatica (radiculopathy)

SECTION 10 ■ SPINE

LUMBAR SPINAL STENOSIS

ICD-9 Code

724.02
Spinal stenosis, lumbar
region

SYNONYMS
None

DEFINITION
Lumbar spinal stenosis is a narrowing of the spinal canal, either centrally or in the lateral aspects such as the foramen, that leads to compression of the neural elements. Narrowing of the canal is most commonly related to acquired pathologies, including degenerative changes of the lumbar spine, spondylolisthesis, and posttraumatic etiologies. Congenital narrowing of the spinal canal is a less common problem and when symptomatic tends to occur in younger patients.

To best understand spinal stenosis, it is important to visualize the three-joint complex of the lumbar spine, consisting of bilateral facet joints and an intervertebral disk. Degenerative processes may begin in any of these sites, but eventually all articulations at each segmental level are involved. Facet joint degeneration with cartilaginous wear followed by joint laxity leads to excessive loads on the disk and eventual loss of structural integrity. Disk bulging and facet joint and ligamentum flavum hypertrophy cause the canal to narrow. Central canal stenosis leads to compression of the cauda equina, whereas lateral canal stenosis causes nerve root compression. These degenerative findings are most common in the lower lumbar spine.

HISTORY AND PHYSICAL FINDINGS
The clinical presentation of lumbar spinal stenosis varies by patient. Some patients may have radiographic findings consistent with narrowing of the lumbar spinal canal and remain asymptomatic. For patients who experience symptoms, the most common are low back pain, neurogenic claudication, and radiculopathy. Neurogenic claudication presents as leg pain, paresthesias, or weakness frequently in a bilateral nondermatomal fashion. It may be accompanied by a more dermatomal radicular component with pain following a specific distribution in the lower extremity. Neurogenic claudication depends on posture, mainly standing and walking, whereas vascular insufficiency to the lower extremity is related to any activity, including cycling in a sitting position. In addition, vascular claudication is not affected by lumbar flexion or extension.

IMAGING STUDIES

Required for diagnosis

Weight-bearing AP and lateral radiographs of the lumbar spine will show spondylotic changes, including diminished disk height, osteophytic spurs, and/or spondylolisthesis, but radiographs cannot evaluate the true dimensions of the spinal canal. MRI is usually required to confirm the diagnosis.

Required for comprehensive evaluation

Axial and sagittal images reveal narrowing of the central canal, and examination of parasagittal images allows for evaluation of the neuroforamen. On axial images, facet joint and ligamentum hypertrophy are the most common causes of spinal stenosis. T2-weighted images will provide the most detail, including loss of cerebrospinal fluid in the thecal sac consistent with narrowing of the canal.

Special considerations

Lumbar myelography is an advanced study that spine specialists often order to further define the severity of spinal stenosis or the presence of lumbar instability. Myelography is used less commonly today given its invasive nature and because of the availability of MRI. Myelography should be considered as an alternative study when MRI is contraindicated. Advantages of myelography include the ability to position the patient prone or standing where dynamic changes of stenosis within the spinal canal are more evident. Lumbar myelography is usually followed by CT to assess more accurately the degree of stenosis and surrounding disk and bone pathology.

Pitfalls

None

Image Description

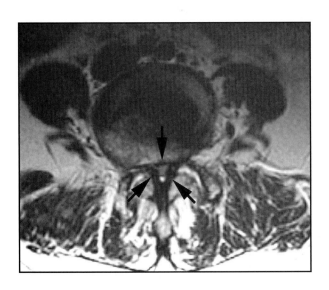

Figure 10-33

Spinal stenosis (lumbar spine)—Axial MRI

Axial MRI scan shows the circumferential nature of spinal canal narrowing (arrows).

Differential Diagnosis

Vascular claudication (no stenosis seen on MRI)

RHEUMATOID ARTHRITIS

SYNONYMS

Atlantoaxial instability
Basilar invagination
C1-C2 instability
Cranial settling
Occipital cervical settling
Odontoid erosion
Subaxial subluxation
Vertical subluxation

ICD-9 Code

720.0
Rheumatoid arthritis of spine
NOS

DEFINITION

Rheumatoid arthritis is a systemic disease of inflammatory synovitis. The etiology is not specifically known, but most cases fit the classic autoimmune mechanism. The patient has characteristic synovial hypertrophy with joint destruction. Women are more commonly affected than men at a ratio of 3:1. The hands and wrists are most commonly affected, with a characteristic ulnar drift at the metacarpophalangeal joints, although all joints of the body can be affected.

Spinal involvement preferentially occurs in the cervical area, given the quantity of synovial-lined bursae in the occipitocervical area, and is seen with more extensive peripheral involvement. In these patients, neck pain is the most common presenting complaint. Other manifestations of rheumatoid disease in the cervical spine include atlantoaxial instability, cranial settling, and subaxial subluxation. Atlantoaxial instability is related to attenuation of the transverse ligament and is seen early in the disease process. Cranial settling refers to vertical subluxation of the dens into the foramen magnum due to cartilage and bony destruction of the occiput, C1, and C2 articular masses. Subaxial subluxation refers to instability below the level of C2 and similarly presents following destruction of the facet and intervertebral articulations. Up to 80% of patients with rheumatoid arthritis demonstrate cervical involvement, although most are asymptomatic. More serious malalignment can affect the spinal cord and cause myelopathy.

HISTORY AND PHYSICAL FINDINGS

Physical examination of patients with rheumatoid arthritis is difficult because most have significant pain and joint deformity that limit neurologic testing. Craniocervical involvement commonly presents with unremitting neck pain that radiates to the occipital area because of irritation of the C2 nerve root and limited neck range of motion. Neurologic examination may reveal weakness, ataxia, and hyperreflexia. Loss of bowel/bladder and sphincter function is a rare finding until late in myelopathy.

IMAGING STUDIES

Required for diagnosis
AP, lateral, open mouth odontoid, and flexion-extension radiographs are required for basic evaluation of the cervical spine in a patient with known rheumatoid arthritis. The flexion-extension views are needed to assess for dynamic instability. Space available for the cord at C1-C2 (measured from the posterior edge of the dens to the anterior edge of the posterior ring of C1) should be > 14 mm. Radiographs should be obtained with the patient in an upright position to fully appreciate the degree of subluxation present.

Required for comprehensive evaluation
MRI is indicated to assess for spinal cord or specific nerve root compression. Brain stem impingement by the odontoid or retro-odontoid pannus is easily identified on this imaging modality. If MRI is not available, CT myelogram would be a reasonable choice.

Special considerations
Patients with acute symptoms of myelopathy, specifically weakness, require immediate radiographs and MRI.

Pitfalls
Severe odontoid erosion and osteopenia make radiographic evaluation difficult. Lateral radiographs of the skull, which center on the craniocervical junction, may help to illustrate anatomy in difficult cases.

IMAGE DESCRIPTIONS

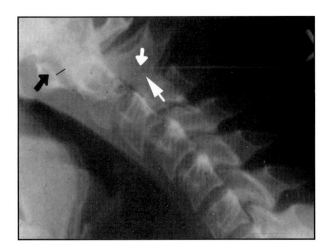

Figure 10-34

Rheumatoid arthritis (cervical spine)— Lateral flexion view

Lateral flexion view of the cervical spine shows atlantoaxial subluxation in a patient with rheumatoid arthritis. Note the abnormal widening between the odontoid and the anterior arch of C1 (black arrow, line). Also note the fusion of the C2 and C3 facet joints (white arrows).

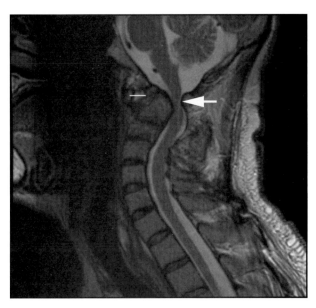

Figure 10-35

Rheumatoid arthritis (cervical spine)— Sagittal T2-weighted MRI

Rheumatoid arthritis with atlantoaxial subluxation causing spinal cord compression. The atlantoaxial subluxation, manifest as widening between the odontoid and the anterior arch of C1 (line), results in the odontoid pressing on the spinal cord (arrow).

DIFFERENTIAL DIAGNOSIS

Gastrointestinal disease (Crohn's disease) (medical history)

Psoriasis (involvement of small joints of the hand)

Trauma (no osteoporosis)

THORACIC DISK DEGENERATION

SYNONYMS

Degenerative disk disease, thoracic spine
Thoracic disk herniation
Thoracic spondylosis

DEFINITION

Idiopathic degeneration of the thoracic disks initiates in the third decade of life, with most thoracic disk herniations occurring in the third to fifth decades. The incidence of degenerative disk disease in the thoracic spine is less common, given the unique stabilizing role of the rib cage in this segment of the spinal column. Most thoracic disk degeneration occurs in the lower third of the thoracic spine, in part due to the increased motion in this region as the transition toward the more flexible lumbar spine. The upper third of the thoracic spine is well protected by the ribs, sternum, and clavicle and hence is much less commonly involved with degenerative processes. The incidence of thoracic disk herniation represents only 1% of all disk herniations. Radiculopathy or myelopathy may occur based on the relationship of the herniated disk to the nerve roots or spinal cord.

HISTORY AND PHYSICAL FINDINGS

Presenting symptoms may include localized pain related to thoracic disk degeneration, radicular pain with radiation to the anterior chest or abdomen, or myelopathy. A history of trauma is present in only 25% of patients. Of the patients with thoracic myelopathy, 25% may have no pain related to the thoracic spine. Neurologic symptoms include urinary urgency, lower extremity weakness, and/or sensory disturbances.

IMAGING STUDIES

Required for diagnosis

AP and lateral radiographs of the thoracic spine will reveal disk space narrowing and end plate spurring, typical of degeneration of the spine. Calcification of the disk space is commonly seen in association with thoracic disk herniation.

SECTION 10 ■ SPINE

Required for comprehensive evaluation

Sagittal MRI will show the loss of disk height and varying degrees of disk dehydration, posterior bulging, or herniation. MRI is also useful to rule out other possible causes of axial thoracic pain such as infection or tumor.

Special considerations

None

Pitfalls

None

IMAGE DESCRIPTIONS

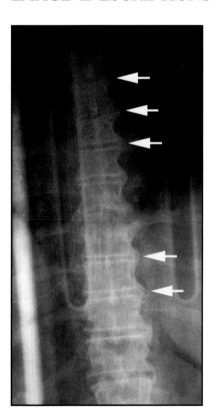

Figure 10-36

Thoracic disk herniation—AP view

AP view of the thoracic spine shows multiple levels of disk space narrowing, subchondral sclerosis, and spurring (white arrows).

SECTION 10 ■ SPINE

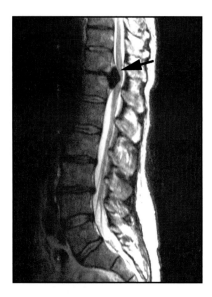

Figure 10-37

Thoracic disk herniation—Sagittal MRI

Sagittal T2-weighted MRI scan of the thoracic spine shows a large posterior herniation of the intervertebral disk material (arrow) extending into the spinal canal, causing cord compression.

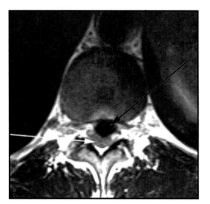

Figure 10-38

Thoracic disk herniation—Axial MRI

Axial T1-weighted MRI scan shows the size and extent of posterior herniation of disk material (black arrow) with loss of the hyperintense cerebrospinal fluid signal normally anterior to the spinal cord and actual deformity of the cord itself (white arrow).

DIFFERENTIAL DIAGNOSIS

Compression fracture (typical wedge-shaped vertebra apparent on lateral radiograph)

Infection (fluid collection seen on MRI)

Scheuermann's disease (end plate irregularity and 5° anterior wedging at three contiguous levels)

Tumor (apparent on MRI)

HEMANGIOMA

SYNONYMS

Arteriovenous hemangioma
Capillary hemangioma
Cavernous hemangioma
Venous hemangioma

ICD-9 Code

228.00
Hemangioma of unspecified site

DEFINITION

Hemangioma of the vertebral body is a benign vascular lesion found in approximately 12% of the population. As a group, hemangiomas constitute only 2% of all benign lesions of the skeletal system. Hemangiomas in vertebral bodies are usually of the capillary type, made up of small vessels. They typically occur in the anterior vertebral body and have a predilection for the thoracic spine. Symptomatic vertebral hemangiomas usually are seen in the third or fourth decade of life and are twice as common in women. Symptoms may be caused by four mechanisms: (1) pathologic fracture, (2) hematoma, (3) an expanding soft-tissue tumor, and (4) "ballooning" of the vertebral body with periosteal stretch. Tumors accompanied by neurologic compromise are more likely to occur in the thoracic spine, have an associated large soft-tissue mass, and are more likely to expand and erode than other hemangiomas. A few cases of consumptive coagulopathy (Kasabach-Merritt syndrome) have occurred as a result of these vascular malformations.

HISTORY AND PHYSICAL FINDINGS

Most hemangiomas of the vertebral body are asymptomatic and are found by serendipity. A history of trauma to the spine with localized pain and tenderness may be present. Lesions in the thoracic spine may result in cord compression with long tract neurologic signs.

IMAGING STUDIES

Required for diagnosis

AP and lateral radiographs of the spine are the initial studies of choice. Vertebral hemangiomas have characteristic coarse, thick, vertical striations that represent thickening of the vertical trabeculae of the vertebra. This is often referred to as "corduroy cloth" or "honeycomb" pattern.

SECTION 10 ■ SPINE

Required for comprehensive evaluation
CT of the affected vertebra will show any fracture. On an axial CT scan, the vertical trabeculae have a characteristic appearance of "polka dots." MRI is effective for demonstrating the soft-tissue extent of the tumor, if present, and the degree of neurologic compression. MRI demonstrates a mottled appearance with high signal intensity on both T1- and T2-weighted images. On T1-weighted images, the high signal intensity is caused by fat within the tumor. On T2-weighted images, it is from the water content of the vascular tumor. CT or MRI should be obtained when significant pain or neurologic symptoms are present.

Special considerations
None

Pitfalls
None

IMAGE DESCRIPTIONS

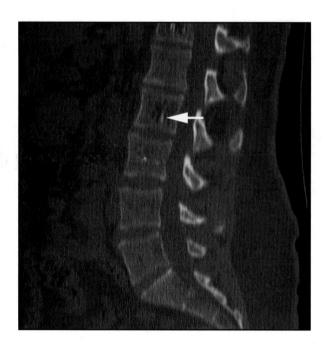

Figure 10-39

Hemangioma (lumbar spine)— Sagittal CT

Sagittal CT reformation of the lumbar spine shows trabecular coarsening through a lytic hemangioma of L2 (arrow).

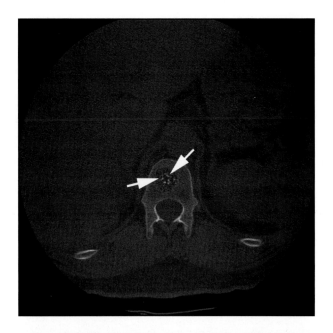

Figure 10-40

*Hemangioma (lumbar spine)—
Axial CT*

Axial CT image of the lumbar spine shows the
corduroy appearance of the thickened
trabeculae (arrows), which is classic in this
lytic hemangioma of L2.

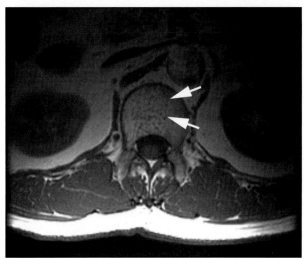

Figure 10-41

*Hemangioma (lumbar spine)—
Axial MRI*

Axial T1-weighted MRI scan shows classic
corduroy appearance of the low signal
intensity thickened trabeculae (arrows) in a
high signal intensity lesion, which is classic
for a hemangioma. Most other lesions,
excluding fat, subacute hemorrhage, and
melanoma, have low signal intensity on T1
weighting.

SECTION 10 ■ SPINE

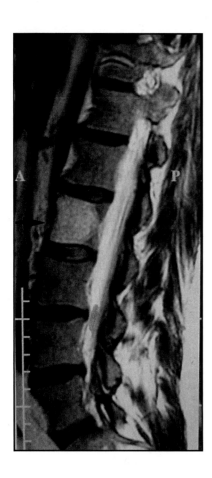

Figure 10-42

Hemangioma (lumbar spine)—
Sagittal MRI

Sagittal T2-weighted MRI scan shows the high signal intensity in a vertebral hemangioma (arrow) due to the vascular content.

DIFFERENTIAL DIAGNOSIS

Metastatic carcinoma (radiolucent appearance)

Myeloma (radiolucent appearance)

Paget's disease (pelvis and hip involvement; dense sclerotic vertebral margins, resulting in a "picture frame" appearance)

METASTATIC VERTEBRAL TUMORS

SYNONYMS

None

DEFINITION

Metastatic disease involving the spine is far more common than primary tumors of the spine and will be the focus of this section. The unique vascularity of the spine predisposes this area of the body to metastatic disease. The most common tumors that metastasize to the spine are lung, prostate, breast, kidney, thyroid, and colon. Multiple myeloma and leukemia can also involve the spine. Metastatic disease to the spine often involves the vertebral body proper and can cause significant collapse and deformity of the spine resulting in severe pain and neurologic deficits.

Hemangioma, eosinophilic granuloma, aneurysmal bone cyst, osteoblastoma, osteoid osteoma, and osteochondroma are the most common benign primary bone tumors of the spine. Giant cell tumor, an aggressive benign tumor, is another tumor that can be found within the spine. Primary malignant tumors found in the spine include osteosarcoma, chondrosarcoma, Ewing's sarcoma, lymphoma, solitary plasmocytoma, and chordoma.

HISTORY AND PHYSICAL FINDINGS

Patients with metastatic disease to the spine will most often report unremitting, progressively worse back pain that frequently occurs at night. Resorption of a vertebral body by tumor can result in a fracture and severe pain without antecedent trauma. Complaints of fatigue, malaise, and weight loss are common. Occasionally, pathologic fracture can be the first presentation of metastatic disease. Patients may also report difficulty initiating urination or overflow from a distended bladder. They also may have weakness or paresthesias at the extremities.

A patient with a history of malignancy who reports a new onset of back pain or neurologic deficit requires a thorough physical examination. Tenderness to palpation or percussion may be noted over an acute fracture secondary to a tumor. Testing of strength and sensation should be carried out immediately. All motor groups of the upper and lower extremities should be tested. Reflexes should be assessed as well, with particular attention to hyperreflexia, clonus, or Babinski's sign. A rectal examination demonstrating absent sphincter tone or sensation should be noted.

ICD-9 Codes

198.5
Secondary malignant neoplasm of other specified sites; bone and bone marrow

733.13
Pathologic fracture of vertebrae

SECTION 10 ■ SPINE

IMAGING STUDIES

Required for diagnosis

Bone scan is essential for evaluating the location and extent of metastases. AP and lateral radiographs generally will show gross vertebral collapse. Radiographs should be obtained with the patient in a standing position, if possible. Sclerosis, a mixed sclerotic and lytic pattern, or a lytic pattern may be seen. Early pedicle destruction is most easily seen as unilateral absence of the pedicle on the AP view (winking owl sign). However, because up to 60% of the vertebral body may need to be resorbed prior to being evident on plain radiographs, MRI is a much more sensitive and specific modality for diagnosis. Soft-tissue extension and spinal canal compromise are well visualized with MRI. The entire spinal axis should be imaged, at least in the sagittal plane, to reveal occult vertebral metastases, in addition to symptomatic ones.

Required for comprehensive evaluation

Sagittal MRI of the entire spine is necessary to visualize other occult metastatic deposits that may be asymptomatic. MRI, however, often overrepresents the amount of bone involvement, which may not always accurately illustrate the structural compromise of the biomechanical function of the vertebra; therefore, CT sometimes is also needed because it is more accurate at representing the degree of bony destruction.

Special considerations
None

Pitfalls
None

IMAGE DESCRIPTIONS

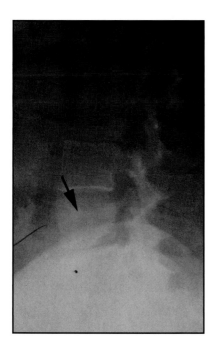

Figure 10-43

Metastatic breast carcinoma—Lateral view

Lateral view of the lumbar spine shows a pathologic fracture of L4 (arrow) secondary to breast carcinoma. The increased density of the abnormal vertebra suggests the presence of metastasis.

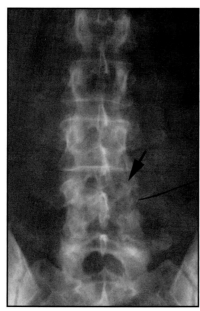

Figure 10-44

Metastatic breast carcinoma—AP view

Unilateral absence of the pedicle (winking owl sign) on the AP view (arrow) is consistent with metastasis.

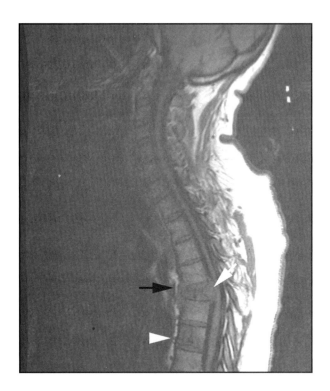

Figure 10-45

Metastatic breast carcinoma— Sagittal MRI

Sagittal T1-weighted MRI scan of the spine shows pathologic collapse of a thoracic vertebra secondary to metastatic disease. Metastases tend to be vertebral-body centered rather than disk-space centered as in pyogenic infection. The superior soft-tissue imaging resolution of MRI allows for excellent delineation of extraosseous tumor spread (black arrow) and epidural spinal cord compression (white arrow). Sagittal image sequences also allow identification of noncontiguous areas of metastatic disease (arrowhead).

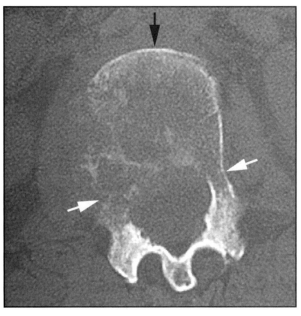

Figure 10-46

Metastatic breast carcinoma— Axial CT

Axial CT scan has excellent bony resolution and most accurately delineates the degree of bone destruction in the vertebra (black arrow) and both pedicles (white arrows).

DIFFERENTIAL DIAGNOSIS

Compression fracture (osteoporotic) (radiographs show generalized osteoporosis)

Paget's disease (hip and pelvic involvement)

Pyogenic infection (centers around disk space symmetrically)

Lymphoma (similar presentation)

DISKITIS

SYNONYMS
Disk space infection
Vertebral osteomyelitis

DEFINITION
Pyogenic infection of the intervertebral disk space may occur by hematogenous spread, direct extension, or through iatrogenic introduction of infection into the disk space during spinal procedures (eg, diskectomy). A remote site of infection also is common. Other risk factors include age, an immunosuppressed state (eg, diabetes), and prior invasive procedures (eg, cystoscopy). Hematogenous infection begins in the vertebral end plate and secondarily spreads to the adjacent disk space. The lumbar spine is most commonly involved, followed by the thoracic and cervical spines. *Staphylococcus aureus* is the most common organism isolated.

HISTORY AND PHYSICAL FINDINGS
The most common symptom on presentation is severe, unremitting back pain that begins insidiously and is relentlessly progressive. About half of patients may report constitutional symptoms such as fever, chills, and night sweats. Radiculopathy also may be present, and in patients with epidural abscess or severe vertebral body destruction and collapse, spinal cord dysfunction with paraparesis or paralysis may occur. Aside from findings on neurologic examination, the most common findings on physical examination are spinal rigidity and tenderness to percussion over the involved area.

IMAGING STUDIES

Required for diagnosis
AP and lateral radiographs of the localized area should be obtained, but they may not show any changes for 3 to 6 weeks following the onset of infection. The earliest changes are loss of disk height and loss of paravertebral soft-tissue shadows. Following these early signs, progressive end plate destruction with loss of end plate cortical integrity may be seen. Both sides of the disk space are commonly involved.

ICD-9 Codes

730.08
Osteomyelitis, periostitis, and other infections involving bone; acute osteomyelitis, other specified sites

730.18
Osteomyelitis, periostitis, and other infections involving bone; chronic osteomyelitis, other specified sites

SECTION 10 ■ SPINE

Required for comprehensive evaluation

MRI is the most sensitive and specific imaging modality and should be obtained when radiographic changes or clinical suspicion for infection exist. MRI will show characteristic changes prior to radiographs. In addition, MRI is the imaging modality of choice to demonstrate epidural abscess formation.

CT will show characteristic fragmentation of the vertebral end plates. The extent of true bony involvement is easily appreciated on CT, whereas MRI may be too sensitive and exaggerate the extent of true bony involvement. CT is imperative for surgical planning.

Special considerations

Patients with quadriparesis or paraparesis require emergent evaluation with MRI. Bone scans have been replaced to a substantial extent by MRI but may be useful in patients in whom MRI is contraindicated, although CT is a more appropriate test.

Pitfalls

None

IMAGE DESCRIPTIONS

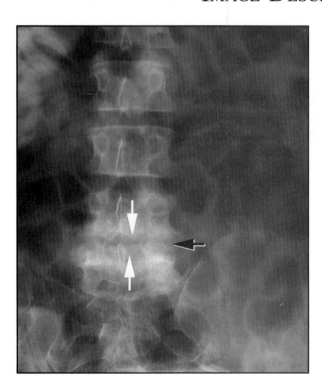

Figure 10-47

Diskitis—AP view

AP view of the lumbar spine shows disk space narrowing (black arrow) and end plate resorption (white arrows), which are the hallmarks of vertebral disk space infection but may take up to 6 weeks to appear on radiographs.

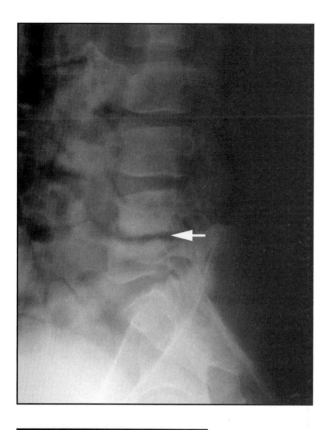

Figure 10-48

Diskitis—Lateral view

Lateral view of the lumbar spine shows disk space narrowing (arrow) with end plate irregularity, a feature of infection.

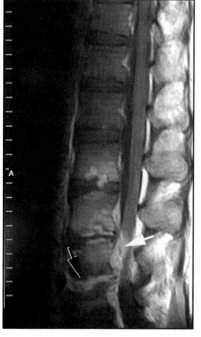

Figure 10-49

Diskitis—Sagittal MRI

Sagittal MRI of multiple-level vertebral osteomyelitis shows abnormal high signal intensity in the disk space (black arrow), characteristic of infection extending posteriorly (white arrow) into the spinal canal as an early epidural abscess. The abscess is producing compression of the thecal sac.

DIFFERENTIAL DIAGNOSIS

Neoplasm (intervertebral disk space destruction not common)

Tuberculosis of the spine (anterior aspect of vertebral body, prevertebral extension, paravertebral mass, more than one segment involved; positive purified protein derivative)

TUBERCULOSIS OF THE SPINE

SYNONYMS

Granulomatous spine infection
Pott's disease
Tuberculous spondylitis

DEFINITION

Tuberculosis of the spine accounts for up to 60% of skeletal
tuberculosis, with one half of the cases occurring in patients
younger than 21 years of age. The lower thoracic and upper lumbar
spine is the preferential site of involvement, with the first lumbar
vertebra the most common. The disease is spread hematogenously
to the spine from a primary focus in the lungs, mediastinum, or
kidneys. Infection may be found in disk spaces and adjacent
vertebrae. Typically two or more adjacent vertebral bodies are
involved. More than 80% of spinal tuberculous infections begin in
the anterior aspect of the vertebral body next to the subchondral
bone plate. The posterior spinal elements are less commonly
involved. Destruction of the vertebrae can result in collapse and
development of an angular deformity referred to as a gibbus. In
approximately 10% of patients the spinal cord may be compressed
or stretched over the gibbus, resulting in paraplegia. Imaging
studies reveal disk space narrowing and destruction of the adjacent
end plates. Tuberculous infections also can spread into adjacent soft
tissues forming a "cold abscess," especially in the psoas muscles.

HISTORY AND PHYSICAL FINDINGS

Classic characteristics include pain, both local and referred; muscle
spasms; night sweats; fever and chills; malaise; and weight loss.
The onset of back pain is insidious. Physical examination will
reveal rigidity caused by muscle spasm. Loss of normal lordosis
will be seen early in the course of the disease, followed by
development of a gibbus deformity. Palpation of the abdomen may
reveal the presence of a mass, which is a sign of a cold abscess.
Neurologic examination may reveal varying degrees of paraplegia.

IMAGING STUDIES

Required for diagnosis
AP and lateral radiographs will show narrowing of the
intervertebral disk space and destruction of the adjacent vertebra.

Required for comprehensive evaluation
MRI is helpful in evaluating intraspinal and paraspinal extension
of the infection. Visualization of posterior element involvement
is also improved.

Special considerations
None

Pitfalls
Tuberculosis may mimic metastatic disease of the spine.

IMAGE DESCRIPTION

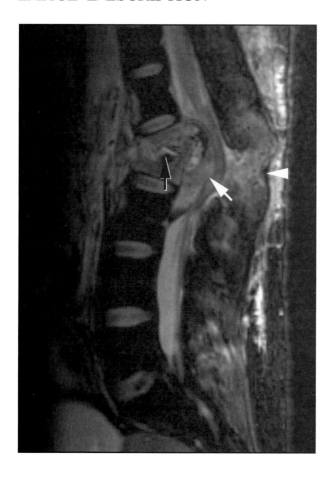

Figure 10-50

*Tuberculosis of the spine—
Sagittal MRI*

Sagittal fat-suppressed T2-weighted MRI scan
shows kyphosis, disk narrowing (black arrow),
and abnormal high signal intensity at L3-4,
consistent with an infection. A large posterior
soft-tissue mass is compressing the spinal cord
(white arrow). This infectious process also
extends into the posterior elements
(arrowhead).

SECTION 10 ■ SPINE

DIFFERENTIAL DIAGNOSIS

Fungal spinal infection (similar to tuberculosis)

Pyogenic spinal infection (involvement of one or more
segments, large calcified paravertebral mass seen with
tuberculosis)

Tumor (disk space may be preserved)

PEDIATRIC ORTHOPAEDICS

Section Editor
John F. Sarwark, MD

Section Co-Editor
Richard M. Shore, MD

Contributors
John M. Flynn, MD
Denise T. Ibrahim, MD
Khristinn Kellie Leitch, MD, MBA, FRCS(C)
David L. Skaggs, MD

IMAGING THE CHILD— AN OVERVIEW

INTRODUCTION

Imaging a child differs from imaging an adult. The adage, "A child is not just a small adult" is evident when viewing radiographs of a skeletally immature patient. Radiographs of the skeletally immature patient present the challenge of not only diagnosing conditions or injuries but also of knowing norms as well. The nonossified, cartilaginous portions of secondary ossification centers are radiolucent, which makes differentiating normal from abnormal difficult at times. Secondary ossification centers and apophyses may be easily confused with fractures, such as at the lesser trochanter of the femur, the base of the fifth metatarsal, or the olecranon. The use of comparison views of the contralateral side is important when there is uncertainty of radiographic findings.

Special knowledge and training are required when ordering and interpreting imaging studies in children. Ultrasound, MRI, and CT have a special place in the evaluation and management of children and can be quite different than in the adult. The indications for their proper use in specific conditions are described below. Remember, though, that despite the relative availability of advanced imaging technology, the utility of plain radiographs should not be forgotten.

When ordering an imaging study, it is important to understand positioning requirements, among other issues. The child's behavior may determine whether sedation is required to obtain an adequate study. Sedating children for MRI or CT is common but requires prior planning, scheduling, and postsedation monitoring.

ANATOMY

Imaging the pediatric musculoskeletal system presents unique challenges. Each long bone consists of four parts: the epiphysis, physis/growth plate, metaphysis, and diaphysis. After birth, the secondary ossification centers appear in the epiphysis at different times and different patterns, depending on the bone. The physis and portions of the epiphysis are not visible on plain radiographs, given their degree of calcification. This fact marks the importance of the clinical examination as an integral part in diagnosing injuries in children because radiographs often appear normal despite an injury to the physis or nonossified epiphysis. Apophyseal centers (nonarticulating ossification centers at the end of bones, ie, the olecranon) often have the reverse problem in which they are overdiagnosed as fractures, given their normal appearance, when in fact they are clinically insignificant. Whenever the diagnosis is in doubt, comparison views should be ordered.

OSSIFICATION CENTERS

These are described in the overviews of the anatomic sections of this text.

SAFETY CONCERNS IN CHILDREN

Parents may occasionally express concern about radiation exposure to children and the potential future harm as a result of radiation exposure. This is a sensitive issue that is best addressed by showing compassion and explaining the relative safety and minimal risk in relation to the importance of the radiograph in the care of the child. It is also helpful to have knowledge of the equipment at the facility and to make comparisons of the relative amount of radiation exposure from one radiograph compared to everyday exposures such as from microwave ovens, television, or travel in an aircraft at 30,000 feet (the latter is equivalent to one chest radiograph.) Such comparisons may be provided by the radiation safety director at the hospital or technicians in the radiology department. The amount of exposure depends on the specific equipment in question (eg, the mini C-arm provides less exposure than does the standard C-arm).

STANDARD IMAGING VIEWS

Radiographs

The standard views are determined by what is being imaged. Typically, AP and lateral views in anatomic positions are routine and required for proper evaluation of a specific bone or joint. Oblique views are useful when imaging the foot or hand and occasionally the lumbar spine. Radiographs of a child in a nonanatomic position may occasionally be required, such as lateral bending views of the thoracic and lumbar spine to assess flexibility of scoliosis or flexion-extension views of the cervical spine to assess segmental stability. Various specialty views can be ordered to address specific problems and require knowledge of the anatomy of the bone or joint in question. For example, an axillary view of the shoulder is one of the most useful views in assessing the humeral head position in relation to the glenohumeral joint and is part of the basic series. It is also a view that may be difficult to perform because of injury or pain. The specifics of different views are discussed with their respective disorders in the anatomic sections of this text.

SECTION 11 ■ PEDIATRIC ORTHOPAEDICS

Computed tomography

CT is highly useful in assessing pediatric musculoskeletal problems. In many instances, it may be even more definitive and of higher utility than MRI, especially when further definition of skeletal morphology is required. CT is commonly requested for definitive assessment of articular fractures and physeal fractures in children as a method to demonstrate the morphology of a fracture pattern and the extent of displacement. CT is used routinely following closed or open reduction of dislocated hips (DDH) in infants and is easily done even with a plaster cast in place. In the spine, CT is often used to assess rotatory displacement of C1-C2 in atlantoaxial rotatory fixation (AARF). The specifics of different indications for CT are discussed with their respective disorders in the anatomic sections of this text.

Magnetic resonance imaging

MRI has become ubiquitous in imaging musculoskeletal problems in both children and adults. This is not to say, however, that its overuse is to be encouraged. In most instances, initial evaluation of clinical problems with radiographs is advised. Additional imaging with MRI follows when further definition of musculoskeletal anatomy or pathology is indicated.

MRI is the procedure of choice for assessment of spine and spinal cord pathology, including infections and benign and malignant lesions. Again, initial assessment with radiographs is required. MRI is useful to define spinal cord involvement by vertebral and disk pathology. However, in spondylolysis, CT remains the imaging modality of choice in defining the skeletal changes and is superior to MRI. In children with potential musculoskeletal infections, MRI is the modality of choice and frequently allows a diagnosis in cases of occult presentations of infections. MRI is also useful in defining joint pathology, including physeal problems (eg, growth arrest) or articular morphology in very young children (eg, bone dysplasias, Legg-Calvé-Perthes disease). The specifics of different indications for MRI are discussed with their respective disorders in the anatomic sections of this text.

EMERGENCIES

In major trauma situations, patients are assessed and stabilized according to the primary survey protocols of Acute Trauma and Life Support (ATLS). Musculoskeletal imaging is an integral component of the secondary survey assessment of initial trauma calls. In other acute, but non-ATLS situations, such as isolated fractures and dislocations, the process of evaluation and imaging requires expert and compassionate care. As a rule, fractures and dislocations *must be splinted* prior to imaging. Reduction and splinting of grossly displaced fractures or dislocations and dressing open wounds are appropriate prior to imaging.

NORMAL VARIANTS

Normal variants are common in pediatric musculoskeletal imaging. Common areas of normal findings or normal variants include synchondroses (areas that are cartilage in childhood but ossify in the preadolescent or teen years—especially in the pelvis and spine), irregular ossification within epiphyses (especially the distal femur), ossicles (especially those around the ankle), and angular problems of the lower extremities that are normal, developmental, and appropriate for age. The specifics of different normal variants are discussed with their respective disorders in the anatomic sections of this text.

IMAGING TIPS

1. Never settle for an inadequate image or poor technique as it can lead to improper diagnosis.
2. Plan accordingly for sedation or general anesthesia if the imaging study requires stillness for quality such as MRI or CT.
3. If a patient requires sedation, ensure that the parents are informed about avoiding oral intake for 12 hours prior to the study (NPO status) or other status based on the needs of the patient.
4. Having a toy, music, or television may be sufficient to distract and relax a child to promote cooperation.
5. Never leave a child unsupervised, especially after sedation.
6. Obtain comparison views when there is uncertainty of normal versus abnormal findings.

SECTION 11 ■ PEDIATRIC ORTHOPAEDICS

Legg-Calvé-Perthes Disease

Synonyms

Aseptic necrosis of the femoral head
Avascular necrosis of the femoral head
Idiopathic osteonecrosis of the femoral head
Juvenile osteochondrosis of the hip

Definition

Legg-Calvé-Perthes disease is an osteonecrosis of the proximal femoral epiphysis occurring in children between the ages of 4 and 8 years. Patients from age 2 years to 12 years can be affected. Legg-Calvé-Perthes disease is four times more common in boys than in girls and occurs bilaterally in approximately 10% of patients. A genetic basis has not been established, nor has a specific cause been established. The disease runs a well-described course over several years through four stages: initial, fragmentation, reossification, and healing. The best prognosis is in children who present before age 6 years and in whom less than half of the proximal femoral epiphysis is involved. The worst prognosis is in children older than age 6 years with involvement of the entire epiphysis, especially if there is subluxation or epiphyseal arrest or if very severe adduction contracture develops. Treatment is directed toward maintenance of motion and containment of the femoral head.

Imaging is an essential part of the management of Legg-Calvé-Perthes disease. At initial presentation, radiographic findings may be subtle, and more advanced imaging studies may be required for diagnosis. Over the active phases of the disease, radiographs are ordered every 6 weeks and are studied for signs of osteochondral fracture, epiphyseal collapse, physeal involvement, and changes in the shape of the femoral head (eg, coxa magna).

History and Physical Findings

Most children present initially with a painless limp. Later in the course of the disease, the child may report hip, thigh, or groin pain. Physical findings include loss of hip range of motion, particularly loss of internal rotation and abduction on the involved side. Trendelenburg gait and a Trendelenburg sign may be observed, and there may be a true or apparent limb-length discrepancy. Children with Legg-Calvé-Perthes disease are somewhat short in stature but otherwise healthy. Muscle atrophy may develop on the involved side, particularly the quadriceps.

ICD-9 Code

732.1
Juvenile osteochondrosis of hip and pelvis

Section 11 ■ Pediatric Orthopaedics

Imaging Studies

Required for diagnosis

Weight-bearing AP and non–weight-bearing frog-lateral views of the pelvis are indicated for initial and follow-up evaluation to assess the proximal femoral epiphysis. Attention is focused on increased radiodensity of the epiphysis, medial joint space widening, and any sign of fragmentation or subchondral fracture (crescent sign).

Required for comprehensive evaluation

If the initial radiographs are normal and the history and physical examination suggest Legg-Calvé-Perthes disease and no other explanation is available for hip pain, advanced imaging is indicated. A technetium Tc 99m bone scan with pinhole (coned-down) images of the hip may show decreased uptake in the epiphysis on delayed phase images, indicative of decreased blood flow to the proximal femoral epiphysis. MRI of the hips may help assess the amount of femoral head involvement and determine the extent of involvement of the epiphysis. Later in the disease, MRI is valuable to visualize the entire cartilaginous morphology of the femoral head, which may extend outside the bony confines of the acetabulum (extrusion).

Special considerations

The ovaries and testes should be shielded for radiographs, being careful not to obscure the hip joint. Sedation or general anesthesia may be necessary for MRI evaluation in younger children.

Pitfalls

Because of decreased range of motion, adequate frog-lateral views may be difficult to obtain. Proper positioning is important; for the AP view, the patient should be standing, with feet at shoulder width and the hips internally rotated. With full-body bone scan images, the epiphysis may not be accurately imaged, given the small size of the femoral head in relation to the body and the potential of the anterior acetabulum to obstruct the view, so pinhole images are required.

IMAGE DESCRIPTIONS

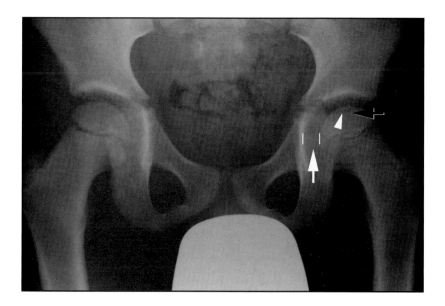

Figure 11-1

Legg-Calvé-Perthes disease (initial stage)—AP view

AP view of the pelvis shows subtly increased radiodensity (black arrow) and medial joint space widening of the left hip (white arrow, lines). A lucent subchondral fracture line (crescent sign) is also seen (arrowhead). These findings are characteristic of the initial stage of Legg-Calvé-Perthes disease.

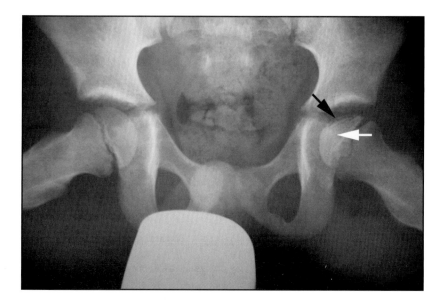

Figure 11-2

Legg-Calvé-Perthes disease (fragmentation stage)— Frog-lateral view

Frog-lateral view shows several classic features of fragmentation-stage Legg-Calvé-Perthes disease in the left hip. Note the crescent sign (black arrow) and increased radiodensity of the epiphysis (white arrow). Also note that in particular, there is a decrease in the anterior epiphyseal height.

SECTION 11 ■ PEDIATRIC ORTHOPAEDICS

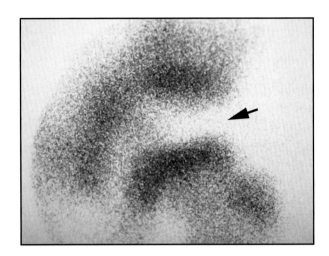

Figure 11-3

*Legg-Calvé-Perthes disease—
Bone scan, pinhole AP view*

Bone scan (pinhole AP view) of the left hip shows decreased uptake in the proximal femoral epiphysis, especially laterally (arrow). This classic finding in Legg-Calvé-Perthes disease demonstrates the avascularity of the femoral epiphysis in the early stages of the disease. Pinhole views of the hip are required images.

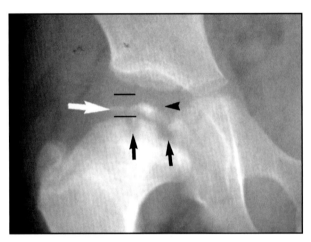

Figure 11-4

*Legg-Calvé-Perthes disease
(late fragmentation/early
reossification stage)—AP view*

AP view of the hip shows Legg-Calvé-Perthes disease in the late fragmentation/early reossification stage. The femoral head appears to be contained within the acetabulum. The femoral neck appears to be relatively foreshortened. Note the cysts in the metaphysis in the juxtaphyseal area (black arrows). Very subtle acetabular changes are present. Note the early reossification (white arrow) and the decreased epiphyseal height (arrowhead, lines).

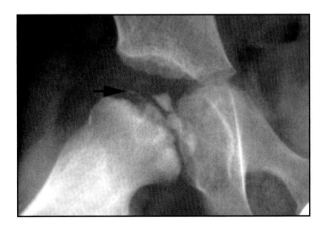

Figure 11-5

*Legg-Calvé-Perthes disease
(late fragmentation/early
reossification stage)—
Frog-lateral view*

Frog-lateral view shows the appearance of Legg-Calvé-Perthes disease in the late fragmentation/early reossification stage. Arrow indicates an area of early reossification.

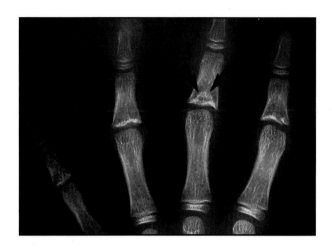

Figure 11-6

Trichorhinophalangeal syndrome—AP view of the hand

AP view of the hand shows chevron-shaped epiphyses (arrows), which can be seen in trichorhinophalangeal syndrome. Children with this syndrome sometimes have proximal femoral epiphyseal changes that mimic Legg-Calvé-Perthes disease.

DIFFERENTIAL DIAGNOSIS

Gaucher disease (systemic skeletal involvement demonstrated on MRI with diffuse marrow changes)

Idiopathic chondrolysis (joint space narrowing on AP view of pelvis without epiphyseal changes)

Meyer dysplasia (irregular ossification of proximal femoral epiphysis on AP view of pelvis)

Multiple epiphyseal dysplasia (bilateral/symmetric involvement of hips with involvement of most other epiphyses on AP view of pelvis; can also develop superimposed changes that resemble Legg-Calvé-Perthes disease)

Osteonecrosis (steroid osteopathy, posttraumatic or iatrogenic osteonecrosis; focal, segmented lesion of femoral epiphysis on AP view of pelvis)

Sickle cell anemia, Sickle cell osteonecrosis (mimics Legg-Calvé-Perthes disease on AP and frog-lateral views of the pelvis, with diagnosis of sickle cell disease)

Transient synovitis (normal findings on AP and frog-lateral pelvis views; ultrasound of hips may demonstrate nonspecific effusion)

Trichorhinophalangeal syndrome (mimics Legg-Calvé-Perthes disease on AP and frog-lateral views of the pelvis; diagnosis is made in conjunction with clinical findings of hair and nail abnormalities; AP view of the hand is diagnostic)

SECTION 11 ■ PEDIATRIC ORTHOPAEDICS

OSGOOD-SCHLATTER DISEASE

ICD-9 Code

732.4
Osgood-Schlatter disease

SYNONYM
Apophysitis of the tibial tubercle

DEFINITION
Osgood-Schlatter disease is a traction apophysitis of the tibial tubercle, typically seen in children between the ages of 10 and 15 years. The condition runs a self-limited course of several months to 2 years, becoming asymptomatic when the tibial tubercle apophysis closes during the teenage years. Persistent signs and symptoms are rare.

HISTORY AND PHYSICAL FINDINGS
The essential physical finding is tenderness over the tibial tubercle on palpation. The tibial tubercle may be prominent on visual inspection. Pain and prominence are often seen on the contralateral side. Knee effusion and other findings of intra-articular pathology are absent, and ligamentous examination is normal. Most individuals with symptomatic Osgood-Schlatter disease will have contracture of the quadriceps and hamstrings.

IMAGING STUDIES

Required for diagnosis
AP, lateral, and axial views of the knee are indicated. In most instances, it is a clinical diagnosis, made without imaging studies. Radiographs, however, are advised to rule out unexpected and rare bone lesions. No other imaging studies are necessary. When bilateral symptoms are present, bilateral AP and lateral views of the knee should be performed.

Required for comprehensive evaluation
Coned-down (pinhole) views of the tibial tubercle may be indicated to better visualize fragmentation of the tubercle. Imaging studies that allow visualization of the soft tissues, such as MRI, are useful.

Special considerations
None

Pitfalls

Failure to obtain images may lead to overlooking other rare causes of pain in the proximal and anterior tibia, such as neoplasm. In cases of sudden pain, tibial tubercle avulsion should be considered as part of the differential diagnosis. Overpenetrated radiographs may not show the tubercle at all. On the axial view, the tibial tubercle fragmentation can be mistaken for a loose body within the knee.

IMAGE DESCRIPTION

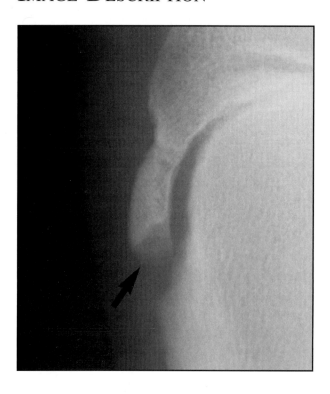

Figure 11-7

Osgood-Schlatter disease— Lateral view

Lateral view of the tibial tubercle in a skeletally immature patient with no history of acute trauma supports the clinical diagnosis of Osgood-Schlatter disease. Note the slight widening of the tibial tubercle apophysis (arrow). There is no evidence of fracture and no significant soft-tissue swelling, which usually is an indicator of acute Osgood-Schlatter disease.

DIFFERENTIAL DIAGNOSIS

Acute fracture of the tibial tubercle (history of acute injury; acute fracture line will be seen)

Patellar fracture (radiographs demonstrate "sleeve" of bone from inferior pole)

Patellar tendinitis (absence of soft-tissue swelling over tibial tubercle)

Primary bone or cartilage neoplasm of the proximal tibia (rare; destructive lesion or new bone formation may be present and is atypical in Osgood-Schlatter disease)

Proximal tibial osteomyelitis (radiographs demonstrate metaphyseal lucency or other changes including periosteal reaction)

Osteochondritis Dissecans of the Knee

ICD-9 Code

732.7
Osteochondritis dissecans

Synonyms

None

Definition

Osteochondritis dissecans (OCD) is a disorder of the subchondral bone. OCD usually involves the knee, but it can also involve the talus (ankle), capitellum (elbow), or other sites. The etiology is unknown, although presumably, repetitive trauma or other factors cause a change in the blood supply of the subchondral bone, leading to osteonecrosis with secondary involvement of the overlying articular cartilage. In its mildest forms, OCD may cause localized discomfort that resolves with time. More advanced forms of the disorder may be associated with complete disruption of the fragment, leading to an osteochondral loose body within the joint and a corresponding large articular defect.

When OCD occurs in the knee, the most common location is the lateral aspect of the medial femoral condyle. This may occur as a result of repetitive trauma, where the tibial spine abuts this area during extension of the knee, resulting in injury to the underlying subchondral bone.

History and Physical Findings

Some cases of OCD of the knee are discovered when a child presents with overuse knee pain. Others are discovered as incidental findings on radiographs of the knee taken for another reason. Tenderness to direct deep palpation over the involved femoral condyle, especially when the knee is fully flexed, may be found. Pain may also be noted when the leg is internally rotated and then extended from a fully flexed position (Wilson's sign). In more advanced cases, especially when there is a loose body, there may be a knee effusion. The remainder of the knee examination is generally normal.

Imaging Studies

Required for diagnosis

AP and lateral views and tunnel (notch) view with the knee flexed 30° are indicated for diagnosis.

Required for comprehensive evaluation

Comparison views of the contralateral knee may be helpful to rule out developmental abnormalities. MRI is indicated to determine the degree of involvement of the overlying articular cartilage. On MRI, a disruption of the articular surface is seen as the presence of joint fluid beneath the subchondral bone in areas of high signal intensity on T2-weighted images. The extent of bone edema will also be apparent on MRI, and the presence and location of loose bodies can be determined. Sometimes MR arthography is required to completely confirm loosening. The use of bone scans for evaluation is not well defined.

Special considerations

Sedation or general anesthesia may be necessary in a younger child who undergoes MRI.

Pitfalls

Normal but irregular ossification patterns in skeletally immature children may mimic OCD of the distal femoral condyle. Contralateral views, along with a history and physical examination, are indicated to make this differential diagnosis.

IMAGE DESCRIPTIONS

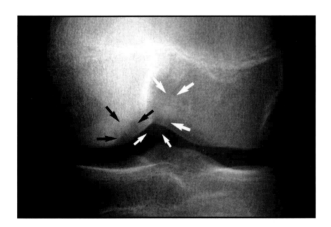

Figure 11-8

Osteochondritis dissecans (knee)— AP view

AP view of the knee of a skeletally immature adolescent shows the outline of an OCD lesion (black arrows) and a detached ossicle from the medial distal femoral condyle (white arrows). Comparing this radiograph with Figure 11-9 demonstrates the importance of ordering a tunnel view in some patients to fully visualize the extent of OCD of the distal femoral condyle.

SECTION 11 ■ PEDIATRIC ORTHOPAEDICS

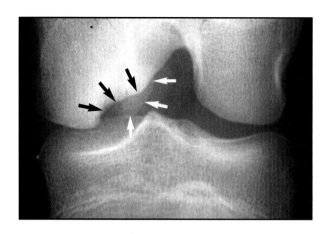

Figure 11-9

Osteochondritis dissecans (knee)— Tunnel view

Tunnel view of the knee in 30° of flexion shows advanced changes of OCD of the lateral portion of the medial femoral condyle (black arrows). Note the large defect in the weight-bearing portion of the medial femoral condyle and a well-circumscribed detached ossicle (white arrows).

DIFFERENTIAL DIAGNOSIS

Osteochondral fracture (lesion is usually patellar in origin with no femoral condylar changes on radiographs; clinical findings indicate injury to the patellar area)

Subacute epiphyseal osteomyelitis (lesion appears more central in the epiphysis on AP and lateral views)

PATELLOFEMORAL MALALIGNMENT SYNDROME

SYNONYMS

Anterior knee pain
Patellofemoral dysfunction
Patellofemoral syndrome

ICD-9 Code
719.46
Pain in joint, lower leg

DEFINITION

Patellofemoral malalignment is a term that describes a developmental condition of abnormal biomechanical relationships at the patellofemoral joint. Patellofemoral malalignment is a very common cause of anterior knee pain, especially in teenage girls. As a girl matures, the pelvis widens, causing biomechanical changes at the anterior knee. This acquired and physiologic alignment change in the anatomic axis of the knee can lead to patellofemoral or anterior knee pain symptoms.

HISTORY AND PHYSICAL FINDINGS

Symptoms are related to overuse. In the typical chronic presentation, the patient reports anterior knee pain that is mechanical in nature, such as when climbing stairs or arising from a chair. In more acute cases, the patient may feel the patella subluxate or dislocate. Physical findings include a positive patellar compression test, an increased Q angle, a positive patellar apprehension test, and quadriceps contracture. Knee effusion, joint line tenderness, or ligamentous instability is usually not present. Tenderness is found along the peripatellar borders. Some notable lateral patellar tilt may be present.

IMAGING STUDIES

Required for diagnosis

AP, lateral, and Merchant axial views of the knee are ordered to make the diagnosis.

Required for comprehensive evaluation

Weight-bearing full-length views of the lower extremities are indicated to assess mechanical or anatomic axis malalignments of the limb in the coronal plane. Following acute patellar subluxation or dislocation with knee effusion, MRI may be indicated to identify loose bodies or other osteochondral injuries related to the acute dislocation.

SECTION 11 ■ PEDIATRIC ORTHOPAEDICS

Special considerations
Tangential views assess the degree of lateral patellar tilt. The patient is prone and the knee is flexed 30°.

Pitfalls
Inaccurately performed tangential views of the patellofemoral joint may fail to reveal the malalignment.

IMAGE DESCRIPTION

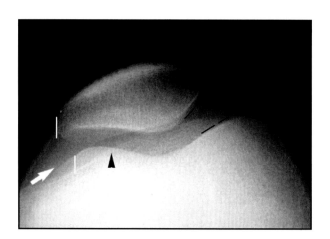

Figure 11-10

Patellofemoral malalignment— Merchant axial view

Merchant axial view of the knee demonstrates typical patellar tilt (black arrow, dashed lines) found in patellofemoral malalignment syndrome. Note the lateral overhang of the patella outside the trochlear groove (white arrow, lines) and the mild underdevelopment of the lateral femoral condyle (arrowhead). No fragmentation or signs of acute injury are apparent.

DIFFERENTIAL DIAGNOSIS

Bipartite patella (radiographs show separate ossification center of the patella)

Patellar tendinitis (radiographs are normal)

Sinding-Larsen–Johansson disease (radiographs show inferior patellar crescent of bone)

Slipped Capital Femoral Epiphysis

Synonyms

SCFE

Slipped epiphysis

Slipped upper femoral epiphysis

ICD-9 Code

732.9
Unspecified
osteochondropathy

Definition

Slipped capital femoral epiphysis (SCFE) is a developmental condition of the proximal femoral physis that typically occurs in adolescence and leads to a progressive displacement of the femoral neck from the proximal femoral epiphysis. In most cases, the femoral neck displaces anteriorly and the femoral epiphysis remains within the acetabulum. Most commonly, this occurs slowly over time. In some cases, it occurs acutely.

Although the exact etiology of SCFE is unknown, it is understood that both mechanical and endocrine factors play a role. Many children with SCFE have relative retroversion of the femur, placing increased stress on the physis. Obesity increases this stress. The condition typically occurs during the period of most rapid adolescent growth (between the ages of 11 and 16 years in boys and 10 and 14 years in girls). SCFE that occurs at a younger age is sometimes due to an endocrinopathy such as hyperthyroidism, hypogonadal endocrinopathy, panhypopituitarism, or renal osteodystrophy. SCFE is about twice as common in boys as in girls. Bilateral involvement occurs in approximately 40% to 50% of patients. In patients who present with one affected hip but go on to experience bilateral SCFE, the second slip occurs within 1 year in about 75% of patients. Presentations include stable SCFE, where the individual is able to bear weight on the involved extremity, and unstable SCFE, where the individual is unable to bear weight in any manner.

History and Physical Findings

In the most common presentation of stable SCFE, the patient reports progressive hip, groin, and sometimes thigh pain lasting weeks to months. Occasionally, the patient reports knee pain; in this case a radiograph of the hip may not be taken, and the diagnosis may be missed. Often the parent will notice a limp or a waddling gait. On physical examination, the patient will be observed to walk with a Trendelenburg gait and the foot turned out. Physical findings include decreased hip internal rotation and pain with internal rotation. A classic finding is obligate external rotation as the hip is flexed from the neutral extended position. In unstable SCFE, the patient is unable to bear weight and will not tolerate any hip range of motion because of discomfort.

IMAGING STUDIES

Required for diagnosis
AP and frog-lateral views are usually sufficient for diagnosis.

Required for comprehensive evaluation
In most presentations of SCFE, additional views are not needed. CT may be used to diagnose mild SCFE, and it also may be required to assess morphology and physeal closure in severe, late-presenting cases. When persistent pain follows internal fixation of SCFE, CT can evaluate the hip for osteonecrosis or penetration of the screw through the cartilage into the joint.

Special considerations
Gonadal shielding is recommended on follow-up radiographs, but care should be taken not to obscure the hips.

Pitfalls
The hip may be difficult to visualize on radiographs of extremely obese individuals (a common scenario). Also, very subtle slips may be overlooked.

IMAGE DESCRIPTION

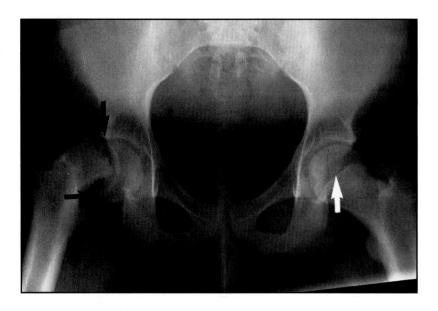

Figure 11-11

Slipped capital femoral epiphysis— AP view

AP view of the pelvis shows a SCFE on the right side (black arrows). The radiographic features suggest medial displacement of the proximal femoral epiphysis in relation to the femoral neck. On the left side, the physis is narrowed (white arrow), and no slip is apparent.

DIFFERENTIAL DIAGNOSIS

Acute type I fracture of the femoral neck (physeal fracture through the proximal femoral physis, no metaphyseal changes on AP hip radiograph)

Endocrinopathy (AP view of the pelvis will demonstrate physeal widening and bilateral changes)

Legg-Calvé-Perthes disease (AP view of the pelvis demonstrates epiphyseal changes without displacement)

TARSAL COALITION

ICD-9 Code

755.67
Anomalies of the foot, not
elsewhere classified

SYNONYMS

Calcaneal bar
Peroneal spastic flatfoot
Rigid flatfoot
Talocalcaneal bar

DEFINITION

Tarsal coalition is a pathologic connection between two or more
tarsal bones that is thought to be embryonic in origin. The
connection can be fibrous, cartilaginous, or bony. Symptoms begin
when the flexible cartilaginous connection begins to ossify during
the adolescent years. This condition is bilateral in 50% to 60% of
patients and occurs in less than 1% of the population. The most
common coalitions are a calcaneonavicular coalition and a
talocalcaneal coalition. Coalitions between other tarsal bones are
much less common. Most symptomatic coalitions can be excised
surgically with good results.

HISTORY AND PHYSICAL FINDINGS

Patients report a gradual onset of unilateral or bilateral foot or
ankle pain, and some report recurrent ankle sprains. Pain may be
localized to the midfoot or the sinus tarsi, or it may be very
difficult to localize. Patients may report that walking on uneven
ground or on hillsides is particularly difficult. Physical examination
reveals decreased or absent subtalar motion (inversion and
eversion). The foot may be in valgus, with apparent tightness or
spasms of the peroneal tendons, leading to the clinical term
peroneal spastic flatfoot.

IMAGING STUDIES

Required for diagnosis

Weight-bearing AP and lateral views and non–weight-bearing
oblique views of the foot will demonstrate the features of many
tarsal coalitions. A calcaneonavicular coalition may be seen best on
a 45° medial oblique view. Talocalcaneal coalitions may be best
seen on the additional Harris axial view (axial view of the subtalar
joint). Weight-bearing AP and lateral views demonstrate the degree
of hindfoot valgus that, if severe, may require correction. A talar
beak, which is a bony protuberance located superiorly on the distal
talus, may be seen on the lateral radiograph in the presence of a
talocalcaneal coalition.

Required for comprehensive evaluation

CT with thin cuts in the coronal and axial planes is indicated for definitive identification of a tarsal coalition. MRI may be useful in visualizing the connection, especially when it is fibrous or cartilaginous.

Special considerations

None

Pitfalls

A tarsal coalition may be missed on radiographs, especially if oblique views are not obtained. Also, sometimes radiographs of the ankle are requested instead of the foot. Non–weight-bearing views may not demonstrate the degree of the valgus deformity. CT is indicated if coalition is suspected but not identified on radiographs.

IMAGE DESCRIPTIONS

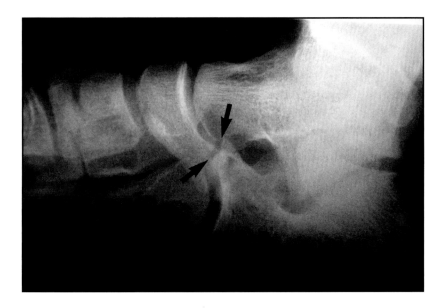

Figure 11-12

Calcaneonavicular coalition— Oblique view

Medial oblique view demonstrates a calcaneonavicular coalition most clearly. Note a very narrow area of segmentation (arrows), indicating a fibrous or cartilaginous connection.

SECTION 11 ■ PEDIATRIC ORTHOPAEDICS

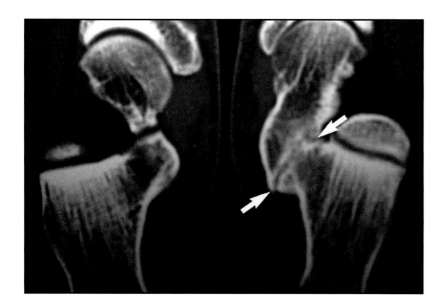

Figure 11-13

Talocalcaneal coalition—Axial CT

Axial CT scan shows a coalition between the talus and calcaneus involving the medial facet (arrows). A normal joint, as seen on the opposite side, is wider, without irregular changes.

DIFFERENTIAL DIAGNOSIS

Juvenile rheumatoid arthritis (can involve the subtalar joint; laboratory studies are indicated)

Rigid flatfoot (flatfoot with a tight heel cord may mimic tarsal coalition, but no coalitions are seen on radiographs in rigid flatfoot)

Stress fracture of the calcaneus (radiographs are normal initially; on follow-up, trabecular healing is seen)

HEMOPHILIC ARTHROPATHY

SYNONYMS
None

ICD-9 Code

286.0
Coagulation defects,
congenital factor VIII disorder

DEFINITION
Hemophilic arthropathy is joint damage associated with hemophilia. Although hemophilia can affect any of the 13 coagulation factors, most musculoskeletal problems are associated with a deficiency of either factor VIII or factor IX. Both factor VIII and factor IX deficiencies are transmitted by sex-linked recessive genes, with males being primarily affected. Hemophilic arthropathy begins when an affected individual experiences several episodes of joint bleeding in a short period of time (6 months to 1 year). As the synovium absorbs the catabolized blood products, iron and other elements lead to the release of factors that initiate articular cartilage damage.

HISTORY AND PHYSICAL FINDINGS
Joints affected by hemarthrosis are painful, warm, and swollen and demonstrate decreased range of motion. Children may experience pain just before the onset of joint bleeding.

IMAGING STUDIES

Required for diagnosis
AP and lateral radiographs of the affected joint may demonstrate findings consistent with articular cartilage changes. The classification of Hilgartner and Arnold is used to radiographically grade the degree of arthropathy. The classification ranges in severity from none (0) to joint ankylosis (V). In some centers, a joint survey (radiographs of major joints) is done annually.

Required for comprehensive evaluation
MRI is not routinely used. However, MRI may be particularly useful to assess articular cartilage erosion and the extent of the hypertrophic synovium. CT and ultrasound are generally not used.

Special considerations
Sedation or general anesthesia may be necessary for MRI evaluation in small children.

Pitfalls
Radiographs that are not orthogonal (perpendicular to the joint) may fail to demonstrate the articular involvement.

IMAGE DESCRIPTIONS

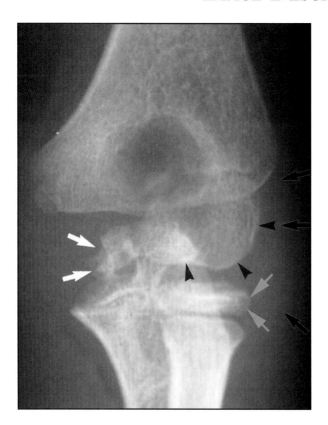

Figure 11-14

Hemophilic arthropathy (elbow)—AP view

AP radiograph of the elbow shows several features suggesting hemophilic arthropathy, including capsular thickening (black arrows) and irregularities of the trochlear portion of the ulna (white arrows). Note the enlargement of the capitellum (arrowheads) and radial epiphysis (gray arrows) in the distal humerus.

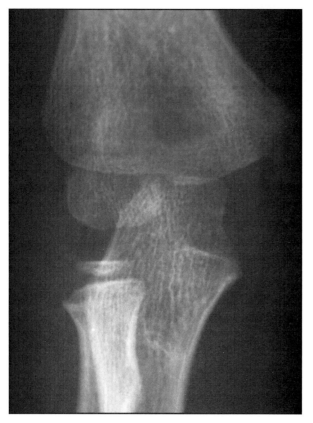

Figure 11-15

Hemophilic arthropathy (normal contralateral elbow)—AP view

In the absence of joint bleeding, there is no radiographic evidence of capsular thickening, no joint narrowing, and no articular enlargement.

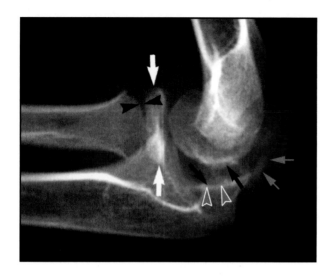

Figure 11-16

Hemophilic arthropathy (elbow)— Lateral view

Lateral view of the elbow of a patient with hemophilic arthropathy shows erosive changes in both the capitellum and the olecranon (black arrows). The entire proximal radius is enlarged (white arrows), and the physis is widened (black arrowheads). Note the fragmentation of the posterior olecranon (gray arrows) and the sclerosis of the subchondral bone of the proximal ulna (gray arrowheads).

DIFFERENTIAL DIAGNOSIS

Juvenile rheumatoid arthritis (similar on radiographs, but the subchondral bone is less sclerotic)

Septic arthritis (similar on radiographs; differentiate by clinical history)

JUVENILE RHEUMATOID ARTHRITIS

ICD-9 Code

714.30
Polyarticular juvenile
rheumatoid arthritis, chronic
or unspecified

SYNONYMS
None

DEFINITION
Juvenile rheumatoid arthritis (JRA) can be classified as pauciarticular (fewer than five involved joints), polyarticular (five or more involved joints), or systemic (fever, rash, hepato-splenomegaly, and polyarticular involvement). JRA is the most common chronic rheumatic disease of childhood and can have multiple musculoskeletal manifestations. The key principles in managing JRA are controlling the musculoskeletal symptoms, screening for iritis (especially in pauciarticular JRA), and managing the systemic manifestations. Joints commonly involved include those in the knee, hand, and ankle. The hip and cervical spine can also be involved.

HISTORY AND PHYSICAL FINDINGS
The clinical presentation depends on the type of JRA. Children with systemic JRA typically present with a high fever; a rash and enlargement of the spleen, liver, and lymph nodes may develop. Pericarditis and/or myocarditis may be present. Polyarticular JRA typically is seen either in the early toddler years or in early adolescence. Pauciarticular JRA is most commonly seen during the early toddler years and may be associated with iridocyclitis. Typical presenting symptoms are joint-related swelling, warmth, and stiffness. Children with pauciarticular JRA rarely have systemic symptoms, but those with polyarticular JRA may have a low-grade fever.

IMAGING STUDIES

Required for diagnosis
AP and lateral views of the affected joint are recommended.

Required for comprehensive evaluation
MRI may be used to evaluate the extent of the synovitis and articular changes. MRI will further detail the articular cartilage changes and meniscal pathology.

Special considerations
Imaging studies are usually confined to the affected joints. Sedation or general anesthesia may be needed for MRI evaluation in very young children.

Pitfalls

Failing to obtain orthogonal, tangential, or weight-bearing views of a lower extremity joint may lead to an inaccurate assessment of joint space narrowing associated with JRA.

IMAGE DESCRIPTIONS

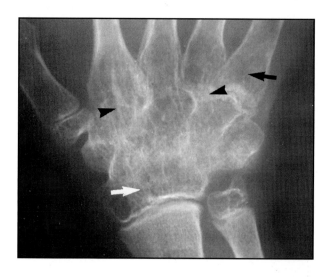

Figure 11-17

Juvenile rheumatoid arthritis (wrist)—AP view

AP view of the wrist of a skeletally immature patient shows generalized osteopenia (black arrow). Note the spontaneous fusion of the carpal bones to each other and to the distal radial epiphysis (white arrow) and the proximal metacarpals (arrowheads).

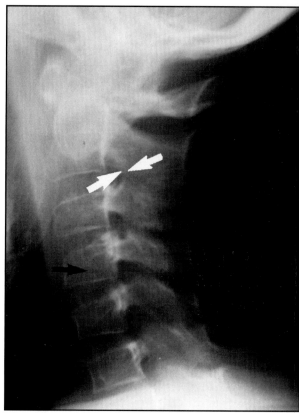

Figure 11-18

Juvenile rheumatoid arthritis (cervical spine)—Lateral view

Lateral view of the cervical spine demonstrates relative osteopenia of the vertebral bodies (black arrow). Note the apparent spontaneous facet joint fusion of C2 and C3 (white arrows).

SECTION 11 ■ PEDIATRIC ORTHOPAEDICS

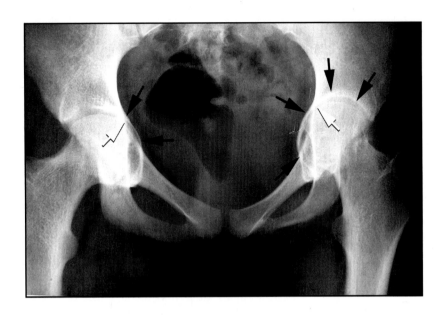

Figure 11-19

Juvenile rheumatoid arthritis (hips and pelvis)—AP view

AP view of the hips and pelvis shows bilateral protrusio acetabulae (medial migration of the femoral head) (black arrows) with axial narrowing of the joint space (white arrows).

DIFFERENTIAL DIAGNOSIS

Hemophilic arthropathy (history of hemophilia)

Reflex sympathetic dystrophy (regional rather than systemic; does not lead to fusion)

Septic arthritis (advanced infections usually demonstrate more metaphyseal destructive changes than does JRA)

Septic Arthritis

Synonyms
Pyogenic arthritis
Septic arthropathy

ICD-9 Code

711.0
Pyogenic arthritis

Definition
Septic arthritis is a bacterial infection, usually of acute hematogenous origin, in a synovial joint. Commonly affected joints include the hip, knee, and ankle. Involvement of the wrist, elbow, or shoulder is rare. Septic arthritis is considered an emergency, with immediate treatment required to prevent destruction of the articular cartilage both by the bacteria and by the host immune response to the bacteria. Septic arthritis of the hip, in particular, is a musculoskeletal emergency. In addition to possible destruction of the articular cartilage, increased pressure within the hip joint may cause vascular embarrassment and can lead to osteonecrosis, femoral head destruction, and physeal arrest.

History and Physical Findings
Children who present with septic arthritis generally appear severely ill. Fever is present, and the child typically refuses to move the involved joint or walk on an affected lower limb. Even short-arc range of motion is resisted.

Imaging Studies

Required for diagnosis
AP and frog-lateral views of the affected joint should be ordered. Views of the contralateral joint may be useful for comparison. Several features may be noted: effusion, metaphyseal bone destruction (suggestive of osteomyelitis), fracture, or other signs of localized change.

Required for comprehensive evaluation
MRI may be valuable to differentiate between juxta-articular metaphyseal osteomyelitis and septic arthritis. Images will show bone changes in the former. MRI of the hip may show concomitant pyomyositis of the adductor or iliopsoas masquerading as septic arthritis. MRI may also be valuable because of its ability to show a localized abscess. Ultrasound may be valuable to evaluate the presence of a hip effusion and to guide aspiration. Hip aspiration and culture are needed for definitive diagnosis. Aspiration usually is done by a radiologist under fluoroscopic control.

SECTION 11 ■ PEDIATRIC ORTHOPAEDICS

Special considerations

Sedation or general anesthesia may be necessary to complete an MRI or to perform an ultrasound- or fluoroscopy-guided aspiration. Gonadal shielding is recommended on follow-up images where appropriate.

Pitfalls

The availability of MRI and ultrasound should not delay the urgent aspiration and analysis of synovial fluid. In most cases, findings on radiographs and joint aspiration will direct treatment.

IMAGE DESCRIPTIONS

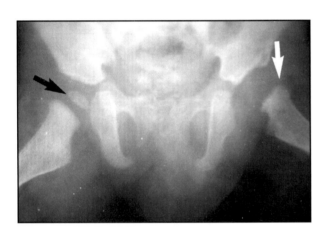

Figure 11-20

Septic arthritis (hip)—AP view of pelvis with hips abducted

AP view of the hips and pelvis in an infant shows a femoral ossific nucleus on the unaffected side (black arrow) but none on the affected side. The femoral metaphysis also appears slightly more laterally displaced (white arrow) compared with the unaffected side, suggestive of an intra-articular collection of fluid or other material.

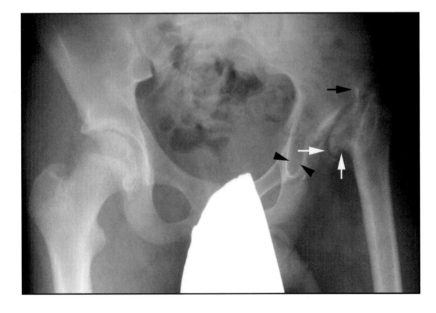

Figure 11-21

Septic arthritis (hip)—AP view of pelvis

AP view shows severe late sequelae of septic arthritis. The left proximal femur is subluxated superiorly (black arrow). There is loss of joint space, coxa breva, and deformation of the femoral head (white arrows). The acetabular teardrop is widened (arrowheads), suggesting that the relationship between the femur and acetabulum has been abnormal for some time.

DIFFERENTIAL DIAGNOSIS

Arthritides (radiographs may show narrowing and involve more than one joint; septic arthritis is generally confined to a single joint and has a more acute and rapidly progressive presentation)

Juxta-articular metaphyseal osteomyelitis (MRI may demonstrate metaphyseal bone involvement but not joint involvement)

Pyomyositis of the adductor, iliopsoas, or periarticular muscles (joint space may be spared; may require aspiration of involved muscle areas for culture and diagnosis)

Transient synovitis (most commonly affects the hip in children age 4 to 8 years; the child will be less ill than with septic arthritis; joint aspirate will show no bacteria and few white cells; radiographs will be normal)

CLUBFOOT

ICD-9 Code

754.70
Talipes, unspecified

SYNONYMS

Congenital talipes equinovarus
Metatarsus varus

DEFINITION

Congenital clubfoot is a complex foot deformity of infancy in which the forefoot is adducted (in varus) and the hindfoot is in equinus and varus. The incidence is about 1:1,000 children, with boys more commonly affected. Inheritance is multifactorial. The underlying cause is unknown, although several types are recognized: intrinsic (probably caused by genetic factors), neuromuscular, syndromic, and extrinsic (caused by fetal molding).

With metatarsus adductus, the forefoot is adducted or medially deviated in the transverse plane, but the hindfoot is in neutral position, in contrast to clubfoot. Molding of the foot due to a cramped intrauterine environment in the third trimester results in a deformation of the forefoot in metatarsus adductus.

HISTORY AND PHYSICAL FINDINGS

Clubfeet vary in severity, flexibility, and correctability. A medial skin crease indicates a more rigid and severe type of clubfoot. The calf on the affected side is generally smaller, and the involved leg may be slightly shorter with an apparent increase in medial tibial torsion. With metatarsus adductus, forefoot adductus alone is noted.

IMAGING STUDIES

Required for diagnosis

A congenital clubfoot is diagnosed by physical examination. AP and lateral radiographs confirm the diagnosis and assess the effectiveness of interventions. In particular, the restoration of the relationships between the talus and calcaneus, talus and navicular, and talus and cuboid may be followed radiographically.

Required for comprehensive evaluation

MRI, ultrasound, and CT are rarely used in the evaluation of congenital clubfoot.

Special considerations

Gonadal shielding is recommended. The foot should be weight bearing or dorsiflexed on AP and lateral views.

Pitfalls

The hindfoot must be positioned properly for the lateral view. A proper lateral image demonstrates the fibula overlapping the posterior tibia.

IMAGE DESCRIPTIONS

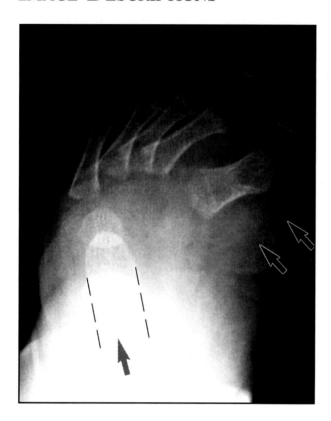

Figure 11-22

Congenital clubfoot—AP view

AP view shows adductus of the forefoot (black arrows) and parallelism between the talus and calcaneus (gray arrow, dashed lines).

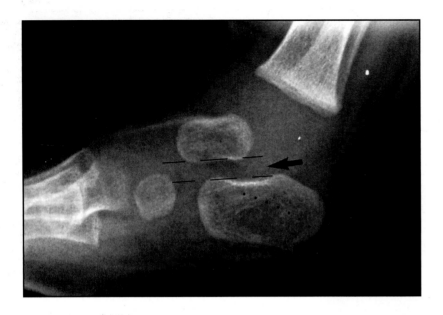

Figure 11-23

*Congenital clubfoot—
Lateral view*

Lateral view shows parallelism between the talus and calcaneus (black arrow, dashed lines). In metatarsus adductus, a normal hindfoot relationship of the talus and calcaneus will be seen. Note also that the calcaneus is in a talipes equinus position: the dotted line shows the expected normal position of the calcaneus. Also note that the fibula is in proper relation to the posterior margin of the tibia in this view.

DIFFERENTIAL DIAGNOSIS

Metatarsus adductus (normal relationship between the talus and calcaneus; appearance of forefoot similar to clubfoot)

Congenital Deformities of the Radius

Synonyms
None

ICD-9 Code
755.53
Radioulnar synostosis

Definition
Radioulnar synostosis is a nontraumatic crossunion that occurs between the radius and ulna in the proximal forearm. This congenital abnormality may not be evident until children start using their hands in a purposeful manner. The forearm muscles, especially the pronators and supinators, and the brachioradialis may be absent. Radioulnar synostosis is usually characterized as one of two types: type I, a complete synostosis of the proximal radius and ulna, or type II, a fusion of the proximal radius to the proximal ulna with dislocation of the radial head. Children with bilateral deformities have the greatest functional deficit. This small group of patients may benefit from surgical correction. Congenital dislocation of the radial head may be isolated or associated with syndromic diagnoses. Parents may note a prominence over the lateral elbow or limitation of forearm rotation.

History and Physical Findings
The principal finding of synostosis on physical examination is decreased rotation of the involved forearm. In patients with unilateral involvement, muscle girth of the forearm may be smaller than the opposite, normal side. The forearm may have a bowed appearance. With congenital dislocation of the radial head, findings are limitation of forearm rotation and a lateral elbow prominence.

Imaging Studies

Required for diagnosis
AP and lateral radiographs of the forearm are indicated to define the extent of synostosis between the radius and ulna.

Required for comprehensive evaluation
CT or MRI may help better define the relationship between the radius and ulna and is useful in preoperative planning.

Special considerations
Sedation or general anesthesia may be required for MRI evaluation in infants and very young children.

Pitfalls

Fibrous synostosis may be present but not apparent on radiographs. This is seen best on MRI.

IMAGE DESCRIPTIONS

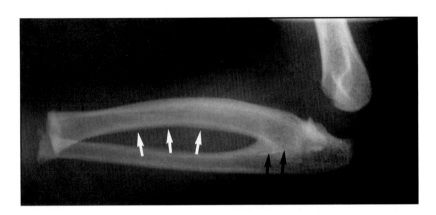

Figure 11-24

Radioulnar synostosis—Lateral view

Lateral view of the forearm and elbow of an infant demonstrates radioulnar synostosis. Note the complete fusion of the proximal radius to the ulna (black arrows) and increased radial bowing (white arrows).

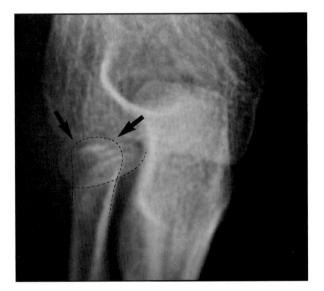

Figure 11-25

Congenital dislocation of the radial head—AP view

AP view of the elbow shows the radial head superimposed on the capitellum (dotted lines), suggesting a posterior dislocation. Note that the radial head has a convex rather than a normal concave shape (black arrows).

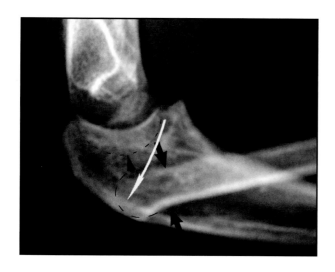

Figure 11-26

Congenital dislocation of the radial head—Lateral view

Lateral view of a congenital dislocation of the radial head demonstrates a relatively small, narrow proximal radius (black arrows). Note that the radial head (white arrow, dashed line) falls posterior to the capitellum (arrowhead).

DIFFERENTIAL DIAGNOSIS

None

POLYDACTYLY

ICD-9 Code

755.00
Polydactyly, unspecified digits

SYNONYM

Extra fingers (or toes)

DEFINITION

Polydactyly is a common congenital abnormality of the hand or foot. Postaxial polydactyly, or duplication of the fifth (or little) finger, is an autosomal dominant trait that is very common. This type of polydactyly is 10 times more common in blacks than in whites.

Preaxial polydactyly, or duplicate thumb, may be associated with congenital heart disease (Holt-Oram syndrome) and Fanconi syndrome. The genetics is usually sporadic.

Central polydactyly (or polysyndactyly) involves the index, middle, and ring fingers or the second or third toes. This condition is almost always bilateral and symmetric and is slightly more common in girls. It is inherited as an autosomal dominant trait.

HISTORY AND PHYSICAL FINDINGS

A family history of the condition is common. Inspection of the affected extremity may reveal that the duplicate digit is a different size and stage of completeness. In some cases, there is a complete equal digit, especially in postaxial polydactyly, while in others there may be as little as a skin tag or a duplicate, fused digit.

IMAGING STUDIES

Required for diagnosis
AP and lateral views of the entire hand or foot are recommended to fully assess the morphology of the digits in two planes.

Required for comprehensive evaluation
MRI is rarely used but may be indicated when the bones of the hand or foot are not ossified and cannot be visualized on radiographs.

Special considerations
Underlying syndromic diagnosis may require genetics consultation.

Pitfalls
Failure to identify an underlying diagnosis as a result of incomplete screening can lead to a delay in diagnosis or to complications relating to surgery and anesthesia, such as Apert syndrome or airway problems.

IMAGE DESCRIPTION

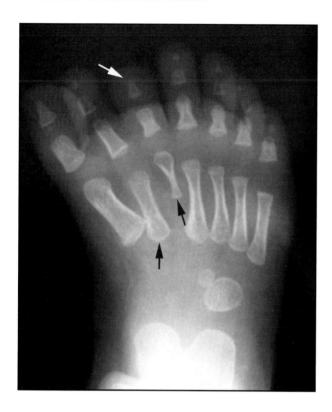

Figure 11-27

Polydactyly (central) of the foot—AP view

AP view of a child's foot shows central polydactyly. Note that there are seven rays, and the two central, abnormal rays (black arrows) are quite different. The more fibular duplicate ray has a short, abnormally shaped metatarsal and an absent distal phalanx (white arrow).

DIFFERENTIAL DIAGNOSIS

None

SECTION 11 ■ PEDIATRIC ORTHOPAEDICS

Radial/Ulnar Club Hand

ICD-9 Code

754.89
Other specified
nonteratogenic anomalies

Synonyms

None

Definition

The term radial club hand describes a spectrum of deficiencies involving the radial aspect of the upper extremity. Problems may range from mild abnormalities of the thumb to complete absence of the radius (the most common manifestation). Associated abnormalities include limited wrist and elbow function, muscle deficiencies, neurovascular deficiencies (absence of the radial artery and superficial radial nerve), and associated anomalies of the cardiovascular, genitourinary, or gastrointestinal systems. Common associations include congenital heart disease (Holt-Oram syndrome), Fanconi syndrome, thrombocytopenia with absent radius (TAR) syndrome, vertebral anomalies (VATER association), and trisomy 17. The incidence of radial deficiency is approximately 1:50,000 live births. The cause is unknown. The term ulnar club hand describes a range of deficiencies along the postaxial or ulnar border of the forearm and hand. About 25% of cases are bilateral. Radial club hand is thought to be about 10 times more common than ulnar club hand.

History and Physical Findings

The range of clinical findings depends on the extent of the deficiency. In the most common form of radial club hand, the radius is completely absent. The wrist is unstable and the elbow is stable, the hand deviates radially, and the thumb may be absent. Range of motion may be decreased in the index and long fingers and in the elbow. Muscles originating from the lateral epicondyle (the extensor muscle mass) may be affected. Thenar muscles may be deficient as well. The radial pulse may be absent, and there may be decreased sensation on the radial side of the hand. In contrast, in ulnar club hand with deficiency of the ulna, the wrist is stable and the elbow is unstable.

Imaging Studies

Required for diagnosis

AP and lateral views of the entire hand and forearm are needed to make the diagnosis.

Required for comprehensive evaluation

MRI may be indicated to assess nonossified tissue, especially for preoperative planning. To diagnose associated syndromes, additional imaging studies, such as a skeletal survey, may be indicated. Echocardiogram and ultrasound of the abdomen and kidneys may be indicated for medical or genetics evaluation.

Special considerations

Sedation or general anesthesia may be necessary for MRI studies.

Pitfalls

Failure to image other systems (cardiac, genitourinary) may result in missed syndromic diagnoses or missed identification of associated anomalies.

IMAGE DESCRIPTION

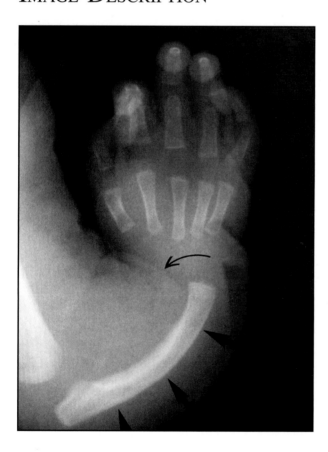

Figure 11-28

Radial club hand—AP view

AP view of the forearm and hand of a child demonstrates a radial club hand, with complete absence of the radius. Note that the ulna is bowed (black arrows) and the carpus is subluxated radially on the distal ulna (curved arrow). The thumb is present in this case.

DIFFERENTIAL DIAGNOSIS

None

SECTION 11 ■ PEDIATRIC ORTHOPAEDICS

SYNDACTYLY

ICD-9 Code

755.10
Syndactyly of multiple and
unspecified sites

SYNONYM
Mitten hand

DEFINITION

Syndactyly is an abnormal connection between digits of the hand or
foot. In simple syndactyly, the digits are connected only by skin. In
complex syndactyly, the digits may be connected by both skin and
bone. Complete syndactyly is characterized by a connection that
spans the commissure to the fingertips, while in incomplete
syndactyly, the connection stops short of the fingertips.

Syndactyly is a common hand abnormality, occurring in about
1:2,000 births. It is more common in whites than in blacks.
Typically, it occurs on the ulnar, rather than the radial, side of the
limb. Although complete syndactyly may have significant functional
consequences, partial syndactyly is usually tolerated quite well. In
complete syndactyly, the connection may cause the longer digits to
angulate toward the shorter digits. These angulation rotation and
flexion abnormalities worsen with growth and can significantly
affect limb function.

HISTORY AND PHYSICAL FINDINGS

The hallmark finding on physical examination is connection
between two adjacent digits. Independent motion should be
observed to assess the functional consequence of the connection.

IMAGING STUDIES

Required for diagnosis
AP and lateral views of the affected extremity are needed to make
the diagnosis.

Required for comprehensive evaluation
Rarely, MRI may be needed to assess cartilaginous and skeletal
involvement.

Special considerations
Sedation or general anesthesia may be required for MRI in infants
and young children.

Pitfalls
Because of the cartilaginous nature of the skeleton of an infant, not
all complex syndactyly morphology may be demonstrable on
radiographs taken at birth. Follow-up radiographs may be needed.

IMAGE DESCRIPTIONS

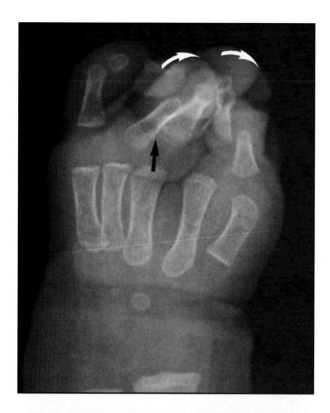

Figure 11-29

Syndactyly (simple) of the hand—AP view

AP view of an infant's hand shows features consistent with simple syndactyly. Note that the central digits are closely spaced but not connected (black arrow), and the affected phalanges are rotated (white arrows).

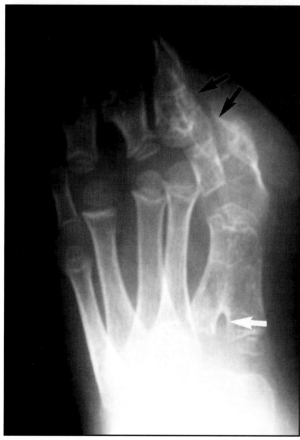

Figure 11-30

Syndactyly (complex) of the foot—AP view

AP view of the foot shows complex syndactyly with synostosis of the phalanges (black arrows). Note that the first metatarsal is bifid proximally (white arrow).

SECTION 11 ■ PEDIATRIC ORTHOPAEDICS

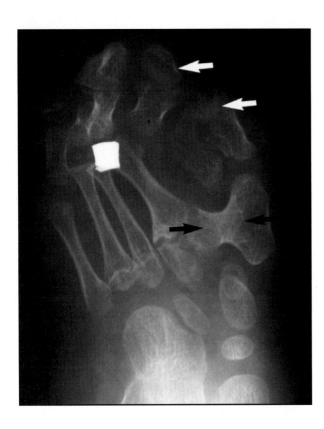

Figure 11-31

Syndactyly (complex) of the foot—AP view

AP view of the foot shows complex syndactyly with synostosis of the first and second rays (black arrows) and marked deformation and malformation of the phalanges of the first and second toes (white arrows).

DIFFERENTIAL DIAGNOSIS

None

TIBIAL BOWING

SYNONYMS

Anterolateral bowing
Posteromedial bowing
Pseudarthrosis of tibia

ICD-9 Code

754.43
Congenital bowing of tibia
and fibula

DEFINITION

Tibial bowing assumes two forms: anterolateral and posteromedial. Anterolateral bowing is associated with congenital pseudarthrosis of the tibia and neurofibromatosis in a large number of cases. When anterolateral bowing progresses to congenital pseudarthrosis, treatment is complex and difficult, and in some cases, the end result is amputation.

Posteromedial bowing, however, is a relatively benign condition caused by fetal deformation noted first at birth. The primary outcome of this abnormality is a limb-length discrepancy ranging from 3 to 7 cm and a calcaneal valgus foot. Posteromedial bowing is not associated with neurofibromatosis. The greater the posteromedial bowing noted at birth, the greater the tibial shortening will be at skeletal maturity. Unlike the complex treatment regimen required for anterolateral bowing, surgical treatment for posteromedial bowing is generally confined to limb equalization, when necessary. The calcaneal valgus foot associated with posteromedial bowing generally resolves with splinting in infancy and with time.

HISTORY AND PHYSICAL FINDINGS

In children with anterolateral bowing, the anterolateral prominence in the lower leg is noted on examination. In associated neurofibromatosis, café au lait spots and axillary freckling may be noted. Ankle and knee range of motion is usually normal, and there may be a small limb-length discrepancy. In more advanced cases, there may be pseudarthrosis through the bowed area. The presence of a medullary canal is a favorable prognostic sign.

Children with posterior medial bowing initially have a posterior medial prominence in the distal tibia and a calcaneal valgus foot. Muscle mass may be slightly smaller on the affected side, and the involved limb may be shorter than the opposite, normal side. A history of fetal constraint or oligohydramnios may be present.

SECTION 11 ■ PEDIATRIC ORTHOPAEDICS

IMAGING STUDIES

Required for diagnosis
Weight-bearing AP and lateral (when appropriate) views of the involved tibia and fibula are required to make the diagnosis.

Required for comprehensive evaluation
MRI may be valuable in assessing the soft-tissue envelope involved with anterior lateral bowing, but it is not used routinely. A scanogram is indicated to assess the extent of the limb-length discrepancy, especially in posterior medial bowing.

Special considerations
Sedation or general anesthesia may be required for MRI in infants and young children.

Pitfalls
None

IMAGE DESCRIPTION

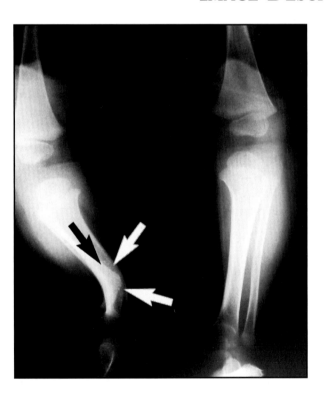

Figure 11-32

Posterior medial tibial bowing— AP view

Weight-bearing AP view shows typical posterior medial bowing of the right leg in a young child. Note that the tibia on the affected side is shorter than that on the opposite, normal side. There is apex posterior bowing of both the tibia and fibula (white arrows), but no other abnormalities are seen. The knee above and the ankle below also appear normal. The medullary canal of the tibia is present and intact (black arrow).

DIFFERENTIAL DIAGNOSIS

Posttraumatic angulation (signs of fracture callus; limb segments equal bilaterally)

Coxa Vara

Synonyms
None

Definition
Coxa vara is a deformity of the proximal femur (hip) in which the neck-shaft angle is smaller than normal. The etiology can be congenital, developmental, traumatic, or metabolic.

Developmental coxa vara is not present at birth but develops gradually in early childhood. With this type of hip deformity, a minor limb-length discrepancy is possible, but few other anomalies are associated with coxa vara. The incidence is approximately 1:25,000 live births. Developmental coxa vara is bilateral in up to half of patients. A percentage of metabolic cases follow an autosomal dominant inheritance pattern.

History and Physical Findings
Children with developmental coxa vara may present as toddlers with an abnormal gait. Other findings on physical examination include decreased hip abduction, a prominent greater trochanter, a positive Trendelenburg test, and a possible associated limb-length discrepancy.

Patients with congenital coxa vara usually have a significant limb-length discrepancy, with the affected side shorter. Hip range of motion, especially abduction, may be decreased.

Imaging Studies

Required for diagnosis
Weight-bearing AP and non–weight-bearing frog-lateral views of the pelvis are needed for diagnosis.

Required for comprehensive evaluation
CT with three-dimensional reconstruction may be useful in better understanding the morphology of the proximal femoral deformity, including identifying subtle acetabular dysplasia, if surgery is being planned.

Special considerations
Gonadal shielding is advised when follow-up radiographs of the pelvis are needed.

Pitfalls
None

Section 11 ■ Pediatric Orthopaedics

IMAGE DESCRIPTION

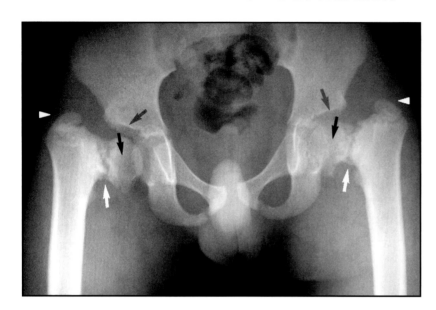

Figure 11-33

Coxa vara (developmental)— AP view

Weight-bearing AP view of the pelvis and hips shows bilateral developmental coxa vara. The neck-shaft angles appear to approach 90° on each side. The proximal femoral physis is nearly vertical on each side (black arrows). Note the classic "inverted Y" radiolucency that appears on both sides (white arrows). The greater trochanter is prominent in both hips and is situated proximal to the center of the femoral head (arrowheads), creating a reduced moment arm for hip abduction strength. There appears to be mild acetabular dysplasia, especially on the right side (gray arrows).

DIFFERENTIAL DIAGNOSIS

Coxa breva from growth arrest (the physis is generally more horizontal)

Developmental Dysplasia of the Hip

Synonyms

Congenital dysplasia of the hip (CDH) (old terminology)
DDH
Hip dysplasia

Definition

The term developmental dysplasia of the hip (DDH) describes a wide spectrum of hip abnormalities, ranging from hip laxity, hip subluxation, and hip dislocation to dysplasia of the acetabulum. In most cases these conditions are present at birth; however, some cases have been well documented to develop after birth, making the term "congenital dysplasia of the hip" inappropriate.

Mechanical, genetic, and epidemiologic factors play a role in DDH. In general, the incidence ranges from 10 to 50 cases per 1,000 live births, but it varies greatly among different ethnic groups. It is more common in girls (80% of cases), first-born infants, infants who have been in a breech position, and infants with a family history of hip dysplasia. The tight intrauterine environment experienced by a first-born infant and the abnormal forces of the breech presentation on the infant's hips both contribute to the increased incidence. Swaddling that forces the infant's hips into adduction and extension also is known to increase the incidence of DDH. Other physical findings associated with a tight intrauterine environment, such as metatarsus adductus and congenital muscular torticollis, may be associated with DDH. Otherwise, there are few common extra-articular manifestations. Most infants with DDH are otherwise healthy.

History and Physical Findings

The physical finding in neonates is the Ortolani sign: when the examiner applies a gentle abduction force, the femoral head can be felt to reduce into the acetabulum. Examination may reveal a sense of increased hip laxity, or the hip may subluxate or dislocate with the Barlow maneuver (adduction in flexion with gentle posterior pressure).

In children older than age 3 months, Ortolani and Barlow maneuvers may be negative. In these children, a positive Galeazzi sign (apparent femoral shortening caused by hip dislocation), decreased hip abduction, or asymmetric gluteal or thigh skinfolds may be indicators of hip dislocation. In the walking child, exaggerated lordosis and a waddling gait may be seen in cases of bilateral hip dislocations.

ICD-9 Codes

754.30
Congenital dislocation of hip, unilateral

754.31
Congenital dislocation of hip, bilateral

754.32
(under 6 months) Congenital subluxation of hip, unilateral

754.33
Congenital subluxation of hip, bilateral

754.35
Congenital dislocation of one hip with subluxation of other hip

Imaging Studies

Required for diagnosis

Hip ultrasound for children between age 6 weeks and 6 months, with or without stress views (Harke technique), is indicated for all female/breech infants or infants with positive physical findings. In children older than age 6 months, a supine AP view of the pelvis with the femurs in internal rotation is the imaging study of choice. After age 1 year, a weight-bearing AP view of the pelvis is indicated to evaluate the status of the hips.

Required for comprehensive evaluation

Arthrography may be used in subluxated or dislocated hips to assess the morphology of the femoral head/acetabulum, the presence of interposed structures between the femoral head and acetabulum, and the hip capsule. CT is indicated after closed reduction to assess congruency of the reduced femoral head to the acetabulum. CT with three-dimensional reconstruction is useful in preoperative planning to assess morphology, including the version of the proximal femur and the acetabulum. In adolescents, a faux profile radiographic view is indicated to identify anterior acetabular deficiency.

Special considerations

A 50% solution of water soluble contrast medium is used for hip arthrograms. Gonadal shielding is recommended when obtaining follow-up radiographs of the pelvis. Sedation or general anesthesia may be necessary for many of these studies.

Pitfalls

Radiographs are unreliable in patients younger than age 3 months because the pelvis is highly cartilaginous. Hip stability may be more accurately assessed using ultrasound in this age group. After age 6 months, hip ultrasound is less reliable but can be attempted if the ossific nucleus is small and does not obstruct visualization of the joint. Infant size and strength may preclude accurate evaluation of hip stability using ultrasound. Unless assessing osteonecrosis, frog-lateral views are of little value.

IMAGE DESCRIPTIONS

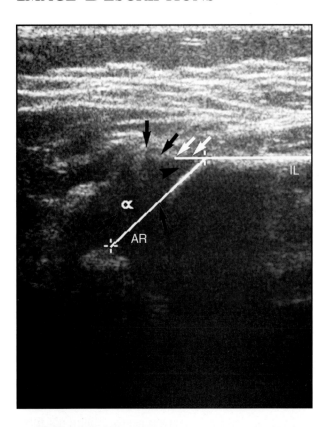

Figure 11-34

Developmental dysplasia of the hip—Coronal ultrasound

Coronal ultrasound demonstrates the cartilaginous femoral head (black arrows), labrum (white arrows), and alpha angle (arrowhead). The alpha angle is formed by the intersection of a line running along the iliac wing (IL) with a line drawn along the bony acetabular roof (AR). The alpha angle should be 60° or greater in a normal hip.

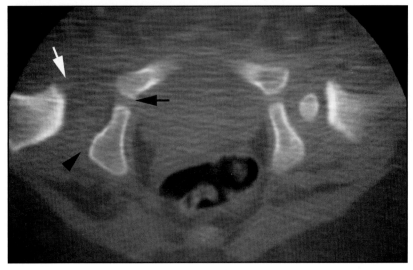

Figure 11-35

Developmental dysplasia of the hip—CT

CT is ordered after a closed reduction or to assess hip morphology. This image shows both proximal femoral metaphyses aimed toward the triradiate cartilage (black arrow). The left hip appears normal. The right hip does not yet have a visible femoral ossific nucleus (white arrow), and the right acetabulum is dysplastic (arrowhead).

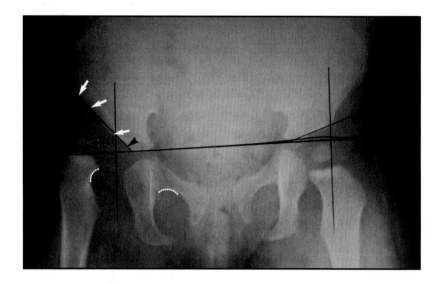

Figure 11-36

Dislocation (DDH) of the hip—AP view

AP view of the pelvis shows a normal left hip and a dislocated right hip. The right femoral ossific nucleus is smaller than the left and is located laterally (black arrow). Note the apparent changes consistent with a false acetabulum on the right side (white arrows). The horizontal line is Hilgenreiner's line; the perpendicular is Perkins line. The angle between Hilgenreiner's line and the line drawn along the acetabulum is the acetabular index. The right acetabulum is very dysplastic (arrowhead). Shenton's line, a curve that can be drawn from the inferior border of the femoral neck to the inferior border of the pubic ramus on an AP view of the pelvis (dotted lines), is disrupted on the right side.

DIFFERENTIAL DIAGNOSIS

None

Genu Valgum

ICD-9 Code
736.41
Genu valgum (acquired)

Synonym
Knock-knees

Definition
Genu valgum, or knock-knees, is commonly seen in children between the ages of 3 and 5 years as a normal phase of physical development. At this age, the tibiofemoral angle is at a maximum valgus and may cause a parent to become concerned. The normal tibiofemoral angle in children of this age can vary widely, from 2° of varus to 20° of valgus. After age 7 years, normal valgus ranges from 0° to 12°. Acquired genu valgum also can be caused by metabolic bone disease (ie, rickets, osteomalacia), skeletal dysplasia (such as spondyloepiphyseal dysplasia), mucopolysaccharidosis type IV (Morquio syndrome), or chondroectodermal dysplasia (Ellis-van Creveld syndrome). It can also follow a proximal tibial fracture producing a growth abnormality in which the valgus resolves with growth.

Of the types listed above, physiologic genu valgum is the most common clinical presentation. After a careful history and physical examination, radiographs generally are not needed, and the parents can be reassured that most cases resolve spontaneously with growth and normal development.

History and Physical Findings
A detailed family history is taken, including the presence of genu valgum in anyone in the family, a nutritional history of reduced calcium intake, and an assessment of the rate of progression of the deformity. Children may report activity-related pain if the valgus is severe.

Physical examination includes coronal measurement of the tibiofemoral angle with a goniometer and assessment of knee stability. Height and weight are obtained to ascertain significantly abnormal short stature or other features that may suggest a syndromic diagnosis. A generalized musculoskeletal examination of the spine and extremities is performed as well.

SECTION 11 ■ PEDIATRIC ORTHOPAEDICS

IMAGING STUDIES

Required for diagnosis

A weight-bearing AP view of both lower extremities on a 14 in. ×
36 in. cassette, including the hips, knees, and ankles, should be
obtained with the patellae facing directly forward to assess the genu
valgum, including both the anatomic axis and the mechanical axis.

Required for comprehensive evaluation

MRI is ordered in younger patients or in children with skeletal
dysplasia to more accurately assess mechanical axis. In certain
skeletal dysplasias, the joint line or articular surfaces may be
indeterminate on radiographs. MRI defines the morphology of the
articular surfaces, which allows assessment of the mechanical axis.

Special considerations

Gonadal shielding is important when obtaining follow-up
radiographs of the pelvis and lower extremities. Images must
include both hips, knees, and ankles so that the mechanical axis can
be assessed. Weight-bearing views are recommended when
developmentally appropriate. The patellae are pointed directly
forward to allow for reproducible images and to avoid a torsion
effect on coronal measurements.

Pitfalls

Non–weight-bearing radiographs or spot radiographs of the knee
only may lead to inaccurate or incomplete assessment of the
coronal mechanical and anatomic axes.

IMAGE DESCRIPTION

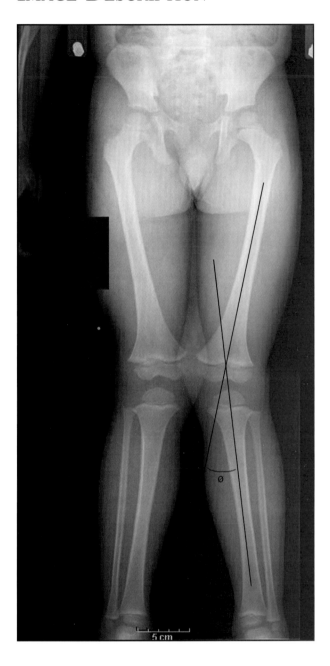

Figure 11-37

Genu valgum—AP view

Weight-bearing AP view of both lower extremities shows a mild to moderately increased tibiofemoral angle (lines) with a mild genu valgus deformity. Note that most of the valgus seems to be centered in the midtibial region. Bone density appears normal, and no other abnormalities are seen.

DIFFERENTIAL DIAGNOSIS

None

SECTION 11 ■ PEDIATRIC ORTHOPAEDICS

Genu Varum

ICD-9 Code

736.42
Genu varum (acquired)

Synonyms

Adolescent tibia vara
Blount's disease
Bowleg
Infantile tibia vara

Definition

Genu varum, or bowlegs, may be a normal developmental phase, a progressive abnormality in juveniles, or a progressive abnormality in adolescents. It also may be associated with skeletal dysplasias or metabolic bone conditions. In most cases it is noticed by parents soon after their children begin to walk. This type of physiologic genu varum resolves with time. In a much smaller percentage of cases, the condition is juvenile tibia vara (Blount's disease), a manifestation of a metabolic bone disease or skeletal dysplasia, or adolescent tibia vara.

The normal tibiofemoral angle is approximately 0° to 5° of varus at walking age. Over the next 1 to 2 years, this varus alignment changes to a valgus alignment. A persistent varus deformity of the tibia after age 2 to 3 years is consistent with a possible diagnosis of Blount's disease rather than a physiologic genu varum.

In some children, varus deformity develops much later (adolescent tibia vara). Although some of these children have a history of genu varum in early childhood, most do not. Most of these patients are obese (above the 95th percentile for body weight).

History and Physical Findings

The history should include questions about family history of skeletal abnormalities, including bowlegs, metabolic bone diseases, or skeletal dysplasias. Physical examination should include assessment of joint range of motion and stability, limb length, and the tibiofemoral angle. The clinical tibiofemoral angle is measured with a goniometer with the child standing and the patellae facing forward. Evaluation of gait as a part of the physical examination is likely to be unremarkable in mild cases or reveal a lateral thrust in severe cases.

IMAGING STUDIES

Required for diagnosis
A weight-bearing AP view of the entire lower extremities from the hips to the ankles, with the patellae facing forward, is necessary to make the diagnosis.

Required for comprehensive evaluation
MRI may be required to assess articular alignment in cases of bone dysplasias where the chondroepiphysis is significantly nonossified and not visible on radiographs.

Special considerations
Gonadal shielding is advised when obtaining full-length views. Sedation or general anesthesia may be required for MRI in young children.

Pitfalls
Non–weight-bearing radiographs or radiographs limited to the knee will not allow an assessment of alignment. Radiographs are not necessary for toddler-age children with physical findings of mild physiologic genu varum.

IMAGE DESCRIPTIONS

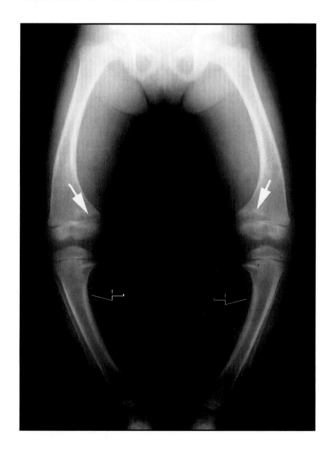

Figure 11-38

Genu varum—AP view

Full-length AP view shows proximal tibial varus deformities in both lower extremities (black arrows) in a patient with rickets. Note the widening of the distal femoral physes (white arrows).

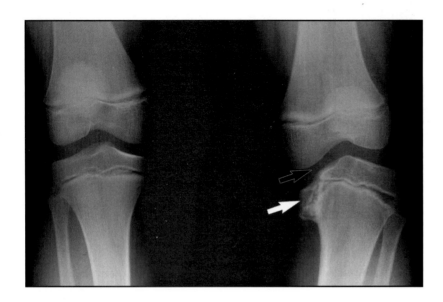

Figure 11-39

Blount's disease (infantile or juvenile tibia vara)—AP view

AP view of both knees in an older child shows a proximal tibial deformity typical of advanced Blount's disease. The left knee shows deformity of the proximal tibial epiphysis (black arrow) and beaking of the metaphysis (white arrow). Note that there are no bony abnormalities in the right knee and no abnormalities of either femur. The abnormal radiographic findings are confined to the proximal tibia, consistent with Blount's disease.

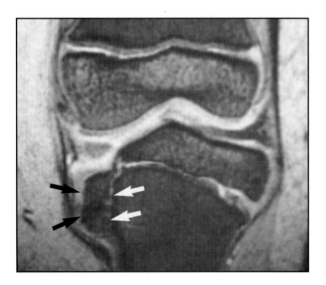

Figure 11-40

Blount's disease (adolescent tibia vara)—MRI

MRI scan of the knee shows a severe proximal tibial epiphyseal deformity and metaphyseal beaking (black arrows), consistent with juvenile tibia vara (Blount's disease). The medial proximal tibial physis appears to be closing (white arrows).

DIFFERENTIAL DIAGNOSIS

Physiologic genu varum (radiographs will be normal for age)

ACHONDROPLASIA

SYNONYMS

Dwarfism

Short-limbed disproportionate dwarfism

ICD-9 Code

756.4
Chondrodystrophy

DEFINITION

Achondroplasia, an inherited autosomal dominant condition that causes failure of enchondral ossification, is considered the most common form of dwarfism. Up to 90% of cases are spontaneous mutations involving fibroblast growth factor type 3. The abnormal enchondral ossification results in disproportionate dwarfism, with proximal limb (rhizomelic) shortening and midfacial hypoplasia. Intramembranous ossification is normal, which explains why the top of the skull appears disproportionately large. Incidence ranges from 1:20,000 to 1:100,000 live births. Intelligence is normal. Developmental milestones may be delayed because of the child's disproportionate stature.

HISTORY AND PHYSICAL FINDINGS

The clinical features of achondroplasia are easily identifiable in infancy, and they can be seen in the fetus by measuring the femur on ultrasound. At birth, these neonates have a characteristic appearance, consisting of obvious shortening of the proximal limbs, normal trunk height, frontal bossing, a flattened nasal bridge, lower rib flaring, and a protruding abdomen. Later, common medical issues include obesity, as well as otitis media secondary to midfacial hypoplasia. In the first years of life, neurologic problems may develop secondary to narrowing of the foramen magnum. Other problems include respiratory insufficiency, hypotonia, apnea, feeding difficulties, quadriparesis, and sudden death. Routine screening protocols for the narrowed foramen magnum have not been established; however, baseline MRI and somatosensory-evoked potential (SSEP) evaluation have been recommended during infancy and are required in the presence of clonus and hyperreflexia. Other findings include trident hand (increased web space between the third and fourth fingers), lack of elbow extension, and genu varum.

A common spine problem requiring intervention is progressive pedicle shortening and spinal stenosis, which may lead to neurologic deficits. Many infants have thoracolumbar kyphosis, which often resolves after they begin to walk. Spine imaging includes upright (sitting or standing) AP and lateral views of the entire spine; MRI, under general anesthesia or sedation, of the brain and cervical spine for foramen magnum stenosis; and MRI of the thoracic and lumbar spine for stenosis.

IMAGING STUDIES

Required for diagnosis

Imaging studies are not required to establish the diagnosis in infancy. The diagnosis is confirmed on clinical examination. A skeletal survey (AP and lateral views of the skull and thoracolumbar spine, AP view of the thoracic cage, AP view of the pelvis, and AP views of the upper and lower extremities) is ordered to support the diagnosis in the initial genetics evaluation by the specialist, either in the nursery or soon afterward by referral to these specialists.

Required for comprehensive evaluation

Weight-bearing bilateral AP views of the entire lower extremities are ordered to assess alignment (excessive genu varum or valgus) on follow-up by the orthopaedic surgeon. AP views of the femur and tibia typically show that the metaphysis is flared and widened, the growth plates are V- or U-shaped, overall limb length is shorter than normal, tibial bowing (eg, genu varum) may be present, and the femoral neck is short relative to the greater trochanter. AP views of the spine will show narrowing of the interpedicular distance, and lateral views of the spine will show posterior scalloping of the vertebral bodies (short, broad pedicles). An AP view of the pelvis will reveal that the iliac bones are rounded (similar to a ping-pong paddle), the acetabular roofs are horizontally oriented, and the sciatic notches are small.

Special considerations

Imaging studies such as MRI are ordered in the first 1 to 2 years of life to assess presence of foramen magnum stenosis. MRI may reveal abnormalities of the cranium, cerebrum, and cervicomedullary junction. Clinical indications in newborns are neurologic findings, severe hypotonia, hyperreflexia, or clonus. MRI is indicated also to assess the extent of stenosis of the lumbar spine in teens and adults.

Pitfalls

Weight-bearing views of the lower extremities are recommended whenever possible to properly assess lower extremity malalignment. Upright (sitting or standing) views of the spine are recommended whenever possible to properly assess spine deformity (usually kyphosis). Rarely, MRI or CT myelogram is used to identify stenosis. CT myelography is performed via cisternal (cervical) puncture rather than a lumbar puncture to avoid neurologic compromise.

IMAGE DESCRIPTIONS

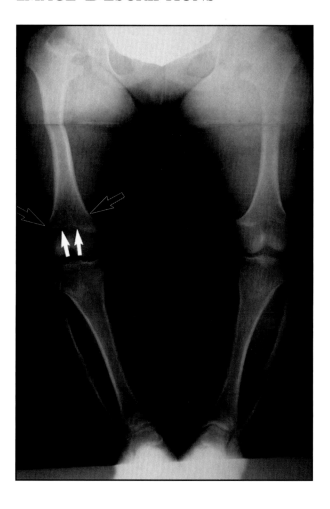

Figure 11-41

Achondroplasia (lower extremities)—AP view

AP view of the lower extremities shows rhizomelic (proximal) shortening of the limbs, flaring of all the metaphyses (black arrows), an inverted-V–shaped configuration of the epiphysis of the distal femur (white arrows), and genu varum (bowing).

SECTION 11 ■ PEDIATRIC ORTHOPAEDICS

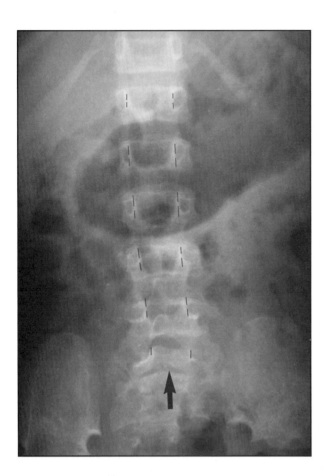

Figure 11-42

Achondroplasia (lumbar spine)— AP view

AP view of the lumbar spine shows the characteristic progressive narrowing of the lumbar interpedicular distances (arrow, lines).

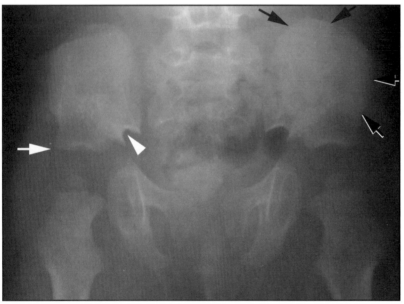

Figure 11-43

Achondroplasia (pelvis)—AP view

AP view of the pelvis shows the circular-shaped (ping-pong-paddle–shaped) iliac wings (black arrows), horizontally oriented acetabular roofs (white arrow), and small sciatic notch (arrowhead).

DIFFERENTIAL DIAGNOSIS

Hypochondroplasia (nonrhizomelic, mostly symmetric shortening of the upper and lower extremities, less lumbar lordosis, less abdominal protrusion, less midfacial involvement)

CAFFEY'S DISEASE

SYNONYM

Infantile cortical hyperostosis

ICD-9 Code

756.59
Osteodystrophies, other

DEFINITION

Caffey's disease is a self-limiting idiopathic infantile condition characterized by abnormal cortical thickening of bone, soft-tissue swelling, irritability, and fever of unknown etiology. The mandible, scapula, clavicle, tubular bones, and ribs are most commonly involved. Multiple bones can be affected, and involvement may be asymmetric.

An iatrogenic cause has been linked to the use of intravenous prostaglandins for treatment of neonatal congenital heart defects. Familial and sporadic forms have been reported. Most patients present at age 9 weeks with the sporadic form of the disease, whereas the familial form is most common prenatally or at birth. The peak age of the sporadic form ranges from 6 weeks to 6 months, and it usually resolves within 6 to 9 months.

HISTORY AND PHYSICAL FINDINGS

Examination is usually characterized by hyperirritability and the presence of a mass, commonly over the mandible (sporadic form). Fever (elevated erythrocyte sedimentation rate and alkaline phosphatase level) resembling infection can occur; however, the mass is not erythematous or warm.

IMAGING STUDIES

Required for diagnosis

AP and lateral views of the involved extremity are required for diagnosis and depend on the presenting symptoms, specifically the affected area. Common findings include periosteal new bone formation of the diaphysis, evidence of soft-tissue swelling, and increased diameter of the diaphysis.

Required for comprehensive evaluation

Skeletal survey allows for a comprehensive evaluation in determining the extent of skeletal involvement. MRI is generally not needed but is sometimes helpful in differentiating the extent of soft-tissue involvement adjacent to the periosteal reaction.

Special considerations

None

Pitfalls
None

IMAGE DESCRIPTIONS

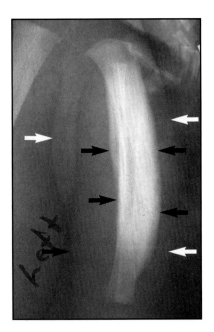

Figure 11-44

Caffey's disease (tibia)—Lateral view

Lateral view of the tibia shows increased bone formation throughout the diaphysis (black arrows) with increased diameter and soft-tissue swelling (white arrows).

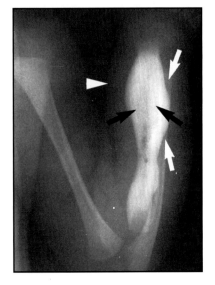

Figure 11-45

Caffey's disease (radius)—Lateral view

Lateral view of the forearm shows increased diameter of the diaphysis in the radius (black arrows), extensive periosteal reaction (white arrows), and soft-tissue swelling (arrowhead).

DIFFERENTIAL DIAGNOSIS

Child abuse (on radiographs, no increase in diaphyseal diameter, multiple bones affected with different stages of healing)

Osteomyelitis (radiographically, no increase in diaphyseal diameter; abnormal laboratory studies)

Scurvy (decreased density and thinned cortices at the knees on radiographs)

CHILD ABUSE

SYNONYMS
Battered child syndrome
Nonaccidental trauma

ICD-9 Code
995.50
Child abuse, unspecified

DEFINITION
According to the Centers for Disease Control and Prevention, 2.8 million cases of alleged child maltreatment are referred to child protective services annually. Almost 25% of cases of abuse that are proved by law involve physical maltreatment. Physical child abuse is the infliction of injury as the result of biting, punching, beating, kicking, shaking, burning, or otherwise physically harming a child. Head trauma (caused by violent shaking) is the leading cause of death and disability among physically abused infants and children. Most victims are younger than 3 years. Fractures found in infants younger than 2 years are highly suggestive of physical abuse. Up to 25% of abused children whose cases are missed will experience further abuse, and 5% risk dying.

HISTORY AND PHYSICAL FINDINGS
Confirming physical abuse with radiographic evidence alone is unreliable. Clinical diagnosis, along with a high index of suspicion, is required. It is important to be systematic during the interview and examination.

It is critical that the history given by the family correlates with the injury. The history and the patient's age are very important factors when evaluating fractures thought to be secondary to abuse.

A general physical examination should include height and weight, a record of developmental milestones, skin findings, and an eye examination for retinal hemorrhage. The musculoskeletal examination includes inspection and palpation of all extremities and the spine. Inspection of the soft tissues is also very important, as there may be bruises or burns in various stages of healing over several parts of the body. Bruising of the buttocks, perineum, trunk, back of the head, legs, and neck; burns (from cigarettes); and symmetric scalding (from bath water) suggest physical abuse.

IMAGING STUDIES

Required for diagnosis

A skeletal survey is ordered in cases of suspected abuse. This series includes AP and lateral views of the skull and thoracolumbar spine, AP view of the thoracic cage, AP view of the pelvis, and AP views of the upper and lower extremities. Findings on radiographs that raise concern of abuse include the following: (1) long bone fractures in infants younger than 2 years; (2) multiple fractures at different stages of healing; and (3) fractures of the ribs, skull, spinous process, metaphyses (corner fractures), or scapula.

Required for comprehensive evaluation

CT of the head may be indicated to rule out cerebral edema and subdural or subarachnoid hemorrhage in the child with unexplained acute or chronic neurologic abnormalities.

Special considerations

Bone scans are useful in identifying occult fractures. A skeletal survey combined with a bone scan increases the yield for identifying occult fractures.

Pitfalls

A babygram (a single body projection of an infant) may lack sufficient detail to identify radiographic signs of physical abuse. Note that radiographic findings alone may not be reliable because some fractures (ie, "toddler fractures," clavicle fractures, and spiral fractures of the femur) have low or no specificity for abuse. Suboptimal radiographic technique may also lead to misinterpretations.

IMAGE DESCRIPTIONS

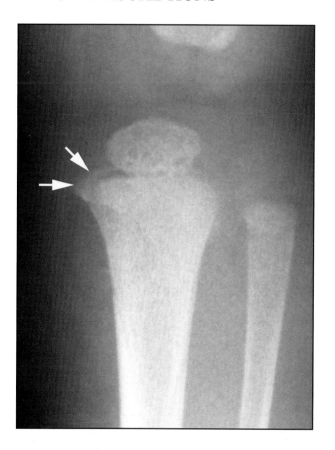

Figure 11-46

Child abuse (corner fracture of the tibia)—AP view

AP view of the proximal tibia in a 3-month-old infant shows a metaphyseal fracture (corner fracture) and evidence of periosteal separation between the physis and metaphysis (arrows), most likely secondary to a forceful downward pulling on the extremity.

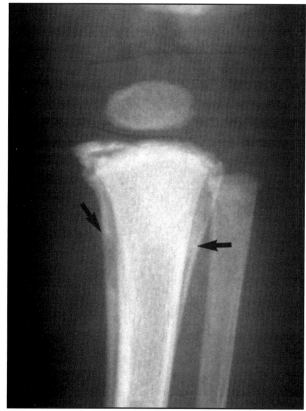

Figure 11-47

Child abuse (new bone formation in the tibia)—AP view

AP view of the same child shown in Figure 11-46 approximately 1 month later shows new periosteal bone formation along the medial and lateral cortices (arrows). Note that the first signs of new periosteal bone can occur as early as 7 to 10 days after the injury.

SECTION 11 ■ PEDIATRIC ORTHOPAEDICS

DIFFERENTIAL DIAGNOSIS

Caffey's disease (periostitis and cortical thickening of diaphyseal and membranous bones, especially the mandible and forearms, with the ulna more commonly affected than the radius; may be difficult to discern from child abuse; often symmetric, whereas child abuse is asymmetric)

Congenital syphilis (chronic osteochondritis, periostitis, or osteitis; destructive lesions usually in the tibial metaphysis; increased density of secondary ossification centers [Wimberger's ring sign]; confirmed by serologic test)

Leukemia (radiolucent metaphyseal bands on radiographs, without fractures)

Osteogenesis imperfecta (blue sclerae, thin cortices, osteopenia, long bone bowing, multiple fractures)

Osteomyelitis (sequestra and involucra, cortical and medullary bone destruction, reactive sclerosis without radiographic evidence of fracture)

Rickets (irregular cupping and widening of the physis; fuzzy cortices; transverse pseudofractures [Looser transformation zones] without radiographic evidence of acute fractures)

Scurvy (increased density adjacent to growth plate [white lines of scurvy]; metaphyseal findings indicate all bones at same stage)

Diastrophic Dysplasia

Synonyms

Diastrophic dwarfism
Hitchhiker's thumb with clubfeet

ICD-9 Code

756.54
Polyostotic fibrous dysplasia
of bone

Definition

Diastrophic (Greek for "crooked" or "twisted") dysplasia is
characterized by rhizomelic skeletal dysplasia, micromelia, and
clubfeet. It has an autosomal recessive inheritance pattern, with
genetic identification on chromosome 5, including a sulfate
transporter gene. The cartilage matrix throughout the entire body is
abnormal, with delayed epiphyseal ossification causing flattening
and irregular bone formation.

History and Physical Findings

Diastrophic dysplasia is diagnosed by clinical examination at birth,
as the neonate will have limbs significantly shorter than normal and
bilateral clubfeet. Characteristic facial features include a narrow
nasal bridge with flared nostrils and full cheeks. Severe short
stature is often accompanied by hitchhiker's thumbs (abducted
thumbs), cauliflower ears, rigid clubfeet, cleft palate (in 50% of
patients), and scoliosis. Patients have normal intelligence. Infants
may have joint contractures with rigid deformities, radial head or
patellar dislocations, symphalangia, and genu valgum. Progressive
kyphoscoliosis usually develops once the child begins walking.

Imaging Studies

Required for diagnosis

Diastrophic dysplasia is a clinical diagnosis in infancy based on
physical examination findings and a skeletal survey (AP and lateral
views of the skull and thoracolumbar spine, AP view of the thoracic
cage, AP view of the pelvis, AP views of the upper and lower
extremities). These studies either are ordered by a specialist in the
nursery or shortly after the infant has been released from the
hospital. The primary care physician should refer the infant to a
clinical geneticist.

Section 11 ■ Pediatric Orthopaedics

Required for comprehensive evaluation

A skeletal survey is recommended upon initial evaluation. AP and lateral upright views of the thoracolumbar spine are recommended to demonstrate the morphology of the vertebrae. AP and lateral views of the cervical spine are recommended to assess for cervical kyphosis. Kyphosis is usually greatest at C2 and C4. When cervical kyphosis is present, MRI is suggested to evaluate spinal cord involvement.

The long bones of the lower extremities are shorter than normal with delayed epiphyseal ossification. Once ossification is complete, irregular epiphyses are evident with flaring, flattening, and a bulbous metaphyseal-epiphyseal region. Genu valgum and patellar dislocations are also frequently present.

AP and lateral radiographs of the upper extremities are ordered to assess shortening of the ulna, a possible cause of ulnar deviation of the hands. AP views of the hands are ordered to assess symphalangia of the proximal interphalangeal joints and triangular-shaped thumb metacarpal physes, which may cause subluxation and an abducted thumb.

AP views of the pelvis are ordered to evaluate coxa vara, hip dislocations, or a saucer-shaped defect of the ossification of the capital femoral epiphysis.

Special considerations

None

Pitfalls

Weight-bearing views of the lower extremities are recommended whenever possible to properly assess lower extremity malalignment. Weight-bearing views of the spine are recommended whenever possible to properly assess spine deformity (usually kyphosis).

IMAGE DESCRIPTIONS

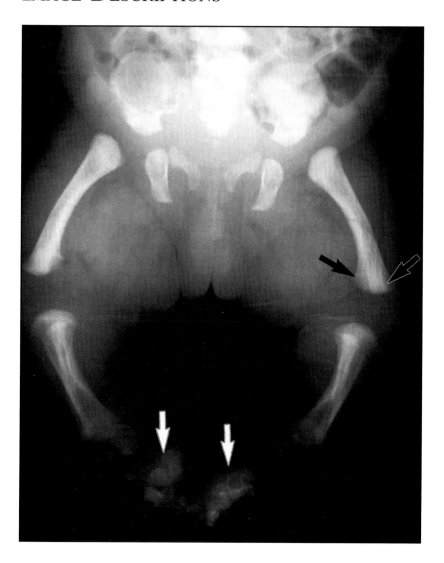

Figure 11-48

Diastrophic dysplasia (lower extremities)— AP view

AP view of the lower extremities in a patient with diastrophic dysplasia shows bulbous-appearing metaphyses in all joints (black arrows), severe equinovarus feet (white arrows), and no evidence of epiphyseal ossification.

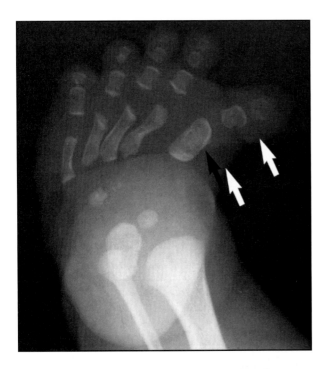

Figure 11-49

Diastrophic dysplasia (foot)— AP view

AP view of a foot in a patient with diastrophic dysplasia shows that the first metatarsal is short and irregular (similar to hitchhiker's thumb) (black arrow) with severe hallux (great toe) varus and medial deviation of the forefoot (white arrows).

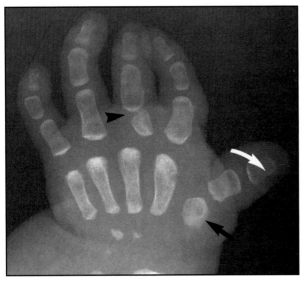

Figure 11-50

Diastrophic dysplasia (hand)— AP view

AP view of a hand in a patient with diastrophic dysplasia shows broad, shortened bones, an irregular and shortened thumb metacarpal bone (black arrow), and a subluxated metacarpophalangeal thumb joint with extreme abduction of the thumb (curved white arrow). Note that the proximal interphalangeal joint of the long finger shows symphalangia (arrowhead).

DIFFERENTIAL DIAGNOSIS

Achondroplasia (more rhizomelic pattern seen on radiographs; lacks rigidity; genu varum)

Arthrogryposis (no limb shortening, but joint deformity with contracture; no radiographic findings of bone dysplasia)

Chondrodysplasia punctata (bilateral cataracts; dry, scaly skin; mild symmetric rhizomelic limb shortening seen on radiographs)

MADELUNG'S DEFORMITY

SYNONYM
Wrist subluxation

DEFINITION
Madelung's deformity is a growth disturbance of the volar-ulnar aspect of the distal radial epiphysis. The ulnar third of the distal radial epiphysis does not ossify, and the ulnar head is prominent with dorsal subluxation. The etiology is unknown; however, it is described most often as congenital and transmitted as an autosomal dominant trait with incomplete penetrance. The deformity is more common in girls and is commonly bilateral.

HISTORY AND PHYSICAL FINDINGS
Patients in middle to late adolescence most commonly present with a perceived dislocation of the ulna or pain over the prominence of the ulnar head as a result of a traumatic event. The pain increases with activity. Until presentation, however, patients may not notice the deformity. A painless wrist deformity (ulnar head prominent dorsally), along with weakness and limited pronation and supination, is also common on initial presentation.

IMAGING STUDIES

Required for diagnosis
AP and lateral views of both wrists in neutral position on the same film are ordered to assess bilaterality and symmetry. The AP view will show that the distal ulna is longer (positive ulnar variance), the radial epiphysis may have a triangular shape, and the volar-ulnar tilt may be severe enough that the physis may not be visualized. On the lateral view, the radius tilts volarly, and the ulna is subluxated or dislocated dorsally.

Required for comprehensive evaluation
CT may be helpful in assessing complex three-dimensional morphology of the deformity and is useful for planning surgery.

Special considerations
None

Pitfalls
None

ICD-9 Code

755.54
Other congenital anomalies of upper limb, including shoulder girdle; Madelung's deformity

SECTION 11 ■ PEDIATRIC ORTHOPAEDICS

IMAGE DESCRIPTION

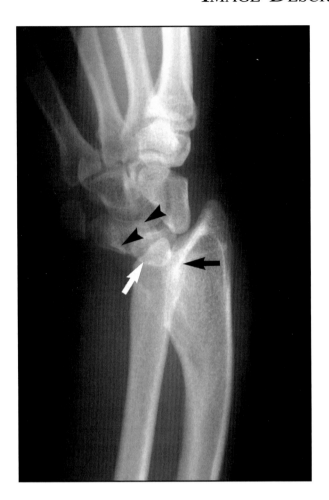

Figure 11-51

Madelung's deformity—AP view

AP view of a wrist with Madelung's deformity shows decreased length of the ulnar aspect of the radius and a triangular-shaped distal radial epiphysis (black arrow). Note also that the carpus is in a triangular configuration with the lunate at the apex (white arrow), and both volar and ulnar radiocarpal subluxation is present (arrowheads).

DIFFERENTIAL DIAGNOSIS

Dyschondrosteosis (radiographically symmetric bilateral Madelung's deformities, mesomelic shortening of the extremities)

Posttraumatic wrist malunion (radiographs may demonstrate evidence of posttraumatic changes)

OSTEOGENESIS IMPERFECTA

ICD-9 Code

756.51
Osteogenesis imperfecta

SYNONYMS

Brittle bone disease
Osteomalacia congenita
Osteoporosis fetalis

DEFINITION

Osteogenesis imperfecta (OI) is a genetic disorder of collagen deficiency that results in bone fragility of varying severity.

HISTORY AND PHYSICAL FINDINGS

Diagnosis is made by history, physical examination, and radiographic findings. The history and physical examination vary depending on the severity and type of OI. Family history is important. Characteristic radiographic findings depend on the type of OI. Infants with severe OI may be stillborn or die shortly after birth and demonstrate evidence of bone fragility on radiographs. Those who survive delivery may have multiple fractures, including skull fractures due to a soft skull. A weak thoracic cage or intracranial hemorrhage may cause death shortly after delivery.

Older children may present with milder types of OI, manifesting as fractures after minimal trauma or a history of multiple fractures with radiographically mild osteopenia.

IMAGING STUDIES

Required for diagnosis

A babygram (AP radiograph of the entire infant) is indicated to identify the type and extent of involvement and possible fractures associated with OI. Characteristic findings may include fractures with generalized osteopenia, osteoporotic-appearing bone with thin cortices, and plastic bowing deformities in long bones secondary to stress fractures and malunions. AP and lateral views of the skull should be ordered to assess for Wormian bones (small ossicles within the suture lines).

Required for comprehensive evaluation
None

Special considerations
Careful positioning of neonates, infants, and severely affected children by both physicians and radiology technicians is advised.

SECTION 11 ■ PEDIATRIC ORTHOPAEDICS

Pitfalls

Radiographic evaluation may suggest a diagnosis of OI but is not definitive. Clinical examination, laboratory studies, and bone/cartilage biopsy may be required for definitive diagnosis.

IMAGE DESCRIPTIONS

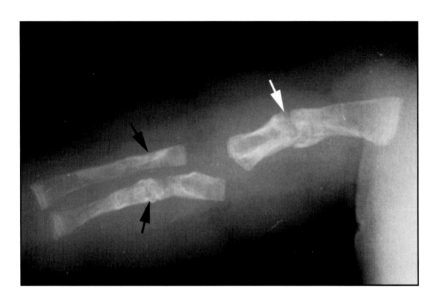

Figure 11-52

Osteogenesis imperfecta—AP view

AP view of a child's humerus, radius, and ulna shows fractures at different stages of healing. Note that the fractures in the radius and ulna have healed (black arrows) and the humerus is healing (white arrow), with evidence of callus formation around the fracture sites. Also note that the bones are osteopenic with thin cortices.

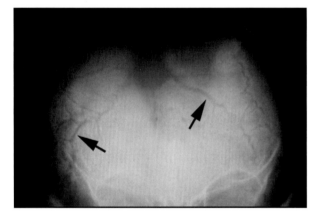

Figure 11-53

Osteogenesis imperfecta—AP view

AP view of the skull in a child shows Wormian bones (arrows) with detached portions of the primary ossification centers.

DIFFERENTIAL DIAGNOSIS

Child abuse (fractured bones not osteopenic, no metaphyseal corner fractures)

Congenital hypophosphatasia (similar to OI on radiographs; laboratory studies needed to differentiate)

Juvenile infantile osteoporosis (radiographically less severe than OI)

Leukemia (osteopenia seen in the metaphyseal regions only)

OSTEOMYELITIS

SYNONYMS

Bone infection
Meningococcemia osteomyelitis
Sickle cell osteomyelitis

ICD-9 Code

730.2x (area affected)
Unspecified osteomyelitis,
(area affected)

DEFINITION

Osteomyelitis is an inflammation of bone secondary to bacterial infection that can be acute, subacute, or chronic. Neonates and patients with immunologic deficiencies are more susceptible to infections leading to osteomyelitis. In children, osteomyelitis is caused predominantly by hematogenous seeding. It occurs during childhood and is more likely to occur in long bones. Boys are most likely to be affected, with peak occurrence at around age 10 years.

Bacteria are believed to infect bone in the following way: the tortuous venous sinusoid vessels in the metaphysis allow bacteria to slow and become trapped within the bone. The physis in children may prevent bacteria from entering the joint; however, this may not be the case in neonates. The hip, radial head, shoulder, and distal tibia/fibula joint capsules attach at the metaphyseal region in neonates, leaving them vulnerable to intra-articular sepsis in the event of metaphyseal osteomyelitis.

Organisms responsible for osteomyelitis vary according to age group. In neonates, likely organisms are group B streptococci, *Staphylococcus aureus*, gram-negative bacilli, and *Neisseria gonorrhoeae*; in infants and young children, *S aureus*, *Streptococcus pneumoniae*, group A streptococci, and *Kingella kingae*; in children older than 5 years, *S aureus* and *Pseudomonas aeruginosa* from puncture wounds; and in young adolescents, *S aureus* and *Neisseria gonorrhoeae*. A number of predisposing conditions may contribute to the bacteriology, including sickle cell (*Salmonella*), meningitis, chickenpox (*Streptococcus*), and otitis media (*Streptococcus* or *Haemophilus influenzae*).

HISTORY AND PHYSICAL FINDINGS

Pain is the most common presenting symptom. An older child can verbalize pain, but a very young child may present with a limp, refusal to move an extremity, or refusal to walk. History of a concomitant infection, recent respiratory infection, rash, swollen lymph nodes, and any reason for compromised immunity are important factors in establishing the diagnosis. Trauma is a potential predisposing factor for osteomyelitis.

SECTION 11 ■ PEDIATRIC ORTHOPAEDICS

Physical examination includes observation for swelling, erythema, loss of skin wrinkles, and pain on palpation, all of which are signs of infection. Patients also may be afebrile. Involvement of the lower extremities may result in a limp or cause a patient to refuse to use the affected limb. Patients also may be irritable, especially during physical examination of the affected limb. The diagnosis is more difficult in neonates because the clinical signs are not as readily apparent as in older children. Irritability and fever may be the only clinical signs; therefore, a high index of suspicion is critical in making the diagnosis in neonates.

IMAGING STUDIES

Required for diagnosis
AP and lateral views of the involved extremity are required for initial assessment. If the exact location is not known, AP and lateral views of the entire extremity should be ordered. Observable changes on radiographs include soft-tissue swelling, bone resorption, and periosteal reaction. Radiographs may be negative, but even these help rule out the presence of a fracture or neoplasm.

Required for comprehensive evaluation
Bone scan may be useful in establishing the diagnosis. Technetium Tc 99m diphosphonate is favored for evaluation in children and has an accuracy rate of approximately 90%. Bone scans are most useful when the infection is difficult to localize. In fact, they are rarely "cold" in patients with infection; decreased uptake usually indicates an abscess.

Special considerations
CT is not required to confirm the diagnosis but is helpful in identifying areas that require needle aspiration. MRI is ordered in most cases in delineating infection, which will appear as decreased signal intensity on T1-weighted images and increased signal intensity on T2-weighted images.

Pitfalls
Normal-appearing radiographs do not rule out infection, and not all positive bone scans indicate infection. Also, bone destruction secondary to infection can be confused with neoplasm on radiographs; if the image is not definitive, MRI and appropriate laboratory studies are indicated. Patients with sickle cell crisis events will also report bone pain and occasionally have a fever, which makes the differential diagnosis difficult.

IMAGE DESCRIPTIONS

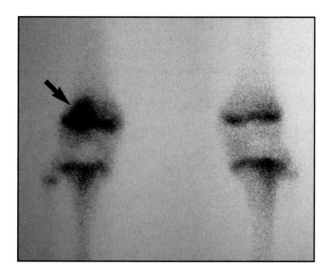

Figure 11-54

Osteomyelitis (knee)—AP bone scan

AP bone scan of both knees in a patient with osteomyelitis shows increased uptake (hot) at the metaphysis of the right distal femur (arrow).

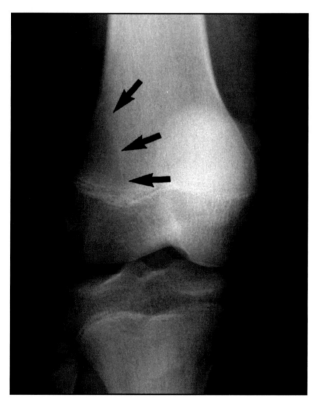

Figure 11-55

Osteomyelitis (knee)—AP view

AP view of a knee in a patient with osteomyelitis shows lucency over the lateral aspect of the distal femoral metaphysis (arrows).

SECTION 11 ■ PEDIATRIC ORTHOPAEDICS

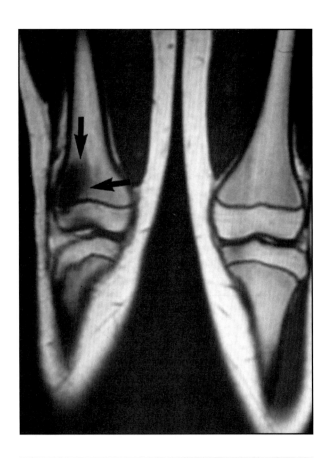

Figure 11-56

Osteomyelitis (knee)—Coronal MRI

Coronal T1-weighted MRI scan of both knees in a patient with osteomyelitis shows decreased signal intensity over the distal femoral metaphysis (arrows).

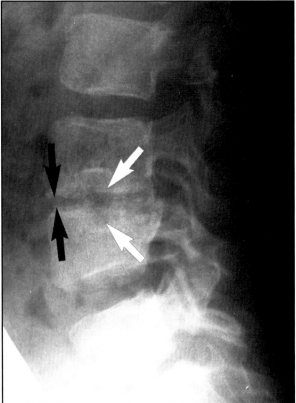

Figure 11-57

Osteomyelitis (spine)—Lateral view

Lateral view of the spine in a 9-year-old child with osteomyelitis shows chronic changes involving the intervertebral space (black arrows). The end plates of the narrowed disk are irregular, lytic, and sclerotic (white arrows), suggesting intervertebral disk involvement.

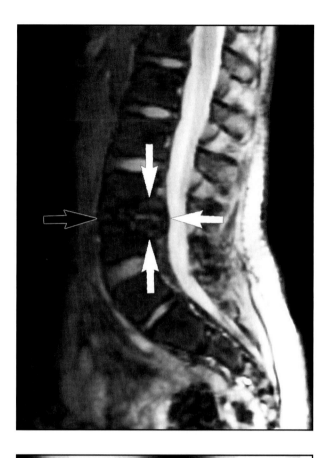

Figure 11-58

Osteomyelitis (spine)—Sagittal MRI

Sagittal MRI scan of a spine in a patient with osteomyelitis shows obliteration of the disk material of L4-L5 (black arrow) and abscess formation in the disk anterior to the posterior longitudinal ligament (white arrows), causing elevation to the ligament.

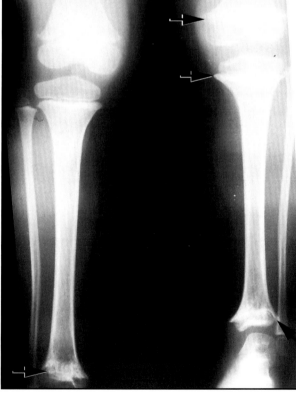

Figure 11-59

Osteomyelitis (tibia)—AP view

Weight-bearing AP view of both tibias in a patient with a history of meningococcemia demonstrates that the left tibia is shorter than the right tibia. The infection resulted in early physeal closure in several sites involving the tibias and distal femur (arrows).

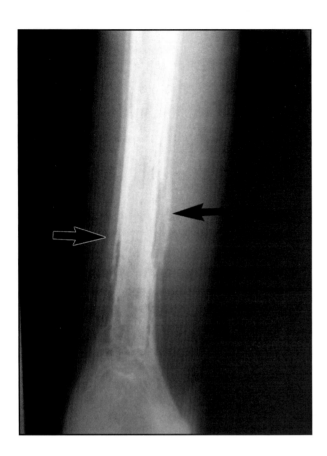

Figure 11-60

Sickle cell anemia (humerus)— AP view

AP view of a humerus in a patient with sickle cell anemia shows periosteal reaction (arrows). Note that when trying to distinguish bony infarction from osteomyelitis in a patient with sickle cell anemia, radiographs can be ambiguous because both conditions show periosteal reaction.

DIFFERENTIAL DIAGNOSIS

Bone infarction (radiographically similar, so biopsy may be needed to confirm diagnosis)

Neoplasia (leukemia, Ewing's sarcoma, eosinophilic granuloma, metastatic neuroblastoma) (radiographically similar)

SPONDYLOEPIPHYSEAL DYSPLASIA

SYNONYMS

SED

Spondyloepiphyseal dysplasia, congenital type

Spondyloepiphyseal dysplasia tarda with progressive arthropathy (progressive pseudorheumatoid dysplasia)

Spondyloepiphyseal dysplasia tarda, X-linked

Spondyloepiphyseal dysplasia with diabetes mellitus (Wolcott-Rallison)

ICD-9 Code

756.54
Polyostotic fibrous dysplasia of bone

DEFINITION

Spondyloepiphyseal dysplasia (SED) is a short-trunk disproportionate form of dwarfism that involves the vertebrae. Two principal types occur: congenital SED and delayed-onset SED (SED tarda). Musculoskeletal characteristics of congenital SED include flattened vertebrae, abnormal epiphyses, and proximal and distal limb shortening at birth, with sparing of the hands and feet. Associated problems include myopia, retinal detachment, cataracts, and deafness. Delayed-onset SED is characterized by growth loss during adolescence due to flattened vertebrae and abnormal epiphyses of the larger proximal joints.

HISTORY AND PHYSICAL FINDINGS

Congenital SED is a clinical diagnosis based on physical and radiographic findings at birth. Examination reveals short stature with disproportionate trunk involvement, a barrel-shaped chest, a flat face, wide-set eyes, a short neck, increased lumbar lordosis, and, occasionally, hip flexion contractures. Cervical myelopathy may occur secondary to a hypoplastic odontoid and atlantoaxial instability presenting with signs of motor delay, respiratory changes, and/or decreased endurance. Scoliosis or kyphoscoliosis may develop in late childhood. Children with SED may demonstrate coxa vara and early osteoarthritis of the hips.

IMAGING STUDIES

Required for diagnosis

A skeletal survey (AP and lateral views of the skull and thoracolumbar spine, AP view of the thoracic cage, AP view of the pelvis, and AP views of the upper and lower extremities) is required for diagnosis.

Required for comprehensive evaluation

When neurologic signs and symptoms are present, MRI of the brain and cervical spine and MRI of the thoracic and lumbar spine are required. In addition, the following radiographic studies are helpful:

Spine Standing or sitting AP and lateral thoracolumbar views will reveal platyspondyly with tonguelike projections from the anterior thoracic bodies and oval lumbar vertebrae.

Cervical spine Active lateral flexion-extension views are helpful to assess atlantoaxial stability.

Pelvis Weight-bearing AP views should be taken with the hips in internal rotation to assess the presence of coxa vara. Signs of coxa vara are evidence of delay of the capital femoral epiphyses, small and short iliac crests, horizontal acetabular roofs, and premature osteoarthritis.

Lower extremities Weight-bearing AP views of the lower extremities will commonly reveal delayed knee epiphyses, flaring of the metaphyses, and coronal malalignment such as genu valgum.

Special considerations

Imaging studies such as MRI are ordered in the first 1 to 2 years of life to assess foramen magnum stenosis. MRI may reveal abnormalities of the cranium, cerebrum, and cervicomedullary junction. Clinical indications in newborns are neurologic findings, severe hypotonia, hyperreflexia, or clonus. MRI is indicated also to assess the extent of stenosis of the lumbar spine in teens and adults.

Pitfalls

None

IMAGE DESCRIPTION

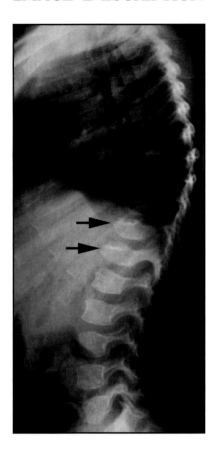

Figure 11-61

Spondyloepiphyseal dysplasia (thoracolumbar spine)—Lateral view

Lateral view of a thoracolumbar spine shows increased thoracic kyphosis, platyspondyly (short, flat vertebrae), oval shape and posterior wedging of the lumbar vertebrae, anterior projections from the thoracic vertebrae (arrows), and abnormal ossification.

DIFFERENTIAL DIAGNOSIS

Kniest's dysplasia (severe kyphoscoliosis; radiographic findings similar to SED, ie, enlarged epiphyses and sclerosis within the epiphysis)

Multiple epiphyseal dysplasia (epiphyseal findings similar to SED but no abnormal findings involving the spine)

CONGENITAL SCOLIOSIS

ICD-9 Code

754.2
Certain congenital
musculoskeletal deformities;
of spine

SYNONYMS

None

DEFINITION

Congenital scoliosis is an embroyologic defect of the formation of vertebrae that occurs during the first 6 weeks of fetal development. Congenital vertebral abnormalities leading to congenital scoliosis include failure of formation, failure of segmentation, or both. On an AP view, the normal spine appears as a series of stacked rectangles (the vertebral bodies) separated by radiolucent disks. Failure of formation (hemivertebrae) appears as a triangle on the AP view. If one or more triangular hemivertebrae are stacked among the square vertebrae, a curvature of the spine results. With failure of segmentation, one or more vertebral bodies may be fused. A unilateral bar is an example of a failure of formation in which multiple vertebral bodies are joined on one side by continuous bone with no growth potential, while on the opposite side there are growth plates with growth potential. A unilateral bar is a severe form of congenital scoliosis, and significant curve progression is likely with growth.

Congenital spinal anomalies are associated with anomalies of the genitourinary system in 25% of patients and the cardiac system in 10% of patients. There is no evidence of a genetic etiology for congenital vertebral anomalies, as these appear to be sporadic events.

HISTORY AND PHYSICAL FINDINGS

Often, the condition is either never detected or is first noted as an incidental finding on radiographs. The natural history of congenital scoliosis is variable.

IMAGING STUDIES

Required for diagnosis

AP and lateral full-body scoliosis views (14 in. x 36 in. cassette, 14 in. x 17 in. cassette in infants and children younger than 5 years) are ordered to establish the diagnosis.

SECTION 11 ■ PEDIATRIC ORTHOPAEDICS

Required for comprehensive evaluation
MRI or CT may be ordered to assess the morphology of vertebral (CT) or spinal cord anomalies (MRI) associated with congenital scoliosis. MRI is ordered to evaluate tethered cord, syrinx, or other abnormalities of the spinal cord such as diastematomyelia. In addition, MRI is ordered to assess the morphology of the growth plates and disks as a method to define the potential for future growth. CT with sagittal reconstructions is quite useful to better define the skeletal morphology of these anomalies. A CT scan with three-dimensional images is useful for surgical planning.

Special considerations
Sedation may be necessary for CT or MRI.

Pitfalls
Radiographs may not show vertebral anomalies in sufficient detail. Also, failure to obtain imaging studies to evaluate genitourinary, cardiac, and other spinal anomalies may lead to delayed diagnosis of these possible associated anomalies.

IMAGE DESCRIPTION

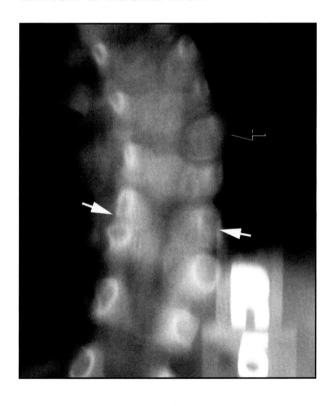

Figure 11-62

Congenital scoliosis— Coronal tomogram

Tomogram in the coronal plane of the thoracic spine demonstrates a hemivertebra on the right side of the spine (black arrow), which causes the scoliosis. Also noted are "butterfly" vertebrae (partial formation of the hemivertebra) (white arrows).

DIFFERENTIAL DIAGNOSIS

Idiopathic scoliosis (no vertebral anomalies will be seen)

IDIOPATHIC SCOLIOSIS

SYNONYMS
None

DEFINITION
Idiopathic scoliosis is a curvature of the spine in the coronal (frontal) plane of at least 10°. There is no known underlying cause. Idiopathic scoliosis most commonly presents during adolescence, though it is uncommonly seen in younger children (infantile and juvenile scoliosis). In contrast to congenital scoliosis, vertebral body development is normal in idiopathic scoliosis. The vertebral bodies at the apex of the curve are rotated toward the convexity of the curve. If such rotation is not present, other causes of scoliosis are likely.

Adult scoliosis is unlikely to progress unless there is substantial curvature. Most patients remain asymptomatic. Individuals may have degenerative low back pain from compensatory processes in the lumbar spine. In addition, degenerative scoliosis may present in adulthood and may be associated with spinal stenosis and lower extremity neurologic symptoms.

HISTORY AND PHYSICAL FINDINGS
Adolescent idiopathic scoliosis is a diagnosis of exclusion. The history and physical examination will focus on identifying an underlying pathology. Idiopathic scoliosis may be identified during a school screening or most commonly during a pediatric/adolescent annual physical examination. Progressive or focal back pain, weakness, bowel or bladder problems, or any neurologic signs or symptoms should alert the physician to the possibility that the scoliosis may be a manifestation of an underlying disease or condition.

Findings on physical examination may include an asymmetry of the trunk, waist, and/or shoulders. When the patient bends forward (Adams forward bend test) with the hands together and legs straight, an asymmetric prominence called a rib or lumbar prominence will present on the back as a result of the rotational asymmetry. A detailed neurologic examination that tests strength, balance, and reflexes should be normal.

Examination of the adult patient with scoliosis includes evaluation of the source or sources of back pain, including disk degeneration, translatory shifts, and facet arthritis. Neurologic evaluation may demonstrate sensory or motor deficits. Adult patients previously treated with posterior spinal fusion and instrumentation may present with symptoms of "flatback" syndrome. These patients report low back pain as a result of loss of lumbar lordosis that worsens throughout the day and with activity. Compensatory hip and knee flexion to maintain an upright posture may lead to lower extremity weakness, fatigue, and pain.

IMAGING STUDIES

Required for diagnosis
Weight-bearing AP and lateral views of the entire spine (14 in. x 36 in. cassette) are required for diagnosis in the adolescent patient. Similar studies are required to assess the adult patient, including flexion-extension radiographs to assess for instability. Preoperative studies also include the additional views of supine right and left side-bending views (14 in. x 36 in. cassette).

Required for comprehensive evaluation
MRI is ordered when there is suspicion of underlying pathology causing a painful scoliosis or when neurologic findings are present to evaluate a tethered cord, syrinx, diastematomyelia, infection, tumor, or other causes. The curvature in adolescent idiopathic scoliosis is characteristically to the right side in the thoracic region (structural curve) and to the left side in the lumbar region (compensatory curve). Many advocate MRI for evaluation of a left thoracic curve and for all significant curves in children younger than 10 years. Adult patients also require MRI or CT myelography to assess for neurologic problems associated with radiculopathy or spinal stenosis.

Special considerations
Approximately 30% of children in early adolescence report some degree of back pain. Children with idiopathic scoliosis generally do not have back pain. Back pain may need to be evaluated if the pain is localized to one specific area, is progressive, or is suspicious in other ways. Most commonly, the pain is the result of spondylolysis or Scheuermann disease.

Pitfalls
Functional scoliosis due to limb-length discrepancy may be confused with idiopathic scoliosis. In functional scoliosis, there is no rotation of the apical vertebra.

SECTION 11 ■ PEDIATRIC ORTHOPAEDICS

IMAGE DESCRIPTION

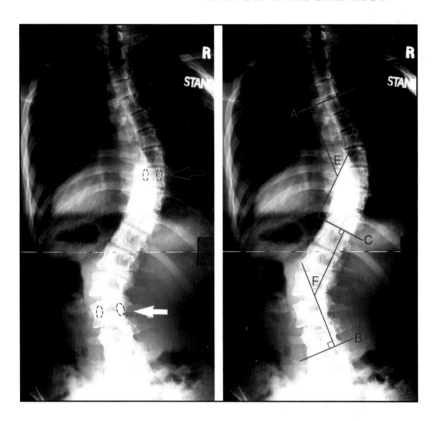

Figure 11-63

Idiopathic scoliosis—AP view

AP radiograph of the spine including C7-S1 shows right thoracic and left lumbar scoliosis. In adolescents, this view is taken on a 14 in. x 36 in. cassette to allow visualization of the entire spine. Note the rotation of the pedicles in the direction of the convexity in the thoracic region (black arrow) and in the opposite direction in the lumbar region (white arrow). The Cobb angles, which measure the maximum arcs within a scoliotic curve, are shown on the image on the right. To measure a Cobb angle, lines are drawn across the end vertebrae of the curve (lines A and B). For a double curve, a single line is also drawn at the midpoint (line C). Lines are then drawn perpendicular to each of lines A, B, and C. The angles formed at the intersection of these lines are the Cobb angles (E and F).

DIFFERENTIAL DIAGNOSIS

Congenital scoliosis (presents at younger age, associated with more acute progressive scoliosis, contains vertebral anomalies)

Neuromuscular Scoliosis

Synonym
Paralytic scoliosis

ICD-9 Code

737.4
Curvature of spine
associated with other
conditions

Definition
This type of scoliosis is associated with neuromuscular conditions, including cerebral palsy, muscular dystrophies, spina bifida, Friedreich's ataxia, Rett syndrome, and poliomyelitis. Its etiology is related to a lack of complex and normal integration of the brain, spinal cord, nerves, and muscle, leading to problems of head, neck, and trunk control.

History and Physical Findings
Because a wide variety of neuromuscular conditions are associated with neuromuscular scoliosis, the history and physical findings will be variable. Children with more severe neuromuscular involvement (ie, nonambulators) are more likely to develop scoliosis. In contrast to idiopathic scoliosis, neuromuscular scoliosis frequently develops before adolescence, and the curves are often longer and C-shaped, sometimes involving the pelvis and causing significant pelvic obliquity, which leads to difficulty in sitting. Pressure sores and skin breakdown may ensue. Patients may need to use their upper extremities for sitting balance, rendering them functionally quadriparetic. Unfortunately, external bracing is generally not effective in providing balance or halting progressive deformity. Surgical stabilization and fusion is commonly required.

Imaging Studies

Required for diagnosis
AP and lateral radiographs of the spine, including the pelvis, taken on a 14 in. x 36 in. cassette, are sufficient for diagnosis.

Required for comprehensive evaluation
Right and left supine side-bending radiographs, taken on a 14 in. x 36 in. cassette, are ordered preoperatively to determine curve flexibility and surgical planning. MRI may be indicated for spine evaluation when intraspinal pathology is suspected, most frequently when the underlying condition has a known association with intraspinal pathology, such as spina bifida. In children with conditions not associated with intraspinal pathology, such as cerebral palsy or muscular dystrophy, MRI is usually not indicated.

Special considerations
Radiographs may be performed with the child in or out of the brace. Consistency is recommended.

Pitfalls
None

IMAGE DESCRIPTION

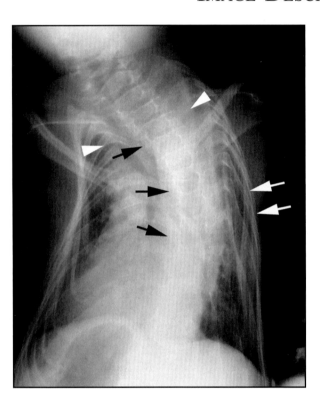

Figure 11-64

Neuromuscular scoliosis—AP view

AP view of a child demonstrates a long, sloping, C-shaped curve (black arrows) characteristic of neuromuscular scoliosis. Note also the narrow, dysplastic thoracic cage with sloping ribs (white arrows), which is also commonly associated with neuromuscular scoliosis. The radiograph shows the decreased thoracic space (arrowheads) available for lung parenchyma and decreased pulmonary function as a result of scoliosis.

DIFFERENTIAL DIAGNOSIS

None

SCHEUERMANN DISEASE

SYNONYMS

Roundback deformity
Scheuermann kyphosis
Scheuermann thoracic kyphosis

ICD-9 Code

732.0
Juvenile osteochondrosis of
spine

DEFINITION

Scheuermann disease is characterized by end plate changes seen in the thoracic, thoracolumbar, and lumbar spine and may be associated with kyphotic deformity. Adolescents may present with an asymptomatic postural thoracic "roundback" or with significant thoracolumbar pain.

HISTORY AND PHYSICAL FINDINGS

Scheuermann disease is often asymptomatic. The patient may present in adolescence because of fatigue in the thoracic or thoracolumbar area or dissatisfaction with cosmetic appearance. The Adams forward bend test will reveal a sharp midthoracic angulation (increased kyphosis) at the point of maximal deformity that demonstrates variable flexibility with hyperextension. This is in contrast to nonstructural postural kyphosis (postural roundback), where normal sagittal alignment is restored with hyperextension.

Patients with thoracolumbar Scheuermann disease may present more commonly with mechanical back pain that increases with activity and is relieved by rest. The deformity is localized to the thoracolumbar junction (apex T11, T12, or L1). Cases may be self-limited and respond to nonsurgical measures such as bracing or physical therapy. Uncommonly, chronic pain may continue into adulthood. Surgical reconstruction is indicated in severe, rigid, and progressive deformities.

IMAGING STUDIES

Required for diagnosis

Imaging studies required are weight-bearing AP and lateral radiographs of the entire spine (14 in. x 36 in. cassette) taken with the arms extended 45° to 60°. The views should include the lumbosacral spine, given an increased incidence of spondylolysis associated with Scheuermann thoracic kyphosis. An AP view of the spine is included initially to assess for accompanying scoliosis.

Classic radiographic manifestations of thoracolumbar Scheuermann disease include end plate irregularities, erosions, sclerosis, disk space narrowing, and Schmorl's nodes, which are

SECTION 11 ■ PEDIATRIC ORTHOPAEDICS

present over multiple contiguous levels. Scheuermann disease in the thoracic spine is defined radiographically as three vertebral segments with anterior vertebral body wedging of 5° or more and a total kyphosis of the thoracic spine greater than 45° to 50°. Discogenic changes described above may also be seen.

Required for comprehensive evaluation

In most instances, no other imaging studies are necessary. MRI or CT with sagittal reformations may help further assess disk, cord, and nerve root morphology.

Special considerations

Gonadal shielding is used on follow-up examinations.

Pitfalls

None

IMAGE DESCRIPTION

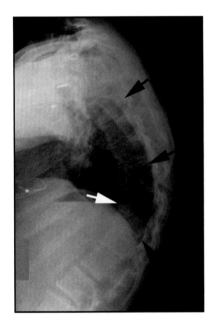

Figure 11-65

Scheuermann disease—Lateral view

Lateral view of the thoracolumbar spine shows exaggerated thoracolumbar kyphosis (black arrows) associated with mild anterior wedging (white arrow) and end plate irregularity of the lower thoracic vertebral bodies.

DIFFERENTIAL DIAGNOSIS

Congenital kyphosis (malformations seen on radiographs include anterior column failure of segmentation, posterior hemivertebrae, or combination of the two)

Eosinophilic granuloma (vertebra plana, or flattening of the vertebra, is seen)

Postural kyphosis (postural roundback) (no radiographic changes of the vertebral bodies)

Spondylolysis and Spondylolisthesis

Synonyms
None

ICD-9 Codes

721.3
Spondylolysis

738.4
Spondylolisthesis

Definition

Spondylolysis is defined as a defect in the pars interarticularis of the posterior elements without vertebral subluxation. Spondylolisthesis is the anterior subluxation of one vertebra on another, most commonly at the lumbosacral junction (L5-S1), and is also associated with a defect of the pars interarticularis. Presentation in children and adolescents is most commonly related to acquired defects in the pars interarticularis and less commonly to dysplastic facet joints. The pars area is at the junction between the superior and inferior facets.

Spondylolysis and spondylolisthesis are seen in approximately 6% to 7% of the general population, making it a common acquired condition. Spondylolysis is due to repetitive hyperextension injuries of the back. A higher incidence of spondylolysis is seen in gymnasts and football players.

History and Physical Findings

Young patients with spondylolysis may present either with an acute onset of pain consistent with a stress injury of the low back or with slowly progressing discomfort related to increasing lysis of the pars. Neurologic examination is normal in these patients. Other findings may include point tenderness and limited lumbar range of motion in extension secondary to pain.

The presentation of spondylolisthesis is variable, depending on the etiology and degree of anterior subluxation. Patients may remain asymptomatic or may have significant symptoms of pain or gait abnormality. Hamstring tightness accompanied by normal neurologic examination is common. Rarely, patients with severe spondylolisthesis from congenital etiology may present with cauda equina syndrome. The treatment of spondylolysis is predominantly nonsurgical. Rest and immobilization are recommended initially. Brace therapy (lumbosacral orthosis) may continue for several months until symptoms resolve. Surgery to repair a defect may be indicated for recalcitrant pain.

Similar management is recommended for spondylolisthesis, including rest and brace immobilization. Surgery is recommended for high-grade symptomatic spondylolisthesis, progressive listhesis in skeletally immature patients, or neurologic symptoms that fail to respond to nonsurgical means of management.

Imaging Studies

Required for diagnosis

Weight-bearing AP, lateral, and two oblique radiographs of the lumbar spine allow visualization of the pars interarticularis. Weight-bearing lateral radiographs of the lumbosacral spine are usually sufficient to diagnose spondylolisthesis.

Required for comprehensive evaluation

Initial radiographic imaging for spondylolysis is often negative, with no identifiable findings. A bone scan with single photon emission computed tomography (SPECT) imaging of the lumbar spine will identify a stress injury of the pars interarticularis. CT with fine cuts and sagittal reformations is the study of choice for radiographically established spondylolysis, defining the skeletal findings of the pars interarticularis defect well.

Special considerations

MRI may be useful in defining the intraspinal morphology, including neural compression in spondylolisthesis with high degrees of severity.

Pitfalls

Radiographs are often negative in the initial and follow-up evaluation of spondylolysis. Also, radiographs that are not weight bearing may fail to reveal the extent of the spondylolisthesis.

Image Descriptions

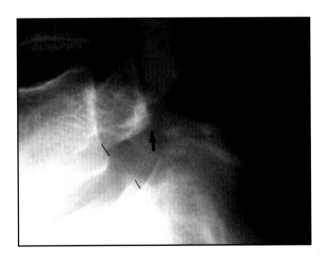

Figure 11-66

Spondylolysis (lumbosacral spine)— Lateral view

Lateral view of the lumbosacral spine demonstrates spondylolysis. Note the defect in the pars interarticularis (arrow). There is a mild (grade 1) spondylolisthesis (lines).

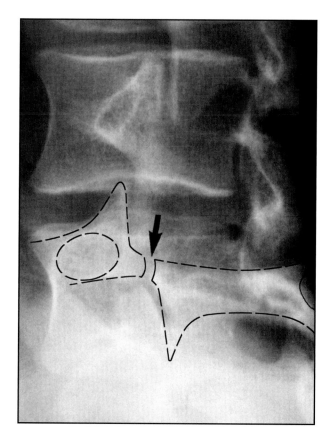

Figure 11-67

Spondylolysis (lumbar spine)—Oblique view

Oblique view of the lumbar spine shows a defect in the pars interarticularis (arrow). A trick to help find this defect on an oblique view of the lumbar spine is to look for a collar on the Scotty dog: Imagine a Scotty dog (outline), with the pedicle as the dog's eye, the superior articular facet as the dog's ear, the inferior articular facet as the dog's front leg, and the pars interarticularis as the dog's neck. A line in the position of the dog's collar (arrow) is a sign of spondylolysis.

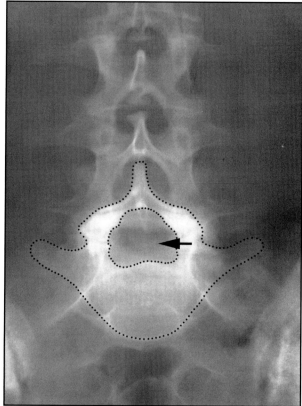

Figure 11-68

Spondylolisthesis (lumbosacral spine)—AP view

AP view of the lumbosacral spine. Note that L5 (dotted line) is viewed in the transverse plane, with the opening of the neural arch clearly seen (arrow). This is seen in high-grade spondylolisthesis where L5 is in excessive lordosis. The L5 vertebral body has the appearance of a "reverse Napoleon's hat."

Section 11 ■ Pediatric Orthopaedics

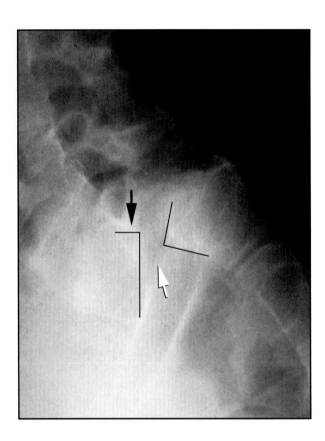

Figure 11-69

Spondylolisthesis (lumbosacral spine)—Lateral view

Lateral view of the lumbosacral spine demonstrates a high grade spondylolisthesis, with 100% anterior slippage of L5 on S1 (black arrow). Note the localized kyphosis between L5 and S1 (white arrow).

DIFFERENTIAL DIAGNOSIS

Low back syndrome (radiographs are normal)

Swayback (radiographs are normal)

FRACTURES IN CHILDREN

DEFINITION

Fractures are disruptions in the continuity of bone or bone-cartilage surfaces. A child's bone is not as strong as an adult's because a child's bone is more plastic and bends or deforms before it breaks, creating different fracture patterns seen in children. For example, torus and greenstick fractures are common in children but rare in adults.

Long bones are those bones that have an intermedullary canal and grow from each end. Fractures of the long bones, with their defining characteristics, are shown in Table 1 below.

Table 1 Fractures of Long Bones in Children	
Fracture type	**Characteristics**
Transverse	Fracture line perpendicular to the shaft of the bone
Oblique	Angulated fracture line
Spiral	A multiplanar and complex fracture line
Torus	An incomplete buckle fracture
Greenstick	An incomplete fracture with angular deformity

Fractures involving the growth plate, or physis, are unique to children and account for approximately 18% of all pediatric fractures. In a child, ligaments are stronger than the growth plate, and the growth plate is more likely to fracture than is the ligament to be injured. These fractures can occur at any growth plate but have common characteristic patterns. The peak age of incidence is 14 years in boys and 11 to 12 years in girls.

The Salter-Harris classification system defines five types of fractures at the growth plate, as shown below.

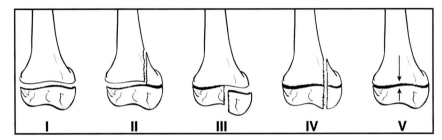

Salter-Harris classification of fractures at the growth plate.
Adapted with permission from Peterson HA: Physeal Fractures: Part 3. Classification. *J Pediatric Orthop* 1994;14:439-448.

Fractures involving the growth plate carry some risk of growth disturbance. Growth arrest may cause an angular deformity or premature shortening of the affected bone. Salter-Harris type III, IV, and V fractures have the highest risk of growth disturbance.

HISTORY AND PHYSICAL FINDINGS

A history of trauma to the affected area of the body is typical. Physical examination reveals tenderness at the site of the fracture, deformity, and swelling. The child may refuse to move the joints in proximity to the injury or bear weight if it involves the lower extremity. If the fracture involves the joint, an associated joint effusion may be present.

IMAGING STUDIES

Required for diagnosis

AP and lateral views of the affected bone are required, and the joints above and below the suspected fracture must be included in the image. If these views do not delineate the fracture, oblique views and/or comparison views of the opposite limb should be considered.

Required for comprehensive evaluation

With Salter-Harris type III, IV, and V fractures, CT with sagittal reformations (1-mm cuts) will more clearly outline the extent of the growth plate injury and the orientation and displacement of the fragments.

Special considerations

None

Pitfalls

A minimum of two orthogonal views must be obtained when there is clinical suspicion of a fracture, as a single view may not reveal a fracture that is displaced 90° to the x-ray beam. Initial radiographs of a type V fracture usually will not reveal an injury because this injury is diagnosed retrospectively. A fracture might not be visible on radiographs if it involves only the physis and if the secondary ossification center has not ossified. Also, failure to image the joints above and below a long bone fracture may fail to identify an associated, anatomically separate intra-articular fracture.

IMAGE DESCRIPTIONS

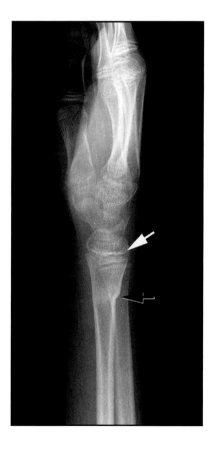

Figure 11-70

Torus fracture (wrist)—Lateral view

Lateral view of a wrist of a child or adolescent shows a torus fracture (black arrow). Note the open distal radial epiphysis (white arrow).

SECTION 11 ■ PEDIATRIC ORTHOPAEDICS

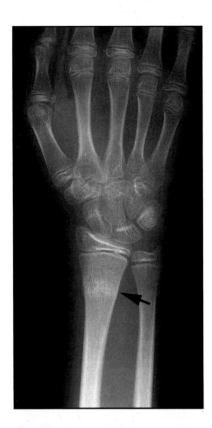

Figure 11-71

Torus fracture (wrist)—PA view

PA view of a right wrist shows a torus fracture of the distal radius (arrow). This is one of the most common locations for a torus fracture.

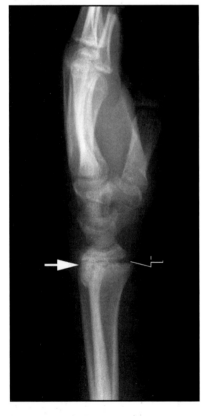

Figure 11-72

Salter-Harris type II fracture (wrist)—Lateral view

Lateral view of a wrist shows a Salter-Harris type II fracture of the distal radial epiphysis. Note the mildly displaced fracture through the distal radial epiphysis (black arrow). Note also the dorsal metaphyseal fragment (white arrow), a defining characteristic of this fracture.

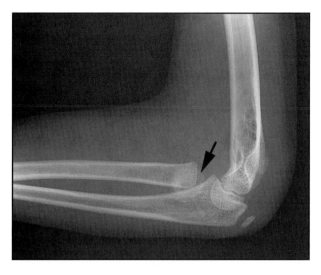

Figure 11-73

Fracture of the radial head (elbow)—Lateral view

Lateral view of a left elbow shows a displaced fracture of the radial head (arrow). It cannot be determined whether this is a Salter-Harris type I or a Salter-Harris type II fracture because, although this is a lateral view, the radial head is viewed end-on, indicating it has rotated 90°. No fat pad sign is visible on this radiograph.

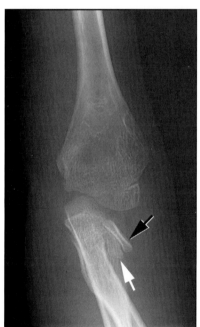

Figure 11-74

Fracture of the radial head (elbow)—AP view

AP view of the elbow shows a displaced Salter-Harris type II fracture of the radial head (black arrow). A fragment of the metaphysis (white arrow) is attached to the radial head, a defining characteristic of a Salter-Harris type II fracture. The fracture has rotated approximately 90°.

SECTION 11 ■ PEDIATRIC ORTHOPAEDICS

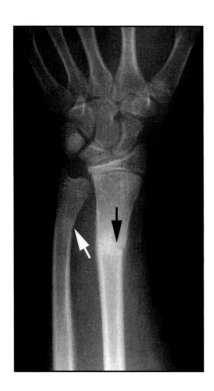

Figure 11-75

Fracture of the distal radius and ulna—PA view

PA view of the distal forearm and wrist shows a healing fracture of the distal radial diaphysis (black arrow) with surrounding callus formation and plastic bowing with a sclerotic fracture line in the distal ulnar diaphysis (white arrow).

DIFFERENTIAL DIAGNOSIS

Bone contusion (marrow changes seen on MRI)

Burn (heat injury) (may result in growth arrest)

Electrical injury (may result in growth arrest)

Frostbite (cold injury) (may result in growth arrest)

Infection (osteomyelitis frequently affects the metaphysis, but it may cross the epiphysis)

Ligament tear (a complete collateral ligament tear of the knee may appear clinically similar to a distal femoral physeal fracture, with the knee opening to varus or valgus stress)

Radiation injury (history of radiation therapy)

Fractures of Both Bones of the Forearm

Synonym
Both-bone fracture of the forearm

ICD-9 Code
813.23
Fracture of the radius with ulna

Definition
Pediatric forearm fractures are common and are treated differently than in adults because of the potential for growth and remodeling in children. Because 75% to 80% of the growth of the radius and ulna depends on the distal growth plates, distal forearm fractures have greater potential for remodeling. Forearm fractures may be complete or incomplete (called greenstick fractures and covered in a separate chapter). Both-bone fractures typically result from indirect trauma such as a fall on an outstretched hand. Open fractures or proximal forearm fractures often result from direct trauma.

History and Physical Findings
A fall on an outstretched arm or a direct blow to the forearm is a typical history for patients with both-bone fractures of the forearm. Pain, swelling, and limited motion, especially pronation and supination, are common symptoms. Physical examination may reveal obvious deformity, swelling, and, less commonly, ecchymosis. Neurologic examination may reveal decreased sensation in the median or ulnar nerve distribution. Careful attention should be paid to checking for compartment syndrome. Pain with passive extension of the fingers is a worrisome sign and warrants special referral. Also, severe pain not controlled with narcotic medication is a red flag for a possible compartment syndrome.

Imaging Studies

Required for diagnosis
AP and lateral views of the forearm are required to assess the extent and angulation of the fracture. The elbow and radiocarpal joint must also be included in each view to best assess possible rotation of the fracture fragments and associated injuries.

Required for comprehensive evaluation
None

Special considerations
Acute fractures should be splinted as part of emergency care, prior to obtaining radiographs.

Pitfalls

Radiographs of any fracture of the ulnar shaft require careful evaluation, particularly of the integrity of the radiocapitellar joint, to rule out a Monteggia fracture.

IMAGE DESCRIPTIONS

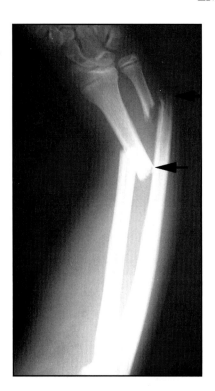

Figure 11-76

Fracture of the forearm (both-bone)—AP view

AP view of the forearm shows transverse fractures of both the radius and ulna with apex ulnar angulation (arrows). Note in this instance that the joints above and below the fracture are not included in the image. The distal radioulnar joint is normal. A separate view of the elbow (not shown) was normal.

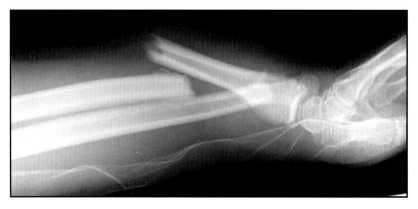

Figure 11-77

Fracture of the forearm (both-bone)— Lateral view

Lateral view of the forearm shows transverse fractures of both the radius and ulna with apex dorsal angulation (arrow). Note in this instance that the joints above and below the fracture are not included in the image but should be. These can be included in a separate view of the elbow (not shown).

Differential Diagnosis

Compartment syndrome (normal radiographs; diagnosis made clinically)

Galeazzi fracture (dislocation of the distal radioulnar joint)

Monteggia fracture (dislocation of the proximal radial head in addition to the ulnar fracture)

FRACTURES OF THE CLAVICLE AND PROXIMAL HUMERUS

ICD-9 Codes

810.00
Fracture of clavicle, closed, unspecified part

812.00
Fracture of humerus, upper end, closed, unspecified part

812.09
Fracture of humerus, upper end, closed, other (epiphysis)

SYNONYMS
None

DEFINITION
Clavicle fractures are among the most common fractures in children. They are described according to where the fracture occurs: in the proximal, middle, or distal third of the bone. Most occur in the middle third of the clavicle. Fractures of the proximal humerus are located distal to the rotator cuff musculature and proximal to the pectoralis major. Physeal fractures in very young children may be transphyseal (Salter-Harris type I), whereas in older children they involve a metaphyseal fragment (Salter-Harris type II). Salter-Harris type III fractures are rare in children; when they occur, they are often associated with shoulder dislocations.

HISTORY AND PHYSICAL FINDINGS
Clavicle fractures commonly occur from a fall on an outstretched arm and are associated with brachial plexopathies. Infants may also sustain these fractures during labor and delivery. Clinically, pain occurs with range of motion at the shoulder and/or direct palpation. In the infant, nondisplaced clavicle fractures may be unrecognized until callus healing with a palpable bump is noted. Fractures of the proximal humerus result from either a birth injury or a torsional force. The child experiences pain and swelling over the lateral aspect of the shoulder. On presentation, the child may refuse to move the affected arm. The pain is localized over the proximal humerus and is exacerbated by rotation of the arm. The patient will be tender over the proximal humerus.

IMAGING STUDIES

Required for diagnosis
An AP view of both clavicles is recommended for diagnosis of fractures of the clavicle. This allows comparison with the opposite clavicle when the acromioclavicular joint must be assessed. AP and apical oblique views of the proximal humerus are required for diagnosis of fractures of the proximal humerus.

Required for comprehensive evaluation

Obtaining an axillary and a transscapular lateral view of the shoulder decreases the risk of missing a fracture. A CT scan of the proximal humerus will delineate the extent, comminution, and articular involvement of the fracture.

Special considerations

MRI is useful if infection is suspected. Acute injuries should be splinted as part of routine care prior to obtaining the radiographs.

Pitfalls

Failure to obtain radiographs of both clavicles may lead to missing an acromioclavicular joint separation or physeal separation. In newborns, the proximal humerus will not yet have ossified, so radiographs may not show a transphyseal fracture. In such cases, an ultrasound is recommended. A high degree of suspicion of infection of the bone or joint is indicated when a neonate does not move an arm.

IMAGE DESCRIPTIONS

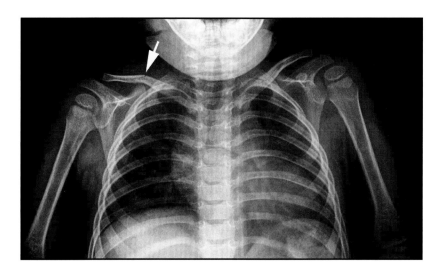

Figure 11-78

Fracture of the clavicle—AP view

AP view of both clavicles demonstrates a fracture in the middle third of the clavicle (arrow).

SECTION 11 ■ PEDIATRIC ORTHOPAEDICS

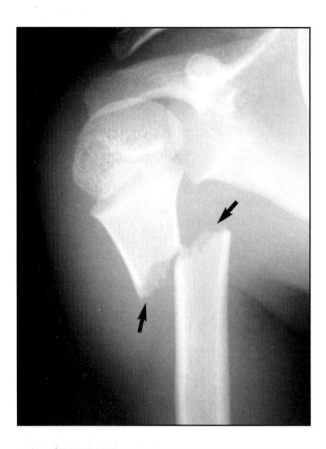

Figure 11-79

Fracture of the proximal humerus—AP view

AP view of the proximal humerus shows fracture displacement at the metaphyseal junction of the proximal humerus (arrows).

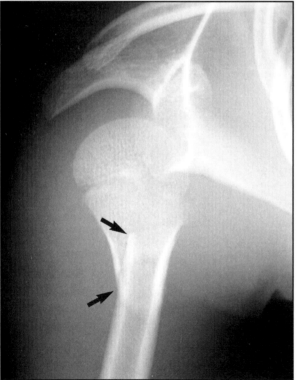

Figure 11-80

Fracture of the proximal humerus— Lateral view

Lateral view of the proximal humerus demonstrates shortening and angulation of the proximal humerus (arrows), indicating a fracture.

DIFFERENTIAL DIAGNOSIS

Brachial plexopathy (clavicle fracture may not be present; clinical correlation required)

Pathologic fracture (presence of destructive lesion in metaphysis)

Rotator cuff tear (no fracture seen on radiographs)

Stress fracture (fracture may not be seen on radiographs)

SECTION 11 ■ PEDIATRIC ORTHOPAEDICS

FRACTURES OF THE FEMORAL SHAFT

ICD-9 Code

821.01
Fracture of femoral shaft,
closed

SYNONYMS
None

DEFINITION
Fractures of the femoral shaft occur between the subtrochanteric and supracondylar regions of the femur and account for almost 2% of all childhood fractures. There is a bimodal distribution of incidence, with the first peak in early childhood and the second in early adolescence. Boys are more than twice as likely to sustain these fractures as are girls. In infants, child abuse is the cause of approximately 40% of femoral shaft fractures in children who are not yet walking, and of 3% of these fractures in children who are walking. In older children, high-velocity injuries are the most likely cause of injury.

HISTORY AND PHYSICAL FINDINGS
Children with these fractures have extreme pain and are unable to walk. Physical examination reveals swelling, tenderness, and crepitus at the fracture site. Deformity is characterized by shortening and angulation of the leg. If the patient has sustained trauma to multiple systems, any associated head, thoracic, or abdominal injuries should be ruled out first.

IMAGING STUDIES

Required for diagnosis
AP and lateral views of the femur that include the hip and knee joints are needed for diagnosis.

Required for comprehensive evaluation
Associated injuries about the hip, distal femoral physis, and proximal tibial physis should be ruled out. A stress fracture may be missed if appropriate imaging is not ordered. MRI or bone scan may be required to identify a torus or stress fracture. The specialist may order CT for surgical planning to assess for limb length.

Special considerations
Splinting should be part of emergency care, prior to radiographs.

Pitfalls
None

IMAGE DESCRIPTIONS

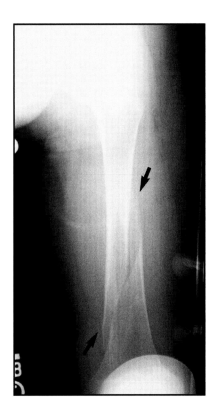

Figure 11-81

Fracture of the femoral shaft—AP view

AP view of the femur in a young (age 2 to 4 years) child shows a spiral fracture of the distal third of the femur with mild lateral displacement (arrows).

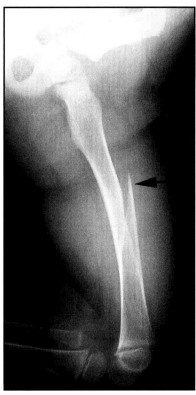

Figure 11-82

Fracture of the femoral shaft—Lateral view

Lateral view of the femur in the same patient shown in Figure 11-81 shows a spiral fracture of the distal third of the femur with mild anterior displacement (arrow).

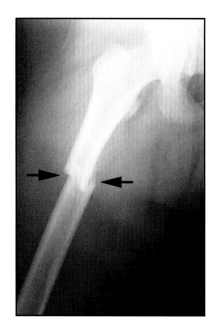

Figure 11-83

Fracture of the femoral shaft—AP view

AP view of the femur in an adolescent shows a transverse fracture of the proximal third of the femur with mild medial displacement (arrows).

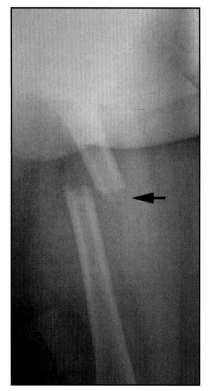

Figure 11-84

Fracture of the femoral shaft—Lateral view

Lateral view of the femur in the same patient shown in Figure 11-83 shows a transverse fracture of the proximal third of the femur with significant posterior displacement (arrow).

DIFFERENTIAL DIAGNOSIS

Muscle contusion (no fracture evident, edema seen on MRI)

Stress fracture (fracture may not be seen on radiographs)

Fractures of the Lateral Condyle of the Elbow

Synonyms
None

ICD-9 Code

812.42
Fracture of the lateral
condyle, closed

Definition
Fractures through the lateral condylar region, which in the immature elbow typically cross the physis and enter the elbow joint, constitute 17% of elbow fractures in children. The most common mechanism of injury is a fall on an outstretched hand.

History and Physical Findings
The main physical finding in children with this fracture is marked swelling over the lateral aspect of the distal humerus. In addition, lateral tenderness at the elbow and a decrease in elbow range of motion are also present. Deformity, which is mainly caused by localized swelling, is less severe than with a supracondylar humeral fracture.

Required for diagnosis
AP, oblique, and lateral views of the elbow are required. The fracture plane is oblique and therefore is best viewed on an oblique radiograph of the elbow from anterolateral to posteromedial.

Required for comprehensive evaluation
The specialist may order an arthrogram, ultrasound, or MRI in an infant or young child to differentiate this fracture from a transphyseal or Salter-Harris type II fracture.

Special considerations
Children may require sedation for the application of a cast. General anesthetic may be required in infants or young children to perform an arthrogram to help differentiate this fracture from a transphyseal fracture.

Pitfalls
The full extent of fracture displacement is often not evident on AP or lateral views. On the AP view, a very thin flake off the lateral distal humerus is diagnostic when seen but may be the only pathology noted.

Section 11 ■ Pediatric Orthopaedics

IMAGE DESCRIPTIONS

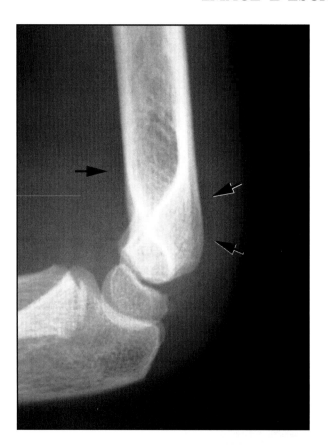

Figure 11-85

Fracture of the lateral condyle (elbow)—Lateral view

Lateral view of the elbow demonstrates minimal findings and positive fat pads (arrows), indicating an intra-articular effusion and possible fracture.

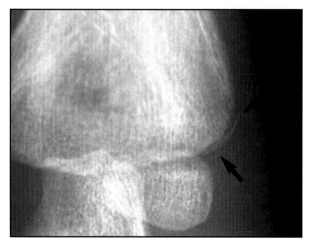

Figure 11-86

Fracture of the lateral condyle (elbow)—AP view

Magnified AP view of the elbow demonstrates a metaphyseal flake off the distal lateral aspect of the humerus, consistent with a lateral condyle fracture (arrows).

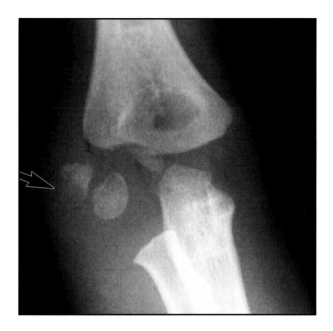

Figure 11-87

Fracture of the lateral condyle (elbow)—AP view

AP view of the elbow shows a fracture and marked displacement of the lateral condyle from the remaining portion of the distal humerus (arrow). The wrist extensor muscles tend to displace this fracture.

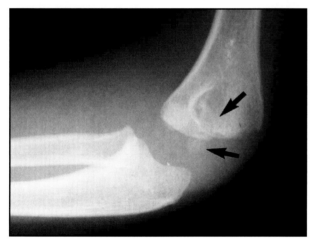

Figure 11-88

Fracture of the lateral condyle— Lateral view

Lateral view of the elbow shows that the distal humerus is irregular and lacks its regular width. Arrows indicate the proximal and distal fragments.

DIFFERENTIAL DIAGNOSIS

Distal humeral physeal separation (involvement of entire physis)

Elbow dislocation (involvement of entire physis)

Supracondylar humerus fracture (involvement of entire physis)

Section 11 ■ Pediatric Orthopaedics

FRACTURES OF THE MEDIAL EPICONDYLE OF THE ELBOW

ICD-9 Code

812.43
Fracture of the medial
condyle, closed

SYNONYMS
None

DEFINITION
Fractures of the medial epicondyle are caused by either a direct blow to the elbow or an avulsion mechanism through the elbow. They constitute 12% of all elbow fractures in children. The peak age of occurrence is 11 to 12 years, with 79% occurring in boys. Up to half of these fractures have associated elbow dislocations.

HISTORY AND PHYSICAL FINDINGS
These injuries usually occur as a result of a fall on an outstretched hand, creating a valgus force on the elbow. Principal findings on physical examination are swelling and tenderness over the medial aspect of the distal humerus. Deformity with this fracture is limited compared to that associated with a supracondylar fracture of the humerus and is well localized over the medial epicondyle. Significant swelling or generalized tenderness suggests an associated elbow dislocation with spontaneous reduction. These injuries may exhibit instability on valgus stress testing. In addition, the ulnar nerve should be tested because it may be injured as well.

IMAGING STUDIES

Required for diagnosis
AP and lateral views of the affected elbow are required, and a comparison view of the opposite, uninjured elbow may aid in making the diagnosis. Widening or irregularity of the apophyseal line may be the only indication of the fracture. On the lateral view, it is important to rule out the possibility that the fragment is incarcerated in the joint.

Required for comprehensive evaluation
CT or MRI may be useful to assess displacement.

Special considerations
Children may require general anesthesia for reduction, particularly for fractures with fragments incarcerated in the joint.

Pitfalls
An incarcerated fragment requiring open reduction may be missed if the physician does not suspect it.

IMAGE DESCRIPTION

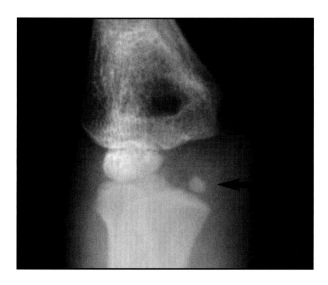

Figure 11-89

Fracture of the medial epicondyle (elbow)—AP view

AP view of the elbow shows a displaced medial epicondylar fragment (arrow) that normally should be at the level of the humerus.

DIFFERENTIAL DIAGNOSIS

Elbow dislocation with medial epicondyle fracture (may or may not have other associated fractures, elbow instability to varus and valgus strain)

Loose body in the elbow joint (the displaced medial epicondyle can simulate an osteochondral body in the elbow joint)

Medial condyle fracture (large medial fragment, elbow instability on valgus strain)

FRACTURES OF THE OLECRANON

ICD-9 Code

813.01
Fracture of the olecranon
process of the ulna, closed

SYNONYMS
None

DEFINITION
Fractures of the olecranon occur through the proximal ulna, either
through the proximal apophysis or through the metaphyseal bone of
the proximal ulna. Apophyseal injuries are extremely rare and are
caused by an avulsion-type mechanism of injury. Approximately
20% of these fractures are associated with another fracture about
the elbow.

HISTORY AND PHYSICAL FINDINGS
Most olecranon injuries are the result of a direct blow to the flexed
elbow. Frequently, there are associated elbow fractures, usually of
the proximal radius or medial epicondyle. Physical examination
reveals swelling and tenderness about the elbow, usually
accompanied by a palpable defect. The child may have weak
extension because of an inefficient triceps mechanism.

IMAGING STUDIES

Required for diagnosis
AP and lateral views of the elbow are needed to establish the
diagnosis.

Required for comprehensive evaluation
An arthrogram, ultrasound, and/or comparison views of the opposite
elbow may be useful to rule out a displaced apophyseal fragment.

Special considerations
Acute fractures should be splinted as part of emergency care, prior
to radiographs.

Pitfalls
An olecranon fracture that is part of a larger constellation of
multiple elbow fractures may be missed.

IMAGE DESCRIPTIONS

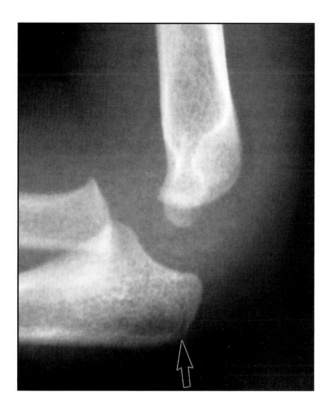

Figure 11-90

*Fracture of the olecranon—
Lateral view*

Lateral view of the elbow shows the fracture line beginning at the posterior tip of the olecranon (arrow).

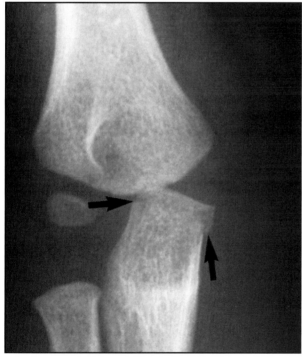

Figure 11-91

Fracture of the olecranon—AP view

AP view of the elbow shows mild medial displacement of the proximal metaphyseal region of the olecranon (arrows).

DIFFERENTIAL DIAGNOSIS

Triceps tear (MRI or ultrasound diagnostic if clinical examination is not conclusive)

FRACTURES OF THE PELVIS

ICD-9 Code

808.8
Fracture of pelvis,
unspecified, closed

SYNONYMS

Fracture of the anterior inferior iliac spine (AIIS)
Fracture of the anterior superior iliac spine (ASIS)
Fracture of the ischial tuberosity (IT)

DEFINITION

Pelvic apophyseal fractures commonly occur at the anterior superior iliac spine (ASIS), the anterior inferior iliac spine (AIIS), and the ischial tuberosity (IT). Avulsion fractures of the ASIS occur as a result of a muscle pull of the sartorius when the hip is extended and the knee is flexed. Avulsion fractures of the AIIS occur as a result of the muscle pull of the direct head of the rectus when the hip is hyperextended and the knee is flexed. Avulsion fractures of the IT occur as a result of the muscle pull of the hamstrings with excessive lengthening. These injuries occur in adolescents and young adults, particularly those participating in soccer, football, track (hurdles), baseball, and gymnastics. They occur from indirect trauma and sudden concentric or eccentric muscle forces, as well as vulnerability of the apophyseal fusion.

HISTORY AND PHYSICAL FINDINGS

A history of immediate pain and weakness in the region of the avulsion during strenuous physical activity is common. Physical examination reveals localized swelling and tenderness at the site of the avulsion. Patients with IT avulsion fractures will also have pain with sitting.

IMAGING STUDIES

Required for diagnosis

AP view of the pelvis is required. It may appear normal or may show displaced pieces of bone or irregularity at the site of the avulsed apophysis.

Required for comprehensive evaluation

CT or MRI may be indicated when radiographs are not diagnostic.

Special considerations

None

Pitfalls

The avulsion may be missed or mistaken for a secondary ossification center; therefore, a comparison view of the contralateral hemipelvis should be obtained. The amount of bone avulsed may be quite small and not seen on radiographs until callus formation weeks later. The changes in the adjacent soft tissues seen on MRI may look like a tumor or infection.

IMAGE DESCRIPTIONS

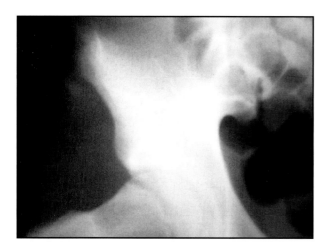

Figure 11-92

Avulsion fracture of the anterior superior iliac spine—AP view

Coned-down AP view of the pelvis shows an ASIS avulsion fracture (arrow) representing avulsion of the sartorius tendon.

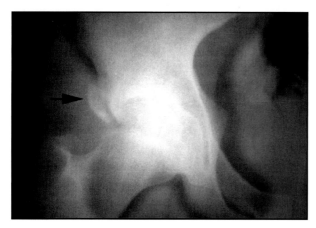

Figure 11-93

Avulsion fracture of the anterior inferior iliac spine—AP view

Coned-down AP view of the pelvis demonstrates an AIIS avulsion fracture (arrow) representing avulsion of the rectus femoris tendon.

SECTION 11 ■ PEDIATRIC ORTHOPAEDICS

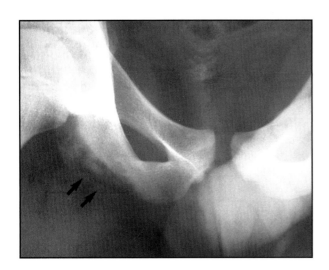

Figure 11-94

Avulsion fracture of the ischial tuberosity—AP view

Coned-down AP view of the pelvis demonstrates avulsed bone displaced distally from the inferior border of the ischium at the origin of the hamstrings (arrows).

DIFFERENTIAL DIAGNOSIS

Muscle strain (no fracture seen on radiographs)

Stress fracture (fracture may not be seen on radiographs)

Tendon tear (no fracture seen on radiographs)

FRACTURES OF THE RADIAL NECK

SYNONYMS
None

ICD-9 Code

813.06
Fracture of neck of radius, closed

DEFINITION
Fractures of the radial neck are much more common in children (age 8 to 10 years), whereas fractures of the radial head are more common in adults. Radial neck fractures occur in one of two locations: 3 to 5 mm distal to the proximal radial epiphyseal plate or through the epiphyseal plate with a metaphyseal fragment (Salter-Harris type II fractures). Most are of the latter type. The epiphyseal plate is weaker than the radial head, which accounts for the increased number of radial neck fractures in children.

HISTORY AND PHYSICAL FINDINGS
A typical history is a fall on an outstretched arm with the arm in supination. On physical examination, swelling over the lateral aspect of the elbow can be seen. Tenderness is localized over the radial head. Pronation and supination of the forearm are more painful and limited than elbow flexion and extension.

IMAGING STUDIES

Required for diagnosis
AP and lateral views of the elbow are needed to establish the diagnosis. The presence of a fat pad sign should be noted.

Required for comprehensive evaluation
AP and lateral views with the arm in both supination and pronation may delineate the fracture. A radiocapitellar view, which is a type of oblique view, may reveal a nondisplaced or minimally displaced fracture of the radial neck.

Special considerations
Oblique views may be helpful to further define the fracture morphology. Acute fractures should be splinted as a part of emergency care, prior to obtaining radiographs.

Pitfalls
A radial neck fracture is frequently a subtle buckle fracture that can be easily overlooked. The presence of an elevated posterior fat pad on a lateral view should encourage careful evaluation of the radial neck. In children younger than 5 years, the radial neck may have a valgus slope of up to 15° and may be mistaken for a fracture.

SECTION 11 ■ PEDIATRIC ORTHOPAEDICS

IMAGE DESCRIPTIONS

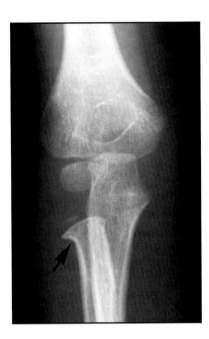

Figure 11-95

Fracture of the radial neck—AP view

AP view of the elbow shows fracture and angulation of the proximal radius (arrow).

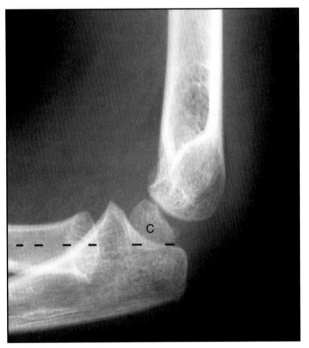

Figure 11-96

Fracture of the radial neck— Lateral view

Lateral view of the elbow shows that the radial head does not line up anatomically with the humeral capitellum, indicating a change or disruption of the normal articulation. A line drawn through the center of the radial shaft must align with the center of the capitellum (C); in this view, it is posterior to the center.

DIFFERENTIAL DIAGNOSIS

Elbow dislocation (associated fractures may or may not be present)

Radial head fracture (fracture does not extend to the radial neck and may be overlooked)

FRACTURES OF THE TIBIAL SPINE

SYNONYMS
None

ICD-9 Code

823.00
Fracture of tibia and fibula; closed fracture of upper end of tibia

DEFINITION
Fractures of the tibial spine (intercondylar eminence) are considered the pediatric version of an anterior cruciate ligament (ACL) tear; fortunately, these are rare injuries in children. While the ACL ligament tears in adults, in children the weak link is the site where the ACL attaches to bone at the tibial spine, resulting in an avulsion.

HISTORY AND PHYSICAL FINDINGS
A typical history is of deceleration, extension, and twisting of the knee. There often is an audible pop that sounds like a gunshot accompanied by pain and swelling that develop within an hour of the injury. Pain and swelling are common as a result of hemarthrosis. Knee range of motion is possible, but patients resist the extremes of motion because of pain.

IMAGING STUDIES

Required for diagnosis
AP, lateral, and tunnel (notch) views of the knee are needed to establish the diagnosis.

Required for comprehensive evaluation
An AP view with the x-ray beam parallel to the posterior slope of the tibial plateau may better reveal the fragment. If the knee joint is swollen and no fracture can be identified on radiographs, MRI should be ordered. The MRI will help identify the fracture and identify associated injuries such as tears of the menisci, collateral ligaments, or posterior cruciate ligament.

Special considerations
None

Pitfalls
A high index of suspicion is needed or an avulsion fracture may be missed on radiographs. The fragment may be primarily cartilaginous and thus not easily seen on a radiograph.

SECTION 11 ■ PEDIATRIC ORTHOPAEDICS

IMAGE DESCRIPTION

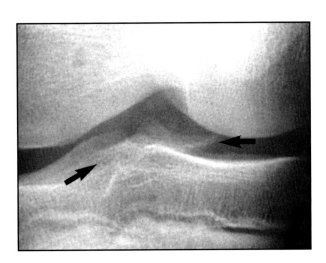

Figure 11-97

Fracture of tibial spine (fragment)—AP view

Coned-down AP view of the knee shows the fragment of a displaced tibial spine fracture (arrows).

DIFFERENTIAL DIAGNOSIS

Anterior cruciate ligament tear associated with a Segond fracture (lateral capsular avulsion off the proximal lateral tibia, avulsion fracture at insertion site on radiographs)

Osteochondral lesion (best seen on MRI, fragments often have smooth edges)

Posterior cruciate ligament tear (sagging of the proximal tibia on the distal femur seen on lateral view with hip and knee flexed)

GREENSTICK FRACTURES

SYNONYMS
None

ICD-9 Code

829.0
Fracture of unspecified
bones, closed

DEFINITION
Greenstick fractures are incomplete fractures in which the cortex and periosteum on one side of the bone remain intact while the opposite side is disrupted. The term "greenstick" comes from the analogy of breaking a fresh green tree branch. When bent, one side of the branch breaks while the other bends but remains intact. Because the cortex on one side remains intact, plastic deformation occurs, resulting in an angular deformity. A common deformity with greenstick fractures of the middle third of the radius and ulna is dorsal angulation of the distal fragments with the apex of the fracture pointed volarly. Greenstick fractures may also involve the distal radius and ulna. These fractures occur almost exclusively in children younger than 10 years and can involve any long bone.

HISTORY AND PHYSICAL FINDINGS
A history of a fall on an outstretched arm is common. Pain, swelling, and possible deformity are common on presentation. Physical examination may reveal deformity, tenderness, and a significant decrease in forearm rotation.

IMAGING STUDIES

Required for diagnosis
AP and lateral views are required to assess the extent and angulation of the fracture. The elbow and radiocarpal joint must be included on each image to assess for possible rotation of the fracture fragments and associated injuries.

Required for comprehensive evaluation
No additional imaging studies are necessary.

Special considerations
Acute fractures must be splinted prior to obtaining radiographs.

Pitfalls
Radiographs of any fracture of the ulnar shaft require careful evaluation, particularly with respect to the integrity of the radiocapitellar joint, to rule out a Monteggia fracture.

SECTION 11 ■ PEDIATRIC ORTHOPAEDICS

IMAGE DESCRIPTIONS

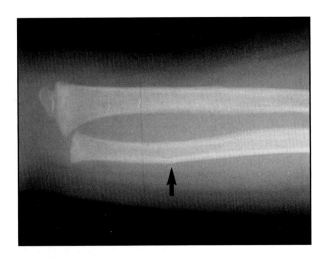

Figure 11-98

Greenstick fracture—AP view

AP view of the distal forearm shows mild ulnar apex angular deformity and plastic deformation of the distal ulna (arrow).

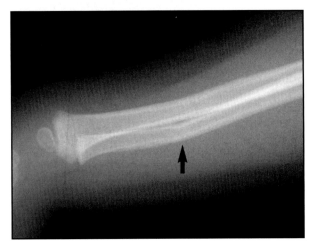

Figure 11-99

Greenstick fracture—Lateral view

Lateral view of the distal forearm shows a volar apex angular deformity of the ulna (arrow).

DIFFERENTIAL DIAGNOSIS

Plastic deformation (no breach in the cortex)

Stress fracture (no displacement on plain radiographs, marrow changes on MRI)

Torus fracture (bone buckles instead of breaking)

JUVENILE TILLAUX FRACTURES

SYNONYMS
Salter-Harris type III distal tibial epiphysis fracture

ICD-9 Code

824.8
Unspecified, closed fracture
of ankle

DEFINITION
Juvenile Tillaux fractures are Salter-Harris type III fractures of the anterolateral portion of the distal tibia, resulting from an epiphyseal avulsion at the site of attachment of the anterior tibiofibular ligament. The mechanism of injury typically is external rotation of the foot. The fibula prevents marked displacement of the fragment; therefore, clinical deformity is usually absent. The location of this fracture is the result of the order of closure of the distal tibial physis (ie, first centrally, then medially, then laterally). Because of this sequence of closure, the medial side is stronger than the lateral until the entire growth plate has fused.

HISTORY AND PHYSICAL FINDINGS
The child may not be able to give an accurate history, but the parent may note that the child is limping. Deformity of the foot and ankle and swelling may be minimal. On physical examination, tenderness to palpation is noted over the anterolateral aspect of the ankle at the joint line.

IMAGING STUDIES

Required for diagnosis
AP, lateral, and mortise views of the ankle are helpful in establishing the diagnosis. The mortise view is essential to obtain a view of the distal tibial epiphysis unobstructed by the fibula. If there is a step-off of the articular surface or if the fracture fragment is displaced 2 mm or more, referral to a specialist for surgical treatment is indicated.

Required for comprehensive evaluation
The extent of this fracture may be missed on radiographs; therefore, CT with sagittal reformations is recommended to evaluate the full extent of articular involvement.

Special considerations
None

Pitfalls
The extent of fracture may be underappreciated on radiographs.

IMAGE DESCRIPTION

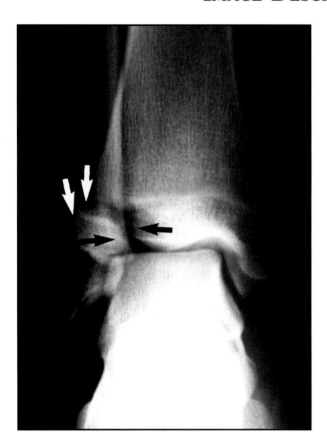

Figure 11-100

Juvenile Tillaux fracture—AP view

AP view of the ankle shows a small anterolateral epiphyseal fragment that is displaced toward the fibula and away from the remaining portion of the epiphysis (black arrows). Note the subtle displacement of the epiphyseal fragment in relation to the metaphysis (white arrows).

DIFFERENTIAL DIAGNOSIS

Anteroinferior tibiofibular ligament avulsion (no fracture seen on radiographs)

Avulsion fracture off the fibula (Wagstaffe's fracture; radiograph shows fracture off the fibula)

PHYSEAL SEPARATION OF THE DISTAL HUMERUS

SYNONYM
Physiolysis of the distal humerus

ICD-9 Code

812.44
Fracture of the condyle(s), unspecified

DEFINITION
Fracture through the growth plate of the distal humerus, most frequently a Salter-Harris type I fracture that does not extend into the metaphysis or epiphysis, may be difficult to diagnose. These fractures most often occur in children younger than 2 years, who may not yet have any ossification of the epiphysis. The mechanism of injury is usually minor or moderate trauma, such as that which occurs during labor and delivery. When the fracture occurs in an infant, often child abuse should be suspected.

HISTORY AND PHYSICAL FINDINGS
A fracture should be suspected when there is a history of injury with pain, swelling, pseudoparalysis, and "muffled" crepitus (which occurs when cartilaginous ends, as opposed to bony ends, rub together) around the elbow. On examination there is tenderness and decreased elbow range of motion. Deformity may be present.

IMAGING STUDIES

Required for diagnosis
AP and lateral views of the elbow (orthogonal views) are needed to establish the diagnosis.

Required for comprehensive evaluation
If radiographs are not definitive, MRI or elbow arthrogram may be required to demonstrate the relationship of the radius and ulna to the cartilaginous distal humeral epiphysis.

Special considerations
Acute fractures should be splinted as part of emergency care, prior to diagnosis.

Pitfalls
These fractures may be unrecognized or misdiagnosed as an elbow dislocation in children with no ossification of the epiphysis. Elbow dislocations are rare in young children.

SECTION 11 ■ PEDIATRIC ORTHOPAEDICS

IMAGE DESCRIPTIONS

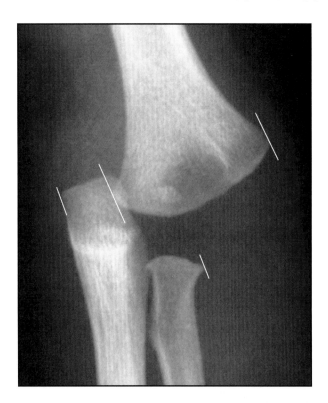

Figure 11-101

Physeal separation (distal humerus)—AP view

AP view of the elbow shows that the ulna and radius maintain their normal alignment, but they are posteromedially translated from the humerus (lines). This is the most frequent direction of displacement.

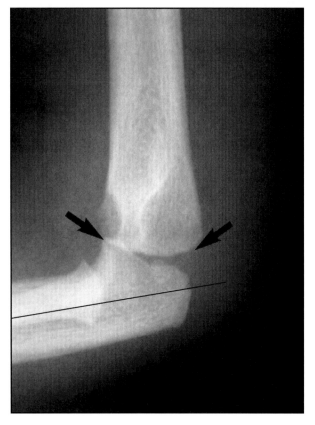

Figure 11-102

Physeal separation (distal humerus)—Lateral view

Lateral view of the elbow shows that the joint space between the humerus and olecranon is not maintained (arrows). Note also that the radius is not in line with the capitellum of the humerus (line).

DIFFERENTIAL DIAGNOSIS

Elbow dislocation (may or may not have an associated fracture)

Lateral condyle fracture (fracture through only a portion of the distal humerus)

Supracondylar humerus fracture (fracture through the thinnest portion of the distal humeral metaphysis)

SUPRACONDYLAR FRACTURE OF THE HUMERUS

ICD-9 Code

812.41
Supracondylar fracture of humerus

SYNONYMS
None

DEFINITION
Fractures through the supracondylar region of the humerus are common childhood injuries, typically occurring in children (primarily boys) between the ages of 5 and 8 years. Most of these fractures displace in an extended position; displacement into a flexed position is rare. The most commonly used system to classify extension-type supracondylar fractures is based on the type of fracture displacement. Type I fractures are nondisplaced; type II fractures show posterior tilting of the distal fragment and an intact posterior hinge. Type III fractures are severe and have no cortex in continuity.

HISTORY AND PHYSICAL FINDINGS
These fractures usually occur as a result of a fall on an outstretched hand. Physical examination is characterized by marked swelling, pain, deformity, tenderness, and decreased range of motion in the elbow. Deformity may be significant, usually in a characteristic "S" shape. Neurovascular assessment is important because both nerves and vessels can be injured in displaced supracondylar fractures. Another characteristic finding is the anterior skin "pucker" sign, which indicates that the proximal fragment has penetrated the dermal layer. The presence of this sign should alert the physician that the fracture may be difficult to reduce.

IMAGING STUDIES

Required for diagnosis
AP and lateral views of the elbow are needed to establish the diagnosis.

Required for comprehensive evaluation
If initial AP and lateral images are poor, additional views may be clinically indicated. Oblique or Jones column views may help visualize a fracture that is difficult to see.

Special considerations
The extremity should be splinted as a part of emergency care, prior to sending the child for radiographs.

Pitfalls

In truly nondisplaced fractures, the fracture line may be difficult or impossible to see on radiographs. If an elevated posterior fat pad is seen on the lateral view, there is a 76% chance that an elbow fracture is present, specifically a nondisplaced supracondylar fracture.

IMAGE DESCRIPTIONS

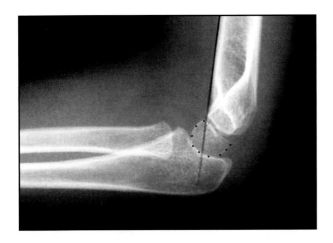

Figure 11-103

Normal elbow—Lateral view

Lateral view of a normal elbow shows that the anterior humeral line passes through the middle third of the capitellum ossification center (dotted line).

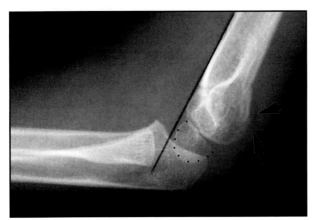

Figure 11-104

Supracondylar humerus fracture, type I—Lateral view

Lateral view of the elbow shows a type I supracondylar humerus fracture. Note that the anterior humeral line does not pass through the middle third of the capitellum ossification center because the distal humerus is displaced into an extended position. Also, note the posterior fat pad sign (arrows).

SECTION 11 ■ PEDIATRIC ORTHOPAEDICS

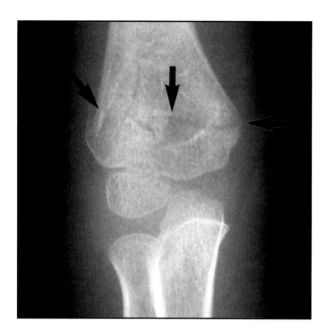

Figure 11-105

Supracondylar humerus fracture, type I—AP view

AP view of the elbow shows a type I supracondylar humerus fracture. Note that the fracture line extends through the supracondylar region (arrows).

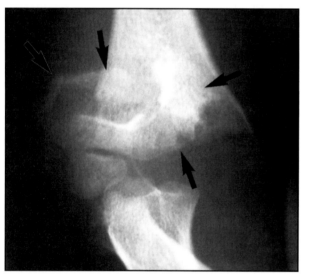

Figure 11-106

Supracondylar humerus fracture, type III—AP view

AP view of the elbow shows a type III displaced supracondylar humerus fracture. Note that the distal supracondylar fragment (arrows) is completely displaced from the humeral shaft.

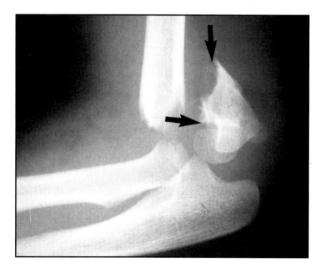

Figure 11-107

Supracondylar humerus fracture, type III—Lateral view

Lateral view of the elbow shows a type III supracondylar humerus fracture. Note that the distal supracondylar fragment (arrows) is completely displaced from the humeral shaft and is in an extended position.

Differential Diagnosis

Distal humeral physeal separation (arthrogram, ultrasound, or MRI will further delineate fracture)

Elbow dislocation (may or may not have associated fractures)

Lateral condyle fracture (unilateral condyle fracture)

TORUS FRACTURES

ICD-9 Code

829.0
Fracture of unspecified bone,
closed

SYNONYM
Buckle fracture

DEFINITION
Torus fractures are longitudinal compression injuries that occur in children from a force that is insufficient to cause a complete disruption of the bone but sufficient to cause the cortex to buckle but not completely break. The most common location for torus fractures is the metaphyseal area of long bones, especially the radius. Other locations for torus fractures include the first metatarsal bone (the bunk-bed injury) and the spine, especially the lamina. Occasionally a torus fracture may occur in combination with a greenstick fracture; this combination is referred to as a "lead pipe" fracture.

HISTORY AND PHYSICAL FINDINGS
A fall on an outstretched hand is a typical mechanism of injury. Because of the lack of deformity, the unwary parent may not suspect a serious injury. However, because of guarding of the extremity, the child is brought to the physician for evaluation. On examination, localized swelling and tenderness are found. Deformity typically is absent. If the radius is involved, wrist motion is limited and painful.

IMAGING STUDIES

Required for diagnosis
AP and lateral views are required to determine the extent and angulation of the fracture. Both the wrist and the elbow joint should be included to assess for radial head dislocation or distal radioulnar disruption.

Required for comprehensive evaluation
None

Special considerations
Plaster splints or casts may obstruct images. Acute fractures should be splinted as part of emergency care, prior to radiographs. Follow-up radiographs are not required.

Pitfalls
This fracture may be misdiagnosed as a wrist sprain as the buckling can be quite subtle.

IMAGE DESCRIPTIONS

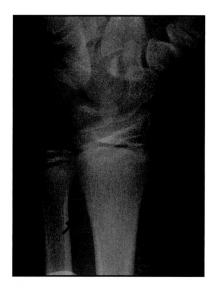

Figure 11-108

Torus fracture—AP view

AP view of the distal forearm and wrist shows a torus fracture. Note the buckling of the distal radius in the metaphyseal region (arrow).

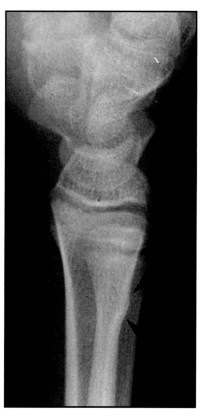

Figure 11-109

Torus fracture—Lateral view

Lateral view of the distal forearm and wrist shows buckling of the distal radius in the metaphyseal region (arrows), consistent with a torus fracture.

DIFFERENTIAL DIAGNOSIS

Greenstick fracture (failure in tension, not compression)

Plastic deformation (no breach in the cortex of either radius or ulna)

TRIPLANE FRACTURES

ICD–9 Code

824.8
Fracture of ankle,
unspecified, closed

SYNONYMS
Marmor-Lynn fracture
Triplanar fracture

DEFINITION
Triplane fractures are complex physeal fractures that have different fracture components (Salter-Harris types III and IV) in all three planes—sagittal, coronal, and transverse planes. These fractures have three principal components: (1) the anterolateral quadrant of the distal tibial epiphysis; (2) the medial and posterior portions of the epiphysis in addition to a posterior metaphyseal spike; and (3) the tibial metaphysis. Triplane fractures most commonly occur in adolescents when they are at the age at which the distal tibial physis is closing.

HISTORY AND PHYSICAL FINDINGS
Triplane fractures are more severe than juvenile Tillaux fractures (anterolateral tibial epiphyseal fractures). Patients report a history of ankle trauma with swelling and deformity. On physical examination, the ankle is swollen and tender to palpation. Active and passive motion is painful. The patient cannot walk on the affected limb.

IMAGING STUDIES

Required for diagnosis
Triplane fractures are easily underappreciated on radiographs if the physician does not carefully examine the tibial epiphysis, growth plate, and metaphysis on AP, lateral, and mortise views. When a fracture line is seen on an AP or mortise view, careful evaluation of the lateral view often reveals a posterior metaphyseal fracture.

Required for comprehensive evaluation
Tomography and/or CT is required to definitively identify the fracture pattern, the number of fragments, the presence of an intra-articular step-off, and the degree of comminution. CT is imperative for assessing fracture alignment and the condition of the articular surface. An articular step-off of greater than 2 mm, or a fracture gap of greater than 2 to 4 mm, is an indication for open reduction.

Special considerations

CT with coronal and sagittal reformations can be done if the patient has a plaster splint or cast in place. These additional views are helpful in determining the adequacy of the reduction in all three planes.

Pitfalls

The extent of fracture displacement may be underappreciated on radiographs; therefore, CT is mandatory.

IMAGE DESCRIPTIONS

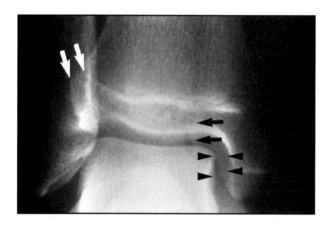

Figure 11-110

Triplane fracture—AP view

AP view of the ankle shows a fracture through the anterior portion of the epiphysis (black arrows). Note the subtle displacement of the epiphysis laterally (white arrows), causing widening of the medial ankle mortise (arrowheads).

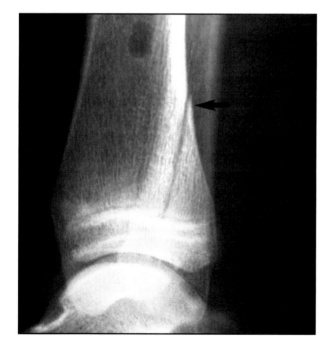

Figure 11-111

Triplane fracture—Lateral view

Lateral view of the ankle shows a posterior metaphyseal fragment (arrow) extending from the physis to the posterior cortex of the tibia. (The lytic lesion in the distal tibial diaphysis is an incidental fibro-osseous lesion.)

DIFFERENTIAL DIAGNOSIS

Metaphyseal fracture of the distal tibia (no involvement of the physis/epiphysis on radiographs)

INDEX OF IMAGES

GENERAL ORTHOPAEDICS

TUMORS

SHOULDER

Elbow and Forearm

Hand and Wrist

HIP AND THIGH

KNEE AND LOWER LEG

FOOT AND ANKLE

SPINE

PEDIATRIC ORTHOPAEDICS

GLOSSARY

Acromial morphology A Y scapular (or transscapular) view outlines the shape of the acromion. Type I is a flat acromion; type II is a curved acromion; and type III is a hooked acromion. Types II and III are implicated in impingement syndrome of the shoulder.

Alpha angle An angle constructed from a coronal ultrasound that is used to study developmental dysplasia of the hip (DDH). The angle is formed by the intersection of a line drawn along the iliac wing with a line drawn along the acetabular roof. This angle is used to assess the coverage of the femoral head and the slope of the acetabular roof. The angle should be > 60°.

Anteroposterior (AP) view Anterior-posterior view in which the x-ray tube is in front and the film cassette is in back. The x-ray beam passes from front to back.

Arthrography A procedure in which a contrast medium is injected into a joint to outline soft tissues such as the meniscus in the knee or a torn structure such as the rotator cuff in the shoulder. MR arthrography is a technique in which a diluted contrast medium such as gadolinium is injected into a joint to improve the delineation of soft tissues and standard MRI is obtained following the injection.

Bamboo spine An appearance of the spine in a patient with ankylosing spondylitis in which the vertebrae may look like "bamboo" related to ossification of the outer anulus fibrosus.

Bankart fracture A small chip fracture off of the anterior and inferior rims of the glenoid that is seen after an anterior dislocation of the shoulder.

Böhler's angle An angle measured on a lateral view of the foot to evaluate the relationship between the talus and calcaneus. The angle is formed by the intersection of two lines: one is drawn from the posterosuperior margin of the calcaneal tuberosity to the tip of the posterior facet of the subtalar joint; the other is drawn from the tip of the posterior facet through the superior margin of the anterior process of the calcaneus. The angle normally ranges between 20° and 40°.

Bone densitometry A procedure used to detect osteopenia in which a special density gradient plate is used to evaluate the comparative density of the spine, femur, or distal radius. Photons from a single- or dual-emitting source are used to measure the density of the bone. These are then compared with normal values for a large patient population based on sex and age.

Bone scan A study used to identify lesions in bone such as fracture, infections, or tumor. A radioisotope is injected into a vein and allowed to circulate through the body. The distribution of radioactivity in the skeleton is measured by a special camera that can detect the emission of gamma rays. Lesions in bone with increased metabolic activity (eg, fracture, tumor, or infection) will show increased uptake of the radioisotope and appear as dark areas in the bone. A bone scan is a very sensitive imaging modality but not very specific in that it cannot distinguish among the various causes of increased uptake. If an infection is suspected, a three-phase bone scan (perfusion, blood pool, delayed) can be helpful. If the perfusion phase is normal, an infection can be ruled out. Also called bone scintigraphy.

Brewerton view A view that profiles the collateral recesses and is helpful for identifying collateral ligament avulsion fractures and other metacarpal head fractures. This view is taken with the metacarpophalangeal joints flexed 65° with the dorsum of the proximal phalanges flat against the cassette and the x-ray beam angled 15° ulnar to radial.

Broden view An oblique tangential view of the foot used to evaluate the subtalar joint. The talofibular joint and the tibiofibular syndesmosis are well visualized on this view.

Carpal tunnel view A tangential view of the volar aspect of the wrist taken with the wrist in maximum dorsiflexion. This view is useful to identify fractures of the hook of the hamate.

Center-edge (C-E) angle of Wiberg A measurement made on an AP view of the pelvis that is useful in evaluating hip dysplasia. The angle is formed by a line (baseline) connecting the centers of the two femoral heads. Two lines are then drawn from the center of the femoral head: one is drawn perpendicular to the baseline; the other is drawn to the superior acetabular lip. Normal values vary with age. From age 5 to 8 years, the lowest normal value is 19°; from age 9 to 12 years, normal values are 12° to 25°; and from age 13 to 20 years, the low normal values range from 26° to 30°. Hip dysplasia is considered present when the measurements fall below the lowest normal values.

Clenched fist view (grip view) An AP view of the hand with the fist clenched tightly, used to identify scapholunate dissociation.

Cobb method A way to measure the degree of curvature in scoliosis. Two lines are drawn: one along the top of the uppermost vertebra in the curve and the other along the bottom of the lowermost vertebra in the curve. Perpendicular lines are then drawn to these two lines. The point of intersection of these two perpendicular lines defines the Cobb angle or degree of curvature.

Codfish vertebra The appearance of a vertebra seen on a lateral view of a spine with advanced osteoporosis. The superior and inferior end plates are depressed in the central portion of the vertebra.

Comparison view A view of the unaffected, opposite side or extremity. Obtaining a comparison view is useful in children, especially in trauma about the elbow. In children, the various ossification centers can be confused with fractures.

Computed tomography (CT, CAT scan) A radiographic modality that allows cross-sectional imaging from a series of x-ray beams. The x-ray tube is rotated 360° around the patient, and the computer converts these images into a two-dimensional axial image. CT is capable of imaging bone in three planes: coronal, sagittal, and oblique. This modality is particularly useful in evaluating fractures and bone tumors.

Crescent sign A crescent-shaped radiolucent space between the subchondral plate and impacted bone of the humeral or femoral head seen on an AP view of the humeral or femoral head with osteonecrosis.

Cross-table lateral view Lateral view of the hip obtained by flexing the opposite hip to avoid patient discomfort when imaging hip fractures.

Discography (diskography) A procedure in which a radiopaque material is injected into a lumbar or cervical intervertebral disk to outline the disk. This procedure is used in conjunction with CT to help identify the source of back pain. The pain produced by the injection is correlated with the patient's symptoms.

Dual-energy x-ray absorptiometry (DEXA) The use of two different x-ray voltages in bone densitometry to correct for soft-tissue density.

Echogenic Description of materials such as bone that give rise to echoes of ultrasound waves.

Fat pad sign (Sail sign) A sign on a lateral view of the elbow with the elbow flexed 90° that indicates swelling within the joint, often from a fracture with hemorrhage. Fat is normally present within the elbow joint, both anteriorly in the coronoid fossa and posteriorly in the olecranon fossa. The posterior fad pad normally is not seen, whereas the anterior fat pad may not be seen or may appear as a straight lucency. An intra-articular hemorrhage forces the fat out of the fossa, resulting in a triangular radiolucent shadow that may be seen both anterior and posterior to the distal humerus.

Fat suppression An MRI technique that suppresses the signal that comes from fat, most commonly used to assess bone marrow edema in subchondral bone. With this technique, fat will appear black on an MRI scan.

Ferguson view An AP view of the pelvis with 30° to 35° cephalad angulation. This view shows fractures of the sacrum and pubic and ischial rami and injury to the sacroiliac joints.

Fleck sign An avulsion injury of the medial aspect of the base of the second metatarsal, indicative of a Lisfranc injury. Also refers to a piece of bone avulsed from the fibula at the site of attachment of the superior peroneal retinaculum.

Fluoroscopy A special type of radiograph that shows continuous motion of the structure, such as wrist motion.

Frog-lateral view An AP view of the hip taken with the hip in abduction and external rotation.

Gilula's lines A guide to assess integrity of the carpal row on a PA view of the wrist. With normal carpal anatomy, three parallel arcs can be drawn: (1) along the proximal margins of the scaphoid, lunate, and triquetrum; (2) along the distal margins of the scaphoid, lunate, and triquetrum; and (3) along the proximal margins of the capitate and hamate. Lack of continuity of any of these arcs indicates a dislocation or fracture-dislocation of one or more carpal bones.

Gradient-echo (GE or GRE) sequence A frequently used pulse sequence in MRI in which a variable radiofrequency pulse is followed by a gradient pulse.

Gun barrel sign An AP view of the foot in a patient with a claw or hammer toe in which the proximal phalanx is seen end-on, similar to looking down the barrel of a gun.

Hallux valgus angle An angle formed by the long axis of the proximal phalanx and the long axis of the first metatarsal.

Harris-Beath view A posterior tangential view of the foot used to evaluate the subtalar joint. The posterior and middle facets of the subtalar joint and the body of the calcaneus are well visualized on this view.

Hawkins sign A radiolucent zone seen beneath the subchondral plate of a talar dome that has normal vascularity in the setting of osteopenia to differentiate from an osteonecrotic talus, which would not have this lucent line.

Hilgenreiner's line (Y line) A line used in the assessment of developmental dysplasia of the hip. The line is drawn through the top of both triradiate cartilages. The intersection of this line with Perkins line (a vertical line drawn from the lateral edge of the acetabulum and perpendicular to Hilgenreiner's line) divides the hip joint into quadrants. If the femoral ossific nucleus is within the lower inner quadrant, the hip is considered reduced.

Hill-Sachs lesion A wedge-shaped impaction fracture of the posterolateral portion of the humeral head seen following anterior dislocations of the shoulder.

Inlet view A view of the pelvis in which the x-ray beam is directed 40° to 60° caudally.

Insall-Salvati ratio A measurement used to identify patella alta. On a lateral view of the knee with the knee flexed 30°, the length of the patellar tendon and the height of the patella are measured. The ratio of the length of the patellar tendon to the height of the patella is the Insall-Salvati ratio. A ratio > 1.3 confirms the diagnosis.

Intermetatarsal (IM) angle An angle formed by the intersection of lines drawn down the center of the first and second metatarsals. Often used to evaluate hallux valgus.

Inversion recovery (IR) sequence A frequently used pulse sequence in MRI that begins with a 180° inverting pulse, followed by a 90° radiofrequency excitation pulse. After the 90° excitation phase, one or more 180° refocusing pulses are applied.

Judet views Oblique views of the pelvis used to evaluate the acetabulum. Anterior (internal) oblique views outline the iliopubic (anterior) column and the posterior acetabular rim. Posterior (external) oblique views outline the ilioischial (posterior) column and the anterior acetabular rim.

Lateral view A view that passes from side to side at 90° to an AP or PA view.

Looser transformation zone (Pseudofracture) A radiolucent defect in cortical bone often seen along the inner femoral neck, axillary margin of the scapula, ribs, and pubic ramus in patients with osteomalacia. This defect results from accumulation of new mineralized osteoid tissue.

Magnetic resonance imaging (MRI) An imaging modality that depends on the movement of protons in hydrogen atoms. When subjected to a magnetic field, protons that are normally randomly aligned become aligned. Radio waves directed at the tissue to be studied are used to change the alignment of these protons. When the radio waves are turned off, the protons emit a signal that is detected and processed by a computer into an image. In the musculoskeletal system, MRI is useful in diagnosing soft-tissue injuries, tumors, stress fractures, and infections.

Merchant view An axial view of the patella in which the patient lies supine on the x-ray table with the knee flexed 45°. The cassette is held perpendicular to the tibia about halfway between the knee and ankle. The x-ray beam is directed caudally through the patella at an angle of 60° from vertical. This view is useful to evaluate subluxation of the patella and patellofemoral arthritis.

Mortise view A view of the ankle in which the ankle is rotated internally so that the medial and lateral malleoli are parallel with the plane of the film. This view is used to assess joint space narrowing.

Myelography A radiographic study in which a water-soluble contrast agent is injected into the subarachnoid space to form a column of opacified fluid that outlines the thecal sac of the spinal cord. Used to assess herniated disks and spinal stenosis. This study has been largely replaced by MRI and CT.

Neck-shaft angle An angle measured on an AP view of the hip that is formed by the intersection of two lines: one is drawn down the center of the femoral head and neck; the other is drawn along the femoral shaft. The normal neck-shaft angle is 115° to 140°.

Neck-shaft anteversion angle An angle measured on a lateral view of the hip that is formed by two lines: one is drawn down the center of the femoral head and neck; the other is drawn along the femoral shaft. The normal neck-shaft anteversion angle is 125° to 130°.

Norgaard view An AP 45° supinated oblique view of both hands used to detect early changes of rheumatoid arthritis. The pisiform bone also can be seen clearly on this view. The original Norgaard view was taken with the fingers extended; the modified Norgaard view is taken with the fingers cupped, as if the patient is trying to catch a ball. Hence, this view is also called the ball catcher's view.

Oblique view A view in which the x-ray beam passes at an angle different from an AP, PA, or lateral view.

Odontoid view An open mouth AP view of the C2 vertebra used to identify fractures of the odontoid (dens) process of C2.

Outlet view A view of the pelvis in which the x-ray beam is directed 40° cephalad. Used to evaluate pelvic fractures.

Outlet view of the shoulder A view to evaluate the morphology of the acromion. With the patient standing, the affected shoulder is placed against the x-ray table and the patient's trunk and opposite shoulder are rotated 20° away from the table. The affected arm is abducted, the elbow flexed, and the hand is resting on the table.

Parallel pitch lines Lines drawn on a weight-bearing lateral view of the os calcis to define a prominent posterior process of the os calcis (Haglund's deformity).

Perkins line A vertical line drawn from the lateral tip of the acetabulum. This line is drawn perpendicular to Hilgenreiner's line. The intersection of these lines divides the hip joint into quadrants. If the femoral ossific nucleus is located in the upper outer quadrant, the hip is considered dislocated.

Posteroanterior (PA) view Posterior-anterior view in which the x-ray beam passes from back to front.

Proton density An MRI study in which the image is dependent on the differences in the density of protons in the imaged tissue. The repetition time (TR) is > 1,000 ms, and the echo time (TE) is < 60 ms.

Pulse sequence A series of radiofrequency and gradient pulses that occur in a predetermined sequence to obtain magnetic resonance images with various contrasts. Three commonly used pulse sequences are spin echo, gradient echo, and inversion recovery.

Quadriceps angle (Q angle) An angle formed by the intersection of two lines: one line is drawn from the anterosuperior iliac spine to the midpatella; the second is drawn from the midpatella to the anterior tibial tuberosity. These lines parallel the quadriceps and patellar tendons.

Radial head-capitellum view of the elbow A view of the elbow that demonstrates the radial head, the capitellum, and the radiohumeral and ulnohumeral articulations. This view is obtained with the patient seated, the affected elbow flexed 90°, the forearm resting on the ulna, and the thumb pointing forward. The x-ray beam is directed at the radial head at an angle of 45° to the forearm.

Radiocapitellar line A line that bisects the proximal radius and intersects the capitellum throughout a full range of motion in the normal elbow. If it does not, the radial head is considered dislocated.

Radiography (X-ray) An imaging modality in which ionizing radiation of a certain wavelength is used to create an image on film. Also referred to as roentgenography.

Ring sign A PA view of the wrist will show a circular density or "ring" in the scaphoid as a result of the horizontal orientation of the scaphoid in patients with scapholunate dissociation and scaphoid rotation.

Risser sign An indication of skeletal maturity based on the appearance of the iliac apophysis. Four grades are identified, with grade 1 the beginning and grade 4 considered skeletal maturity.

Robert view An AP view of the thumb with the forearm pronated and the dorsum of the thumb metacarpal and phalanges resting on the cassette. With this view, the carpometacarpal joint of the thumb is well visualized, which is helpful in diagnosing osteoarthritis.

"Rugger jersey" spine White and black stripes similar to those of an athletic jersey seen on radiographs of the spine in patients with renal osteodystrophy or hyperparathyroidism.

Scaphoid nonunion advanced collapse (SNAC) wrist A nonunion of the scaphoid seen on a PA view of the wrist, along with a radioscaphoid arthritis and later a capitolunate arthritis.

Scapholunate advanced collapse (SLAC) wrist A pattern of carpal injury and secondary osteoarthritis seen on a PA view of the wrist. Following a scapholunate dissociation, osteoarthritis develops between the radius and the scaphoid and later between the capitate and lunate.

Scapular Y view (Transscapular view) A lateral view of the shoulder taken so that the blade of the scapula, the coracoid process, and the spine of the scapula form a "Y." Used to evaluate anterior and posterior glenohumeral shoulder dislocations.

Scintigraphy Another name for a nuclear scan such as a bone scan.

Scotty dog sign An oblique view of the lumbar spine in patients with spondylolysis and spondylolisthesis shows the outline of what looks like a Scotty dog. The collar of the dog is the lysis or fracture of the pars interarticularis, the eye is the pedicle, and the nose is the transverse process. The lamina forms the body and the posterior spinous process the tail.

Shenton's line A continuous curved line that starts at the lesser trochanter, runs along the medial aspect of the femoral neck, and ends at the top of the obturator foramen. In a dislocated hip, this line is broken.

Spin-echo (SE) sequence A commonly used pulse sequence in MRI in which a 90° (typically) radiofrequency pulse is followed by a 180° refocusing pulse. Fast spin-echo (FSE) sequences use a 90° radiofrequency pulse, but unlike a typical SE sequence, FSE is followed by multiple 180° refocusing pulses.

Stryker notch view A special view of the shoulder used to demonstrate a Hill-Sachs lesion (a compression fracture of the humeral head on the posterolateral aspect of the articular surface) seen after recurrent anterior dislocations of the shoulder. This view is taken with the patient supine, the hand of the affected shoulder on the top of the head, and the x-ray beam directed 10° cephalad.

Sunrise view An axial view of the patella in which the patient lies prone with the knee flexed 115°. The x-ray beam is directed through the patella at an angle of 10° to 15° cephalad. This view shows the patellofemoral joint but is not as useful in diagnosing patellar subluxation as the Merchant view.

Superior labrum anterior to posterior (SLAP) lesion A tear of the superior labrum in the shoulder.

Swimmer's view A lateral view of the cervical spine taken with one arm held overhead and the other arm pulled down. Used for suspected cervical spine trauma when C7 cannot be seen on a lateral view.

T1-weighted image An MRI image in which the image is determined by the longitudinal relaxation time called T1. The repetition time (TR) is < 600 ms, and the echo time (TE) is < 20 ms. Fat has a high signal intensity (appears bright) on a T1-weighted image.

T2-weighted image An MRI image in which the image is influenced by the transverse magnetic relaxation time called T2. The repetition time (TR) is > 2,000 ms and the echo time (TE) is > 80 ms. Fluid has a high signal intensity (appears bright) on a T2-weighted image.

Teardrop (acetabulum) This characteristic shape is seen on an AP view of the acetabulum. The inner border of the acetabulum forms the outer border of the teardrop, whereas the outer wall of the pelvis adjacent to the inferior acetabulum forms the inner border.

Terry-Thomas sign A widened space between the scaphoid and lunate seen on a PA view of the wrist in a patient with a scapholunate dissociation. A gap > 2 mm is abnormal. The appearance has been compared with the gap seen between the front teeth of the late British comedian Terry-Thomas.

Tomography A radiographic modality that allows visualization of lesions or tissues that are obscured by overlying structures. Structures in front of and behind the level of tissue to be studied are blurred, which allows the object to be studied to be brought into sharp focus. Tomography has been used to evaluate the degree of fracture healing and to evaluate tumors such as osteoid osteoma. Increasingly, CT has replaced tomography as the imaging modality of choice in these circumstances.

Tunnel view A view in which the patient is prone with the knee flexed 40° and the x-ray beam directed caudally toward the knee joint at an angle 40° off vertical. Both the intercondylar notch and the posterior aspect of the femoral condyles are well visualized on this view. Also called a notch or intercondylar view of the knee.

Ultrasound (Ultrasonography) An imaging modality in which images are created from high-frequency sound waves (7.5 to 10 MHz [1 MHz = one million cycles per second]) that reflect off of different tissues. The reflected sound waves are recorded and processed by a computer and then converted into an image. Ultrasound is used to evaluate infant hip disorders and tears of the rotator cuff.

West Point axillary view An axillary view of the shoulder in which the patient is prone on the x-ray table with a pillow placed under the affected shoulder, the arm abducted 90°, and the forearm hanging off the edge of the table. The cassette is placed against the top of the shoulder, and the x-ray beam is then directed at the axilla, angled 25° toward the table surface and 25° toward the patient's midline. Useful to visualize potential damage to the anterior glenoid rim and Hill-Sachs lesions after an anterior dislocation.

Windshield wiper sign A radiolucent zone about the tip of a total joint prosthesis caused by the back-and-forth movement of the tip in a loose prosthesis.

Winking owl sign A unilateral absence of the pedicle on an AP view of the spine, often indicative of a tumor.

Y Scapular view A view taken tangential to the scapula. Normally, the humeral head sits in the convergence of the "Y," which comprises the scapula, acromion, and coracoid. Useful view to identify anterior and posterior dislocations of the glenohumeral joint.

Zanca view A view in which the patient is standing with the arm at the side and the x-ray beam is directed 15° cephalad toward the clavicle. Useful view to evaluate the acromioclavicular joint.

INDEX

Page numbers in *italics* indicate figures.

A

Abdominal aneurysms, 725
Accessory navicular, 574-576, *575, 576,* 596
Accessory ossicles, 682
Accessory scaphoid, 574
Accessory sesamoids, 600
Acetabular dysplasia, 455
Acetabular fractures, 427-430, *428-430*
  differential diagnosis, 426, 435, 444
Achilles bursitis, 571
Achilles tendinitis, 557, 571, 640-641, *641*
Achilles tendon rupture, 557
Achilles tendon tear, 641
Achondroplasia, 809-812, *811-812,* 822
Acquired adult flatfoot, 653
Acromioclavicular (AC) joint
  arthritis, 203, 216, 221, 225, 232, 237, 243, 247, 253
  instability, 177-179, 181, 184, 195, 205
  osteoarthritis, 210-213, *212, 213*
  separation, *178, 179*
  sepsis, 203, 221
Acromioclavicular ligament disruption, 177
Acromioclavicular sepsis, 225, 228, 232
Acromion fractures, 193
Acroosteolysis, finger, *75*
Acute lymphoblastic leukemia, *139*
Adductor muscle pyomyositis, 781
Adhesive capsulitis, 209, 216, 221, 225, 228, 232, 237, 243
Adolescent tibia vara, 806
Agressive fibromatosis, 152
ALARA principle, 29
Albright's syndrome, 116
Allergic reactions to contrast medium, 20
Amyloidosis, differential diagnosis, 106
Aneurysmal bone cysts, 120, 132, 149
Aneurysms, 409, 725. *see also* Pseudoaneurysms
Angulated fractures, *40*
Ankle
  fracture-dislocations, 577
  fractures, 577-583
  imaging overview, 560-563
  instability, 642-647, *645-647,* 652
  normal syndesmotic relationships, *643*
  synovial sarcoma, *167*
  synovitis, 573

triplane fractures, *893*
Ankylosing spondylitis, 47, 461, 713-716, *715*
  differential diagnosis, 357, 392
Anterior cruciate ligament (ACL)
  disruption, 546
  function, 475
  Segond fractures and, 514
  tears, 502, 547, *548,* 877, 878
Anterior inferior iliac spine (AIIS)
  fractures, 414, 872, *873*
Anterior interosseous nerve syndrome
  paralysis, 318
Anterior knee pain, 765
Anterior lateral impingement syndrome, 652
Anterior pelvic ring injuries, 421-423
Anterior superior iliac spine (ASIS)
  fractures, 414, 872, *873*
Anterior tibiofibular ligament ruptures, 642
Anteroinferior tibiofibular ligament
  avulsion, 882
Anterolateral bowing, 795
Apophyseal centers, in children, 750
Apophysis, differential diagnosis, 590
Apophysitis of the tibial tubercle, 760
Arm, fractures, 185. *see also* Forearms; Humerus; Radius
Arteriovenous hemangiomas, spinal, 735
Arthritis. *see* Juvenile rheumatoid arthritis; Osteoarthritis; Psoriatic arthritis; Rheumatoid arthritis
Arthritis mutilans, 634
Arthritis of inflammatory bowel disease, 392
Arthrography, 19-22
  contraindications, 21
  CT, 9
  indications, 21
  knee, 476
  lower leg, 476
  rotator cuff tear, *241*
Arthrogryposis, 822
Arthroscintigraphy, 93
Aseptic loosening
  differential diagnosis, 94, 103
  THA components, *98*
  total joint replacement and, 95-100, *98-99*
Aseptic necrosis, 468. *see also* Osteonecrosis
  femoral head, 468, 755

lunate, 399
scaphoid, 403
talus, 616
Atlanto-occipital dislocation, 707
Atlantoaxial instability, 729
Atlantoaxial rotatory subluxation and
  dislocation, 700
Atlas, fractures, 699-700, *700,* 707
Atopic dermatitis, 632
Avascular necrosis (AVN). *see also* Osteonecrosis
  femoral head, 755
  hip and thigh, 468
  humeral head, 218
  knee, 543
  lunate, 399
  scaphoid, 403
Aviator's astragalus, 603
Aviator's fractures, 603
Avulsion fractures
  distal phalanx, 368
  fibula, *577,* 882
  navicular tuberosity, 576
  proximal lateral tibia, 514
  tuberosity, 589, 611
Avulsions, 308, 317-318, *318*

B

Baker's cysts, 167
Bamboo spine, 713
Bankart fractures, *183, 184,* 196, 197, *199*
Barton's fractures, 337, *340*
Basal joint arthritis, 383
Baseball finger, 368
Basilar invagination, 729
Battered child syndrome, 815
Bayonetted fractures, 40
Benign nerve sheath tumors, 150-151, 709
Bennett's fractures, 358, *360-361*
Biceps anchor tear, 251
Biceps tendons
  anchor, 251
  distal, 308-310, *309, 310*
  rupture, 245-247, *247,* 308-310, *309*
  tear, 245
  tendinitis, 216, 232, 250, 253
Bimalleolar fracture-dislocations, *582,* 647
Bimalleolar fractures, 577, *579, 581*
Bipartite patella, 493, *497,* 766
Bipartite sesamoid, 602, *602*
Black disk disease, 722
Blastic lesions, 109-110

Humerus. *see also* Distal humerus
  fractures; Proximal humerus
  fractures
    distal physeal separation, 883-885
    fracture/dislocation, *192*
    osteogenesis imperfecta, *826*
    osteomyelitis, *832*
    periprosthetic fractures, *103*
    supracondylar fractures, 886-889,
      887-889
    unicameral bone cyst, *132*
Hutchinson's fractures, 337
Hydroxyapatite deposition disease
  (HADD), 229
Hygromas, 155
Hypercalcemia of malignancy, 75
Hyperostosis, sternoclavicular, 213
Hyperparathyroidism, 73-75
  brown tumor of, 120
  differential diagnosis, 72, 122, 143,
    146
  hand, *75*
Hypochondroplasia, 812
Hypoxia, gas gangrene and, 54

I

Idiopathic chondrolysis, 759
Idiopathic osteonecrosis of the femoral
  head, 755
Idiopathic scoliosis, 837, 838-840, *840*
Iliac wing fractures, 441
Iliopsoas bursitis, 420
Iliopsoas muscle pyomyositis, 781
Imaging overviews
  elbow, 257-259
  hand, 312-315
  hip, 414-417
  imaging children, 750-753
  knee, 475-477
  lower leg, 475-477
  shoulder, 171-175
  spine, 679-683
  tumors, 108-111
Impaction fractures, *41*
Impingement syndromes, 233-237
  anterior lateral, 652
  differential diagnosis, 203, 213, 216,
    225, 232, 244, 247, 250, 253
  hook-shaped acromion, *236*
  subacromial spur, *235*
  supraspinatus tendinosis, *236, 237*
Implant synovitis, 104
Infantile cortical hyperstosis, 813
Infantile rickets, 76
Infantile tibia vara, 806

Infections
    after THA, 94
    arthrography contraindications, 21
    differential diagnosis, 42, 100, 103,
      106, 120, 854
    disk space, 743
    fracture nonunion and, 36, 38
    hip and thigh, 420, 448, 451, 472
    laboratory findings, 92
    osteomyelitis, 827
    spine, 734
    total joint replacement and, 91-94
Infectious arthritis, 61, 292, 301, 540
Infectious diskitis, 716
Infectious inflammatory granulomas, 124
Inflammation
    fracture healing, 33
    pubic symphysis, 423
Inflammatory arthritis
    foot and ankle, 608, 633, 636, 659,
      661, 666, 676
    in patients with psoriasis, 390
    rheumatoid, 222
Inflammatory arthropathies, 461-464,
  467
Inflammatory bowel disease, arthritis,
  392
Inflammatory synovitis, 104
Infraspinatus tear, 238
Insertional Achilles tendinitis/tendinosis,
  570, 573, 639
Insufficiency fractures, 50, 449, 516,
  620. *see also* Stress fractures
Intercondylar fractures, 269
Interdigital neuritis, 669
Internal derangement of the hip, 419
Intertrochanteric fractures, 435, 442-
  444, *443-444,* 454
Intra-articular bodies. *see* Loose bodies
Intra-articular fractures, *41*
Intracortical Brodie's abscesses, 130
Intramuscular myxomas, 151, 159
Intraosseous ganglion, 402
Ischemic calcification, 167
Ischial tuberosity fractures, 872, *874*
Ischium fractures, 421, 423
Isolated shaft fractures, 262, 282-284

J

Jefferson fractures, 682, 699
Jersey finger, 317
Joint effusion, 524, 527-528, *528*
Joint mouse, 506
Joints, arthrography, 19-22
Jones fractures, 589, 610-611, *611*
Jumper's knee
    differential diagnosis, 480

extensor injuries, 486
MRI results, 487, *488*
radiographs, 487
Juvenile chronic arthritis, 393
Juvenile infantile osteoporosis, 826
Juvenile osteochondrosis, 455, 607,
  755, 843
Juvenile rheumatoid arthritis (JRA),
  776-778
    cervical spine, *777*
    differential diagnosis, 772, 775
    hips, *778*
    pelvis, *778*
    polyarticular, 461
    wrist, *777*
Juvenile tillaux fractures, 881-882, *882*
Juxta-articular metaphyseal
  osteomyelitis, 781
Juxtacortical chondromas, 49

K

Kienböck's disease, 376, 396, 399-402,
  400-402
Knees
    acute lymphoblastic leukemia, *139*
    anterior knee pain, 765
    chondrocalcinosis, *71*
    congenital deformity, 493
    contusions, 484
    hereditary multiple exostoses, *128*
    imaging overview, 475-477
    loose bodies in, 506-509
    nerve sheath sarcomas, *165*
    nonossifying fibromas, *122*
    normal variants, 476-477
    osteolysis after TKA, *100*
    osteomyelitis, *829-830*
    periprosthetic fractures, 101
    scurvy, 814
Kniest's dysplasia, 835
Knock-knees, 803
Köhler's disease, 607
Kyphosis, Scheuermann's, 843

L

Labral tears, 419-420, *420*
Lachman test, 514, 546
Langerhans histiocytosis, 137
Lap belt injuries, 693
Lateral capsular sign, 514
Lateral collateral ligaments (LCLs)
    disruption, 546
    function, 475
    tears, 547, *549*

Osteomyelitis
  bone scans, *63*
  differential diagnosis, 53, 137, 139,
    149, 624, 814, 818
  foot and ankle, 676
  juxta-articular metaphyseal, 781
  knee, 543
  metatarsal head, 608
  pediatric patients, 827-832, *829-832*
  proximal tibia, 761
  subacute epiphyseal, 764
  vertebral, 743
Osteonecrosis (ON), 218-221
  differential diagnosis, 209, 216, 225,
    228, 759
  early, *470*
  end stage, *472*
  foot and ankle, 602
  hip and thigh, 451, *470-471*
  humeral head, *220, 221*
  knee, *544-545*
  late, *471*
  metatarsal head, 607
  scaphoid, 403-404, *404*
  sickle cell, 759
  spontaneous, 543-545
  transient osteoporosis and, 468-474
Osteopenia, *14,* 106
Osteophyte formation, *300*
Osteoporosis, 79-81
  compression fractures, 742
  differential diagnosis, 78
  spine, *81*
  transient, 468-474, *472*
Osteoporosis fetalis, 825
Osteoporotic compression fractures, 710
Osteosarcomas, 124, 132, 147-149, *148*

P

Paget's disease, 82-85, *84,* 146, 738,
  742
Pantrapezial arthritis, *386*
Paralytic scoliosis, 841
Parathyroid hormone (PTH), 73
Parosteal osteosarcoma, 49
Particle disease, 95-100
Particle synovitis, 104
Patella
  chondromalacia, 483
  ossification centers, 476-477
Patellar dislocation, 487, *491-492, 508*
Patellar fractures, 493-498, *495-497*
  differential diagnosis, 521, 761
  stress, 483
Patellar tendons
  rupture, 486
  subluxation, 481

tears, 487, *489*
tendinitis, 766
tendinosis, 480, 487, *488*
Patellofemoral joints
  anatomy, 475
  dysfunction, 765
  instability and malalignment, 481-
    483
  malalignment, 480, *482-483,* 492,
    498, 765-766, *766*
Pathologic fractures, *41,* 186, 192, 861
Pectoralis major tendon rupture, 248-
  250, *250*
Pediatric patients
  coronal ultrasound of hip, *24*
  fracture nonunion, 36
  imaging overview, 750-753
  lateral condylar variants, 476
  medial condylar variants, 476
  radiation safety, 27
  septic arthritis, *63, 64*
  transient synovitis of the hip, 64
Pelvic fractures, 421, 427, 439
  differential diagnosis, 426
  multiple, *423*
  pediatric, 872-874
  stress-related, 449-451
Pelvic ring
  fractures, 430
  injuries, 421-423
  instability, 445-448, *447-448*
Pelvis
  achondroplasia, *812*
  anatomy, 414
  benign nerve sheath tumors, *151*
  imaging overview, 414-417
  juvenile rheumatoid arthritis, *778*
  Legg-Calvé-Perthes disease, *757-758*
  metastatic carcinoma, *143*
  multiple exostoses, *127*
  ossification centers, 415
  osteoid osteomas, *130*
  osteomalacia/rickets, *77*
  secondary chondrosarcoma, *134*
  septic arthritis, *780*
Pelvospondylitis ossificans, 713
"Pencil in a cup" deformities, 633
Periarticular muscle pyomyositis, 781
Perilunate dislocation, 372, *375*
Perilunate instability and dislocation,
  372-376
Periosteal chondromas, 128
Periosteal chondrosarcomas, 128
Periosteal osteosarcomas, 49
Peripheral nerve entrapment, 725
Peripheral nerve sheath tumors, benign,
  150-151

Periprosthetic fractures, 87, 101-106,
  102-103
Perirectal abscesses, 432
Permeative lesions, 110, *110,* 111
Peroneal spastic flatfoot, 770
Peroneal tendons, 648-652, *650*
Pes anserine bursitis, 522, *524*
Phalanges, fractures, 349-352, *350-352,*
  597-598, *598*
Physeal fracture of the medial clavicle,
  206
Physiologic genu varum, 808
Physis, injury in children, 750
Piedmont fractures, 279
Pigmented villonodular synovitis, 106,
  509, 533-534, *534*
Pilon fractures, 577, *581*
PIP joints. *see* Proximal interphalangeal
  joints
Pisiform bone fractures, 353-354, *354*
Pisotriquetral arthritis, 334, 344, 354, 382
Plantar fasciitis, ruptured, 568
Plantar fibromatosis, 568
Plantar interdigital neuromas, 669
Plantar nerve lesions, 669
Plantar plate disruption, 602
Plantaris tendon tears, 555, *557*
Plasmacytoma, 141
Plastic deformation, 880, 891
Plexiform neurofibroma, 155, 159
Podagra, 625
Polyarticular juvenile rheumatoid
  arthritis, 461, 776
Polydactyly, 788-789, *789*
Polyethylene wear, 95-100, *100*
Polymyositis, 411
Polyneuropathy, 144
Polyostotic fibrous dysplasia of bone,
  819, 833
"Popeye" sign, 245
Popliteal cysts, 522, *523-524,* 557
Positron-emission tomography (PET),
  16, 109
Posterior cruciate ligaments (PCLs)
  disruption, 546
  function, 475
  tears, 547, *549,* 878
Posterior inferior iliac spine (PSIS), 414
Posterior malleolus fractures, *580*
Posterior tibial tendinitis, 653
Posterior tibial tendon dysfunction, *655*
Posterior tibial tendons, 653-655
Posterolateral corner injuries, 547, *550*
Posteromedial bowing, 795
Posttraumatic angulation, 796
Posttraumatic arthritis, 289, 295, 301,
  638
Posttraumatic diskitis, 716

Posttraumatic myositis ossificans, 47
Posttraumatic toe deformity, 664, 668
Posttraumatic wrist malunion, 824
Postural kyphosis, 844
Pott's disease, 746
Pregnancy, radiation safety, 27
Prehallux, 574
Prepatellar bursitis, 522, *523*
Pretendon bursitis, 569
Primary osteoarthritis, 464
Progressive systemic sclerosis, 410
Pronation-eversion fractures, *647*
Prostate cancer, metastatic, 85
Proximal biceps tendinitis, 216, 232,
    250, 253
Proximal biceps tendon tear, 245
Proximal humerus
    endochondroma, *115*
    osteosarcoma, *148*
Proximal humerus fractures, 181, 187-
    192, *189-192*
    differential diagnosis, 184, 186, 195,
        201, 209, 216, 221, 232, 247, 250
    greater tumerosity, *191-192*
    pediatric, 858-861, *860*
    surgical neck, *189-190*
Proximal interphalangeal (PIP) joints
    Boutonnière deformity and, 319-321
    claw toes, 662
    dislocations, *329*
    fracture-dislocations, *330*
    hammer toe, 667
    rheumatoid arthritis, 636
    scleroderma, *411*
Proximal lateral tibia, 514
Proximal phalanx, fractures, 379
Proximal plantar fasciitis (PPF), 565,
    567
Proximal radius fractures, 276
Proximal tibia
    fractures of, 499
    Hohl classification of fractures, *499*
    osteomyelitis, 761
    primary neoplasms of, 761
Proximal ulnar fractures, 273
Pseudoaneurysms, 409
Pseudoarthrosis, 36, 38, 795
Pseudogout syndrome, 68, 525
Pseudomonas aeruginosa, 61
Pseudotumors, 163
Psoriasis
    differential diagnosis, 731
    foot and ankle, 628, 633
    pigmented villonodular synovitis
        and, 533

Psoriatic arthritis, 390-392, *391, 461,*
    535-537
    calcaneus, *634*
    differential diagnosis, 389
    foot and ankle, 633-635
    hand and wrist, 395
    knee, *536-537,* 539
    metatarsals, *634*
    spine, 716
Psoriatic arthropathy, 535
Pubic rami fractures, 435
Pubic symphysis inflammation, 423
Pulled muscles, 555
Pump bump, 569-570
Pyemic arthritis, 61
Pyogenic arthritis, 61, 540, 779
Pyogenic infections, 742, 747
Pyomyositis, 781

Q
Quadriceps tendons
    rupture, 486
    tears, 487, 490-491
    tendinosis, 487, *490*

R
RA. *see* Rheumatoid arthritis
Radial collateral ligament tear, 379
Radial head, congenital dislocation,
    786-787
Radial head fractures, 276-278, *278*
    differential diagnosis, 265, 272, 275,
        286, 295, 310, 876
    pediatric, *853*
Radial neck fractures, 875-876, *876*
Radial nerve entrapment, 304
Radial nerves, 386
Radial shaft fractures, 279, 281
Radial/ulnar club hands, 790-791
Radiation injuries, 854
Radiation safety, 27-29, *28*
Radiation therapy, HO and, 88
Radiculopathies, 209, 213, 216, 221,
    225, 228, 237, 244, 250, 253
Radiocapitellar arthritis, 304
Radiocapitellar dislocation, 263
Radiocarpal arthritis, 342, 396
Radiography, 3-7
    cautions, 5
    contraindications, 5
    detection limits, 3
    imaging children, 751
    imaging with, 3-7
    indications, 5
    screening views, *6*

Radiohumeral arthritis, 278
Radiohumeral dislocations, 263
Radiohumeral osteoarthritis, 293
Radiopharmaceuticals, 16-17
Radioscaphoid arthritis, 357, 396
Radioulnar dislocations, 281
Radioulnar synostosis, 785, *786*
Radius
    both-bone fractures, 261-262, *262,*
        855-857, *856*
    Caffey's disease, *814*
    congenital deformities, 785-787
    isolated shaft fractures, 262, 282-284
    Monteggia fractures, 285-286
    osteogenesis imperfecta, *826*
    pediatric fractures, *854*
    torus fractures, *891*
Reactive arthritis, 539
Reactive periosteal response, 110, 111,
    111
Rectal carcinomas, 432
Rectus femoris strain, *556*
Reflex sympathetic dystrophy, 778
Reiter's syndrome, 461
    differential diagnosis, 64, 213, 357,
        392
    foot and ankle, 635
    spine, 716
Renal failure, 139
Renal osteodystrophy, 72, 85
Reticulum cell sarcomas, 140
Retinacular ganglions, 405
Retrocalcaneal bursitis, 570, 571-573,
    572, 641
Reverse Monteggia fractures, 279
Reverse Barton's fractures, 337
Rhabdomyosarcomas, 163
Rheumatism. *see* Rheumatoid arthritis
Rheumatoid arthritis, 222-225, 299-301,
    461
    cervical spine, *731*
    classification, 223
    differential diagnosis, 64, 72, 106,
        207, 209, 213, 217, 221, 228,
        232, 237, 244, 247, 292
    elbow, *300, 301*
    foot and ankle, 628, 632, 635, 636-
        639, *638-639*
    hand and wrist, *4,* 389, 393-395,
        394-395
    hips, *463-464*
    knee, 357, 532, 538-539, *539*
    periprosthetic fractures and, 101
    polyarticular juvenile, 461
    shoulder, *224*
    spine, 704, 716, 729-731

Rheumatoid factor—positive
arthropathy. *see* Rheumatoid arthritis
Rhizomelic spondylitis, 713
Rickets
active, 76
differential diagnosis, 818
genu varum, *807*
vitamin D—resistant, 76
Rigid flatfoot, 770, 772
Rolando's fractures, 358, *359-360*
Rotator cuff disease, 233
Rotator cuff tear arthropathy, 226-228,
227, 228
differential diagnosis, 225
Rotator cuff tears, 238-244, *240-243*
differential diagnosis, 179, 192, *201,*
213, 217, 225, 232, 237, 247,
250, 253, 861
Rotator cuff tendinitis, 233
Roundback deformity, 843
"Rugger jersey" spine, 74, 713
Ruptured plantar fasciitis, 568

S

Sacral fractures, 432
Sacroiliac joints, 439-441, *448*
Sacroiliitis, 445, *447*
Sacrum fractures, 439-441, *441, 450*
"Salt and pepper" skull, 74
Salter-Harris classification, *850, 852*
Sarcomas, low grade, 153
Scaphoid
fracture, 355-357, *356,* 398
osteonecrosis, 403-404
Scaphoid-trapezium-trapezoid (STT)
arthritis, 386
Scapholunate advanced collapse
(SLAC) wrist, 251-253, *253,* 396-
398, *398*
chondrocalcinosis and, 69, *72*
differential diagnosis, 213, 232, 237,
244, 247, 386
Scapholunate dissociation, 342, *374-
375,* 402
Scapholunate ligament disruption, *20*
Scapular fractures
body, 184, 193
coracoid process, 179
differential diagnosis, 192, *201,* 205
nonarticular, 193-195, *194*
Scapulothoracic dislocations, 195
Scapulothoracic dissociations, 204-205,
205
Scheuermann's disease, 843-844, *844*
differential diagnosis, 734
Sciatic nerve
benign nerve sheath tumors, *151*

nerve sheath sarcoma, *165*
sciatica, 420, 725
Scintigraphy. *see* arthroscintigraphy;
Bone scintigraphy
Scleroderma, 67, 72, 395, 410-411, *411*
Sclerosis, tibial, *517*
Scoliosis
congenital, 836-837, *837*
idiopathic, 838-840
neuromuscular, 841-842
Scurvy, differential diagnosis, 139, 814,
818
Seat belt injuries, 693, 712
Segmental fractures, *41*
Segond fractures, 514-515, *515,* 878
Separated shoulder, 177
Sepsis
differential diagnosis, 203, 209, 213,
217, 221, 225, 228, 232
sternoclavicular joint, 207
total joint replacement and, 91-94
Septic arthritis, 61-64
differential diagnosis, 775
foot and ankle, 628
hips, *780*
knee, 540-542, *541-542*
laboratory tests, 62
metatarsophalangeal joints, 609
pediatric patients, 778, 779-781
pelvis, *63*
Septic joints, 321, 352, 464, 526
Seronegative arthropathies, 213, 217,
448
Seronegative spondyloarthropathies,
390, 633, 639
Seropositive arthritis. *see* Rheumatoid
arthritis
Sesamoid fractures, 599-602, *600-601*
Shin-splints, 516, 519
Shoulder girdle injuries, 204
Shoulders
calcific tendinitis, *231*
dislocation of, 177, 196
fractures, 182, 187-192
imaging overview, 171-175
impingement syndrome, *235-237*
neuropathic, 208-209
osteoarthritis, 214-217
rheumatoid arthritis, *224*
rotator cuff tear, *240*
rotator cuff tear arthropathy, *227,
228*
subluxation of, 196
Sickle cell disease, 139, 759, *832*
Sickle cell osteomyelitis, 827
Sickle cell osteonecrosis, 759
Silicone synovitis, 104-106, *106*
Sinding-Larsen-Johansson disease, 766

Single-photon emission computed
tomography (SPECT), 16
Skier's thumb, 377
Skin lacerations, 56
Skull
multiple myeloma, *146*
osteogenesis imperfecta, *826*
SLAP lesions. *see* Superior labrum
anterior to posterior lesions;
Slipped capital femoral epiphysis
(SCFE), 767-769, *768*
Smith's fractures, 337
Soft tissue calcification, 65-68
Soft tissue contractures, 289
Soft-tissue tumors, 292, 524
Spina bifida occulta, 682
Spinal canal
differential diagnosis, 441
function, 679
lumbar, 726-728, *728*
pain characteristics, 685
stenosis, *688, 689*
Spine, *see* Vertebrae
achondroplasia, *812*
fractures, 439
imaging overview, 679-683
juvenile rheumatoid arthritis, *777*
metastatic carcinoma, 142
osteomyelitis, *830-831*
osteoporosis, *81*
Paget's disease, *85*
spondylopeiphyseal dysplasia, *835*
Spiral fractures, *41, 849*
Spondylitis, tuberculous, 746
Spondyloarthropathy, seronegative, 390
Spondylolisthesis
adult, 685-689
anterolisthesis, *688*
CT myelogram, *687*
lumbar spine, *687*
of the pars interarticularis of C2,
705
pediatric patients, 845-848, *846,
847-848*
spinal stenosis, *689*
Spondylolysis, pediatric patients, 752,
845-848, *846-847*
Spondylopeiphyseal dysplasia (SED),
833-835, *835*
Spondylosis
cervical, 717-721, *718-720*
lumbar, 722
thoracic, 732
Spontaneous osteonecrosis, 543-545
Sprains
ankle, 619, 641

differential diagnosis, 42
foot, 624
Sterner's tumor, 47
Sternoclavicular (SC) joints
dislocation, *207*
hyperstosis, 213
instability, 181, 184, 195, 205, 206-207
osteoarthritis, 207, 210-213, *212*
separation/dislocation, 206
sepsis, 207
Straddle injuries, 421
Strains
ankle, 642
extremity muscles, 725
hamstring, *556*
hips, 451
knee and lower leg, 555-557
muscle injuries, 555-557, *556-557*, 725, 874
myotendinous, 555
rectus femoris, *556*
Stress fractures, *41*, 50-52
bone scan, *17*
calcaneus, 566, 568, 772
diaphyseal, 611
differential diagnosis, 864, 874, 880
fibula, *518*
foot, 620-624, 670
hip and pelvis, 449-451
hip and thigh, 448, 472
knee and lower leg, 485, 492, 513, 532, 554, 557
lower leg, 516-519
metatarsal, *622-623*, 624
navicular, 594, *596*
patellar, 483, 493, 494, *496-497*
pediatric, 861
periprosthetic, 101
tibial plateau, *519*
Stress-reactive lesions, 130
Subacromial bursitis, 233
Subacromial impingement, 233
Subacromial septic bursitis, 221, 225, 228, 232
Subacromial spurs, *235*
Subacute epiphyseal osteomyelitis, 764
Subaxial subluxation, 729
Subchondral sclerosis, *544, 631*
Subdeltoid subacromial bursitis, 233
Subscapularis tear, 238
Subtalar joints, 606, 652
Subtalar ligament injuries, 652
Subtrochanteric fractures, 438, 452-454, *453-454*
Superior glenoid labrum tear, 251-253

Superior labrum anterior to posterior (SLAP) lesions, 251-253, *253*
differential diagnosis, 213, 232, 237, 244, 247
Superior peroneal retinaculum injuries, 648-649, *650*
Supracondylar fractures, *102*, 269, 438
Supracondylar humeral fractures, 186, 867, 885, 886-889
Supraspinatus tear, 238
Supraspinatus tendinosis, *236, 237*
Surface osteosarcomas, 128
Sway back, 848
Symphisis pubis disruption, 421
Syndactyly, 792-794, *793-794*
Syndesmosis, 583, 644, *644*
Synovial chondromatosis, 296, 534
Synovial cysts, 405, 522
Synovial pseudoarthrosis, 38
Synovial sarcomas, 163, 166-167
Synoviomas, 166
Synovitis, 104-106, 573
Synovitis syndrome, 609
Systemic lupus erythematosus, 395, 411, 461
Systemic sclerosis, progressive, 410

T

T condylar fractures, 269
Tailbone fractures, 431
Tailor's bunion, 660
Talocalcaneal coalition, *772*
Talus
fractures, 603-606, *605-606*
gout, *628*
osteochondral fracture, 606
osteochondral lesions, 616-619
osteonecrosis, 603
Tarsal coalition, 655, 770-772
Tarsal navicular fractures, 593
Tarsometatarsal fracture-dislocations, 612
Tendon injuries, 409, 583, 606, 874. *see also* specific tendons
Tennis elbow, 302
Tennis fractures, 589, *590*
Tennis leg, 555
Teres minor tear, 238
Thighs
calcification of soft tissues, *67*
desmoid tumor, *153*
imaging overview, 414-417
lipoma, *158*
malignant fibrous histocytoma, *163*
myositis ossificans, *49*
myxoid liposarcoma, *161*

necrotizing fasciitis, *60*
Thoracic disk degeneration, 732-734
Thoracic disk herniation, 732, *733-734*
Thoracic kyphosis, Scheuermann, 843
Thoracic spondylosis, 732
Thrombocytopenia with absent radius, 790
Thumb
carpometacarpal arthritis, 383-386
metacarpal fractures, 358-362, *359-361*
ulnar collateral ligament injury, 377-379, *378-379*
Tibia. *see also* Proximal tibia
Caffey's disease, *814*
child abuse, *817*
fibrous dysplasia, *118*
fracture of fibula and, 514
ossification centers, 475
osteomalacia/rickets, *78*
osteomyelitis, *831*
Salter-Harris type II distal epiphysis fracture of, 881
stress fractures, *17, 52, 516, 517, 518, 519*
Tibia vara, 806
Tibial apophysitis, 479
Tibial bowing, 795-796, *796*
Tibial plateau
depressed fractures, *501*
fractures, 499-502, 505, 521
split fractures, *502*
stress fractures, *519*
Tibial shaft fractures, 503-505, *504-505*
Tibial spine fractures, 877-878, *878*
Tibial tubercles
apophysitis, 760
fractures, 761
Tibialis tendinitis, 653
Tibiotalar joints, gout, *628*
Toes
deformities, 664-665
fibrous dysplasia, *110*
polydactyly, 788, *789*
Torus fractures, *41*
in children, *849*
differential diagnosis, 880
pediatric patients, 890-891, *891*
wrist, *851-852*
Total joint replacement
dislocation/subluxation, 86-87
heterotopic ossification, 88-90
infection, 91-94
osteolysis, wear and loosening, 95-100
periprosthetic fractures, 101-106
silicone synovitis, 104-106